Comprehensive Respiratory Therapy Exam Preparation Guide

Second Edition

Edited by

CRAIG L. SCANLAN, EDD, RRT, FAARC
Professor Emeritus
School of Health Related Professions
Rutgers, the State University of New Jersey
Newark, New Jersey

ALBERT J. HEUER, PHD, MBA, RRT, RPFT
Program Director, Masters of Science in Health Care Management
Associate Professor, Respiratory Care Program
School of Health Related Professions
Rutgers, the State University of New Jersey
Newark, New Jersey

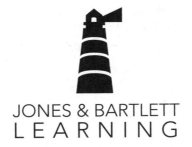

JONES & BARTLETT
LEARNING

World Headquarters
Jones & Bartlett Learning
5 Wall Street
Burlington, MA 01803
978-443-5000
info@jblearning.com
www.jblearning.com

Jones & Bartlett Learning books and products are available through most bookstores and online booksellers. To contact Jones & Bartlett Learning directly, call 800-832-0034, fax 978-443-8000, or visit our website, www.jblearning.com.

Substantial discounts on bulk quantities of Jones & Bartlett Learning publications are available to corporations, professional associations, and other qualified organizations. For details and specific discount information, contact the special sales department at Jones & Bartlett Learning via the above contact information or send an email to specialsales@jblearning.com.

Production Credits
Executive Publisher: William Brottmiller
Publisher: Cathy L. Esperti
Associate Acquisition Editor: Teresa Reilly
Production Editor: Jill Morton
Marketing Manager: Grace Richards
VP, Manufacturing and Inventory Control: Therese Connell
Composition: Cenveo Publisher Services
Cover Design: Theresa Day
Cover Image: © VikaSuh/ShutterStock, Inc.
Printing and Binding: Courier Companies
Cover Printing: Courier Companies

To order this product, use ISBN: 978-1-2840-2903-1

Library of Congress Cataloging-in-Publication Data

Certified respiratory therapist exam review guide.
  Comprehensive respiratory therapy exam preparation guide / edited by Craig L. Scanlan, Albert J. Heuer. — Second edition.
      p. ; cm.
  Preceded by Certified respiratory therapist exam review guide / edited by Craig L. Scanlan, Albert J. Heuer, Louis M. Sinopoli.
  Includes bibliographical references and index.
  ISBN-13: 978-1-284-02892-8
  ISBN-10: 1-284-02892-5
  I. Scanlan, Craig L., 1947- editor of compilation. II. Heuer, Albert J., editor of compilation. III. Title.
  [DNLM: 1. Respiratory Therapy—methods—Examination Questions. WB 18.2]
  RC735.I5
  615.8'36—dc23
                                                                2013022891

6048
Printed in the United States of America
17 16 15 14   10 9 8 7 6 5 4 3 2

Contents

Contributors	*xi*
Reviewers	*xiii*
Introduction	*xv*

SECTION I

NBRC Exams Shared Topical Content — **1**

CHAPTER 1

Review Existing Data in the Patient Record — **3**

Objectives	**3**
What to Expect on this Category of The NBRC Exams	**3**
Pre-Test	**3**
What You Need to Know: Essential Content	**4**
Patient History	5
Physical Examination	5
Lab Results	7
Sputum Analysis	7
Pulmonary Function Testing Results	7
ABG Results	9
Imaging Studies	11
Monitoring Data	11
Maternal History and Perinatal and Neonatal History	14
Data Pertaining to Sleep Disorders (RRT-Specific Content)	16
Common Errors to Avoid	**18**
Sure Bets	**18**
Pre-Test Answers and Explanations	**19**
Post-Test	**20**

CHAPTER 2

Collect and Evaluate Pertinent Clinical Information — **21**

Objectives	**21**
What to Expect on this Category of The NBRC Exams	**21**
Pre-Test	**22**

What You Need to Know: Essential Content	**25**
Assess a Patient's Overall Cardiopulmonary Status by Inspection	25
Neonatal Inspection	27
Assess a Patient's Overall Cardiopulmonary Status by Palpation	30
Assess a Patient's Overall Cardiopulmonary Status by Percussion	33
Assess a Patient's Overall Cardiopulmonary Status by Auscultation	33
Integrating Physical Examination Findings	34
Interviewing the Patient	34
Review and Interpret the Chest Radiograph	44
Review Lateral Neck Radiographs	47
Obtaining and Interpreting a 12-Lead ECG	47
Bedside Assessment of Ventilation	49
Lung Mechanics and Ventilator Graphics	51
Monitoring Peak Expiratory Flow Rates	51
Assessing Spirometry at the Bedside	53
Conducting Pulmonary Function Laboratory Studies	55
Exhaled Nitric Oxide Analysis (RRT-Specific Content)	56
Blood Gases and Related Measures	59
Apnea Monitoring	60
Overnight Pulse Oximetry	61
Titration of CPAP or BiPAP During Sleep	62
6-Minute Walk Test	63
Cardiopulmonary Exercise Testing	66
Oxygen Titration with Exercise	68
Hemodynamic Monitoring	68
Common Errors to Avoid	**77**
Sure Bets	**77**
Pre-Test Answers and Explanations	**78**
Post-Test	**80**

CHAPTER 3

Recommend Procedures to Obtain Additional Data — **81**

Objectives	**81**
What to Expect on this Category of The NBRC Exams	**81**

Pre-Test 82
What You Need to Know:
Essential Content 83
Radiographic and Other Imaging Studies 83
Diagnostic Bronchoscopy 83
Bronchoalveolar Lavage 85
Sputum Gram Stain, Culture, and Sensitivity 85
Blood Tests (RRT-Specific Content) 85
Pulmonary Function Tests 85
Lung Mechanics 86
Blood Gas Analysis, Pulse Oximetry,
    and Transcutaneous Monitoring 88
Capnography 90
Electrocardiography 90
Hemodynamic Monitoring 90
Sleep Studies 91
Thoracentesis (RRT-Specific Content) 92
Common Errors to Avoid 92
Sure Bets 93
Pre-Test Answers and Explanations 93
Post-Test 94

CHAPTER 4
Manipulate Equipment by Order or Protocol 95

Objectives 95
**What to Expect on this Category
    of The NBRC Exams** 96
Pre-Test 96
What You Need to Know:
Essential Content 99
Gas Cylinders, Reducing Valves,
    Flowmeters, and O_2 Blenders 99
Air Compressors 100
Portable O_2 Systems (RRT-Specific Content) 101
Oxygen Administration Devices 101
He/O_2-Delivery Systems
    (RRT-Specific Content) 110
Humidifiers, Nebulizers, and Mist Tents 111
Aerosol Drug-Delivery Systems 114
Incentive Breathing Devices 121
Mechanical Devices Used to
    Aid Airway Clearance 121
Resuscitation Devices 121
Artificial Airways 123
Ventilators, CPAP Devices,
    and Breathing Circuits 123
Vacuum/Suction Systems 134
Pleural Drainage Systems 136
Manometers 138
O_2, He, CO, and Specialty Gas Analyzers 140
Bedside Pulmonary Function Devices 140
ECG Monitors 145

12-Lead ECG Machines 145
Point-of-Care Blood Gas Analyzers 148
Noninvasive Oximetry Monitoring Devices 149
Hemodynamic Monitoring Devices
    (RRT-Specific Content) 151
Bronchoscopes 153
Common Errors to Avoid 154
Sure Bets 155
Pre-Test Answers and Explanations 155
Post-Test 158

CHAPTER 5
Ensure Infection Control 159

Objectives 159
**What to Expect on this
    Category of The NBRC Exams** 159
Pre-Test 159
What You Need to Know:
Essential Content 161
Key Terms and Definitions 161
Ensure Equipment Cleanliness 161
Properly Handle Biohazardous Materials 164
Adhere to Infection Control
    Policies and Procedures 165
Adhere to the Ventilator-Associated
    Pneumonia Protocol 168
Implement Specific Infectious
    Disease Protocols 169
Common Errors to Avoid 171
Sure Bets 171
Pre-Test Answers and Explanations 172
Post-Test 173

CHAPTER 6
Perform Quality Control Procedures 174

Objectives 174
**What to Expect on this Category
    of The NBRC Exams** 174
Pre-Test 174
What You Need to Know:
Essential Content 175
Key Terms and Definitions 175
Laboratory Blood Gas and
    Hemoximetry Analyzers 175
Point-of-Care Analyzers 180
Pulmonary Function Test Equipment 181
Mechanical Ventilators 183
Gas Analyzers 186
Noninvasive Monitors 187
Gas Delivery and Metering Devices 188
Common Errors to Avoid 189
Sure Bets 189

Pre-Test Answers and Explanations 189
Post-Test 190

CHAPTER 7

Maintain Records and Communicate Information 191

Objectives 191
What to Expect on this
Category of The NBRC Exams 191
Pre-Test 191
What You Need to Know:
Essential Content 193
Accept and Verify Patient Care Orders 193
Record Therapy and Results 194
Communicating Information 199
Applying Computer Technology to
Medical Record Keeping 199
Explaining Planned Therapy and
Goals to Patients 201
Communicating Results of Therapy and
Altering Therapy According
to Protocol(s) 201
Educating the Patient and Family 202
Common Errors to Avoid 206
Sure Bets 206
Pre-Test Answers and Explanations 207
Post-Test 208

CHAPTER 8

Maintain a Patent Airway/ Care of Artificial Airways 209

Objectives 209
What to Expect on this
Category of The NBRC Exams 209
Pre-Test 209
What You Need to Know:
Essential Content 210
Position Patients Properly 210
Insert Oropharyngeal and
Nasopharyngeal Airways 210
Endotracheal Intubation 213
Tracheotomy 216
Tracheal Airway Cuff Management 220
Troubleshooting Tracheal Airways 221
Alternative Emergency Airways 222
Maintaining Adequate Humidification 228
Perform Extubation 231
Common Errors to Avoid 232
Sure Bets 232
Pre-Test Answers and Explanations 233
Post-Test 234

CHAPTER 9

Remove Bronchopulmonary Secretions 235

Objectives 235
What to Expect on this
Category of The NBRC Exams 235
Pre-Test 235
What You Need to Know:
Essential Content 237
Selecting the Best Approach 237
Postural Drainage, Percussion, Vibration,
and Turning 237
Provide Instruction in and Encourage
Bronchopulmonary Hygiene Techniques 239
Mechanical Devices to Facilitate
Secretion Clearance 241
Clearance of Secretions via Suctioning 245
Administer Aerosol Therapy with
Prescribed Medications 250
Common Errors to Avoid 251
Sure Bets 251
Pre-Test Answers and
Explanations 252
Post-Test 253

CHAPTER 10

Achieve Adequate Respiratory Support 254

Objectives 254
What to Expect on this Category
of The NBRC Exams 254
Pre-Test 254
What You Need to Know:
Essential Content 257
Instruct Patients in Deep
Breathing/Muscle Training 257
Initiate and Adjust Mechanical Ventilation 259
Noninvasive Ventilation 269
Elevated Baseline Pressure
(CPAP, PEEP, EPAP, P_{low}) 271
Selecting Ventilator Graphics 273
Applying Disease-Specific
Ventilator Protocols 275
Initiating and Adjusting
High-Frequency Ventilation 276
Initiate and Modify Weaning Procedures 279
Administer Medications 281
Treating and Preventing Hypoxemia 287
Common Errors to Avoid 289
Sure Bets 289
Pre-Test Answers and
Explanations 290
Post-Test 292

CHAPTER 11

Evaluate and Monitor the Patient's Objective and Subjective Responses to Respiratory Care — 293

Objectives — 293
What to Expect on this
  Category of The NBRC Exams — 293
Pre-Test — 293
What You Need to Know:
  Essential Content — 297
  Recommend and Review Chest Radiographs — 297
  Obtaining Blood Samples — 298
  Obtaining a Capillary Blood Sample — 301
  Arterial Blood Gas Interpretation — 301
  Evaluating CO-Oximetry Results — 304
  Obtaining and Interpreting Pulse
    Oximetry Data — 305
  Obtaining and Interpreting
    Capnography Data — 306
  Interpreting Transcutaneous
    Monitoring Data — 308
  Hemodynamic Assessment — 309
  Measuring and Recording Vital Signs — 309
  Monitoring Cardiac Rhythms — 310
  Evaluating Fluid Balance — 312
  Interpreting Bronchoprovocation Studies — 312
  Recommending Blood Tests — 312
  Observing and Interpreting
    Changes in Sputum Characteristics — 312
  Auscultating the Chest and
    Interpreting Breath Sounds — 313
  Observing for Patient–Ventilator Asynchrony — 313
  Adjusting and Checking Alarm Systems — 314
  Measuring FIO_2 and Liter Flow — 317
  Monitoring and Assessing Airway Pressures — 317
  Interpreting Ventilator Graphics — 321
Common Errors to Avoid — 325
Sure Bets — 326
Pre-Test Answers and Explanations — 326
Post-Test — 328

CHAPTER 12

Independently Modify Therapeutic Procedures Based on the Patient's Response — 329

Objectives — 329
What to Expect on this
  Category of The NBRC Exams — 329
Pre-Test — 329
What You Need to Know:
  Essential Content — 333

Terminating Treatment Based on the Patient's
  Response to Therapy — 333
Modifying Treatment Techniques — 333
Ventilator Waveform Evaluation — 348
Weaning from Ventilatory Support — 351
Common Errors to Avoid — 351
Sure Bets — 352
Pre-Test Answers and Explanations — 352
Post-Test — 354

CHAPTER 13

Recommend Modifications in the Respiratory Care Plan — 355

Objectives — 355
What to Expect on this
  Category of The NBRC Exams — 355
Pre-Test — 355
What You Need to Know:
  Essential Content — 359
  Recommending and Modifying
    Bronchial Hygiene Therapy — 359
  Recommending Changes in
    Patient Positioning — 359
  Recommending Insertion or Modifications of
    Artificial Airways — 359
  Recommending Treatment of
    a Pneumothorax — 359
  Recommending Adjustment in Fluid Balance — 362
  Recommending Adjustment of
    Electrolyte Therapy — 362
  Recommending Initiation and
    Modification of Drug Therapy — 362
  Recommending Sedation and
    Neuromuscular Blockade — 362
  Recommending Changes in Oxygen Therapy — 365
  Recommending Changes in
    Mechanical Ventilation — 365
Common Errors to Avoid — 374
Sure Bets — 374
Pre-Test Answers and Explanations — 375
Post-Test — 378

CHAPTER 14

Determine Appropriateness of the Prescribed Respiratory Care Plan and Recommend Modifications — 379

Objectives — 379
What to Expect on this
  Category of The NBRC Exams — 379
Pre-Test — 379
What You Need to Know:
  Essential Content — 381

Analyzing Available Data to Determine
Pathophysiological State 381
Reviewing Prescribed Therapy to
Establish a Therapeutic Plan 381
Determining the Appropriateness of
Prescribed Therapy and Goals 381
Recommending Changes in the Therapeutic
Plan When Indicated Based on Data 383
Performing Respiratory Care Quality
Assurance 383
Developing, Monitoring, and
Applying Respiratory Care Protocols 385
Examples of Protocol Algorithms 385
Protocol Monitoring and Quality Assurance 385
Common Errors to Avoid **386**
Sure Bets **387**
Pre-Test Answers and Explanations **387**
Post-Test **389**

CHAPTER 15

Initiate, Conduct, or Modify Respiratory Care Techniques in an Emergency Setting 390

Objectives **390**
What to Expect on this
Category of The CRT Exam **390**
Pre-Test **390**
What You Need to Know:
Essential Content **391**
Basic Life Support 391
Advanced Cardiac Life Support (ACLS) 392
Pediatric and Neonatal Emergencies 395
Treat a Tension Pneumothorax 395
Patient Transport 398
Medical Emergency Teams 402
Disaster Management 402
Common Errors to Avoid **405**
Sure Bets **406**
Pre-Test Answers and Explanations **406**
Post-Test **407**

CHAPTER 16

Act as an Assistant to the Physician Performing Special Procedures 408

Objectives **408**
What to Expect on this
Category of The NBRC Exams **408**
Pre-Test **408**
What You Need to Know:
Essential Content **410**
Common Elements of Each Procedure 410
Assisting with Endotracheal Intubation 410

Assisting with Bronchoscopy 416
Assisting with Tracheotomy 418
Assisting with Thoracentesis 419
Assisting with Chest Tube Insertion
(Tube Thoracostomy) 420
Assisting with Cardioversion 421
Assisting with Moderate
(Conscious) Sedation 422
Assisting with Pulmonary Artery
Catheterization (RRT-Specific Content) 423
Common Errors to Avoid **425**
Sure Bets **425**
Pre-Test Answers and
Explanations **426**
Post-Test **427**

CHAPTER 17

Initiate and Conduct Pulmonary Rehabilitation and Home Care 428

Objectives **428**
What to Expect on this
Category of The NBRC Exams **428**
Pre-Test **428**
What You Need to Know:
Essential Content **430**
Pulmonary Rehabilitation 430
Respiratory Home Care 432
Common Errors to Avoid **443**
Sure Bets **443**
Pre-Test Answers and
Explanations **443**
Post-Test **444**

SECTION II

Clinical Simulation Exam (CSE) Preparation 445

CHAPTER 18

Preparing for the Clinical Simulation Exam 447

CSE Content **447**
CSE Topical Coverage 447
CSE Content by Disease Category 449
CSE Structure **452**
Overall Structure and Sections 452
Relationship Between Information
Gathering and Decision Making 453
Relationship Between NBRC Topics
and CSE Skills 454
Disease Management and
Diagnostic Reasoning 454

Summary of CSE Preparation
Do's and Don'ts 455
Do's 455
Don'ts 456

CHAPTER 19

Taking the Clinical Simulation Exam 457

CSE Computer Testing Format
and Option Scoring 457
Scenario Guidance 459
Information Gathering Guidance 460
Do's and Don'ts 460
"Always Select" Choices 460
Selecting Respiratory-Related Information 461
Selecting Pulmonary Function
and Exercise Test Information 461
Selecting Laboratory Tests 462
Selecting Imaging Studies 462
Information Needs in Cases Involving
a Cardiovascular Disorder 463
Information Needs in Cases Involving a
Neurologic or Neuromuscular Disorder 463
Analysis: The Missing Link between
Information Gathering
and Decision Making 464
Decision-Making Guidance 464
Do's and Don'ts 464
Decision Making Based on Physical
Assessment Findings 464
Decision Making Based on Problems
with Secretions and/or Airway Clearance 465
Decision Making Based on Problems
Involving Acid–Base Imbalances 465
Decision Making Based on Problems
Involving Disturbances of Oxygenation 465
Pacing Yourself When Taking The CSE 467
Summary Guidance and Next Steps 467

CHAPTER 20

Clinical Simulation Exam
Case Management Pearls 468

Chronic Obstructive
Pulmonary Disease 468
Assessment/Information Gathering 468
Treatment/Decision Making 468
Trauma 470
Chest Trauma 470
Head Trauma (Traumatic Brain Injury) 472
Spinal Cord Injuries 473
Burns/Smoke Inhalation 475

Hypothermia 477
Cardiovascular Disease 479
Congestive Heart Failure 479
Coronary Artery Disease and
Acute Coronary Syndrome 481
Valvular Heart Disease 483
Cardiac Surgery 483
Neuromuscular Disorders 487
Neuromuscular Disorders with
Acute Manifestations (Guillain-Barré
Syndrome and Myasthenia Gravis) 487
Muscular Dystrophy 487
Tetanus 491
Pediatric Problems 492
Croup (Laryngotracheobronchitis)
and Epiglottitis 492
Bronchiolitis 492
Childhood Asthma 495
Cystic Fibrosis 499
Neonatal Problems 501
Delivery Room Management 501
Apnea of Prematurity 503
Infant Respiratory Distress Syndrome 504
Bronchopulmonary Dysplasia 505
Critical Congenital Heart Defects 506
Other Medical or Surgical
Conditions 508
Drug Overdose and Poisonings 508
Obesity–Hypoventilation Syndrome 509

APPENDIX A

Test-Taking Tips and Techniques 511

How to Fail your NBRC Exam 511
How to Pass your NBRC
Written Exam 512
Know Your Enemy 512
Working in the NBRC Hospital 514
Develop Test-Wiseness 515
Taking Your Test 533
Be Familiar with the Exam Format 533
Strategies to Employ During the Test 533

APPENDIX B

Cardiopulmonary Calculations 535

Ventilation Calculations 535
Oxygenation Calculations 535
Calculations Involving
Pulmonary Mechanics 535
Pulmonary Function Calculations 535
Cardiovascular Calculations 541

Equipment Calculations **541**
Formulas and Example Problems
for Mechanical Ventilation
Time and Flow Parameters **541**
Drug Calculations **541**

APPENDIX C
Selected Sources **547**

General Sources **547**
Books 547
Guidelines and Consensus Statements 547
Chapter-Specific Sources **551**
Chapter 2 551
Chapter 4 552
Chapter 5 552
Chapter 6 552
Chapter 7 552
Chapter 8 552
Chapter 9 552
Chapter 10 553
Chapter 12 553
Chapter 14 553

Chapter 15 553
Chapter 16 553
Chapter 17 553
Chapter 20 553

APPENDIX D
What's Online **556**

Accessing The Companion Website **556**
Online Resources **556**
Chapter Post-Tests 556
Mock CRT and WRRT Exams 556
CSE Practice Problems 556
Web Resources 557
Updated Mock Exam, Topical Content,
and Practice Exercises 557

APPENDIX E
RTBoardReview.com **558**

Index **559**

Contributors

Second Edition

Narciso E. Rodriguez, BS, RRT, NPS, ACCS, RPFT, AE-C
Program Director and Assistant Professor
Rutgers, the State University of New Jersey
Newark, NJ

First Edition

Salomay R. Corbaley, MBA, RRT, NPS, AE-C
Professor, Respiratory Care Program
El Camino College
Torrance, CA

Sandra McCleaster, MA, RRT, NPS
Adjunct Faculty
Bergen Community College
Paramus, NJ

Roy Mekaru, BS, MHA, RRT, NPS
Director of Clinical Education
El Camino College
Torrance, CA

Narciso E. Rodriguez, BS, RRT, NPS, ACCS, RPFT, AE-C
Assistant Professor, Department of Primary Care
School of Health Related Professions
University of Medicine and Dentistry of New Jersey
Newark, NJ

John A. Rutkowski, MBA, MPA, RRT, FACHE
Assistant Professor, Department of Primary Care
School of Health Related Professions
University of Medicine and Dentistry of New Jersey
Newark, NJ

Brian X. Weaver, MS, RRT, RPFT, NPS
Director of Respiratory Therapy
The University Hospital
University of Medicine and Dentistry of New Jersey
Newark, NJ

Robert L. Wilkins, PhD, RRT, FAARC
Clinical Professor, Department of Respiratory Care
University of Texas Health Science Center
San Antonio, TX

Kenneth A. Wyka, MS, RRT, FAARC
Cardiopulmonary Clinical Specialist
Anthem Health Services
Albany, NY

Reviewers

Thomas D. Baxter, EdD
Dean–Allied Health; Program Director–Respiratory Care
St. Johns River State College
St. Augustine, FL

Charity Bowling, MA, RRT
Associate Profession, Program Chair Respiratory/Polysomnography
Ivy Tech Community College–Central
Indianapolis, IN

Sharon Hatfield, PhD, RRT, CPFT, AE-C, COPD Educator
Chair of Community Health Sciences, RT Faculty
Jefferson College of Health Sciences
Roanoke, VA

Joanne Jacobs, MA RRT, AE-C
Professor, Program Director
Community College of Rhode Island
Lincoln, RI

Tammie Jones, BS, RRT
Assistant Professor, Clinical Coordinator of Respiratory Care
Kansas City Kansas Community College
Kansas City, KS

Chris Kallus, MEd, RRT
Professor and Program Chair
Victoria College
Victoria, TX

Debra Kasel, MEd
Associate Professor
Northern Kentucky University
Highland Heights, KY

Becky Renfrow, MS, RRT, CPFT, CHT
Clinical Coordinator, Respiratory Care
Angelina College
Lufkin, TX

Chris Trotter, MH, BS, RRT
Assistant Professor
Marshall University/St. Mary's Center for Education
Huntington, WV

Introduction

Using This Book and Online Resources: Your Roadmap to Success

Craig L. Scanlan

To obtain a license to practice and become a Registered Respiratory Therapist (RRT), you currently must pass three National Board for Respiratory Care (NBRC) exams: the certification examination (CRT), the written registry exam (WRRT), and the clinical simulation exam (CSE).* Preparing for and passing these exams is no small task. Each year, despite intensive schooling, many candidates fail one or more of these exams, often requiring multiple attempts to achieve their goal. And because most states require that you pass the CRT exam to become licensed, you simply cannot afford to do poorly on that portion of your boards.

To accomplish any major task, you need the right plan and the right tools. This book provides you with both. Our plan is based on decades of experience in helping candidates pass their board exams. Underlying our plan is a set of tried-and-true tools that have helped thousands of candidates become licensed and get registered. Follow our plan and you, too, can obtain the NBRC credentials you desire!

BOOK OVERVIEW

This book and its online resources provide you with everything you need to pass the NBRC exams. Following this introduction, Section I provides 17 chapters covering the *topical content* tested on all three NBRC exams (see the accompanying box). Each chapter in Section I covers the corresponding NBRC exam topic. This approach lets you concentrate on the exact knowledge tested in each area. Organizing these chapters by NBRC topic also is helpful if you have to retake a written exam. The best way to ensure success when retaking the CRT or WRRT exam is to focus your efforts on those topics where you previously did poorly. To do so, simply review your NBRC written exam score report to identify the topics where you scored lowest, and then focus your work on the corresponding text chapters.

Because the same 17 major topics underlie the CSE exam, Section I also is useful in preparing for that portion of the NBRC test battery. However, due to the CSE's unique structure and case-management approach, the text provides a separate three-chapter section on preparing for and taking this exam.

Section I: Shared Topical Content (Chapters 1–17)

Chapter Objectives and What to Expect

Each chapter begins with a set of *Objectives* and a brief description of what to expect on the corresponding section of the NBRC exams. Chapter objectives delineate the specific knowledge you need to master. Objectives always cover the topics *shared* across all three NBRC exams (CRT, WRRT, and CSE). Where applicable, separate objectives are provided to cover *RRT-specific* exam topics—that is, those topics appearing only on the WRRT or the CSE. By highlighting RRT-specific topics, we help you focus your study efforts when preparing for these advanced exams.

---

*Beginning in 2015 there will be one written exam with two different cut scores. Candidates attaining the lower score will earn the CRT credential, while those meeting the higher score requirement will be eligible for the CSE. Text updates reflecting these and other NBRC credentialing exam changes can be accessed via the JB Learning companion website described in Appendix D.

Topical Content Areas Common to the CRT, WRRT, and CSE Exams

I. Patient Data Evaluation and Recommendations

    A. Review Data in the Patient Record

    B. Collect and Evaluate Additional Pertinent Clinical Information

    C. Recommend Procedures to Obtain Additional Data

II. Equipment Manipulation, Infection Control, and Quality Control

    A. Manipulate Equipment by Order or Protocol

    B. Ensure Infection Control

    C. Perform Quality Control Procedures

III. Initiation and Modification of Therapeutic Procedures

    A. Maintain Records and Communicate Information

    B. Maintain a Patent Airway, Including the Care of Artificial Airways

    C. Remove Bronchopulmonary Secretions

    D. Achieve Adequate Respiratory Support

    E. Evaluate and Monitor the Patient's Objective and Subjective Responses to Respiratory Care

    F. Independently Modify Therapeutic Procedures Based on the Patient's Response

    G. Recommend Modifications in the Respiratory Care Plan Based on the Patient's Response

    H. Determine the Appropriateness of the Prescribed Respiratory Care Plan and Recommend Modifications When Indicated by Data

    I. Initiate, Conduct, or Modify Respiratory Care Techniques in an Emergency Setting

    J. Act as an Assistant to the Physician Performing Special Procedures

    K. Initiate and Conduct Pulmonary Rehabilitation and Home Care

---

    Each chapter's *What to Expect* descriptions specify the number and level of questions you will encounter on the current exams. This knowledge is intended to help you set your study priorities. For example, there are proportionately twice as many questions on the current CRT exam covering topic II-A (Manipulate Equipment by Order or Protocol) than on the WRRT exam. Based on this knowledge, you would logically give more attention to this area when preparing for the CRT exam than when studying for the WRRT.

    Because chapter length roughly corresponds to the topical emphasis on the NBRC exams, you also can use this information to help set study priorities. For example, Chapter 2 (Collect and Evaluate Additional Pertinent Clinical Information) is among the longest not only because topic I-B constitutes a large proportion of CRT and WRRT exam content, but also because this topic underlies the information gathering skills needed to succeed on the CSE. In contrast, Chapter 16 (Assisting the Physician with Special Procedures) is among our shortest chapters because the current NBRC written exams contain only two questions in this category. Thus you can gauge the needed exam prep time by the relative length of our chapters.

Pre-Test Questions with Answers and Explanations

All 17 topical chapters begin with a short pre-test and end with the answers to these questions and their explanations. Like chapter length, the number of questions on each pre-test varies according to the relative topical emphasis on the CRT and WRRT exams. In total, the 17 chapter pre-tests provide more than 270 practice questions to help you prepare for the NBRC written exams. Because the same topics are covered on the CSE, your mastery of this knowledge can help you succeed on that exam as well.

    A word of warning: Some candidates try to memorize as many questions and answers as possible in hopes that doing so will help them pass the NBRC exams. *This is a huge mistake and a waste of your time*. The likelihood of seeing the exact same questions from any source on the NBRC exams is small. Instead, we recommend that you take our chapter pre-tests to assess your knowledge of each topic. This information will help you (1) identify high-priority topics and (2) adjust the amount of time you spend on each chapter.

In terms of study priorities, *use the pre-tests to help differentiate between the concepts you have mastered and those for which you need further study*. For example, if you consistently get questions on ventilator peak and plateau pressures wrong, you do not fully understand the mechanics of ventilation. You should then review the relevant content, including (in this example) the measurement of total impedance, airway resistance, and compliance.

In general, the first source for reviewing a pre-test question is the explanation provided at the end of the chapter. You should thoroughly review these explanations until you understand *why* the answer is the right choice. If you are still unclear about a concept after reviewing its explanation, seek out the more detailed information provided in the chapter or the supplemental online resources.

What You Need to Know: Essential Content

The *Essential Content* section is the "meat" of each Section I chapter. We have distilled this content down to what we consider the essential *need-to-know* information most likely to appear on the NBRC exams, with an emphasis on bulleted outlines and summary tables.

Common Errors to Avoid

One of the unique aspects of this text is its use of prior candidates' common testing mistakes (obtained by analysis of question statistics from online testing). The *Common Errors to Avoid* section of each chapter provides a short summary of these common errors. You can improve your NBRC exam scores by avoiding these mistakes!

Sure Bets

Although you probably have been told to watch out for "always" answers, a few relative certainties apply when responding to NBRC test questions. We highlight these *Sure Bets* at the end of each chapter. As with avoiding common mistakes, knowing what consistently is the right choice can add extra points to your score!

Section II: Clinical Simulation Exam (CSE) Preparation (Chapters 18–20)

Most candidates know that the CSE has a unique structure. What most candidates fail to appreciate—and the reason why so many fail the CSE—is that the skills assessed on this exam also differ significantly from those tested on the CRT and WRRT. Yes, the CSE shares the same topical content with the multiple-choice exams. However, mastering topical content alone will not get you a passing score on the CSE, because the CSE also tests your *case-management abilities*.

Section II of the text helps you prepare for the CSE by emphasizing case-management preparation. Chapter 18 reviews the seven disease categories from which current CSE cases are drawn and outlines a specific review strategy that focuses on disease management skills. Chapter 19 discusses the different reasoning needed to do well on the information gathering and decision-making sections of CSE problems, while also recommending both general Do's and Don'ts and specific choices likely to help you boost your scores. Chapter 20 completes the CSE section with over two dozen sets of case-management pearls covering the clinical problems most likely to appear on the CSE.

Appendices

Supplementing these chapters are two useful appendices—one on "Test-Taking Tips and Techniques" (Appendix A), and one on "Cardiopulmonary Calculations" (Appendix B). Additional appendices provide a list of the selected sources supporting this book (Appendix C), a description of the supplemental resources provided online by Jones & Bartlett Learning (Appendix D), and information on RTBoardReview.com (Appendix E), the online review program from which this book evolved.

Robust Online Resources

To enhance this text, Jones & Bartlett Learning provides a set of online resources to further support your preparation for the NBRC exams. To access these resources, point your browser to **go.jblearning.com/respexamreviewCWS**.

These resources include a post-test for each of the 17 Section I chapters, mock CRT and WRRT exams, and seven practice clinical simulation problems. Also available online is the latest information on the exam changes the NBRC plans for 2015, including—where applicable—new custom content and representative new practice questions. In addition, this site provides access to regularly updated Web resources covering both the NBRC topical content and disease management guidelines, provided courtesy of RTBoardReview.com.

TEST PREPARATION STRATEGY

Written Test Preparation (CRT and WRRT Exams)

The following figure (next page) outlines the strategy we recommend you follow to prepare for the CRT and WRRT exams. *You should devote at least 6 weeks to this process.* One of the most common reasons why candidates fail the NBRC written exams is hasty or last-minute preparation. Do yourself a favor and follow a deliberate and unhurried process. Remember—it was the slow-and-steady tortoise who won the race, not the rushing hare!

Some of you will implement this strategy on your own, while others may be guided in their preparation while still in a respiratory therapy program. In either case, it is important to proceed systematically through each chapter and not to move forward until you have mastered the relevant content.

For Those Who Have Not Been Successful

If you purchased this text because you failed an NBRC exam, you are not alone. For example, approximately 1 in 5 candidates is unsuccessful in passing the CRT exam the first time around, with nearly 3 out of 4 repeaters not passing subsequent attempts. Although you likely are unhappy with your test results, such an event gives you an advantage over those who have never taken the exam. First, you know what to expect regarding the testing procedures. Second, your score report tells you where you did well and where you did poorly. Based on this information, we recommend you compute the percentage of correct questions for each of the 17 topical subscores on your NBRC score report. For example, if you correctly answered 11 of 22 questions on section II-A of the NBRC CRT exam, you would compute your percentage correct as $11/22 = 0.50$ or 50%. We *recommend that you flag any section on which you scored less than 75%.* You should then focus your attention on these flagged topics and their corresponding book chapters in preparing to retake the exam. Of course, you should still review chapters in areas where you scored more than 75%, *but only after attending to your high-priority needs.*

Topical Chapter Review Process

For this strategy to succeed, it is essential that you proceed systematically through each chapter. As delineated in **Figure 1**, this normally involves the following steps:

1. Take and score the chapter pre-test.
2. Review the pre-test to determine your shortcomings.
3. Prioritize chapter content based on identified shortcomings.
4. Review the applicable chapter content.
5. Take and pass the online chapter post-test.
6. Repeat steps 1 to 5 for each chapter.

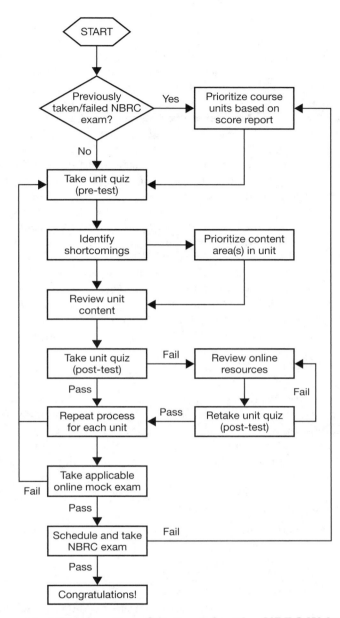

Figure 1 Recommended Preparation Strategy for the NBRC Written Exams.

In regard to step 5 (taking and passing chapter post-tests), we recommend you set a goal of achieving at *least 80% correct* on each chapter post-test. In addition, your post-test scores generally should be higher than your pre-test scores. The greater this difference, the more you have learned!

What if you fail a chapter post-test? Your first job should be to review the question explanations. If you are still unsure of the concept being tested, review the applicable chapter content yet again. If that does not suffice, you should go online to access and review any applicable Web resources related to the topic with which you are having difficulty.

Take the Applicable Mock Exam

The CRT and WRRT mock exams are intended to simulate the corresponding NBRC test. Like the chapter pre-tests and post-tests, these online exams give you feedback on each and every question, including the correct answers and their corresponding explanations.

With this feedback, our mock exams become a critical learning tool in your path to success on the NBRC written exams. First, your overall score on these exams tells you how well you have mastered the content covered in the book and on the applicable test. Second, careful review of the question explanations should enhance your understanding of the concepts likely to be tested on the exam for which you are preparing. Finally, review of these explanations can help you identify any remaining areas of weakness you need to address before scheduling your exam date.

Because the mock exams serve as a bridge between the book and the applicable NBRC written exams, we recommend that you take them only after completing all 17 of the book's topical content chapters, including passing each of their post-tests. We also recommend that you complete the applicable mock exam *at least 2 weeks* before you are scheduled to take the corresponding NBRC exam. This way, you will have enough time to review any persistent areas of misunderstanding and can avoid the anxiety that last-minute cramming always creates.

We also recommend that you track your time when taking our mock exams. *Based on the number of questions included and the NBRC time limits, you will need to complete approximately one question per minute.* If you find yourself taking significantly longer on each question, you will need to increase your testing pace before taking the actual NBRC exam.

What if you do not score well on our mock exams? If you carefully follow the strategy we outline here, it is highly unlikely that you will do poorly on our exams. In the unusual case where you score less than 75%, it's "back to the books." In this case, careful review of the test items you got wrong on our mock exams should help you identify the content areas and book chapters that need additional review.

Schedule and Take the Exam

After successfully completing all topical chapters, their post-tests, and the applicable mock exam, it is time to schedule and take the real exam. If you have not already done so, we strongly recommend you use some of the time you have set aside before sitting for your written NBRC exam to review Appendix A (Test-Taking Tips and Techniques). Also, consider taking a practice trip to and from your NBRC testing center, ideally at the same time your exam is scheduled. This run-through can help you gauge travel time and iron out little details where you will park and where you can get a cup of coffee before the exam.

What if you do not pass an NBRC written exam? There are several Do's and Don'ts associated with a failed attempt on the exam. First the Don'ts:

- Don't get disheartened or give up.
- Don't immediately reschedule a retake.

Instead, take a proactive approach. Do the following:

- Do carefully analyze your NBRC score report.
- Do use your score report to prioritize content areas needing further study.
- Do revisit the key content area resources we provide in the book and online.
- Do give yourself adequate time to implement your new study plan (at least 3–4 weeks).

Last, if you want or need access to regularly updated content, additional practice written tests based on larger pools of NBRC-like questions, and more CSE practice problems, we recommend that you consider the RTBoardReview.com online review courses described in Appendix E. Purchasers of this book are eligible for discounted RTBoardReview.com enrollment fees.

CSE Test Preparation

As emphasized in Chapter 18, we strongly recommend that you *schedule the CSE only after you have passed the WRRT exam* and devote at least 3 to 4 weeks preparing for it (beginning in 2015, you will not be able to take the CSE on the same day with the new single written exam). Besides avoiding the anxiety caused by last-minute preparation, this approach lets you apply your WRRT results to your study plan.

As previously discussed, the CSE shares the same topical content as is covered on the CRT and WRRT. Consequently, preparation for the CSE should begin with a review of all 17 Section I book chapters. As discussed in Chapter 18, you should use your CRT and WRRT results to identify the topics needing the most attention, and then proceed with their review.

However, topical review should *not* be the primary focus for your CSE preparation. Why? There are three reasons. First, to be eligible for the CSE, you already had to demonstrate topical content mastery, by passing at least the CRT exam. Second, *the primary focus of the CSE is case management, not topical knowledge*. Third, the CSE's structure requires that you develop and apply special test-taking skills specific to its unique test format.

In terms of case management, we recommend you devote the majority of your time to reviewing the medical management of specific cases likely to appear on the CSE. Chapter 18 applies this important information and outlines our recommendations on the resources you should use to strengthen your case management knowledge.

In regard to test-taking proficiency, the unique format of the CSE requires a different set of skills from those needed to succeed on multiple-choice exams (the test-taking tips covered in Appendix A). For this reason, we provide a separate chapter designed to help you develop CSE-specific testing proficiency (Chapter 19). You should review these tips before working through the online practice simulation problems.

The online practice problems are designed to give you experience with the CSE format and help you apply the case management and CSE test-taking skills reviewed in Chapters 18 and 19. If you score poorly on any individual practice problem or consistently have difficulty with either information gathering or decision making, we recommend you review the test-taking skills in Chapter 19 and the corresponding disease management "pearls" provided in Chapter 20. You also may want to access and review the disease management resources available online at the companion Jones & Bartlett Learning website. Then retake the applicable practice problems until you achieve passing scores for both information gathering and decision making.

After completing the practice problems and applying their results to your exam preparation, it is time to schedule and take the CSE. The same general guidance we recommend for scheduling and taking NBRC written exams applies to the CSE. Again, although you currently can schedule the WRRT and the CSE for the same day, we *strongly* recommend against doing so. Besides the fact that 6 hours of testing is bound to cause fatigue and likely compromise your performance, you will miss the opportunity to apply your WRRT results to help prioritize your topical review.

SECTION I

NBRC Exams Shared Topical Content

CHAPTER 1

Review Existing Data in the Patient Record

Albert J. Heuer
(previous version co-authored with Sandra McCleaster)

The medical record contains vital information on the patient's past medical history, physical examinations, lab and imaging test results, and other respiratory-related monitoring data—all of which are needed to support good decision making. Therefore, before providing care, you should always review the medical record to verify the doctors' orders, to familiarize yourself with the patient's overall condition, and to consider all data needed to make decisions or recommendations. For these reasons, the NBRC exams will assess your ability to both locate relevant patient information in the record and apply it to optimize care.

OBJECTIVES

In preparing for the shared NBRC exam content, you should demonstrate the knowledge needed to:

1. Review and determine the relevancy of data in the patient record, including:
   a. Past and present medical history
   b. Physical exams, including vital signs and physical findings
   c. Lab studies such as PFTs, CBC, coagulation studies, sputum tests, and arterial blood gases
   d. Imaging studies, including chest x-rays, MRI and CT scans
   e. Data relating to pulmonary mechanics, noninvasive monitoring, and fluid balance
   f. Other specialized procedures including ECGs and hemodynamics
   g. Maternal, perinatal, neonatal history and data

In preparing for the RRT-specific NBRC exam content, you should demonstrate the knowledge needed to:

2. Review and assess data relating to the diagnosis and treatment of sleep disorders

WHAT TO EXPECT ON THIS CATEGORY OF THE NBRC EXAMS

CRT exam: 4 questions; all recall
WRRT exam: 5 questions; about 20% recall, 80% application
CSE exam: indeterminate number of questions; however, exam I-A knowledge is a prerequisite to success on CSE Information Gathering sections

PRE-TEST

Carefully respond to each of the following questions. After completing the pre-test, compare your answers to those provided at the end of this chapter. Then thoroughly review each answer's explanation to help understand why it is correct.

1-1. Which of the following tests would be most useful in diagnosing a pulmonary emboli?

A. Chest x-ray
B. Pulmonary function test (PFT)
C. Ventilation–perfusion scan (V/Q scan)
D. Arterial blood gas (ABG)

1-2. While examining a patient in the ICU, you note that he appears somewhat edematous, and the nurse has indicated that the patient's urine output is "minimal." In which section of the record would you find the patient's fluid balance (intake versus output)?
   A. Physician orders
   B. Consent form
   C. Laboratoy results
   D. Nurses' notes and flow sheet

1-3. Which of the following physical findings would you expect to see in an alert but anxious patient with asthma early in the course of an attack?
   A. Respiratory acidosis
   B. Respiratory alkalosis
   C. Clubbing
   D. Cor pulmonale

1-4. In the lab results section of a patient's record, the overall WBC count is shown as 22,000 for a febrile patient who appears acutely ill and in moderate respiratory distress. What is the most likely diagnosis?
   A. Bacterial pneumonia
   B. Emphysema
   C. Pulmonary embolus
   D. Pulmonary fibrosis

1-5. A PET scan would be most useful in the diagnosis of which of the following conditions?
   A. Bronchogenic carcinoma
   B. Chronic bronchitis
   C. Pulmonary fibrosis
   D. Smoke inhalation

1-6. Negative inspiratory force (NIF) is most useful in the determination of which of the following?
   A. Airway resistance
   B. Functional residual capacity
   C. Respiratory muscle strength
   D. Sustained maximal inspiration

1-7. A 23-year-old fire fighter is admitted with suspected smoke inhalation. You place him on a nonrebreathing mask. What is the most appropriate method of monitoring his oxygenation?
   A. Arterial blood gas analysis
   B. CO-oximetry
   C. Pulse oximetry
   D. Calculation of $P(A-a)O_2$

1-8. Which of the following notes in the maternal medical and/or obstetric history increases the likelihood of a high-risk pregnancy?
   A. Weight gain
   B. First pregnancy
   C. Regular exercise
   D. Tobacco smoking

1-9. Sputum culture and sensitivity would be indicated in the evaluation of which of the following clinical conditions?
   A. Pulmonary edema
   B. Bacterial pneumonia
   C. Bronchiectasis
   D. Empyema

1-10. A polysomnography report for a patient with a history of excessive daytime sleepiness indicates an average of 25 apnea/hypopnea events per hour, with most events showing continued efforts to breathe. Which of the following statements is most consistent with this observation?
   A. The findings confirm a diagnosis of a moderate central sleep apnea.
   B. The findings confirm a diagnosis of mild obstructive sleep apnea.
   C. The findings confirm a diagnosis of moderate obstructive sleep apnea.
   D. The findings confirm a diagnosis of severe obstructive sleep apnea.

WHAT YOU NEED TO KNOW: ESSENTIAL CONTENT

The patient record contains a variety of clinical information. Today, such records typically are maintained at least in part in both "paper" form and as electronic records. Although the actual organization and formatting of data within the sections of a record may vary among institutions, there is reasonable uniformity in how such information is organized. **Table 1-1** lists the major sections of the typical patient record and the information that may be found in each section.

Table 1-1 Where to Find Clinical Information in the Patient Record*

Section of Record	Information Located in That Section
Admitting sheet/face sheet	Patient's next-of-kin, address, religion, and employer; health insurance information.
Informed consent	Consent forms signed by the patient (and witness) for various diagnostic and therapeutic procedures, such as bronchoscopy and surgery.
DNR/advanced directives	Properly signed and witnessed do-not-resuscitate (DNR), do-not-intubate (DNI), and/or advanced directives.
Patient history	Past/present family, social, and medical history; medications and demographics.
Physician's orders	Doctors' diagnostic and therapeutic orders, including those pertaining to respiratory care. (Note: Incomplete/unclear orders must be clarified with the prescribing physician.)
Laboratory results	WBC/RBC counts, ABGs, electrolytes, coagulation studies, and culture results (e.g., sputum, blood, urine); may include PFTs and sleep study results.
Imaging studies (e.g., x-rays/ CT, MRI, ultrasound)	X-ray, CT, MRI, PET, V/Q scan reports; may also include ultrasound and echocardiography results.
ECGs	The results of electrocardiograms (ECG/EKGs).
Progress notes	Discipline-specific notes on a patient's progress and treatment plan by physicians and other caregivers.
Therapy (respiratory)	Respiratory therapy charting; may include ABGs, PFTs, and sleep study results.
Nurses' notes and flow sheet	Nurses' subjective and objective record of the patient's condition, including vital signs, fluid intake/output (I/O), and hemodynamic monitoring.

*A neonate's medical record may have a section dedicated to birth history, or it may be included in the *patient history* section.

While a complete review of the medical record is important to many aspects of respiratory therapy, the NBRC expects you to be especially familiar with selected patient data. This critical information includes the patient history and physical, pulmonary function tests (PFTs) and arterial blood gas (ABGs) results, imaging tests, and (for RRT exams) sleep studies.

Patient History

Your review of patient demographics and history can provide important clues relating to the patient's chief complaint(s). This review may also uncover information relevant to the patient's current illness, including past medical conditions or surgeries, occupational or environmental exposures, or a history of tobacco and/or alcohol/drug use. **Table 1-2** summarizes areas to emphasize when reviewing a patient's history. More detail on the occupational history is provided in Chapter 2.

Physical Examination

The physical exam portion of the record typically provides vital signs data and the results of chest inspection, palpation, percussion, and auscultation. This information usually is found in the *admission*, *progress notes*, or *respiratory* sections of the record, with subsequent ongoing vital signs trends recorded in the *nurses' notes* or *flow sheet*.

In regard to vital signs, the NBRC expect you to know the normal reference ranges by major age group, as delineated in **Table 1-3**. Remember that single "point" values are generally less informative than trends over time.

Table 1-2 Chart Elements Related to Patient History

Element	Importance
Demographic Data	Factors such as a patient's place of residence and age may be relevant in that some respiratory conditions tend to be more common in certain age groups, in specific geographic locations, and among certain ethnic groups.
History of Present Illness	The patient's chief complaint, description of symptoms, frequency, duration, quality, severity, onset, and features that aggravate or alleviate discomfort are often important in diagnosis and treatment.
Past Medical History	Surgeries, treatments for cancer and heart disease, and congenital and childhood conditions also may be relevant.
Medication History	Complete knowledge of medications, including their dosages and frequencies, that the patient has been taking is essential when implementing new prescriptions.
Family Disease History	The health status of blood relatives that may be useful in considering diseases with hereditary tendencies.
Occupational History/Environmental Exposures	Work history and past environmental exposures (e.g., mining, chemical production, and work involving asbestos) may be linked to respiratory dysfunction.
Social History	Smoking and tobacco usage may contribute to respiratory disorders and should be noted along with alcohol or drug use, social activities, hobbies, recreational activities, and pets.
Patient Education History	Knowledge of prior patient/caregiver education regarding the medical condition and treatment can help in planning future efforts.

In regard to the physical exam of the chest, key aspects to look for are summarized here:

- *Inspection*: to identify scars, chest contour, and abnormalities including increased AP diameter, pectus excavatum, and kyphoscoliosis.
- *Palpation* of the chest: to evaluate symmetry, expansion, and fremitus (vibrations felt at the chest wall).
- *Percussion*: to evaluate underlying soft tissue, most notably the lung and diaphragm. The following sounds are most clinically significant:
  - Normal resonance (moderately low-pitched sound, commonly heard over normal lung tissue)
  - Dull note (high pitched, short duration, not loud, heard over consolidation or atelectasis)
  - Hyperresonance (low pitched, loud, longer duration heard over hyperinflated lungs from asthma or COPD [bilateral] or pneumothorax [unilateral])

Table 1-3 Reference Ranges for Vital Sign Measurements

Vital Sign	Adult	Child (Preschool Age)	Infant
Temperature	98.6°F (37°C)	37.5°C	37.5°C
Pulse	60–100/min	80–120/min	90–170/min
Respiratory rate	12–20/min	20–25/min	35–45/min
Blood pressure	< 120/80 mm Hg	94/52 mm Hg	84/52 mm Hg
Pulse oximetry	95-98%	95-95%	> 92%

- *Auscultation*: to determine the presence of adventitious breath sounds, which may signify clinical abnormalities such as the following:
  - ○ Wheezing (bronchial obstruction, inflammation, asthma)
  - ○ Rhonchi (presence of secretions)
  - ○ Misplaced bronchial sounds (pneumonia)
  - ○ Crackles/rales (pulmonary edema, atelectasis [late inspiratory])
  - ○ Diminished breath sounds with prolonged expiration (COPD or asthma)

Lab Results

Pertinent lab data that you need to assess include both hematology and clinical chemistry test results. **Table 1-4** lists common lab reference ranges for adult patients for the tests likely to appear on NBRC exams as well as the significance of their results. Following are some common examples of abnormal findings:

- Elevated overall white blood cell (WBC) count and differential WBC values such as neutrophils and bands suggest an acute bacterial infection.
- Abnormal red blood cells (RBCs) impact the O_2-carrying capacity of the blood. Increased RBCs (polycythemia) may be associated with chronic hypoxemia, whereas decreased levels may be associated with bleeding or anemia.
- Low serum potassium (hypokalemia) may lead to certain dysrhythmias, such as PVCs, and may be associated with respiratory muscle weakness. *Certain respiratory medications, such as albuterol, may lower serum potassium.*
- Low platelet counts or abnormally long prothrombin time (PT), International Normalized Ratio (INR), and partial thromboplastin time (PTT) indicate a potential for excessive bleeding with procedures causing tissue or blood vessel trauma such as ABG sampling, thoracentesis, or bronchoscopy.
- Cardiac markers such as CK-MB and troponin I can help confirm the occurrence of acute myocardial infarction, while B-type natriuretic peptide (BNP) levels can help diagnose congestive heart failure (CHF).

Sputum Analysis

The characteristics of a patient's sputum, including the amount, color, consistency, and odor, may provide important clinical clues. For example, thick, green, foul-smelling secretions may indicate the presence of a bacterial lung infection. If you detect abnormal sputum, consider recommending a sputum Gram stain and culture and sensitivity (Chapter 3).

Sputum characteristics are often found in the *respiratory therapy* section of the medical record, with the results of microbiological analysis generally found in the *laboratory* section of the chart. Sputum assessment is discussed in more detail in Chapters 2.

Pulmonary Function Testing Results

Pulmonary function test results may include those derived from spirometry, static lung volumes and capacity measurements, and diffusion studies. Results generally can be found either in the laboratory or respiratory sections of the record. These results typically provide information useful in diagnosing the type of condition present (obstructive versus restrictive), the degree of impairment, and the likely prognosis.

Most pulmonary diseases are categorized as restrictive, obstructive, or mixed. **Table 1-5** summarizes the primary features of these categories. Predicted PFT values are primarily a function of a patient's height, sex, and age. The degree of impairment is determined by comparing actual PFT

Table 1-4 Reference Ranges and Significance of Selected Laboratory Tests (Adult Values)

Test	Reference Ranges*	Significance
Hematology		
Red blood cells (RBC)	M 4.6–6.2 × 10⁻⁶/mm³ F 4.2–5.4 × 10⁻⁶/mm³	• Oxygen transport • Response to hypoxemia • Degree of cyanosis
Hemoglobin	M 13.5–16.5 g/dL F 12.0–15.0 g/dL	• Oxygen transport • Response to hypoxemia • Degree of cyanosis
Hematocrit	M 40–54% F 38–47%	• Hemoconcentration (high) or polycythemia (high) • Hemodilution (low)
White blood cells (WBC)	4500–11,500/mm³	• Infection (high)
Platelets	150,000–400,000/mm³	• Slow blood clotting (low) • Check before ABG
Prothrombin time (PT)	12–14 seconds	• Slow clotting (high) • Check before ABG
International Normalized Ratio (patient PT/mean normal PT)	0.8–1.2 (2.0–3.0 for patients on anticoagulants)	• Slow clotting (high) • Check before ABG
Partial thromboplastin time (PTT)	25–37 seconds	• Slow clotting (high) • Check before ABG
Clinical Chemistry		
Sodium	137–147 mEq/L	• Acid–base/fluid balance
Potassium	3.5–4.8 mEq/L	• Metabolic acidosis (high) • Metabolic alkalosis (low) • Cardiac arrhythmias (low)
Chloride	98–105 mEq/L	• Metabolic alkalosis (low)
Blood urea nitrogen (BUN)	7–20 mg/dL	• Renal failure (high)
Creatinine	0.7–1.3 mg/dL	• Renal disease (high)
Glucose	70–105 mg/dL	• Diabetes/ketoacidosis (high)
Total protein	6.3–7.9 g/dL	• Liver disease; malnutrition (low)
Albumin	3.5–5.0 g/dL	• Liver disease; malnutrition (low)
Cholesterol	150–220 mg/dL	• Atherosclerosis (high)
Lactate acid	0.4–2.3 mEq/L	• Tissue hypoxia, shock (high)
Cardiac Biomarkers		
Total creatine kinase (CK)	50–200 U/L	• Acute myocardial infarction (AMI)/various skeletal muscle disorders (high)
Creatine kinase isoenzyme (CK-MB)	< 4–6% total CK	• AMI (rises 4–6 hours after insult, peaks at 24 hours, returns to normal in 2–3 days)
Troponin I	< 0.4 µg/L	• AMI/acute coronary syndrome (rises 3–6 hours after insult, peaks at 12 hours, can persist 7 days)
B-type natriuretic peptide (BNP)	< 20 pg/mL	• < 100 pg/L rules out diagnosis of congestive heart failure (CHF) • > 500 pg/mL help rules in diagnosis of CHF

*Reference ranges vary by institution.

Table 1-5 Restrictive Versus Obstructive Disease

Category of Disorder	Examples	Impact on Flows and Volumes	Typical Measurements
Restrictive	Neuromuscular, pulmonary fibrosis	↓ volumes	FVC, IRV, ERV, RV, TLC
Obstructive	Asthma, COPD	↓ flows	FEV_1, FEV_1% (FEV_1/FVC), PEFR, FEF_{25-75}
Mixed (combined restrictive and obstructive)	Cystic fibrosis	↓ volumes and ↓ flows	As above

results with predicted values, expressed as percent predicted. Results generally can be categorized as follows:

Normal: 80–120%
Mild: 65–80%
Moderate: 50–65%
Severe: < 50%

For obstructive disorders, the degree of reversibility is judged by pre/post bronchodilator testing. An increase in flows of 12–15% or more after bronchodilator therapy suggests significant reversibility.

In addition to measures of flow and volume, the record of some patients may include assessment of diffusing capacity. Diffusing capacity is measured via the inhalation of a trace amount of carbon monoxide (CO) and abbreviated as DLco. The commonly cited reference range for patients with normal lungs is 25–30 mL/min/mm Hg. A low DLco is observed in disorders such as pulmonary fibrosis and emphysema, whereas higher than normal values may occur in polycythemia.

ABG Results

Analysis of ABG samples provides precise measurement of acid–base balance and of the patient's ability to oxygenate and remove CO_2 from the blood. ABG results typically are found with other lab results or in the respiratory section of the record. The following are some considerations you should keep in mind while reviewing ABG results.

Normal Ranges

To review ABG results, you first need to know the common adult reference ranges as listed in **Table 1-6**. We recommend that you first interpret the acid–base status, then evaluate oxygenation separately.

Table 1-6 Arterial Blood Gas Reference Ranges

Parameter	Normal Range
pH	7.35–7.45
$Paco_2$	35–45 torr
Pao_2	80–100 torr*
HCO_3	22–26 mEq/L (mmol/L)
BE	0 ± 2
Sao_2	95–98%*
*Breathing room air.	

Interpreting Primary Acid–Base Disturbances

To quickly determine the basic acid–base status, you need consider only two parameters: pH and $Paco_2$.

As indicated in **Figure 1-1**, you first determine whether the pH is normal (7.35–7.45), low (< 7.35; acidemia), or high (> 7.45; alkalemia). After judging the pH, you then assess the $Paco_2$. A normal $Paco_2$ in the presence of a normal pH indicates normal acid–base balance. If the pH is low, the primary disturbance must be either respiratory acidosis ($Paco_2$ > 45 torr) or metabolic acidosis ($Paco_2 \leq 45$ torr). With a high pH, the primary disturbance must be either respiratory alkalosis ($Paco_2$ < 35 torr) or metabolic alkalosis ($Paco_2 \geq 35$ torr). Confirm metabolic involvement (either primary or compensatory) by assessing the base excess (BE), with values greater than +2 indicating metabolic alkalosis and values less than −2 indicating metabolic acidosis.

Interpreting Severity of Hypoxemia

You categorize the severity of hypoxemia as follows:

Mild: Pao_2 60–79 torr
Moderate: Pao_2 40–59 torr
Severe: Pao_2 < 40 torr

Of course, this interpretation depends in part on whether the patient is breathing supplemental O_2. For example, if a patient's Pao_2 is less than 60 torr when breathing a high F_IO_2 (≥ 0.60), most clinicians would categorize this level of hypoxemia as severe. You also should note that as an alternative to the Pao_2 or Sao_2, it is common to monitor oxygenation noninvasively via pulse oximetry, as described later in this chapter.

Common Abnormal Patterns

More detail on assessing acid-based balance and oxygenation is provided in Chapter 11. In terms of NBRC expectations in reviewing the patient record, you should be able to recognize at least the common abnormal patterns of acid–base balance and oxygenation described in **Table 1-7**.

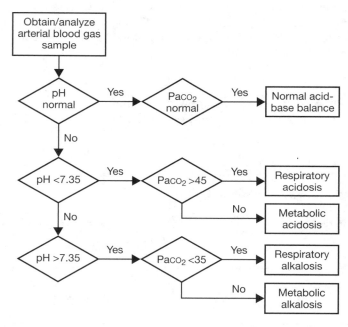

Figure 1-1 Interpretation of Simple Acid–Base Disturbances.

Source: Courtesy of Strategic Learning Associates, LLC, Little Silver, New Jersey.

Table 1-7 Common ABG Abnormalities

Underlying Disorder	Typical ABG Result	Interpretation
Moderate to severe COPD with CO_2 retention	pH 7.36 $Paco_2$ 58 torr Pao_2 62 torr (air) HCO_3 34 mEq/L BE ±7	Fully compensated respiratory acidosis with mild hypoxemia.
Pneumonia, asthma attack, pulmonary emboli, or any other condition associated with moderate or severe hypoxemia	pH 7.53 $Paco_2$ 27 torr Pao_2 53 torr (2 L/min cannula) HCO_3 22 mEq/L BE −7	Uncompensated respiratory alkalosis with moderate hypoxemia. The alkalosis may be a result of hyperventilation associated with hypoxemia.
Uncontrolled diabetes with ketoacidosis	pH 7.32 $Paco_2$ 28 torr Pao_2 108 torr (air) HCO_3 14 mEq/L BE −10	Partially compensated metabolic acidosis with normal oxygenation.
Cardiopulmonary arrest	pH 7.05 $Paco_2$ 60 torr Pao_2 39 torr (air) HCO_3 16 mEq/L BE −8	Combined respiratory and metabolic acidosis with severe hypoxemia (likely causing lactic acidosis).

Imaging Studies

There is usually a separate section in the record for x-ray results or imaging studies. The most common imaging study for most pulmonary patients is the chest x-ray. Chest x-rays are useful in identifying pulmonary conditions such as emphysema, pneumonia, and respiratory distress syndrome (as detailed in Chapters 2 and 11). In addition to the chest x-ray, the NBRC expects you to be familiar with selected other imaging tests results that may be found in the record, as summarized in **Table 1-8**.

Monitoring Data

Additional information related to the pulmonary status of the patient can be found throughout the medical record. With the exception of fluid balance (usually located in the nurses' notes and flow sheet), you will find most of this supplemental information in the respiratory or progress notes sections of the record.

Fluid Balance (Intake and Output)

A patient's fluid balance is the relationship between fluid intake, mainly from drinking and IV infusion, and output, primarily from urination. Normally intake equals output, with each being about 2–3 liters per day. A positive fluid balance results from excessive intake (e.g., IV fluid resuscitation) or decreased output (e.g., renal insufficiency) and may contribute to pulmonary or peripheral edema and/or hypertension. A negative fluid balance is generally due to insufficient hydration and/or excessive urine output from medications such as diuretics or xanthines (theophylline); it may lead to hypotension and low cardiac output.

Table 1-8 Specialized Imaging Studies

Imaging Test	Description
CT scan (computerized tomography)	Facilitates evaluation of abnormalities of the lungs, mediastinum, pleura, and chest wall as well as diagnosis of pulmonary emboli.
MRI (magnetic resonance imaging)	Highly detailed imaging for identifying pathology of the heart, major vessels, mediastinum, lungs, and chest well. Contraindicated in morbidly obese patients and in patients with certain implanted metallic devices.
PET (positron emission tomography)	Creates "metabolic images" of body tissue via uptake of a radioactive tracer injected into the patient. Detects metabolic cellular changes and can identify rapidly growing cells such as those found in lung cancer.
Angiography	By injection of contrast medium, permits evaluation of arterial abnormalities such as arterial aneurysm or pulmonary embolism (now performed mainly via CT scan).
Ventilation–perfusion (V/Q) scan	Angiography to examine lung perfusion and an image of the distribution of ventilation via inhalation of radio-labeled gas (xenon-133); used in diagnosing pulmonary emboli but being replaced by CT angiography.

I/O data normally are found in the nurses' notes and flow sheet section of the record. In assessing output, you should note that urine is usually 60% of the total (1200–1500 mL/day), equivalent to a rate of at least 50 mL/hr. Because 25 mL/hr is considered the minimum output needed to excrete metabolic waste products, values below that level are considered abnormal, and typically described using the term oliguria.

Respiratory Monitoring Parameters

Bedside respiratory monitoring data also may be found in the record, typically in the respiratory section. This information usually appears for patients at risk for developing respiratory failure or those being assessed for weaning from mechanical ventilation. **Table 1-9** summarizes the commonly cited adult reference ranges for these key measures, as well as the critical threshold values that indicate a patient's inability to maintain adequate spontaneous breathing.

Among these measures, the respiratory rate and rapid shallow breathing index have been shown to be the best indicators of whether a patient can tolerate spontaneous breathing. The MIP/

Table 1-9 Respiratory Monitoring Thresholds

Parameter	Common Adult Reference Range	Critical Threshold*
Tidal volume (V_T)	5–8 mL/kg PBW	< 4–5 mL/kg PBW or < 300 mL
Respiratory rate/frequency (f)	12–20/min	> 30–35/min
Minute volume/ventilation ($V\dot{}_E$)	5–6 L/min	> 10 L/min
Rapid shallow breathing index (f/V_T)	20–65	> 100 (SB)
Deadspace/tidal volume ratio (V_D/V_T)	0.25–0.40	> 0.6
Vital capacity (VC)	56–75 mL/kg PBW	< 15 mL/kg PBW
Maximal inspiratory pressure (MIP)/ negative inspiratory force (NIF)	80–100 cm H_2O (negative)	< 30 cm H_2O (negative)
PBW = predicted body weight; SB = spontaneous breathing without CPAP. *Indicating likely inability to maintain adequate spontaneous ventilation.		

NIF and VC measures are less frequently obtained, being used primarily to monitor patients with neuromuscular disorders for changes in respiratory muscle strength and function. Actual measurement of the V_D/V_T ratio (via the Bohr equation) is uncommon; however, this parameter can be estimated via capnography.

Pulmonary Mechanics and the Work of Breathing

Pulmonary mechanics data appearing in a patient's record may include measures of lung and thoracic compliance and airway resistance. These measures may be reported along with other PFT data from labs with body plethysmograph capability. Alternatively, these parameters may be estimated for patients receiving mechanical ventilation, and are usually found on the ventilator flow sheets.

Total (lung plus thoracic) compliance measured via body plethysmography normally is about 100 mL/cm H_2O. Normal values obtained during mechanical ventilation typically are lower, in the range of 40–80 mL/cm H_2O. In mechanically ventilated patients, a reduction in compliance is indicated by rising plateau pressures (see Chapter 11). **Table 1-10** outlines the common causes of decreased lung and thoracic compliance, both acute and chronic. Note that due to loss of elastic tissue, lung compliance typically increases in patients with emphysema.

Normal airway resistance measured via body plethysmography is in the range of 1–3 cm H_2O/L/sec. During mechanical ventilation, the artificial airway adds at least 4–6 cm H_2O/L/sec to the total resistance. Thus, levels significantly above 5–9 cm H_2O/L/sec are associated with airway obstruction (Table 1-10). In mechanically ventilated patients, an increase in inspiratory airway resistance is associated with a widening of the difference between the peak and plateau airway pressures (Chapter 11).

Work of breathing (WOB) is a measurement of the energy used to breathe. The normal reference range for healthy adults is 0.5–0.7 joules/L, obtained by computing the area of an esophageal pressure-versus-volume curve during spontaneous breathing. Any condition that decreases overall compliance or increases airway resistance will increase WOB (Table 1-10).

Estimates of the WOB and its trending can be obtained during mechanical ventilation using the pressure–volume graphics display (Chapter 11). Alternatively, you can estimate the inspiratory work of breathing during controlled mechanical breaths using the area under the airway pressure curve (the pressure–time product). More commonly, you can surmise that a patient likely is experiencing increased WOB based on the clinical signs of tachypnea and accessory muscle use.

Capnography

Capnography measures exhaled carbon dioxide. The most common measure provided is the end-tidal P_{CO_2}, or P_{ETCO_2}. In patients with normal lungs, the P_{ETCO_2} provides a good estimate of the arterial P_{CO_2}, typically running 2–5 torr below the normal ABG value, or between 30 and 43 torr. As with the Pa_{CO_2}, increases in P_{ETCO_2} indicate hypoventilation, while decreases in P_{ETCO_2} signify hyperventilation. Moreover, if the Pa_{CO_2} is known, abnormal increases in the *difference* between the arterial and end-tidal value (the Pa_{CO_2} – P_{ETCO_2} gradient) indicate an increase in physiologic deadspace.

Table 1-10 Common Causes of Abnormal Pulmonary Mechanics

Decreased Lung Compliance	Decreased Thoracic Compliance	Increased Airway Resistance
Pulmonary fibrosis (C)	Kyphoscoliosis (C)	Bronchospasm (I + E)
Pulmonary edema/ARDS (A)	Obesity (C)	Small airway closure (E)
Atelectasis/mainstem intubation (A)	Pectus excavatum (C)	Increased secretions (I + E)
Pneumothorax (A)	Fibrothorax (C)	Peribronchial edema (I + E)
Large pleural effusion (A or C)	Chest wall tumor (C)	Airway tumors (I + E)
Surfactant deficiency (A)		Artificial airway occlusion (I + E)
A = acute; C = chronic; I = inspiratory; E = expiratory.		

Chapter 3 outlines the indications for capnography, Chapter 6 provides details on the setup and calibration of capnographs, and Chapter 11 focuses on the interpretation of basic capnography data.

Pulse Oximetry

Pulse oximetry measurements (SpO_2) are used to noninvasively monitor arterial hemoglobin saturation with oxygen. SpO_2 values typically appear in the progress, respiratory, or nursing notes. The reference range for adults breathing room air is 95–98%, with values below 88–90% on any FIO_2 indicating arterial hypoxemia. Because the relationship between SpO_2 and PaO_2 is often misunderstood by clinicians, we recommend application of the "40-50-60/70-80-90" rule of thumb—that is, PaO_2 values of 40, 50, and 60 torr roughly correspond to saturation values of 70%, 80%, and 90% respectively. Also critical in assessing SpO_2 values is the knowledge that standard pulse oximetry is *not* accurate in victims of carbon monoxide (CO) poisoning, and understanding that readings may be affected by movement artifacts, skin pigmentation, and peripheral circulation.

CO-Oximetry

CO-oximetry uses the principle of spectrophotometry (multiple light waves) to measure relative blood concentrations of oxyhemoglobin, carboxyhemoglobin, methemoglobin, and reduced hemoglobin. Look for these measurements in place of pulse oximetry in cases of suspected CO poisoning.

Transcutaneous Monitoring

Transcutaneous monitoring continuously measures diffusion of oxygen and carbon dioxide through the skin. Although it was originally used primarily for neonates, newer technology has emerged for such monitoring in adults. Transcutaneous diffusion occurs through the use of a heated electrode applied to the skin and maintained at 43–44°C. Readings should be validated against arterial blood gas values.

Cardiovascular Data

The patient record also provides data related to the patient's cardiovascular status. This information may include relevant vital signs, electrocardiograms (ECGs), echocardiograms, results of exercise testing, and hemodynamic monitoring data. ECG "strips" provide information on the patient's heart rate and rhythm. Echocardiograms provide noninvasive indices of cardiac performance (e.g., ejection fraction, cardiac output) and estimates of flows and pressures in the great vessels. If the patient's hemodynamic status is being monitored invasively through a central venous or pulmonary artery (PA) catheter, these values—including central venous pressures (CVP), PA pressures, PA wedge pressures (PAWP), and cardiac output—generally are found in a flow sheet designed for that purpose maintained by nursing staff. **Table 1-11** lists the hemodynamic reference values for adults. Details on the interpretation of hemodynamic data are provided in Chapter 2.

Maternal History and Perinatal and Neonatal History

Maternal Data

The medical record of a pregnant woman is similar to that of other patients, with much of the information located in the sections described in Table 1-1. However, some of the data may be unique. A good example is information used to estimate the gestational age of the fetus, including time since last menses, ultrasound measurement of the fetus's crown-to-rump length, and biochemical analysis of amniotic fluid to obtain levels of chemical indicators of fetal lung maturity. See Chapter 2 for details on interpreting these and other measures of gestational age.

Another example of how the maternal record is somewhat unique is the type of information recorded in the *patient history* section. Proper prenatal care requires thorough documentation of maternal history, including factors that may place the mother or neonate at risk. Common factors associated with high-risk pregnancies include the following:

- Socioeconomic factors
  - Low income and poor housing
  - Unwed status, especially adolescent (younger than 16 years)

Table 1-11 Common Hemodynamic Parameter Reference Values (Adults)

Parameter	Reference Values[a]
Systolic blood pressure	< 120 mm Hg
Diastolic blood pressure	< 80 mm Hg
Mean arterial blood pressure	70–105 mm Hg
Central venous pressure (CVP)	2–6 mm Hg
Right atrial pressure	2–6 mm Hg
Right ventricular pressure, systolic	15–30 mm Hg
Right ventricular pressure, diastolic	2–8 mm Hg
PA pressure, systolic	15–30 mm Hg
PA pressure, diastolic	8–15 mm Hg
PA pressure, mean	9–18 mm Hg
PA wedge pressure (PAWP), mean	6–12 mm Hg
Cardiac output (CO)	4.0–8.0 L/min
Cardiac index (CI)	2.5–4.0 L/min/m^2
Stroke volume (SV)	60–130 mL/beat
Stroke index (SI)	30–50 mL/m^2
Ejection fraction (EF)	65–75%
Systemic vascular resistance (SVR)[b]	900–1400 dynes-sec/cm^5
Pulmonary vascular resistance (PVR)[b]	110–250 dynes-sec/cm^5

[a]Normal values and ranges vary by laboratory, norms used, and/or reference source.
[b]To convert resistance measures from dynes-sec/cm^5 to mm Hg/L/min, divide by 80.

- - Minority status
  - Obese or underweight prior to pregnancy
- Obstetric history
  - History of infertility
  - History of infant malformation or birth injury
  - History of miscarriage, stillbirth, or ectopic pregnancy
  - High parity (many children)
  - History of premature or prolonged labor
  - History of low-birth-weight infant
- Maternal medical history
  - Cardiac, pulmonary, or renal disease
  - Diabetes or thyroid disease
  - Gastrointestinal or endocrine disorder
  - History of hypertension or seizures
  - History of venereal and other infectious diseases
  - Weight loss greater than 5 pounds
- Current obstetric status
  - Surgery during pregnancy
  - Absence of prenatal care
  - Rh sensitization or maternal anemia
  - Excessively large or small fetus
  - Preeclampsia or premature labor
  - Premature membrane rupture or vaginal bleeding
  - Postmaturity

- Habits
  - Smoking
  - Regular alcohol intake
  - Drug use or abuse

Perinatal and Neonatal Data

At birth, a separate medical record is established for the newborn. Some of the information from the mother's record, such as her history, is transferred into the neonate's chart. Other data are reflective of the delivery and the clinical status of the neonate at birth and will be included in the *birth history* or *patient history* section of the neonate's chart. Birth and delivery information recorded in this section of the chart includes the delivery position, presence of meconium, and the baby's initial color, muscle tone, and heart rate. Based on these and other factors, the neonate will often be classified generally as either "vigorous," with a favorable initial assessment, or "nonvigorous" if in distress. Any unusual interventions or treatment immediately following the birth, such as resuscitative efforts, also will be noted.

At 1 and 5 minutes after birth, the status of the newborn is determined using the Apgar score. As detailed in Chapter 2, the Apgar score is based on five variables, each rated from 0–2, with scores ranging from 10 for a stable, responsive neonate to a minimum of 0 if stillborn. Although this score generally is not used to dictate medical intervention, it is helpful in documenting a newborn's clinical status and somewhat predictive of clinical outcomes.

Data Pertaining to Sleep Disorders (RRT-Specific Content)

Sleep disorders or **dyssomnias** are widespread, with obstructive sleep apnea (OSA) being the most common form. As a result, you frequently will encounter patients for whom related diagnostic tests and treatments have been ordered. Common to all dyssomnias is the symptom of excessive daytime sleepiness, usually assessed using the Epworth Sleepiness Scale (ESS). The ESS is a simple eight-item questionnaire that assesses the likelihood of a patient dozing off in several common situations. Scores range from 0–24, with the threshold value of 10 indicating the need for further evaluation.

In addition to the assessment for daytime sleepiness, the record may include information relevant to assessing the patient's risk for sleep disorders. Risk factors for OSA include male gender, obesity, hypertension, excessive alcohol or sedative use, upper airway or facial abnormalities, smoking, a family history of OSA, large neck circumference, and certain endocrine and metabolic disorders. These risk factors are generally documented in the *history and physical* section.

For patients deemed to be at risk for sleep disorders such as OSA, tests such as overnight oximetry or the more definitive polysomnogram (sleep study) may be ordered to help make the diagnosis. The order for such a test is reflected in the *physician's orders* section. A polysomnogram is a continuous recording of multiple physiological variables that measure sleep stage and cardiopulmonary function during sleep. Some of the major variables measured during such a test include the electroencephalogram (EEG), the electro-oculogram (EOG), the electromyogram (EMG), SpO_2, nasal airflow, and chest, abdominal, and leg movements. **Figure 1-2** provides a sample polysomnography report, like that usually found in either the laboratory or respiratory therapy section of the record.

Full interpretation of a sleep study report requires the expertise of a physician trained in sleep disorders. However, application of the basic definitions provided in **Table 1-12** can facilitate your understanding of these reports and help you assess the presence and severity of a patient's sleep disorder.

Based on generally accepted guidelines, the severity of the disorder is judged according to the frequency of either AHI or RDI events as follows:

0–4/hr	Normal range
5–14/hr	Mild sleep apnea
15–30/hr	Moderate sleep apnea
> 30/hr	Severe sleep apnea

Date: 3/19/2013	Patient: Jane Doe	Patient ID: 1234567

Exam: Standard attended laboratory PSG measuring 2 EEG channels, 2 EOG channels, chin EMG, ECG, leg activity, O_2 saturation, thoraco-abdominal movements, and nasal airflow

Summary Data	
Bedtime: 22:38 Time in bed (min): 465.5 Total sleep time (min): 387.5 Sleep efficiency: 83.4% Wake before sleep (min): 15 Wake during sleep (min): 59.5 Wake after sleep (min): 3 Number of arousals: 8 % Stage wake: 16.6%	% Stage 1: 4.3% % Stage 2: 63.7% % Stage 3–4: 4.9% % Stages REM: 27.1% Latency to stage 1 (min): 10 Latency to stage 2 (min): 19 Latency to persistent sleep (min): 16.5 Latency to stage REM (min): 104

ECG: Usual heart rate in wake was 76, in sleep 70.

EEG: Percentage of REM sleep was increased versus normal and REM latency was longer than normal.

EMG: There were occasional increases in muscle activity in sleep with abnormal respiratory events.

Respiration: There were 110 abnormal respiratory events (17/hour sleep), with 70% being primarily obstructive apneas/hypopneas and the rest respiratory effort-related arousals (RERAs). Waking O_2 saturation was 95%. During apnea/hypopnea events the Spo_2 declined to 89% in NREM sleep and 86% in REM sleep. Audio monitoring revealed snoring during REM respiratory events. Sao_2 was below 88% for < 2 min/hour sleep.

Medications: None.

Interpretation: Moderate obstructive sleep apnea syndrome (OSAS) (ICD Code: 780.53-0).

Figure 1-2 Data Pertaining to Sleep Disorders.

If a patient is diagnosed with a sleep disorder, several treatment options are available. The most common treatment is continuous positive airway pressure (CPAP) or its variant known as bilevel positive-pressure ventilation. Such therapy would need to be ordered by a physician and recorded in the *physician's orders'* section of the medical record. Chapter 17 contains more details on the treatment of sleep disorders in the home.

Table 1-12 Definitions Related to Sleep Studies

Term	Definition
Obstructive apnea	A cessation of airflow (> 80% reduction in flow) for at least 10 seconds, during which there is continued effort to breathe
Central apnea	A cessation of airflow (> 80% reduction in flow) for at least 10 seconds, during which there is no effort to breathe
Hypopnea	A reduction in airflow of at least 30% from baseline lasting at least 10 seconds and associated with significant oxygen desaturation (> 3–4%)
Apnea–hypopnea index (AHI)	The average number of apneas and hypopneas occurring per hour of sleep
Respiratory effort–related arousal (RERA)	A 10-second or longer sequence of breaths with increasing respiratory effort leading to an arousal from sleep
Respiratory disturbance index (RDI)	The average number of apneas, hypopneas, and RERAs occurring per hour of sleep

COMMON ERRORS TO AVOID

You can improve your score by avoiding these mistakes:

- Never proceed with therapy until after you review the patient's record, including the physician's orders.
- Do *not* follow any order if an error is apparent; instead, contact the physician and clarify and correct the order.
- Never make recommendations based on information in one section of the chart; instead, review and interpret all relevant data to do so.
- Avoid reviewing only the most recent clinical data; instead, review data over time, looking for trends.
- Avoid using clinical data that appear erroneous (e.g., SpO_2 of 80% for a patient resting comfortably) or grossly inconsistent with other results.
- Never initiate or continue resuscitative efforts for a patient with a properly executed and current DNR order or advance directive indicating the patient's desire not to be resuscitated.
- Never review a patient's medical record solely for the purpose of confirming orders. Instead, be mindful that potentially valuable patient data can be found in all sections of the patient's chart.

SURE BETS

In some situations, you can always be sure of the right approach to a clinical problem or scenario:

- Always review the medical record before performing respiratory procedures to ensure the physician's order has been written and to become familiar with the patient's condition and potential contraindications.
- Always clarify incomplete or unclear orders with the prescribing physician.
- Always review trends in vital signs and other clinical data to gain insight regarding the patient's response to therapy and to monitor overall progress (or lack thereof).
- In reviewing clinical data, always remember that the normal ranges often vary by age. For example, the normal heart rate for an adult is 60–100/min, while that for a newborn is 90–170/min.
- When reviewing PFT results, always keep in mind that a *restrictive disorder* is characterized by a reduction in volumes and capacities, and an *obstructive disorder* is associated with reduced flows.
- Always remember that if the record indicates an increase in ventilatory plateau pressures, a decrease in compliance is the likely cause; increased airway resistance is revealed by data showing a widening of the difference between the peak and plateau airway pressures.
- Always remember that the normal fluid intake and output for adults is 2–3 L/day and that a urine output less than 25 mL/hr is abnormal.
- If a patient has excessive secretions, always note the amount, consistency, color, and odor of such secretions and consider recommending a Gram stain and culture and sensitivity.
- Always recognize that an adult respiratory rate greater than 30–35/min or a rapid-shallow breathing index greater than 100 is inconsistent with maintenance of adequate spontaneous breathing.
- Always be aware that trending of VC measurements less than 15 mL/kg PBW or NIF values less than 20–25 cm H_2O negative indicate decreasing respiratory muscle strength and the potential need for mechanical ventilation.
- Always try to recognize the cluster of clinical signs and symptoms associated with certain conditions. For example, a patient with moderate emphysema will often present as barrel chested, with dyspnea on exertion and an ABG that reflects a compensated respiratory acidosis.
- Always consider that when reviewing a chest x-ray report, radiolucency is seen as darkness on the image and is associated with the presence of air. Opacities are seen as whiteness

and generally mean the absence of air (solid tissue or fluid); they may be associated with atelectasis, consolidation, ARDS, or a tumor.

- Always take into account that certain conditions, such as acute asthma or pneumonia, may cause hyperventilation due to hypoxemia, resulting in an uncompensated respiratory alkalosis (increased pH and decreased $Paco_2$). With appropriate oxygen therapy, hyperventilation will often subside and $Paco_2$ normalize.
- Always remember that the Apgar score is used to assess and document the status of the newborn at 1 and 5 minutes after birth, with scores ranging from 10 for a stable, responsive neonate to a minimum of 0 if stillborn. In contrast, during the first few hours or days of life, the neonate's gestational age is estimated using either the Dubowitz or Ballard tools.
- Always recognize that the diagnosis of a sleep disorder is confirmed primarily via a polysomnogram record indicating five or more apneas and hypopneas per hour of sleep (the apnea–hypopnea index [AHI]).

PRE-TEST ANSWERS AND EXPLANATIONS

Following are this chapter's pre-test answers and explanations. Be sure to review each answer's explanation thoroughly to help you understand why it is correct. If the explanation is still unclear to you, review the chapter content.

1-1. **Correct answer: C.** Ventilation–perfusion scan (V/Q scan). A chest x-ray and an ABG would not specifically detect a pulmonary embolus. Standard PFTs will not reveal the perfusion problems occurring with an embolus. A V/Q scan would show a lack of blood flow in the affected region of the pulmonary circulation. Ventilation to lung regions would be shown as well.

1-2. **Correct answer: D.** Nurses' notes and flow sheet. A patient's fluid balance normally is recorded in the *nurses' notes* and *I&O flow sheet*. A positive fluid balance results from excessive intake and/or decreased output and may contribute to edema and hypertension. A negative fluid balance generally is due to insufficient hydration and/or excessive urination from medications such as diuretics and may lead to hypotension/ low cardiac output.

1-3. **Correct answer: B.** Respiratory alkalosis. Early in the course of an attack or worsening of symptoms, patients with asthma typically present with respiratory alkalosis. Shortness of breath and accompanying hypoxemia cause the patient to increase the rate of breathing, so that alkalosis occurs. Once hypoxemia is relieved by the administration of O_2, the patient's $Paco_2$ and pH may normalize.

1-4. **Correct answer: A.** Bacterial pneumonia. The elevated WBC suggests a bacterial infection. The respiratory distress further points to a respiratory infection such as bacterial pneumonia. The other choices are not infectious processes, and therefore you would not likely see an elevated WBC.

1-5. **Correct answer: A.** Bronchogenic carcinoma. A PET scan is a nuclear imaging technique used in the diagnosis and staging of tumors such as bronchogenic carcinoma.

1-6. **Correct answer: C.** Respiratory muscle strength. Negative inspiratory force (NIF/MIP) is used for the bedside assessment of respiratory muscle strength and is a measurement of pressure.

1-7. **Correct answer: B.** CO-oximetry. In the case of smoke inhalation, carbon monoxide binds to hemoglobin in place of oxygen. CO-oximetry will detect this state, but ABGs, standard pulse oximetry, or an A-a gradient calculation will not.

1-8. **Correct answer: D.** Tobacco smoking. In terms of medical history, any coexisting cardiac, pulmonary, renal, gastrointestinal, or endocrine disorder can increase the risk of pregnancy, as can a history of smoking and alcohol or drug abuse. Regarding the obstetric history, high parity (many children) and prior miscarriages, stillbirths, and premature births all increase pregnancy risk.

1-9. **Correct answer: B.** Bacterial pneumonia. Sputum culture and sensitivity are used to identify microorganisms and their most appropriate drug therapy.

1-10. **Correct answer: C.** The findings confirm a diagnosis of moderate obstructive sleep apnea. In adults, a diagnosis of obstructive sleep apnea is confirmed if the apnea–hypopnea index (AHI) is greater than 5/hour and the events are mainly obstructive in nature. The severity of sleep apnea is graded as follows: mild: AHI = 5–14; moderate: AHI = 15–30; severe: AHI > 30.

POST-TEST

To confirm your mastery of this chapter's topical content, you should take the chapter post-test, available online at http://go.jblearning.com/respexamreview. A score of 80% or higher indicates that you are adequately prepared for this section of the NBRC written exams. If you score less than 80%, you should continue to review the applicable chapter content. In addition, you may want to access and review the relevant Web links covering this chapter's content (courtesy of RTBoardReview. com), also online at the Jones & Bartlett Learning site.

CHAPTER 2

Collect and Evaluate Pertinent Clinical Information

Craig L. Scanlan
(previous version co-authored with Robert L. Wilkins)

Respiratory therapists (RTs) must be proficient in patient assessment. Obtaining pertinent clinical information at the bedside helps you determine the patient's condition, develop good treatment plans, and evaluate the patient's response to the therapy. For this reason, the NBRC exams include numerous questions about collecting and interpreting data for patients with cardiopulmonary disease. Your success on these exams depends heavily on your knowledge in this area.

OBJECTIVES

In preparing for the shared NBRC exam content, you should demonstrate the knowledge needed to:

1. Assess the patient's overall cardiopulmonary status by inspection, palpation, percussion, and auscultation
2. Integrate common physical examination findings
3. Interview the patient to obtain essential information regarding the patient's:
   a. Level of consciousness, pain, ability to cooperate, and emotional state
   b. Cough and sputum production, breathing difficulties, and exercise tolerance
   c. Nutritional status and activities of daily living
   d. Social history and occupational/environmental exposures
   e. Advance directives
   f. Learning needs
4. Review and interpret chest and lateral neck radiographs
5. Perform and interpret the results of diagnostic procedures, including:
   a. Noninvasive and invasive monitoring of respiration and gas exchange
   b. Bedside and laboratory testing of pulmonary function, lung mechanics, and airway reactivity
   c. Assessment of exercise tolerance and cardiac/pulmonary limitations to exercise
   d. Evaluation of cardiac and hemodynamic status
   e. Titration of CPAP/NPPV therapies
   f. Measurement and adjustment of tracheal tube cuff pressures (covered in Chaper 8)

In preparing for the RRT-specific NBRC exam content, you should demonstrate the knowledge needed to:

6. Review a chest radiograph to determine the quality of imaging
7. Perform and interpret the results of exhaled nitric oxide measurement
8. Select, obtain, and interpret ventilator graphics (covered in Chapter 11)
9. Detect auto-PEEP (covered in Chapter 11)

WHAT TO EXPECT ON THIS CATEGORY OF THE NBRC EXAMS

CRT exam: 18 questions; about 35% recall, 60% application, and 5% analysis
WRRT exam: 18 questions; about 10% recall, 10% application, and 80% analysis
CSE exam: indeterminate number of questions; however, exam I-B knowledge is a prerequisite to success on CSE Information Gathering sections

PRE-TEST

Carefully respond to each of the following questions. After completing the pre-test, compare your answers to those provided at the end of this chapter. Then thoroughly review each answer's explanation to help understand why it is correct.

2-1. Which of these conditions is associated with jugular venous distension?
  A. Cor pulmonale
  B. Pneumonia
  C. Simple pneumothorax
  D. Septic shock

2-2. You palpate the patient's neck and notice that the trachea is shifted to the patient's left. Which of the following conditions could explain this finding?
  A. Left ventricular enlargement
  B. Left upper lobe collapse
  C. Right lower lobe collapse
  D. Pleural effusion on the left

2-3. On reviewing the results of the attending physician's physical examination of a patient's chest, you note "a dull percussion note and bronchial breath sounds—LLL." All of the following are potential problems *except*:
  A. Infiltrates
  B. Atelectasis
  C. Consolidation
  D. Pneumothorax

2-4. You hear bronchial breath sounds over the patient's right middle lobe. Which condition is probably present?
  A. Emphysema
  B. Asthma
  C. Pneumonia
  D. Pleural effusion

2-5. Upon exam of an acutely dyspneic and hypotensive patient, you note the following (all limited to the left hemithorax): reduced chest expansion, hyperresonance to percussion, absence of breath sounds and tactile fremitus, and a tracheal shift to the right. These findings suggest:
  A. Left-sided pneumothorax
  B. Left-sided consolidation
  C. Left lobar obstruction/atelectasis
  D. Left-sided pleural effusion

2-6. During an interview with your patient, you determine that she is disoriented to time, place, and person. What may explain this finding?
  A. Respiratory alkalosis
  B. Severe hypoxemia
  C. Metabolic acidosis
  D. Hyperthermia

2-7. To assess the level of pain that a 2-year-old child is experiencing during a procedure, you would do all of the following *except*:
  A. Look for facial grimacing
  B. Ask for the mother's judgment
  C. Use a numeric pain scale
  D. Observe for crying

2-8. During an interview with your patient, you discover that he gets short of breath at night when he lies down, so he often sleeps with several pillows propping his head up. Which symptom is present?
  A. Apnea
  B. Orthopnea
  C. Platypnea
  D. Orthodeoxia

2-9. A patient complains that she has a chronic cough usually accompanied by sputum production. This information indicates that the patient probably has which of the following conditions?
  A. Acute asthma
  B. Chronic bronchitis
  C. Pulmonary emphysema
  D. Pulmonary fibrosis

2-10. All of the following are associated with a patient being at risk for malnutrition *except*:
  A. Recent weight gain
  B. Being significantly underweight
  C. Having poor dietary habits
  D. Inability to prepare own food

2-11. Which of the following aspects of a patient's history is most important in the diagnosis of lung disease?
   A. Marital status
   B. Cultural background
   C. Education
   D. Occupational history

2-12. You come upon an elderly patient who is unresponsive and is not breathing. You had heard from her nurse that she had discussed with her physician having a do not resuscitate (DNR) order in her chart. What should you do?
   A. Check the patient's chart for a DNR order/advance directive
   B. Immediately call a code and begin resuscitation efforts
   C. Contact the nurses' station and ask how best to proceed
   D. Call a "slow code" (i.e., apply basic CPR, but not ACLS)

2-13. What is the best way to determine whether a patient has learned the information needed to understand how her disease affects lung function?
   A. Have the patient take a multiple-choice quiz
   B. Discuss the information with the patient's family
   C. Have the patient "teach" the information back to you
   D. Have the patient perform a return demonstration

2-14. You note on inspection of an anterior–posterior (AP) chest radiograph that the right hemidiaphragm is elevated above normal. Which of the following is the most likely cause of this abnormality?
   A. Right pleural effusion
   B. Right tension pneumothorax
   C. Right phrenic nerve paralysis
   D. Right lower lobe pneumonia

2-15. An AP x-ray of a 3-year-old child with wheezing and stridor shows an area of prominent subglottic edema, but the lateral neck x-ray appears normal. What is the most likely problem?
   A. Croup
   B. Foreign body

   C. Epiglottitis
   D. Cystic fibrosis

2-16. On reviewing an ECG printout, you note widened QRS complexes. Which of the following is the most likely cause of this problem?
   A. Atrial fibrillation
   B. First-degree heart block
   C. Sinus arrhythmia
   D. Bundle branch block

2-17. A 150-lb patient is breathing at a frequency of 20/min, with a tidal volume of 550 mL. What is his estimated *alveolar* ventilation per minute?
   A. 11.00 L/min
   B. 8.00 L/min
   C. 3.00 L/min
   D. 14.00 L/min

2-18. Early in a spontaneous breathing (weaning) trial, you observe a 170-lb, 6-foot-tall male patient breathing at a rate of 35/min with a minute volume of 8.75 L/min. Which of the following conclusions can you draw from this finding?
   A. The patient's alveolar ventilation is normal for his size and weight
   B. The patient is in acute hypoxemic respiratory failure
   C. The patient likely cannot sustain prolonged spontaneous ventilation
   D. The patient has weakened respiratory muscle strength

2-19. You inspect a chest radiograph and observe the medial borders of the scapulae in the upper lung fields, the ribs positioned horizontally, and the thoracic spine about 5 cm to the left of the sternum. Which of the following best describes this radiograph?
   A. Anterior–posterior (AP) view, improperly rotated
   B. Anterior–posterior (AP) view properly aligned
   C. Posterior–anterior (PA) view, improperly rotated
   D. Posterior–anterior (PA) view, properly aligned

2-20. A patient's bedside spirometry results (as compared to normal) are as follows: FVC decreased, FEV_1 normal, and $FEV_1\%$ increased. What is the most likely diagnosis?
- **A.** An obstructive disorder
- **B.** Poor patient effort
- **C.** A restrictive disorder
- **D.** Within normal limits

2-21. A patient has a vital capacity of 3200 mL, a functional residual capacity of 4500 mL, and expiratory reserve volume of 1200 mL. What is her residual volume (RV)?
- **A.** 8900 mL
- **B.** 2000 mL
- **C.** 3300 mL
- **D.** 5700 mL

2-22. A patient with a confirmed diagnosis of asthma who is prescribed daily inhaled steroids has an exhaled nitric oxide reading of 72 ppb. This could indicate:
1. The presence of a comorbidity with similar symptoms, such as cardiac disease.
2. The need to increase the dosage of the inhaled steroid or add a beta agonist.
3. Poor compliance with drug regimen or improper inhaler technique.
- **A.** 1 only
- **B.** 1 and 2
- **C.** 2 and 3
- **D.** 1, 2, and 3

2-23. An apnea monitor on a premature infant indicates an abnormal *decrease* in respiratory rate and an abnormal *increase* in heart rate. What is the most likely cause of this problem?
- **A.** Hypoxemia
- **B.** Apnea of prematurity
- **C.** Periodic breathing
- **D.** Motion/activity artifact

2-24. In analyzing overnight oximetry data, a desaturation event represents a decrease in SpO_2 of which amount?
- **A.** 2% or more
- **B.** 3% or more
- **C.** 4% or more
- **D.** 5% or more

2-25. You conduct a 6-minute walk test (6MWT) on four patients before and after participation in a pulmonary rehabilitation program. Based on the 6-minute walking distance (6MWD) data provided here, for which of these patients has the program been effective in improving their functional capacity?

Patient	Pre-program 6MWD	Post-program 6MWD
A.	200 m	210 m
B.	150 m	200 m
C.	250 m	270 m
D.	400 m	430 m

2-26. As measured on the Borg Scale, which of the following exertion levels is appropriate for titrating a COPD patient's O_2 flows to support exercise?
- **A.** Weak/light exertion (rating of 2)
- **B.** Somewhat strong exertion (rating of 4)
- **C.** Very strong exertion (rating of 7)
- **D.** Maximal exertion (rating of 10)

2-27. To assess gas exchange at the tissues, you would sample blood from which of the following?
- **A.** Systemic artery
- **B.** Central vein
- **C.** Pulmonary artery
- **D.** Peripheral vein

2-28. A patient has a pulmonary artery wedge pressure (PAWP) of 20 mm Hg. All of the following are potential causes for this finding *except*:
- **A.** Hypovolemia
- **B.** Mitral valve stenosis
- **C.** Positive end-expiratory pressure
- **D.** Left ventricular failure

2-29. Based on the results of cardiopulmonary exercise testing, which of the following patients most likely has a ventilatory limitation to exercise?

Patient	Vo2max	Anaerobic Threshold	Breathing Reserve
A.	Decreased	Decreased	Normal
B.	Decreased	Normal	Normal
C.	Normal	Increased	Increased
D.	Decreased	Normal	Decreased

2-30. A patient undergoing CPAP titration during sleep exhibits three obstructive apnea events during a 5-minute observation interval at a pressure of 8 cm H_2O. What would be the appropriate action at this time?

A. Switch the patient to BiPAP with EPAP = 8 cm H_2O and IPAP = 12 cm H_2O

B. Increase the CPAP to 10 cm H_2O for 5 minutes and continue observation

C. Discontinue the titration trial and place the patient on nasal O_2 at 2 L/min

D. Decrease the CPAP to 6 cm H_2O for 5 minutes and continue observation

WHAT YOU NEED TO KNOW: ESSENTIAL CONTENT

Assess a Patient's Overall Cardiopulmonary Status by Inspection

In regard to inspection, the NBRC expects you to be proficient in evaluating a patient's general appearance, examining the airway, and evaluating cough and sputum production. In addition, you should understand the use of gestational age assessment, Apgar scoring, and transillumination in assessing infants' cardiopulmonary status.

General Appearance

Table 2-1 summarizes the major observations arising from patient inspection.

A key point often tested on the NBRC exams is the distinction between central and peripheral cyanosis. Central cyanosis indicates low arterial hemoglobin (Hb) saturation associated with poor oxygenation of the blood by the lungs, usually evident as a bluish discoloration of the mucous membranes of the lips and mouth. Assuming normal Hb content, central cyanosis generally appears when Sao_2 drops below 80%, or a Pao_2 of about 45–50 torr. Peripheral cyanosis or *acrocyanosis* is due to poor blood flow; it can occur in the presence of normal Hb saturation, and tends to appear *only* in the extremities. *When observed together with coolness of the extremities, peripheral cyanosis suggests circulatory failure.* Regardless of type, the intensity of cyanosis increases with the amount of Hb in the blood. For this reason, patients with high Hb content (polycythemia) can be cyanotic yet still have adequate O_2 content. Conversely, patients with low Hb content (anemia) can be severely hypoxic before cyanosis ever appears.

Airway Assessment

Assessment of the airway can help determine the cause of other physical or history findings, such as snoring and sleep apnea. Airway assessment also can help you determine whether special procedures or equipment will be needed for insertion of an artificial airway. To assess the airway, you should follow these steps:

1. Inspect the patient's external nose, noting any asymmetry or deformities.
2. Test for nasal patency by occluding each nostril in turn and asking the patient to breathe in.
3. Inspect the nasal cavities (use a nasal speculum and penlight if needed) for a deviated septum, polyps, edema, erythema, bleeding, or lesions.
4. With the patient's mouth open widely and the tongue extended, look for dentures or other dental appliances and inspect the tongue, hard/soft palate, uvula, tonsillar pillars, and other features.
5. Inspect the neck for length and circumference; have the patient flex and extend the neck as far as possible while you view the motion from the side.

Table 2-2 outlines the potential significance of the most common observations associated with the assessment of a patient's airway.

Table 2-1 Signs Observed During Patient Inspection and Their Implications

Sign	Observation	Potential Implications
General		
Body habitus	Weak/emaciated (cachexia)	General ill health/malnutrition
Position	Sitting/leaning forward	Respiratory distress
	Always elevated with pillows	Orthopnea, congestive heart failure
Respiratory rate	Tachypnea	Respiratory distress, restrictive disease
Breathing pattern	Prolonged exhalation	Expiratory obstruction (asthma, chronic obstructive pulmonary disease [COPD])
	Prolonged inspiration	Upper airway obstruction (croup, epiglottitis)
	Rapid and shallow	Loss of lung volume (atelectasis, pulmonary fibrosis, adult respiratory distress syndrome [ARDS], acute pulmonary edema)
	Kussmaul's breathing (deep and fast)	Diabetic ketoacidosis
	Biot's breathing (irregular breathing with periods of apnea)	Increased intracranial pressure
	Cheyne Stokes breathing (waxing and waning)	Central nervous system (CNS) diseases or severe congestive heart failure (CHF)
Speech pattern	Interrupted	Respiratory distress
Skin	Diaphoretic (sweating)	Fever, increased metabolism, acute anxiety
Facial expression	Anxious	Fear, pain
Personal hygiene	Poor	Illness affecting patient's daily activities
Sensorium	Depressed	Poor cerebral oxygenation, degenerative brain disorders, drug overdose
Head/Neck		
Nose	Nasal flaring (especially in infants)	Increased work of breathing
Lips/oral mucosa	Central cyanosis	Arterial hypoxemia
Lips	Pursed-lip breathing	Expiratory airway obstruction
Jugular veins	Distended	Right heart failure (cor pulmonale)
Thorax		
Configuration	Barrel chest	COPD
	Kyphoscoliosis	Severe restrictive lung defect
Muscle activity	Accessory muscle use	Increased work of breathing, loss of normal diaphragm function
	Abdominal paradox	Diaphragmatic fatigue or paralysis, increased work of breathing
	Retractions	Reduced lung volume, low lung compliance, increased work of breathing
Extremities		
Digits	Clubbing	Bronchogenic carcinoma, COPD, cystic fibrosis, chronic cardiovascular disease
Capillary beds	Peripheral cyanosis	Poor perfusion

Table 2-2 Inspection of the Airway

Area	Observation	Significance
Nostrils/nasal cavity	Broken, misshapen, swollen nose; occluded nasal passages; deviated septum	Compromised nasal route for O_2 or airway insertion
Oral cavity and pharynx	Dentures or dental appliances present	Potential aspiration risk; may need to be removed for airway access
	Macroglossia (large tongue)	Associated with difficult intubation and may impair aerosol delivery via the mouth
	Mallampati classification of pharyngeal anatomy: Class 1: Full visibility of tonsils, uvula, and soft palate Class 2: Visibility of hard and soft palate, upper portion of tonsils, and uvula Class 3: Soft and hard palate and base of the uvula are visible Class 4: Only hard palate visible	Class 4 is associated with difficult intubation as well as a higher incidence of sleep apnea
Neck	Short/thick	Difficult endotracheal intubation; difficult tracheostomy tube fit
	Poor range of motion (patient cannot touch tip of chin to chest and/or cannot extend neck)	Difficult bag-valve-mask (BVM) ventilation; difficult endotracheal intubation

Cough and Sputum Production

Table 2-3 describes some of the common types of cough and their likely causes. As indicated in Table 2-3, several conditions are associated with production of sputum, such as COPD, infections, bronchiectasis, lung abscess, and asthma. Sputum assessment should be included in patient history taking and also be conducted whenever secretion clearance takes place. Typically you evaluate the volume, color, consistency, and odor of sputum.

When inquiring about sputum volume, help patients by using familiar measures such as a teaspoon (about 5 mL), tablespoon (about 15 mL), or shot glass full (about 1 oz or 30 mL). More precise quantification can be obtained using a calibrated sputum cup. *As a rule of thumb, sputum production greater than 30 mL/day indicates the need for airway clearance.*

In terms of color, sputum is typically described as being either clear/white, pinkish, red, yellow, or green. Consistency is typically described as being thin/watery, frothy, or thick/viscous. Regarding odor, foul-smelling or *fetid* sputum indicates tissue necrosis. In combination, these characteristics help classify the sputum "type" as being mucoid, mucopurulent, purulent, or bloody and indicate the likely disorder (**Table 2-4**).

Neonatal Inspection

The NBRC expects you to be proficient in basic fetal/neonatal assessment methods, including Apgar scoring, gestational age, and transillumination.

Table 2-3 Common Types of Coughs with Likely Causes

Description	Likely Causes
Acute (< 3 weeks)	Postnasal drip, allergies, and infections (especially common cold, bronchitis, and laryngitis)
Chronic (> 3 weeks) or recurrent (adults)	Postnasal drip, asthma, gastroesophageal reflux, chronic bronchitis, bronchiectasis, COPD, tuberculosis (TB), lung tumor, angiotensin-converting enzyme (ACE) inhibitors, CHF
Recurrent (children)	Viral bronchitis, asthma, allergies
Barking	Epiglottitis, croup, influenza, laryngotracheal bronchitis
Brassy or hoarse	Laryngitis, laryngeal paralysis, laryngotracheal bronchitis, pressure on laryngeal nerve, mediastinal tumor, aortic aneurysm
Wheezy	Bronchospasm, asthma, cystic fibrosis, bronchitis
Dry	Viral infections, inhalation of irritant gases, interstitial lung diseases, tumor, pleural effusion, cardiac conditions, nervous habit, radiation or chemotherapy
Dry progressing to productive	Atypical pneumonias, Legionnaires' disease, pulmonary embolus, pulmonary edema, lung abscess, asthma, silicosis, emphysema (late phase), smoking, AIDS
Chronic productive	Bronchiectasis, chronic bronchitis, lung abscess, asthma, fungal infections, bacterial pneumonias, TB
Paroxysmal (especially at night)	Aspiration, asthma, CHF
Positional, especially when lying down	Bronchiectasis, CHF, chronic postnasal drip or sinusitis, gastroesophageal reflux with aspiration
Associated with eating or drinking	Neuromuscular disorders affecting the upper airway, esophageal problems, aspiration

Adapted from: Wilkins RL, Sheldon RL, Krider SJ. *Clinical assessment in respiratory care* (5th ed.). St. Louis, MO: Mosby; 2005.

Apgar Score

The Apgar score (**Table 2-5**) is used to assess neonates, usually at 1 and 5 minutes after birth. The score's five dimensions (**A**ppearance, **P**ulse, **G**rimace, **A**ctivity, **R**espirations), are rated from 0 to 2, with a maximum score of 10 (stable, responsive) and a minimum score of 0 (stillborn).

An Apgar score of 7–10 is normal. Babies scoring 4–6 typically need more intensive support, while those scoring 0–3 usually undergo resuscitation. *Needed interventions should never be delayed to obtain the Apgar score.*

Table 2-4 Sputum Assessment

	Color and Consistency	Likely Conditions
Mucoid	Clear/white, thin to thick	Asthma
Mucopurulent	Clear to yellowish, thick	Chronic bronchitis, cystic fibrosis, pneumonia (blood streaked)
Purulent	Yellow to green, thick	Aspiration pneumonia, bronchiectasis (fetid/foul smelling, may separate into layers), lung abscess (fetid/foul smelling, may separate into layers)
Bloody	Pink to red/dark red, thin (unless coagulated)	Tuberculosis (red), lung cancer (red), pulmonary infarction (red), pulmonary edema (pink, watery, frothy)

Adapted from: MacIntyre NR. Respiratory monitoring without machinery. *Respir Care.* 1990;35:546–553.

Table 2-5 Apgar Score

Parameter	Acronym	0	1	2
Color	Appearance	Blue or pale	Pink body with peripheral cyanosis (acrocyanosis)	Completely pink
Heart rate	Pulse	Absent	< 100 beats/min	> 100 beats/min
Reflex irritability	Grimace	Unresponsive	Grimace when stimulated*	Active movement, crying, coughing
Muscle tone	Activity	Flaccid, limp	Some flexion of extremities	Active movement
Respiratory effort	Respirations	Absent	Slow, irregular, weak, gasping	Crying, vigorous breathing
*Catheter in nares or tactile stimulation.				

Gestational Age

Normal gestation lasts 38–42 weeks. Knowledge of gestational age can help clinicians anticipate perinatal problems and establish sound care plans. **Table 2-6** summarizes the methods commonly used to estimate gestational age before birth. After birth, clinicians determine gestational age by careful assessment of selected neuromuscular and physical characteristics using methods developed by Dubowitz and Ballard. Although RTs normally do not conduct this assessment, you should be familiar with their components.

Figure 2-1 depicts the Ballard Gestational Age Assessment and scoring system. Scores are summed across both components to yield a composite score. A composite score of 10 or less indicates significant prematurity (≤ 28 weeks' gestation). An infant born at full term (38–42 weeks) typically scores in the 35–45 range, with higher values indicating a post-term baby.

Transillumination of Chest

Transillumination uses high-intensity fiberoptic light applied to the chest wall to detect pneumothoraces in infants. You should recommend transillumination for high-risk infants (especially those receiving mechanical ventilation) with clinical signs of pneumothorax—that is, retractions, tachypnea, cyanosis, hypotension, and asymmetrical chest motion.

The accompanying box (on next page) outlines the basic procedure. Normally only the skin approximately 1 cm around the light will illuminate, forming a halo. If the chest "lights up," a pneumothorax is likely. Note that transillumination can miss small pneumothoraces and may be of

Table 2-6 Methods Used to Estimate Gestational Age Before Birth

Method	Measurement	Comments
Time since last menses	Weeks since end of last normal menstrual period + 2	Traditional but unreliable
Ultrasonography	1. Crown to rump length up to 14 weeks (table lookup)	Accurate and reliable
	2. Fetal head diameter (biparietal diameter) between 14 and 20 weeks' gestation (table lookup)	
Biochemical analysis (measurement of amniotic fluid phospholipid levels)*	1. Lecithin/sphingomyelin (L/S) ratio > 2.0	Fetal maturity indicated by L/S ratio > 2; presence of PG; or L/A ratio > 40.0 mg/g
	2. Presence of phosphatidylglycerol (PG)	
	3. Lecithin/albumin (L/A) ratio ≥ 40.0 mg/g	
*Used primarily to indicate fetal lung maturity and/or predict infant respiratory distress syndrome.		

Neuromuscular Maturity

	−1	0	1	2	3	4	5
Posture							
Square Window (wrist)	>90°	90°	60°	45°	30°	0°	
Arm Recoil		180°	140°–180°	110°–140°	90°–110°	<90°	
Popliteal Angle	180°	160°	140°	120°	100°	90°	<90°
Scarf Sign							
Heel to Ear							

Maturity Rating

Score	Weeks
−10	20
−5	22
0	24
5	26
10	28
15	30
20	32
25	34
30	36
35	38
40	40
45	42
50	44

Physical Maturity

Skin	Sticky; friable; transparent	Gelatinous; red; translucent	Smooth; pink; visible veins	Superficial peeling and/or rash; few veins	Cracking; pale aeas; rare veins	Parchment; deep cracking; no vessels	Leathery; cracked; wrinkled
Lanugo	None	Sparse	Abundant	Thinning	Bald areas	Mostly bald	
Plantar Surface	Heel-toe 40–50 mm: −1 <40 mm: −2	>50 mm; no crease	Faint red marks	Anterior transverse crease only	Creases ant. 2/3	Creases over entire sole	
Breast	Imperceptible	Barely perceptible	Flat areola; no bud	Stippled areola; 1–2 mm bud	Raised areola; 3–4 mm bud	Full areola; 5–10 mm bud	
Eye/ear	Lids fused loosely: −1 tightly: −2	Lids open; pinna flat; stays folded	sl. curved pinna; soft; slow recoil	Well-curved pinna; soft but ready recoil	Formed and firm; instant recoil	Thick cartilage; ear stiff	
Genital Male	Scrotum flat; smooth	Scrotum empty; faint rugae	Testes in upper canal; rare rugae	Testes descending; few rugae	Testes down; good rugae	Testes pendulous; deep rugae	
Genitals Female	Clitoris prominent; labia flat	Prominent clitoris; small labia minora	Prominent clitoris; enlarging minora	Majora and minora equally prominent	Majora large; minora small	Majora cover clitoris and minora	

Figure 2-1 Ballard Gestational Age Assessment.

Modified from: Ballard JL, Novak KK, Denver M. A simplified score for assessment of fetal maturation in newborn infants. *J Pediatr.* 1979;95:769–774.

limited value in large babies. For this reason, if the transillumination test is negative but the infant still exhibits symptoms of pneumothorax, you should recommend an immediate chest x-ray.

Transillumination Procedure

1. Place the infant in the supine position and switch on the light.

2. Hold the light against the skin along the midaxillary line about halfway down the chest on the affected side.

3. Observe whether the chest illuminates (lights up).

4. Repeat the assessment on the same side at the midclavicular line halfway down the chest.

5. Repeat the assessment on the opposite side of the chest to compare the degree of illumination.

Assess a Patient's Overall Cardiopulmonary Status by Palpation

You palpate a patient for five purposes: (1) evaluate heart rate, rhythm, and force; (2) assess tracheal position; (3) evaluate vocal/tactile fremitus; (4) estimate thoracic expansion; and (5) assess the skin and tissues of the chest and extremities.

Heart Rate, Rhythm, and Pulse Strength

To evaluate a patient's heart's rate, rhythm, and force, you should palpate both peripheral and apical pulses (over the precordium). You palpate the peripheral pulse to measure a patient's heart rate, typically using the radial artery. Other peripheral pulse locations include the carotid, brachial, femoral, and popliteal (behind the knee) arteries. You palpate the apical pulse to assess the location and strength of the heart's point of maximum impulse (PMI).

Normal references ranges for heart rates by age group are specified in Chapter 1. Based on this knowledge, you determine whether the rate is normal or whether the patient has tachycardia or bradycardia. **Table 2-7** outlines the most common causes of tachycardia and bradycardia.

To detect if the pulse is regular or irregular, you may need to palpate it for a full minute. Minor irregularities are common, particularly in children (sinus arrhythmia). If you detect an irregularity, repeat your assessment with a second clinician simultaneously measuring the apical rate via palpation or auscultation. If the apical rate exceeds the peripheral rate, a *pulse deficit* exists. A pulse deficit usually indicates a cardiac arrhythmia, such as atrial fibrillation or flutter, PVCs, or heart block.

Careful assessment of the peripheral pulse also can reveal variation in strength. **Table 2-8** summarizes the most common findings and their likely causes.

For apical pulse assessment, you locate and palpate the heart's point of maximum impulse (PMI), normally at or near the fifth intercostal space, midclavicular line. Variations in PMI strength or position indicate abnormalities. A weak impulse may indicate hyperinflation (as with COPD) or decreased cardiac contractility. Abnormally strong pulsations or a shift in the PMI downward and to the left suggests left ventricular hypertrophy. Also, the PMI moves when the mediastinum is displaced. For example, the PMI tends to shift *toward* areas of atelectasis, and *away from* space-occupying lesions such as pneumothoraces or pleural effusions.

Tracheal Position

Normally, the trachea lies in the midline of the neck. Because it is connected to mediastinum structures, abnormal deviations are due to the same problems causing PMI shifts. Thus, the trachea tends to shift *toward areas of collapse/atelectasis* and *away from space-occupying lesions* such as pneumothoraces.

Fremitus

Fremitus refers to vibrations that you can feel on the chest wall. There are two types of fremitus: rhonchial fremitus and vocal fremitus.

Table 2-7 Common Causes of Abnormal Heart Rates

Tachycardia	Bradycardia
Fever	Vasovagal reflex
Hypoxemia	Cardiac arrhythmias
Pain	Increased intracranial pressure
Shock	Hypothyroidism
Anemia	Hypothermia
Cardiac arrhythmias	Electrolyte imbalances
Hyperthyroidism	Drug effects: beta-adrenergic blockers; calcium-channel blockers; digoxin; antiarrhythmic agents
Thyrotoxicosis	
Drug effects: beta-adrenergics; cholinergic blockers (e.g., atropine); stimulants (e.g., nicotine, caffeine); illicit drugs (e.g., amphetamines, cocaine)	

Table 2-8 Summary of Pulse Findings

Type	Description	Causes
Strong	Easy to palpate	Increased stroke volume (e.g., exercise)
Weak or thready	Hard to palpate	Decreased cardiac contractility; decreased blood volume; loss of vascular tone (e.g., septic shock); aortic stenosis
Bounding	Rapid/strong initial pressure rise followed by a quick fall-off	Aortic insufficiency; patent ductus arteriosus; atherosclerosis
Pulsus alternans	Pulse alternates in strength from beat to beat	Left-sided heart failure/CHF
Pulsus paradoxus	Pulsations vary with the breathing cycle (weaker pulses during inspiration)	Severe airway obstruction (status asthmaticus); cardiac tamponade

Rhonchial fremitus is associated with the presence of excess secretions in the large airways and detected by placing the flat of your hand on the chest to either side of the sternum. Typically, rhonchial fremitus diminishes or clears with coughing or after suctioning.

Vocal fremitus is the result of voice sounds being transmitted to the chest wall. You assess vocal fremitus by having the patient repeat the word "ninety-nine" while you palpate the chest. Conditions increasing lung tissue density (such as pneumonia and atelectasis) increase vocal fremitus. In contrast, vocal fremitus decreases in obese patients and those with COPD. Vocal fremitus also decreases whenever the lungs separate from the chest wall, as with pneumothorax and pleural effusion. In addition, vocal fremitus decreases over areas where the underlying lung lobe or segment is obstructed by a mucus plug or foreign body.

Thoracic Expansion

Palpation can help determine if chest expansion is equal on both sides. Anteriorly, you place your hands over the lower lateral chest wall, with the thumbs extended along the lower rib margins. Posteriorly, you position your hands over the lateral chest with the thumbs meeting at about the eighth thoracic vertebra. When the patient takes a full, deep breath, each thumb should move equally about 1–2 inches from the midline. Lesser or unequal movement is abnormal. Bilateral reductions in chest expansion are seen in COPD patients and those with neuromuscular disorders. Unilateral reductions in chest movement (on the affected side) occur with lobar pneumonia, atelectasis, pleural effusion, pneumothorax, and unilateral (right or left) phrenic nerve paralysis.

Skin and Soft Tissues

You can palpate the skin and soft tissues to determine temperature and assess for crepitus, edema, capillary refill, and tenderness.

When blood flow is poor, blood vessels in the extremities constrict to help direct flow to the vital organs. With less blood flow, the extremities tend to cool. For this reason, cold hands and feet usually indicate poor perfusion.

Especially in patients receiving positive-pressure ventilation, gas can leak into the tissues around the head, neck, and chest, forming subcutaneous bubbles, a condition called *subcutaneous emphysema*. When palpated, these bubbles produce a crackling sensation called *crepitus*. Although subcutaneous emphysema itself is harmless, it often occurs in conjunction with a pneumothorax. For this reason, *if you detect crepitus, assess the patient for a pneumothorax and immediately communicate your findings to the patient's physician*. Many clinicians recommend a chest x-ray whenever crepitus occurs in mechanically ventilated patients.

Many patients with chronic heart failure exhibit gravity-dependent tissue edema, typically in the feet and ankles (pedal edema). Firmly pressing on edematous tissue with a finger causes it to "pit" or indent. The degree of pitting is usually rated on a 3-point scale, with +3 being the most serious. In general, the farther up the legs the edema can be detected, the more severe the heart failure.

You assess capillary refill by pressing firmly on a patient's fingernails, then releasing the pressure and noting how quickly blood flow returns. When cardiac output is reduced and digital perfusion is poor, capillary refill is slow, taking 3 seconds or longer.

You palpate the abdomen for evidence of distension and tenderness. Abdominal distension and pain can restrict diaphragmatic movement, impair coughing and deep breathing, and contribute to respiratory insufficiency. Typically, the right upper quadrant of the abdomen is palpated for tenderness and to estimate the size of the liver. Abdominal tenderness and an enlarged liver (hepatomegaly) may be seen in patients with chronic cor pulmonale.

Assess a Patient's Overall Cardiopulmonary Status by Percussion

In a complete thoracic exam, you should percuss the lung fields on both sides of the chest, being sure to avoid bony structures and female breasts. To move the scapulae out of the way for posterior percussion, have the patient raise his or her arms.

Percussion over normal air-filled lung tissue produces a low-pitched hollow sound, called *normal resonance*. A percussion sound that is louder and lower pitched than normal is referred to as *increased resonance* and typically occurs in patients with hyperinflation (acute asthma, COPD) or a pneumothorax. A percussion note that is short, muted, and higher pitched than normal is termed *dull* or *flat*. Dull percussion notes occur over areas of increased tissue density, as observed in patients with pneumonia, atelectasis, or lung tumors. Decreased resonance also occurs if there is fluid in the pleural space.

Percussion over the lower posterior thorax can help determine the position of the diaphragm and its range of motion. As you percuss downward over the lower lung fields, the sound changes from a normal to a dull note, indicating the level of the diaphragm. The difference between the maximum inspiratory and expiratory levels represents the full range of diaphragm motion, which in adults ranges from 5–7 cm. Diaphragm motion typically is decreased in patients with neuromuscular disorders and severe hyperinflation.

Assess a Patient's Overall Cardiopulmonary Status by Auscultation

You auscultate the thorax with a stethoscope to identify lung and heart sounds. In general, you should use the stethoscope's diaphragm for auscultation of higher-pitched breath sounds, whereas the bell is recommended to listen to lower-pitched heart sounds.

Breath Sounds

Table 2-9 summarizes the characteristics of normal breath sounds, *which are considered normal only if noted at the specified location*. Normal sounds identified at abnormal locations are abnormal! For example, bronchial breath sounds are abnormal when heard over the lung periphery. They tend to replace normal vesicular sounds when lung tissue increases in density, as in atelectasis and pneumonia/consolidation.

Table 2-9 Normal Breath Sounds

Breath Sound	Description	Normally Heard at (Location)
Vesicular	Low-pitched soft sounds; heard primarily during inhalation, with only a minimal exhalation component	Periphery of lungs
Bronchial	High-pitched loud, tubular sounds with an expiratory phase equal to or longer than the inspiratory phase	Over trachea
Bronchovesicular	Moderate pitch and intensity; equal inspiratory and expiratory phases	Around upper sternum (anterior); between scapulae (posterior)

Breath sounds are diminished when the patient's breathing is shallow or slow. A decrease in breath sound intensity also occurs when airways are obstructed or the lung is hyperinflated, as in asthma or COPD. Air or fluid in the pleural space and obesity can reduce breath sounds as well.

Abnormal or *adventitious* breath sounds include crackles (rales), rhonchi, wheezes, and stridor. Chapter 11 provides details on the characteristics and causes of these adventitious sounds.

Heart Sounds

Heart sounds are generated when the heart valves close. The first heart sound (S_1) signals closure of the mitral and tricuspid valves, while the second heart sound (S_2) occurs with closure of the pulmonic and aortic valves. You listen to heart sounds to assess the apical heart rate and to identify gross abnormalities in structure or function.

When the peripheral pulses are difficult to palpate, you should assess the *apical rate* by direct auscultation at the PMI. As with palpation, you also can use auscultation to compare the apical rate to that palpated at a peripheral artery to determine if a pulse deficit is present.

Heart sound intensity diminishes in conditions that impair sound transmission between the heart and the exterior chest wall, such as pulmonary hyperinflation, pleural effusion, pneumothorax, and obesity. Heart sounds also decrease in heart failure, hypotension, and shock. In contrast, heart sound intensity can increase with partial obstruction to outflow from the ventricles, as in mitral stenosis (affecting S_1) and pulmonary hypertension (affecting S_2). Heart sounds may also be louder than normal in children and thin-chested patients. Variation in the intensity of heart sounds, especially S_1, occurs with cardiac arrhythmias that alter ventricular filling, such as atrial fibrillation and complete heart block.

You will sometimes hear a third heart sound (S_3) occurring just after S_2. The presence of this extra sound creates a galloping pattern, often equated with the saying the word "Kentucky." S_3 can be heard in normal children and also in well-conditioned athletes. Its presence in older patients usually indicates CHF.

Cardiac murmurs indicate turbulent flow through a valve, which occurs when either the valve fails to properly close (causing backflow or regurgitation) or outflow is obstructed (stenosis). Systolic murmurs are heard when either an atrioventricular (AV) valve allows backflow or a semilunar valve restricts outflow. Diastolic murmurs occur with semilunar valve regurgitation or AV valve stenosis.

Auscultatory Assessment of Blood Pressure

You use auscultation to noninvasively measure blood pressure. As you deflate the cuff, you listen for the *Korotkoff sounds*, which are caused by turbulent flow through the partially obstructed artery. The pressure at which the Korotkoff sounds first appear is the systolic pressure, while the point at which these sounds suddenly become muffled and disappear is the diastolic pressure.

In patients with normal blood pressure, auscultation of these sounds is relatively easy and provides accurate data. However, several situations deserve special consideration when using auscultation for noninvasive blood pressure measurement, as summarized in **Table 2-10**.

Integrating Physical Examination Findings

When reviewing a patient's physical exam findings, you need to integrate the results of inspection, palpation, percussion, and auscultation. **Table 2-11** summarizes the major physical findings associated with various common clinical disorders.

Interviewing the Patient

Interviewing provides essential information about a patient's (1) level of consciousness, ability to cooperate, and emotional state; (2) experience of pain; (3) breathing difficulties; (4) activities of daily living and exercise tolerance; (5) social history; and (6) advance directives.

Table 2-10 Special Considerations in Noninvasive Measurement of Blood Pressure

Problem	Caused by	Solution
Inaudible blood pressure	Poor technique	Use proper technique.
	Severe hypotension or shock	Consider arterial line monitoring.
	Venous engorgement (due to repeated measurements)	Remove the cuff and have the patient raise his or her arm over the head for 1–2 minutes before repeating the measurement.
Irregular cardiac rhythms	Atrial fibrillation, frequent PVCs, heart block	Make several measurements and use the average.
Auscultatory gap	A silent interval between systolic and diastolic sounds that can result in underestimating systolic pressure or overestimating diastolic pressure; usually caused by hypertension	Measure and record three pressures: (1) the opening systolic or "snap" pressure, (2) the pressure at which continuous pulses again are heard, and (3) the diastolic pressure.
Paradoxical pulse (pulsus paradoxus)	A larger than normal drop (more than 6–8 mm Hg) in systolic pressure during inspiration in patients with severe airway obstruction (such as acute asthma) or conditions that impair ventricular filling (such as cardiac tamponade)	To measure paradoxical pulse, slowly deflate the cuff until you hear sounds only on exhalation (point 1). Then reduce the pressure again until you can hear sounds throughout the breathing cycle (point 2). The difference in pressures between points 1 and 2 is the paradoxical pulse measurement.

Table 2-11 Physical Findings Associated with Various Common Clinical Disorders

Abnormality	Inspection	Palpation	Percussion	Auscultation
Asthma	Use of accessory muscles	Reduced expansion	Increased resonance	Expiratory wheezing
COPD	Increased AP diameter; use of accessory muscles	Reduced expansion	Increased resonance	Diffuse decrease in breath sounds; early inspiratory crackles
Consolidation (pneumonia or tumor)	Inspiratory lag	Increased fremitus	Dull note	Bronchial breath sounds; crackles
Pneumothorax	Unilateral expansion	Decreased vocal fremitus	Increased resonance	Absent breath sounds
Pleural effusion	Unilateral expansion	Absent vocal fremitus	Dull note	Absent breath sounds
Atelectasis	Unilateral expansion	Absent vocal fremitus	Dull note	Absent breath sounds
Diffuse interstitial fibrosis	Rapid shallow breathing	Often normal; increased fremitus	Slight decrease in resonance	Late inspiratory crackles
Upper airway obstruction (e.g., croup, foreign body)	Labored breathing	Often normal	Often normal	Inspiratory and/or expiratory stridor

Level of Consciousness, Ability to Cooperate, and Emotional State

To quickly assess patients for their level of consciousness or "sensorium," ask them what the time of day is, where they are, and who they are. Alert patients are well oriented to time, place, and person—that is, "oriented × 3." The most common reasons for a patient not being oriented include neurologic injury, sedation, and severe hypoxemia or hypercapnia. *In general, only alert patients can fully cooperate and participate in their own care.*

You also should try to assess the emotional state of alert patients. A normal emotional state is evident when patients respond with changing facial expressions suitable to the conversation, describe themselves as appropriately concerned about their condition, and appear either relaxed or moderately anxious. Patients in an abnormal emotional state typically appear depressed, overly anxious, or irritable. They may also have difficulty focusing and exhibit breathlessness, dizziness, trembling, palpitations, or chest pain. In general, patients in an abnormal emotional state will be difficult to manage until their anxiety can be resolved.

Whenever encountering patients who are not alert, you should objectively assess their level of consciousness using the Glasgow Coma Scale (**Table 2-12**). To apply this scale, you assess the patient's eye, verbal, and motor responses and assign a numeric value to each component. The three values are summed to yield a composite score, with the lowest possible value being 3 (deep coma) and the highest possible value being 15. Relative impairment is interpreted as follows:

- Mild impairment: 13–15
- Moderate impairment: 9–12
- Severe impairment (coma): < 8

Experience of Pain

To determine if an alert patient is experiencing pain, ask the question, "Are you having any pain or discomfort now?" If the patient answers yes, then he or she is in pain. To quantify pain with alert adults, have them rate its severity on a scale ranging from 0–10, where 0 signifies "no pain" and 10 represents "the worst possible pain." Patients can use the same scale to pinpoint their maximum tolerable level of pain. For young children or those persons unable to express themselves, you can interview family members to get information about behaviors the patient typically exhibits with pain and activities that may cause or worsen it. Without such information, you may have to rely on observing behaviors such as moaning or looking for facial expressions such as grimacing or tearing.

After you determine the severity of pain, you should assess how much it interferes with the patient's daily activities. A similar 10-point scale can be used to make this assessment, with 0 signifying "no interference" and 10 signifying "unable to carry out usual activities." *Whenever a patient rates an interference level greater than 4, you should report this finding to the patient's physician.*

Table 2-12 Glasgow Coma Scale

	1	2	3	4	5	6
Eyes	Does not open eyes	Opens eyes in response to painful stimuli	Opens eyes in response to verbal stimuli	Opens eyes spontaneously	N/A	N/A
Verbal	Makes no sounds	Incomprehensible speech	Utters inappropriate words	Confused, disoriented	Oriented, converses normally	N/A
Motor	Makes no movements (flaccid)	Extension to painful stimuli	Abnormal flexion to painful stimuli	Flexion/withdrawal to painful stimuli	Localizes painful stimuli	Obeys commands

Breathing Difficulties

The evaluation of patients' dyspnea, orthopnea, work of breathing, and exercise tolerance is a critical skill for all RTs. Dyspnea and orthopnea are clinical *symptoms* that must be evaluated by interviewing the patient. In contrast, the work of breathing and exercise tolerance are clinical *signs* that must be detected and quantified by the health professional.

Dyspnea and Orthopnea

Dyspnea is a patient's sensation of breathlessness. *Orthopnea* is the patient's sensation of uncomfortable breathing when lying down, which typically is relieved by sitting or standing up. Both dyspnea and orthopnea are associated with cardiac or pulmonary disorders.

The most common method used to quantify a patient's dyspnea is the modified Borg Scale (**Table 2-13**). Like the pain scale, the Borg Scale is a 0–10 point numeric scale, with 0 representing no sensation and 10 representing maximal sensation. As indicated in Table 2-13, the Borg Scale can be used to assess a patient's dyspnea *or* degree of exertion and is always applied in association with a predefined level of activity (e.g., exercise test level, end of a 6-minute walk). To administer the Borg Scale, have the patient stop the activity, review the scale ratings, and select the number corresponding to his or her degree of breathing difficulty being experienced at that moment.

Work of Breathing

Abnormal work of breathing is a clinical *sign*. In combination, the following observations should indicate to you that a patient is experiencing an abnormally high work of breathing:

- Tachypnea
- Thoracic–abdominal dysynchrony ("seesaw" motion)
- Use of accessory muscles

Exercise Tolerance

The gold standard for assessing a patient's exercise tolerance is a graded cardiopulmonary exercise test. A less rigorous but very useful alternative method for evaluating exercise tolerance is the 6-minute walk test. Both of these tools are discussed later in this chapter.

A simpler measure used to assess exercise tolerance is the American Thoracic Society (ATS) Breathlessness Scale (**Table 2-14**). This scale helps quantify the point at which a patient develops

Table 2-13 Modified Borg Scale

Rating	For Rating Dyspnea	For Rating Exertion
0	Nothing at all	Nothing at all
0.5	Very, very slight (just noticeable)	Very, very weak (just noticeable)
1	Very slight	Very weak
2	Slight	Weak (light)
3	Moderate	Moderate
4	Somewhat severe	Somewhat strong
5	Severe	Strong (heavy)
6		
7	Very severe	Very strong
8		
9	Very, very severe (almost maximal)	Very, very strong (almost maximal)
10	Maximal	Maximal

Table 2-14 American Thoracic Society Breathlessness Scale

Grade	Degree	Description of Breathlessness
0	None	Not troubled with breathlessness except with strenuous exercise
1	Slight	Troubled by shortness of breath when hurrying on level ground or walking up a slight hill
2	Moderate	Walks slower than people of the same age on level ground because of breathlessness or has to stop for breath when walking at own pace on level ground
3	Severe	Stops for breath after walking about 100 yards or after a few minutes on level ground
4	Very severe	Too breathless to leave the house or breathless when dressing and undressing

dyspnea during common activities. By inquiring as to when the patient first notices breathlessness, you can assign a grade of 0–4 to the symptom, with a descriptive term indicating the degree of impairment.

Nutritional Status

Nutritional assessment usually is conducted by a clinical nutritionist or the patient's doctor. However, because nutritional status can affect the response to respiratory care, RTs should at least be able to assess a patient's risk for malnutrition. Obvious physical signs associated with severe malnutrition include a weak or emaciated appearance (*cachexia*); generalized edema (*anasarca*); cracked lips (*cheilosis*); dry, scaly skin; and listlessness. For patients lacking obvious signs of malnutrition, you should try to gather the following basic information:

- The patient's weight and weight history
- The types of foods the patient eats, the number of meals per day, and recent changes in appetite
- The approximate amount of fluid the patient takes in daily
- Whether the patient is able to afford and obtain the desired/needed foods and who prepared them
- Whether the patient has any problem with chewing or swallowing
- The patient's perception of his or her own nutritional status

Based on this information, you should be able to identify patients at risk for malnutrition. This would include any patient who matches one of the following descriptions:

- Is significantly underweight (less than 90% predicted body weight)
- Has had recent weight loss of 10% or more of usual body weight
- Has poor dietary habits or inadequate food intake (due to any cause)
- Is impoverished, isolated, or unable to prepare own food

If you identify a patient at risk for malnutrition, you should share this information with the patient's doctor or refer the patient to a dietitian or clinical nutritionist.

Activities of Daily Living

Activities of daily living (ADLs) represent the basic tasks of everyday life. Measurement of ADLs is important because they are predictive of both healthcare use (such as hospital admissions) and outcomes (such as mortality).

Table 2-15 Basic Activities of Daily Living

Category	Description	Independent? Yes	Independent? No
1. Bathing	Receives no assistance or assistance in bathing only part of body	☐	☐
2. Dressing	Gets clothed and dresses without assistance except for tying shoes	☐	☐
3. Toileting	Goes to toilet room, uses toilet, and returns without any assistance (may use cane or walker for support and may use bedpan or urinal at night)	☐	☐
4. Transferring	Moves in and out of bed and chair without assistance (may use cane or walker)	☐	☐
5. Continence	Controls bowel and bladder completely by self (without occasional accidents)	☐	☐
6. Feeding	Feeds self without assistance (except for cutting meat or buttering bread)	☐	☐

Adapted from: Katz S, Downs TD, Cash HR, et al. Progress in the development of the index of ADL. *Gerontologist.* 1970;10:20–30.

The simplest measure of basic ADLs is depicted in **Table 2-15**, which addresses an individual's degree of independence with common self-care activities. Each of the six questions is answered as a "yes" or "no," with the scale score being the number of "yes" answers out of a possible 6. A score of 6 indicates full function; a score of 4, moderate impairment; and a score of 2 or less, severe impairment. Patients unable to perform these activities usually require daily caregiver support.

Because the basic ADLs in Table 2-15 do not assess the full range of activities needed for independent living, a separate set of "instrumental" ADLs (IADLs) was developed. The IADL categories include handling personal finances, meal preparation, shopping, mode of transportation, doing laundry, housekeeping, using the telephone, and taking medications. Patients receive a score of 1 for each of the 8 categories if they exhibit at least minimally acceptable function on one or more specific activities within each category, making the maximum score 8 (high function, independent). The lower the score, the higher the level of dependence.

Social and Occupational History

A complete interview should gather information about a patient's social and occupational history, to include questions addressing the following key elements:

- Marital status and family relationships
- Cultural and religious influences
- Living situation and social support
- Education, employment, and finances
- Occupational/environmental exposures
- Diet, exercise, and other habits
- Social activities, hobbies, and recreation
- Tobacco, alcohol, or drug use (substance abuse)
- Satisfaction/stress with life situation

Due to its importance in diagnosis, the occupational and environmental exposure history is often considered a separate category of interview. The accompanying box outlines the key areas for questioning patients regarding their occupational and environmental exposure history.

Outline of Occupational and Environmental Exposure History

Part 1. Exposure Survey

A. Exposures

- Current and past exposure to metals, dust, fibers, fumes, chemicals, biologic hazards, radiation, or noise
- Typical workday (job tasks, location, materials, and agents used)
- Changes in routines or processes
- Other employees or household members similarly affected

B. Health and Safety Practices at Work Site

- Ventilation
- Personal protective equipment (e.g., respirators, gloves, and coveralls)
- Personal habits (Smoke and/or eat in work area? Wash hands with solvents?)

Part 2. Work History

- Description of all previous jobs including short-term, seasonal, part-time, and military service
- Description of present jobs

Part 3. Environmental History

- Present and previous home locations
- Jobs of household members
- Home insulating and heating/cooling system
- Home cleaning agents
- Pesticide exposure
- Water supply
- Recent renovation/remodeling
- Air pollution, indoor and outdoor
- Hobbies (e.g., painting, sculpting, ceramics, welding, woodworking, automobiles, gardening)
- Hazardous wastes/spill exposure

Adapted from: Carter W, et al. *Taking an exposure history.* Atlanta, GA: U.S. Department of Health and Human Services, Agency for Toxic Substances and Disease Registry; 2000.

Tobacco Use/Smoking History

You should obtain the smoking history of all patients, including whether the habit involves primarily cigarettes, cigars, or pipe smoking. For former smokers, determine how long ago they quit. For current or former cigarette smokers, quantify their smoking history in *pack-years* as follows:

Pack-years = daily packs of cigarettes smoked × number of years smoking

Example: A 38-year-old patient has been smoking 1-1/2 packs per day for 20 years.

Pack-years = 1.5 × 20 = 30 pack-years

The number of cigarettes smoked per day (1 pack = 20 cigarettes) also is a good indicator of nicotine dependence, along with how soon after waking the patient begins smoking. Patients who smoke more than one pack a day and must have their first cigarette upon waking are heavily nicotine dependent.

Substance Abuse

Substance abuse consists of any harmful use of a drug or chemical (including alcohol) that results in adverse social consequences. People can abuse illegal drugs, over-the-counter drugs, prescription medications, and common chemicals such as alcohol or glue. According to the *Diagnostic and Statistical Manual for Mental Disorders* (DSM-IV-TR), symptoms of substance abuse include one or more of the following:

- Substance use resulting in a recurrent failure to fulfill work, school, or home obligations (e.g., work absences, substance-related school suspensions, neglect of children)
- Substance use in physically hazardous situations such as driving or operating machinery
- Substance use resulting in legal problems such as drug-related arrests
- Continued substance use despite negative social and relationship consequences

Other signs and symptoms of substance abuse depend on the specific drug class. For example, amphetamine abuse is associated with a rapid heartbeat, elevated or depressed blood pressure, dilated pupils, weight loss, inability to sleep, confusion, and occasional paranoid psychotic behavior.

To help identify substance abuse, you should ask the following two questions:

- Have you felt you wanted or needed to cut down on your drinking or drug use in the past year?
- In the past year, have you ever drunk or used drugs more than you meant to?

A positive response to either of these two questions indicates current substance abuse.

Advance Directives and DNR Orders

Unless otherwise informed, you should presume that your patients want life-saving treatment. Indeed, *whenever in doubt or when written orders are not present, you should always initiate emergency life support when needed.* However, to ensure that your actions match your patients' desires, you always should determine whether advance directives have been established.

An advance directive specifies the healthcare choices a patient wants should he or she be unable to make informed decisions. Because you are legally obliged to follow advanced directives, you need to know if your patient has made these arrangements, usually via either a living will or durable power of attorney. A living will specifies the level of care that patients desire should they become incapacitated. A durable power of attorney (also called a *proxy directive*) gives another individual the legal authority to make healthcare decisions for the patient. Normally, these advance directives are obtained upon admission to the hospital and can be found in the patient's chart (see Chapter 1).

Do not resuscitate (DNR) orders are a special type of advance directive in which patients specify that no resuscitation should be attempted should they suffer cardiorespiratory arrest. This request can come from the patient or from his or her legal proxy. After obtaining informed consent from the patient or proxy, the attending physician places the DNR order in the chart.

Patients can change or revoke a DNR order at any time, as long as they are able to communicate their wishes clearly. Although such changes normally are made in writing, patients can communicate their desires orally to medical personnel or to family members or friends. Should a patient or the patient's surrogate ask you to change or revoke an advance directive or DNR order, you must *immediately* notify the attending physician, who must either cancel the DNR order or have the new request replace any prior documentation.

Assess the Patient's Learning Needs

The provision of effective patient education is a standard of The Joint Commission, the accrediting body for hospitals. According to The Joint Commission, patient education should be designed to foster healthy behaviors and increase patients' involvement in their healthcare decisions.

Assessment of a patient's learning needs, abilities, and readiness to learn is the first step in patient education. Normally, this is performed via a comprehensive educational assessment conducted upon admission to a care unit and documented in the patient's chart. **Figure 2-2** provides an example of a patient educational documentation form.

Patient/Family Education Record

Teaching/Learning Assessment	Assessment of Patient Ability to Learn	Assessment of Patient Readiness to Learn
Speaks English? ☐Y ☐N If no, primary language _____ Preferred learning method: ☐ Listening ☐ Television ☐ Doing ☐ Demonstration ☐ Reading ☐ Other (specify) _____	☐ No barriers noted ☐ Cannot assess Specific barriers noted: ☐ Physical ☐ Emotional ☐ Cognitive ☐ Motivational ☐ Cultural ☐ Language ☐ Religious ☐ Developmental ☐ Other:_____	Receptive to learning? Patient: ☐Y ☐N ☐NA Other ☐Y ☐N ☐NA (specify) _____ Capable of learning? Patient: ☐Y ☐N ☐NA Other ☐Y ☐N ☐NA

Date	What Was Taught	To Whom	How (Method)	Response	Signature

Acceptable Abbreviations

What	D/C = discharge instruction; EQ = equipment; REHAB = rehabilitation techniques; MED = drugs
To Whom	PT = patient; SP = spouse; PR = parent; SO = significant other (e.g., other family member, partner)
How	D = demonstration; T = television/video; V = verbal instructions; W = written materials
Response	AV = attentive verbal response; RD = return demonstration; DI = seems disinterested; NR = needs reinforcement

Figure 2-2 Example of a Patient/Family Educational Documentation Form. Typically such forms include assessment of the patient's learning ability and needs, as well as documentation of the education provided to meet those needs.

Courtesy of: Strategic Learning Associates, LLC, Little Silver, New Jersey.

As indicated on this form, you first determine whether any language barrier is present. If so, you may need to enlist an English-speaking family member for assistance or secure a translator.

You then determine the patient's preferred learning method. To do so, have patients tell you about something they recently learned and how they learned it, or how they would have liked to learn it. Hints as to preferred ways of learning also can be gleaned from questions about the patient's work and hobbies.

The next step is to identify any barriers affecting learning, as revealed by chart review or patient interview. **Table 2-16** outlines the most common barriers to patient learning and suggests ways to address them. Note the importance of gaining family assistance in overcoming many of these barriers.

After identifying barriers to learning, you should assess the patient's readiness to learn. Especially useful in this regard is the desire of patients to learn more about their condition. When patients are ready to learn, they tend to express discomfort with their current situation.

The last step is to determine the patient's learning needs as related to the care you will provide. To do so, you should ask the following questions, using language appropriate to the patient's ability to understand:

- Does the patient understand his or her current condition?
- Is the patient knowledgeable about his or her medications?
- Is the patient familiar with the procedures you will implement?
- Is the patient familiar with the equipment you plan to use?

If answers to any of these questions indicate a shortcoming or "knowledge gap," you have identified a learning need. In addition to identifying needs, you should try to discover the patient's

Table 2-16 Accommodating Common Barriers to Patient Learning

Barrier to Learning	Accommodations
Age (young child)	Keep teaching/learning episodes short Use "fun and games" approach Enlist family assistance
Reduced level of consciousness	Postpone until the patient becomes alert Apply methods that don't require cooperation
Presence of pain	Recommend analgesia Postpone until pain management is effective
Presence of anxiety	Postpone until anxiety management is effective Enlist family assistance Recommend anxiolytic (anti-anxiety) therapy
Physical limitations	Ascertain specific limitations Apply methods that circumvent the limitations Enlist family assistance
Educational level (low)	Emphasize oral (versus written) instruction Adjust language level as appropriate Provide written materials at fifth- to eighth-grade reading level
Potential language barrier	Enlist family assistance Secure a translator
Cultural or religious factors	Ascertain key factors affecting care Modify to accommodate Enlist family assistance
Vision difficulty	Have the patient wear glasses Emphasize sound and touch Enlist family assistance
Hearing difficulty	Have the patient use a hearing aid Emphasize visualization and touch Enlist family assistance

"wants"—that is, any specific things the patient desires to learn. In combination, these needs and wants provide the basis for setting mutually agreed-upon education goals.

After implementing any patient learning activity, you need to evaluate the results and document the intervention in the chart. As outlined in **Table 2-17**, how you evaluate a patient's learning depends on whether your focus was on improving knowledge, developing skills, or changing attitudes.

Table 2-17 Evaluating Patient Learning

Change That You Are Evaluating	Method to Evaluate the Change
Patient knowledge	Teach-back (patients to repeat in their own words the information you are trying to get them to understand)
Patient skill level	Return demonstration (patients perform the procedure after you have demonstrated it to them)
Patient attitudes	Discussion with patient and/or family or observation of behavioral change

Like all patient interventions, patient education episodes should be documented in the medical record. Such documentation must include who was taught (patient and/or family), what was taught, how it was taught, and what relevant outcomes were achieved (Figure 2-2).

Review and Interpret the Chest Radiograph

Chapter 1 outlines the various imaging studies used in the diagnosis and management of respiratory disorders. Chapter 11 specifies the characteristics of the common abnormalities seen on chest radiographs. Here we outline the process of reviewing a chest x-ray, including what to look for during assessment. The accompanying box outlines the basic steps in reviewing a chest x-ray.

Basic Steps in Review of a Chest X-Ray

1. Obtain image; verify identification (patient, date), orientation (using side marker), and image quality.
2. Identify the view of the film (AP or PA).
3. Review the entire film for symmetry and identify:
    a. Clavicles, scapulae, and ribs
    b. Spinal column (note whether it is midline)
    c. Lungs, right and left
    d. Level of hemidiaphragms and costophrenic angles (sharp or blunted)
    e. Gastric air bubble
    f. Breast shadows
4. Trace the outline of each rib, noting the angle and any fractures or other abnormalities.
5. Observe the tracheal position.
6. Identify the carina and the mainstem bronchi.
7. Examine the hila for size and position.
8. Identify the lung markings.
9. Identify the aortic knob and the heart shadow.
10. Estimate the cardiothoracic ratio.
11. Note the presence and position of any artificial airways or catheters.
12. State an overall impression of the film.

Image Orientation and Quality (RRT-Specific Content)

When reviewing an x-ray, you first need to verify the identification information (patient, date) and assess image orientation and quality. As outlined in **Table 2-18**, you can use the mnemonic R-I-P-E to assess image orientation and quality.

Position of or Change in Hemidiaphragms

Table 2-19 summarizes key findings related to the position or appearance of the hemidiaphragms.

Tracheal Position

As visualized on x-ray, the trachea should lie in the midline of the neck, overlying the spinal column on the AP view. In general, the trachea can be seen on x-ray shifting *toward* areas of collapse/atelectasis and *away from* space-occupying lesions such as pneumothoraces, large effusions, and tumors.

Position of Endotracheal or Tracheostomy Tubes

Taking an AP chest x-ray is the most common method used to confirm proper placement of an endotracheal (ET) or tracheostomy tube. Ideally, the tube tip should be positioned 4–6 cm above the carina. This normally corresponds to a location between thoracic vertebrae T2 and T4, or about the same level as the superior border of the aortic knob.

Table 2-18 R-I-P-E Mnemonic for Assessing Chest Radiograph Quality

R	Rotation	*The patient's shoulders should be perfectly perpendicular to the x-ray beam* (i.e., not rotated left or right). The patient is aligned "straight" if the thoracic spine aligns in the center of the sternum and equally between the medial end of each clavicle.
I	Inspiration	*A good inspiration is needed to properly visualize lung structures, especially at the bases.* Inspiration is adequate if diaphragm is at the level of the tenth posterior rib (eighth to ninth posterior ribs in AP films) or sixth anterior rib on the right.
P	Position	*Verify anterior–posterior (AP) versus posterior–anterior (PA) view.* • The AP view is most common in bedridden patients. In the typical AP view, the medial borders of scapula are seen in the upper lung fields, ribs appear more horizontal, and the heart appears more magnified. • In the typical PA view, the borders of the scapula are clear of the upper lung fields, ribs are angled downward, and the heart appears less magnified. *Verify left versus right sides of film.* If not labeled with a side marker, both the gastric bubble (upright posture only) and the apex of a normal heart should appear on the right side of the film (patient's left side). *Verify proper angulation* (head/toe). In the AP view, the clavicle should be at about the level of the third rib.
E	Exposure	*Verify proper intensity of the x-ray beam passing through the patient.* In a good exposure, the intervertebral disks should just be visible through the heart and the costophrenic angles should be well defined (assuming proper inspiration and no effusions). Overexposed = too dark; underexposed = too white.

Table 2-19 Abnormalities Associated with Changes in the Position or Appearance of the Hemidiaphragms

Appearance or Position	Likely Problem
Blunted costophrenic angles (affected side)	Lower-lobe pneumonia, pleural effusion
Flattened (affected side)	Hyperinflation, tension pneumothorax
Elevated (affected side)	Phrenic nerve paralysis, hepatomegaly
Air under diaphragms (differentiate from normal gastric air bubble)	Perforated gastrointestinal tract

Lung Fields

Because a radiograph is a negative, areas of increased whiteness or *radiopacity* indicate high-density objects, such as bone or consolidated tissue, whereas areas of darkness or *radiolucency* indicate low-density matter such as air. **Table 2-20** lists the most common causes of radiopacity and radiolucency seen on an x-ray. Details on the specific findings associated with these abnormalities are provided in Chapter 11.

Position of Indwelling Tubes, Catheters, and Foreign Objects

Objects visible on a chest radiograph not coming from the patient are *foreign bodies*. Foreign bodies include those appearing by accident or trauma—such as an aspirated tooth or bullet—as well as purposefully placed medical devices. Aspiration of small objects is the most common source of accidental foreign body ingestion, especially in children. This possibility always should be considered when encountering airway obstruction in children and justifies recommending both a chest *and* lateral neck x-ray.

Other than some plastics, most foreign bodies are denser than human tissues. Thus these objects appear radiopaque, with their shape often helping identify their origin. For example, an

Table 2-20 Common Pulmonary Abnormalities Altering the Density of the Lung Fields on a Chest Radiograph

Increased Radiopacity	Increased Radiolucency
Atelectasis	Pulmonary emphysema
Consolidation	Pneumothorax
Interstitial lung disease	Pneumomediastinum
Pulmonary infiltrates/edema	Pneumopericardium
Pleural effusion	Subcutaneous emphysema
Lung/mediastinal tumors	Pulmonary interstitial emphysema
Calcification	

aspirated coin will appear as a solid white, round object on a radiograph. Likewise, devices such as surgical staples are easily identifiable by their shape and position.

In contrast, low-density plastic devices, such as ET tubes and vascular catheters, are more difficult to visualize on an x-ray. For this reason, radiopaque markers are embedded in these devices. **Table 2-21** outlines common medical devices that may be visualized on a chest radiograph.

Table 2-21 Medical Devices Visualized on the Chest Radiograph

Devices	Comments
Extrathoracic	
ECG leads	Three electrodes and lead wires typically are visible.
Clamps, syringes, and other instruments	May be on top of or under the patient but can appear to be "inside" the thorax and thus confuse interpretation.
Ventilator circuits, heating wires, temperature sensors	Adult circuits normally exhibit typical corrugated appearance; wires/sensors may be confused with intrathoracic devices such as pacemakers.
Breast implants	Either unilateral or bilateral; shadows can be confused with lung pathology.
Intrathoracic	
Thoracostomy (chest) tubes	To evacuate air (pneumothorax), the tube normally is positioned antero-superiorly; to evacuate fluid, it is positioned posteroinferiorly.
Endotracheal tubes	The tube tip should be 4–6 cm above the carina, or between T2 and T4.
Nasogastric or feeding tubes	Visualized passing through the mediastinum and diaphragm into the stomach. Misplacement high in the esophagus or in the trachea can result in massive aspiration.
Central venous catheter	Should be seen in the superior vena cava or right atrium.
Pulmonary artery (PA) catheter	The catheter tip should appear in the lower lobe, ideally posteriorly. Improper placement can result in false PAWP readings.
Implanted cardiac pacemakers and cardioverter/defibrillators	The pulse generator is usually visualized below clavicle; one or two pacing wires should appear coursing through the superior vena cava into the heat chamber(s).
Sternal wires	Appear on the chest radiograph as several opaque "tied" loops running up and down the sternum (in patients after median sternotomy for cardiac surgery).
Cardiac valve replacements (prostheses)	Appear in the same location as what they replace (mitral and aortic being the most common).
Intra-aortic counterpulsation balloon device (IACB or IABP)	Consists of an inflatable balloon about 25 cm long, the tip of which normally can be visualized just distal to the left subclavian artery in the descending thoracic aorta.

Review Lateral Neck Radiographs

When used together with a chest radiograph, lateral neck x-rays are useful in assessing for upper-airway obstruction, especially in children. The most common causes of upper-airway obstruction in children are aspirated foreign bodies and infection. As indicated previously, high-density aspirated objects are readily visualized on x-ray. Some plastic objects may be more difficult to identify and often require laryngoscopy or bronchoscopy to confirm and resolve.

In terms of serious upper-airway infections in pediatric patients, croup and epiglottitis are the most commonly encountered diseases. **Table 2-22** compares the typical radiographic findings in these two conditions.

Table 2-22 Radiographic Findings: Croup Versus Epiglottitis

View	Condition	
	Croup	**Epiglottitis**
Chest film (AP)	"Steeple sign" (i.e., narrowed and tapering airway below larynx due to subglottic edema); tracheal dilation may be present if film was taken during expiration	Usually appears normal (little or no evidence of subglottic involvement)
Lateral neck film	May appear normal (little or no evidence of supraglottic involvement)	"Thumb sign" due to prominent shadow caused by swollen epiglottis

Obtaining and Interpreting a 12-Lead ECG

The 12-lead ECG is used to assess rhythm disturbances, determine the heart's electrical axis, and identify the site and extent of myocardial damage. Chapter 4 provides details on the use and troubleshooting of ECG machines. The accompanying box outlines the basic procedure for obtaining a 12-lead ECG.

Basic 12-Lead ECG Procedure

1. Turn on the machine (plug it into an outlet if AC powered); run the self-test/calibration process.

2. Place the patient appropriately in supine or semi-Fowler's position.

3. Have the patient remove all jewelry or metal and relax completely.

4. Apply clean limb electrodes to muscular areas of the arms and legs.

5. Place chest leads in the proper locations:

   V1: Fourth intercostal space, right sternal margin

   V2: Fourth intercostal space, left sternal margin

   V3: Midway between V2 and V4

   V4: Fifth intercostal space, left midclavicular line

   V5: Fifth intercostal space, left anterior axillary line

   V6: Sixth intercostal space, left midaxillary line

6. Ensure patient comfort and respect patient privacy and modesty.

7. Run the 12-lead ECG to obtain a good tracing (stable isoelectric baseline, no extraneous noise/AC interference).

The NBRC expects all candidates for all its exams to be proficient in identifying common abnormalities from an ECG rhythm strip. To do so, you systematically assess the rate, rhythm, P waves, the PR interval, QRS complex, QT interval, ST segment, and T waves. The easiest way to estimate heart rate is to use the "rule of 300," as depicted in **Figure 2-3**. **Table 2-23** summarizes key findings defining major abnormalities in rhythm, P waves, the PR interval, QRS complex, QT interval, ST segment, and T waves, as well as their most common causes.

Table 2-23 Major ECG Rhythm Abnormalities and Their Common Causes

Abnormal ECG Findings	Common Causes
P waves—abnormal	Left or right atrial hypertrophy, PACs
P waves—absent	Atrial fibrillation
P-P interval—variable	Sinus arrhythmia
PR interval—prolonged (> 0.20 sec)	First-degree or Mobitz-type I A-V block
QRS complex—widened (> 0.12 sec)	PVC, R or L bundle branch block, ventricular fibrillation, hyperkalemia
QT interval—prolonged (> 0.45 sec)	Myocardial ischemia/infarction, electrolyte imbalance, antiarrhythmics, tricyclic antidepressants
QT interval—shortened (< 0.30 sec)	Electrolyte imbalance, digoxin
R-R interval—shortened (< 0.60 sec)	Tachycardia (R-R < 0.60 sec or rate > 100/min)
R-R interval—prolonged (> 1.00 sec)	Bradycardia (R-R > 1.00 sec or rate < 60/min)
R-R interval—variable (> 0.12 sec or > 10% variation)	Sinus arrhythmia; atrial fibrillation; second-degree heart block (Type I)
ST segment—depressed (chest leads)	Myocardial ischemia/infarction, ventricular hypertrophy, conduction disturbances, hyperventilation, hypokalemia, digoxin
ST segment—elevated (chest leads)	Myocardial ischemia/infarction, conduction disturbances, ventricular hypertrophy, hyperkalemia, digoxin
T wave—tall	Hyperkalemia, acute myocardial infarction, conduction disturbances, ventricular hypertrophy
T wave—small, flattened, or inverted	Myocardial ischemia, hyperventilation, anxiety, left ventricular hypertrophy, digoxin, pericarditis, pulmonary embolism, conduction disturbances, electrolyte imbalances
U wave—prominent	Hypokalemia, hypomagnesemia, ischemia

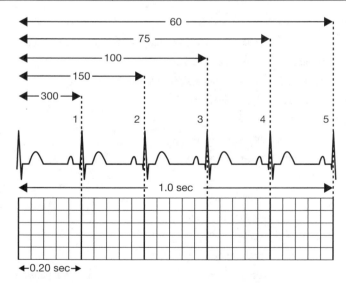

Figure 2-3 Using the Rule of 300. At the standard recording speed of 25 mm/sec, each little 1 mm box represents 0.04 sec, with each large box representing 5 × 0.04 or 0.20 sec. Therefore, if a QRS complex were to occur with *each large box*, then the R-R interval would be 0.20 sec, and the rate would be 5 beats/sec × 60 sec/min or 300 beats/min. As long as the rhythm is regular, dividing 300 by the number of big boxes spanned by the R-R interval provides a good estimate for any cardiac rate. For example, if the R-R interval spans three large boxes, the rate would be about 300 ÷ 3 = 100/min.

Courtesy of: Strategic Learning Associates, LLC, Little Silver, New Jersey.

In addition to rhythm assessment, the NBRC RRT-level exams require *basic* knowledge of 12-lead ECG interpretation, including the ability to ascertain axis deviation, confirm hypertrophy, and identify the presence of myocardial ischemia or myocardial infarction (MI). **Table 2-24** summarizes the common 12-lead ECG findings associated with these problems. *The most common pattern in patients with chronic lung disease is right axis deviation/right ventricular hypertrophy.* Also important is your understanding that the 12-lead ECG alone cannot diagnose an MI. Other clinical data, including patient presentation and cardiac biomarkers (Chapter 1), are needed to establish this diagnosis. Moreover, the distinction between ST-segment elevation MI (STEMI) and non-ST-segment elevation MI (NSTEMI) is essential because treatment of the two conditions differs substantially. Patients with STEMI typically undergo thrombolytic therapy and/or angioplasty, whereas those with NSTEMI typically receive antiplatelet drugs and anticoagulants.

Bedside Assessment of Ventilation

Bedside assessment of ventilation involves measurement of a patient's tidal volume, rate of breathing, minute volume, vital capacity, and maximum inspiratory and expiratory pressures. **Table 2-25** defines these common measures, and provides both the approximate adult normal and critical values for each. You should recommend measuring these parameters when the need exists to perform the following assessments:

- Assess the progress of diseases affecting respiratory muscle strength (e.g., neuromuscular disorders)
- Evaluate a patient's potential need for mechanical ventilation

These measures have also been used to assess whether a patient is ready to be removed from ventilatory support or "weaned" from mechanical ventilation. However, new evidence-based guidelines have established different criteria to assess a patient's readiness to wean (Chapter 13).

Table 2-24 Common 12-Lead ECG Findings

Abnormality	12-Lead ECG Findings
Axis Deviation (normally QRS is positive in leads I and aVF)	
Left axis deviation	QRS is positive in lead I but negative in lead aVF*
Right axis deviation	QRS is negative in lead I but positive in lead aVF
Extreme right axis deviation	QRS is negative in leads I and aVF
Hypertrophy	
Left ventricular hypertrophy (Sokolow-Lyon index)	Left axis deviation (up to −30° is normal)
	Lead V1 S wave + lead V5 or V6 R wave ≥ 35 mm
	Lead aVL R wave ≥ 11 mm
Right ventricular hypertrophy	Right axis deviation (> 100°)
	Increase in voltage in V1, V5, and V6
	R waves in lead V1 > 7 mm
	R waves > S waves in lead V1 or R waves < S waves in leads V5 or V6
Myocardial Ischemia/Infarction*	
Ischemia/NSTEMI	ST-segment depression (horizontal or downsloping ≥ 0.5 mm)
	T-wave flattening or inversion ≥ 1 mm
Acute STEMI	ST-segment elevation ≥ 2 mm (men) or ≥ 1.5 mm (women) in two contiguous precordial leads
	Pathological (deep/prolonged) Q waves
	Prominent R waves in V1–V2
STEMI = ST-segment elevation myocardial infarction; NSTEMI = non-ST-segment elevation myocardial infarction. *Electrical events occurring in the leads "facing" the damage; may vary according to time since insult.	

Table 2-25 Bedside Ventilation Parameters

Measure (Abbreviation)	Definition	Approximate Adult Normal	Critical Adult Value*
Tidal volume (VT)	Volume inhaled or exhaled on each breath	5–7 mL/kg predicted body weight (PBW)	< 4-5 mL/kg or < 300 mL
Rate (f)	Number of breaths inhaled or exhaled in 1 min	12–20/min	> 30–35/min
Minute volume (V̇E)	Total volume exhaled per minute; equals rate times tidal volume (f × VT)	5–10 L/min (depends on body size/metabolic rate)	< 4 L/min or > 10 L/min
Slow vital capacity (SVC)	Maximum volume exhaled after a maximum inhalation measured during a slow exhalation	70 mL/kg PBW	< 10–15 mL/kg
Maximum inspiratory pressure (MIP, NIF, PI$_{max}$)	Maximum pressure generated against airway occlusion at or near residual volume (RV) after successive inspiratory efforts for 15–25 sec	−80 to −120 cm H_2O	0 to −20 cm H_2O
Maximum expiratory pressure (MEP, PE$_{max}$)	Maximum pressure generated by forced exhalation against airway occlusion at or near total lung capacity (TLC)	> +150 cm H_2O	< +60 cm H_2O

*Critical values represent the threshold below which patients likely cannot maintain adequate spontaneous ventilation.

In combination, VT and rate (f) affect the efficiency of ventilation. You typically obtain these measurements in spontaneously breathing patients using a respirometer attached to a one-way valve, as described in Chapter 4. Over a 1-minute interval, you measure the accumulated volume and count the frequency of respirations. To compute the tidal volume, you divide the minute volume by the frequency (i.e., $VT = \dot{V}E \div f$). For example, the tidal volume of a patient breathing at a rate of 38/min with a minute volume of 11.4 L/min would be computed as follows:

$$VT = 11.4 \text{ L/min} \div 38 \text{ breaths/min} = 0.3 \text{ L or } 300 \text{ mL}$$

A different and more useful measure called the *rapid shallow breathing index* (RSBI) can be computed using the same data. You compute the RSBI by dividing the patient's rate of breathing by the average tidal volume *in liters*: $RSBI = f \div VT$ (L). For example, the RSBI for a patient breathing spontaneously at a rate of 38/min with a tidal volume of 300 mL, would be computed as follows:

$$RSBI = f \div VT \text{ (L)}$$
$$RSBI = 38 \div 0.3$$
$$RSBI \approx 127$$

Unlike the individual measures in Table 2-25, the RSBI is a good predictor of a patient's ability to be weaned from mechanical ventilation. In general, *when the RSBI exceeds 105 early in a spontaneous breathing trial, the attempt is likely to fail.* In the preceding example, the patient's RSBI is significantly greater than 100, indicating that successful weaning is unlikely.

Fast and shallow breathing also increases deadspace ventilation, which is evident in the formula for alveolar minute ventilation—a point *commonly tested on the NBRC exams*. Alveolar minute ventilation (V̇A) is the volume of "fresh" gas reaching the alveoli per minute. To compute V̇A, you multiply a patient's breathing frequency (f) by the *difference* between the tidal volume (VT) and the physiologic deadspace per breath (VD):

$$\dot{V}A = f \times (VT - VD)$$

Unless otherwise indicated, *you should assume a deadspace of approximately 1 mL per pound of predicted body weight*. Using the preceding formula and assuming a 125-lb patient breathing at a rate of 15/min with a tidal volume of 400 mL, you would compute this patient's alveolar minute volume as follows:

$$\dot{V}_A = f \times (V_T - V_D)$$
$$\dot{V}_A = 15 \times (400 - 125) = 4125 \text{ mL}$$

In this case, approximately 70% of the patient's ventilation per minute is fresh gas, with the remaining 30% being deadspace ventilation. Thirty percent deadspace ventilation is considered roughly normal.

To demonstrate the effect of rapid shallow breathing, let's double the patient's rate but halve her tidal volume, keeping her minute ventilation constant at 6000 mL/min:

$$\dot{V}_E = 30 \times 200 \text{ mL} = 6000 \text{ mL/min}$$
$$\dot{V}_A = 30 \times (200 - 125) = 2250 \text{ mL}$$

Even though the patient's $\dot{V}_E$ remains unchanged, the rapid shallow breathing pattern has doubled her deadspace ventilation per minute. Now only about 40% of the patient's $\dot{V}_E$ consists of fresh gas. Because the alveolar P_{CO_2} is directly proportional to the amount of deadspace ventilation, this patient's arterial P_{CO_2} will rise. As a rule of thumb, *high rates and low tidal volumes result in the highest deadspace ventilation per minute, while low rates and high tidal volumes waste the least amount of ventilation per minute.*

The vital capacity indicates how well the entire ventilatory "pump" is working, including both lung/chest wall interaction and respiratory muscle function. For this reason, along with the pressure measures discussed subsequently, the vital capacity is a good indicator of the progress of diseases affecting respiratory muscle strength, such as neuromuscular disorders. You measure the slow vital capacity (SVC) using either a mechanical respirometer or an electronic spirometer. To obtain the SVC, have the patient inhale as deeply as possible (*deeper, deeper, deeper, . . .*) and then exhale slowly and completely for as long as possible (*more, more, more, . . .*) or until no volume change occurs for at least 2 seconds. This procedure should be performed at least three times to ensure maximum effort and repeatability. Obviously, the SVC can be obtained only with alert and cooperative patients.

The maximum pressure measurements assess the patient's inspiratory and expiratory muscle strength. As such, these measures are good indicators of how various disorders affect respiratory muscle strength. You measure maximum inspiratory pressure (MIP) using a manometer attached to a one-way valve configured to allow exhalation but not inspiration. With this setup, the patient "bucks down" toward RV on each successive breath, at which point a maximum effort is ensured (the patient need not be conscious). Given that this outcome can cause anxiety in alert patients, you should provide a careful and reassuring explanation. Measurement of maximum expiratory pressure (MEP) also is obtained with a manometer but does not require the valve. However, unlike the MIP, you can obtain a MEP only with an alert and cooperative patient.

Lung Mechanics and Ventilator Graphics

More sophisticated measures of ventilatory mechanics can be provided on patients being supported by critical care ventilators equipped with graphic displays. These measures include estimates of total compliance and airway resistance and plotting of pressure–volume and flow–volume loops during breathing. Details on these advanced monitoring tools are provided in Chapter 11.

Monitoring Peak Expiratory Flow Rates

A patient's peak expiratory flow rate (PEFR) is the maximum flow generated on forced expiration, and is a simple measure used to assess for airway obstruction. However, because the PEFR is highly effort dependent, it is not used for definitive diagnosis but instead is considered a supplemental monitoring tool. For this reason, the PEFR is used primarily for the following purposes:

- Monitoring the effect of bronchodilator therapy (using pre- and post-test measures)
- Assessing the severity of asthma symptoms
- Detecting early changes in asthma control that require adjustments in treatment

Often the patient makes these measurements at home and records them in a log. Inspection of this log can help RTs assess the pattern of a patient's symptoms and response to therapy.

Typically, you measure a patient's PEFR with a mechanical peak-flow meter or electronic spirometer and report the value in liters per second (L/sec) or liters per minute (L/min) body temperature pressure, saturated (BTPS). *To convert L/sec to L/min, multiply by 60; to convert L/min to L/sec, divide by 60.*

To make this measurement, the patient must be able to follow simple instructions and coordinate breathing with use of the measurement device. Data needed for interpretation include the patient's gender and height. In addition, you should ascertain the patient's smoking history and current medications, including bronchodilators and steroids. Key points needed to ensure valid measurement include the following:

- If using a mechanical meter, it must be set to zero and properly positioned (some devices must be held level).
- Ideally the patient should sit or stand up straight and inhale fully to TLC.
- The mouthpiece should be inserted above the tongue, with the patient forming a tight lip seal.
- The patient should exhale in a sharp burst with maximum force (full exhalation is not needed).
- The measurement should be repeated until three values are obtained that vary by less than 10%.
- Record the highest of the three values.
- If assessing bronchodilator therapy:
  - Allow the drug to reach its full effect before the post-test (usually 20–30 minutes).
  - Compute the pre-test to post-test percent change.

Table 2-26 lists the common cited PEFR reference ranges by patient age and sex. If using an electronic spirometer to measure PEFR, inputting of the patient's gender and height will provide the predicted value, from which the percent predicted is computed. As with all pulmonary function tests, a patient's percent predicted value is computed as follows:

$$\% \, predicted = \frac{actual}{predicted} \times 100$$

In general, *PEFR values less than 80% of predicted indicate expiratory flow obstruction.* However, because the test is so dependent on patient effort and starting lung volume, you should always consider the possibility of either poor effort or poor technique whenever a patient's PEFR is significantly below normal.

In asthma management, we often substitute the patient's *personal best* value for the predicted value in computing the percent predicted measure. A patient's personal best PEFR is the highest value achieved over a 2-week asymptomatic period.

Table 2-26 Reference Ranges for PEFR

Patient Category	Common Reference Ranges	
	L/min	L/sec
Adult males	450–750 L/min	8–12 L/sec
Adult females	350–530 L/min	6–9 L/sec
Children (depends on height)	150–450 L/min	3–8 L/sec

Table 2-27 Severity of Disease and Recommended Therapy for Asthma Based on PEFR Measurement

% Predicted *or* % Personal Best	Severity (Including Symptoms)	Recommended Therapy
> 80%	Mild	Short-acting beta agonist (SABA) bronchodilator Vital sign monitoring
50–80%	Moderate	O_2 to keep saturation > 90% SABA Consider anticholinergic + oral steroids
< 50%	Severe	Admit to hospital O_2 to keep saturation > 90% SABA + anticholinergic + oral steroids Consider epinephrine Frequent vital sign monitoring

As indicated in **Table 2-27**, when a patient presents to the emergency department with a history of asthma and corresponding symptoms, the percent predicted PEFR can help determine the severity of the exacerbation and the proper course of therapy.

Assessing Spirometry at the Bedside

Bedside spirometry involves the measurement of the forced vital capacity and related measures (e.g., PEFR, FEVt, FEF_{25-75}) at the bedside using a portable electronic spirometer. Chapter 4 provides details on the selection, use, and troubleshooting of bedside spirometers. Here we focus on performing spirometry and interpreting its results.

As with peak flow, forced expiratory volume measurements depend on proper patient performance, as instructed and coached by the clinician. The accompanying box outlines a basic procedure designed to help ensure accurate and reproducible results.

Bedside Spirometry Procedure

1. Turn the spirometer on and connect a new mouthpiece or sensor (some sensors require inputting individual calibration data).
2. Input all requested patient data accurately (e.g., age, sex, height, ethnicity).
3. Remove candy, gum, or dentures from the patient's mouth; loosen any tight clothing.
4. Have the patient sit or stand, but be consistent and record the patient's position.
5. Demonstrate the procedure using your own mouthpiece/sensor, being sure to emphasize the following points:
   a. How to hold the sensor steady and avoid jerky motions (can cause flow or start-of-test errors)
   b. How deeply to inhale
   c. How to correctly place the mouthpiece on top of the tongue
   d. How fast and long to exhale (at least 6 seconds)
6. Use nose clips to prevent patient leaks.
7. Have the patient perform the maneuver while you carefully observe test performance:
   a. Ensure that the patient breathes in as deeply as possible (to full TLC).
   b. Coach the patient to forcibly blast the breath out, as fast and as long as possible (at least 6 seconds; patients with severe COPD may take up to 15 seconds to fully exhale).
   c. Carefully observe the patient for poor technique and correct as needed.
8. Repeat the procedure until you have three acceptable maneuvers.
9. Print and review the results.

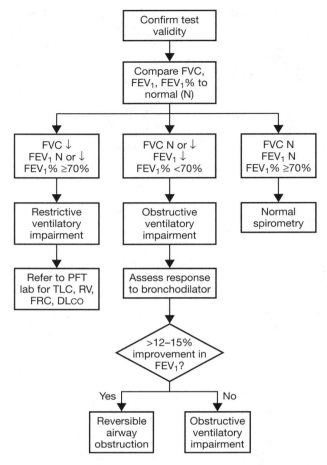

Figure 2-4 Basic Procedure for Interpreting the Results of Bedside or Ambulatory Spirometry.

Adapted from: Barreiro TJ, Perillo I. An approach to interpreting spirometry. *Am Fam Physician.* 2004;69:1107–1114.

Figure 2-4 outlines the basic process for interpreting spirometry results. Because the results require proper patient performance, the first step is always to assess test validity, as described in Chapter 6. Assuming valid test results, you first compare the patient's FVC, FEV_1, and $FEV_1\%$ to the patient's computed reference ranges. In general, the FVC and FEV_1 are considered normal if the patient's values are at least 80% of those predicted. *A normal $FEV_1\%$ ($FEV_1/FVC \times 100$) is 70% or more for all patients.* As indicated in **Table 2-28**, by comparing these three values, you can immediately categorize the type of impairment present.

Graphic analysis should always supplement numeric assessment. Depending on the spirometer used, the FVC graph may be volume versus time or flow versus volume. **Figure 2-5** compares the typical normal, obstructive, and restrictive patterns seen on these two types of spirograms.

Table 2-28 Bedside Spirometry Categorization of Pulmonary Function Impairment

Parameter	Normal	Obstructive	Restrictive	Mixed
FVC (% predicted)	N	↓ or N	↓	↓
FEV_1 (% predicted)	N	↓	↓ or N	↓
$FEV_1\%$ (N ≥ 70%)	N	↓	↑ or N	↓
Notes: N = normal; ↓ = decreased; ↑ = increased. For obstructive impairments, judge severity by either % predicted FVC or FEV_1 as follows: 65–80%, mild; 50–65%, moderate; < 50%, severe.				

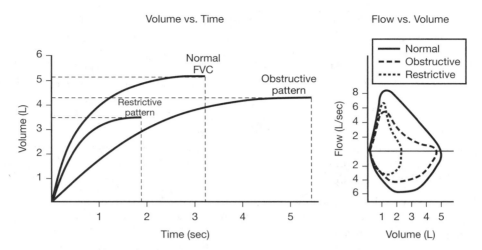

Figure 2-5 Typical Volume Versus Time (left) and Flow Versus Volume (right) Spirograms. Normal subjects can forcibly exhale the vital capacity (FVC) in about 3 seconds, whereas patients with obstructive conditions may require 6 seconds or longer for complete exhalation. Patients with restrictive conditions typically have reduced expiratory volumes, but may exhibit near normal expiratory flows. Their absolute FEV_1 values usually are below normal, but their FEV_1% may be normal or even high.

Courtesy of: Strategic Learning Associates, LLC, Little Silver, New Jersey.

If the analysis indicates an obstructive impairment, you should recommend assessing the patient's response to bronchodilator therapy, with repeat spirometry timed to correspond to the peak response time of the drug, usually after 20–30 minutes. You then compute the % change as follows:

$$\% \ change = \frac{post - pre}{pre} \times 100$$

where "post" is the patient's FEV_1 after bronchodilator and "pre" is the FEV_1 before bronchodilator.

If the patient's FEV_1 improves by at least 12–15% (and by 200 mL or more in adults), then the obstruction is classified as reversible, as in asthma. Lesser improvement indicates that the obstruction is not reversible, as in most forms of COPD.

If analysis indicates a restrictive or mixed impairment, you should recommend that the patient undergo a full evaluation in the pulmonary laboratory, to include measurement of static lung volumes and diffusing capacity. In combination, these tests will help differentiate among the various causes of restriction.

Conducting Pulmonary Function Laboratory Studies

Pulmonary function laboratory studies include the same FVC measurements assessed at the bedside, plus static lung volumes (TLC, FRC, VC, IC, ERV, and RV) and sometimes the diffusing capacity. Additionally, some labs may measure airway reactivity via bronchial provocation testing or expired nitric oxide analysis.

Static Lung Volumes

The key static lung volume from which the others are derived is the functional residual capacity (FRC). If the FRC is known, both the RV and TLC are computed as follows:

RV = FRC – ERV
TLC = FRC + IC

Table 2-29 describes the three methods most commonly used to measure FRC in pulmonary function laboratories. Note that whereas the helium dilution and nitrogen washout methods both measure actual FRC (lung volume communicating with the airways), body plethysmography measures total thoracic gas volume (TGV). Normally the FRC and TGV are equal. *A TGV that exceeds FRC indicates the presence of "trapped" gas that is not in communication with the airways, as in seen in bullous emphysema.*

Diffusing Capacity

The diffusing capacity of the lung (DLco) is assessed by measuring the transfer of carbon monoxide (CO) from the lungs into the pulmonary capillaries. The *single breath* test is the most common procedure, key elements of which include the following:

- The patient exhales completely to RV.
- The patient inspires from RV to TLC, inhaling a mixture of 21% O_2, 10% He, and 0.3% CO.
- The patient performs a 10-second breath hold.
- The first portion of the patient's exhalation (anatomic deadspace) is discarded.
- Thereafter, a sample of 0.5–1.0 L of expired gas is collected and analyzed for % He and % CO.
- The test is repeated after at least a 4-minute wait until results are within 5% or 3 mL/min/mm Hg.
- Reported measures include the DLco in mL/min/mm Hg (Hb and HbCO corrected), the alveolar volume (VA, an estimate of TLC), the ratio of DLco to VA, and the inspiratory VC.

Prediction equations based on age, gender, height, and weight are used to compute the patient's reference range, with the "typical" normal single-breath DLco ranging between 25 and 30 mL/min/mm Hg. The DLco is low in conditions that impair alveolar–capillary diffusion (as in pulmonary fibrosis) or decrease surface area (as in emphysema). The DLco also is low when Hb levels, pulmonary capillary blood flow, or alveolar volumes are reduced. Increases in DLco occur with increased Hb (as in secondary polycythemia), pulmonary blood flow, and alveolar volume, and during exercise.

The severity of impairment in pulmonary diffusion capacity is judged against the patient's predicted normal value, with values in the 65–80% range representing mild impairment, between 50% and 65% being moderate abnormality, and less than 50% of normal indicating a severe problem.

Interpreting and Applying PFT Test Results

Once the results of the FVC, static lung volume, and diffusing capacity tests are known, the nature of the impairment can be determined. **Figure 2-6** provides an algorithm for interpreting pulmonary lab test results based on the FEV_1%, SVC, TLC, and DLco. You assess the FEV_1% first, followed by the VC, TLC, and then (if needed) the DLco.

A low FEV_1% indicates either an obstructive disorder or a mixed obstructive and restrictive disorder. For obstructive disorders, the DLco differentiates between emphysema (low DLco) and other forms of airway obstruction—such as asthma or chronic bronchitis—in which the DLco is normal. To differentiate asthma from chronic bronchitis, you should recommend a pre-/post-bronchodilator assessment or (in advanced labs) a methacholine challenge.

If the FEV_1% is at or above normal, the patient has either normal pulmonary function or a restrictive disorder. The disorder is restrictive if the TLC is low. Again, the DLco helps differentiate the two most common types of restrictive disorders, with a normal or high value suggesting a chest wall or neuromuscular problem and a low value consistent with interstitial lung diseases that limit diffusing capacity, such as pulmonary fibrosis.

Exhaled Nitric Oxide Analysis (RRT-Specific Content)

Nitric oxide (NO) is a chemical mediator that appears in the exhaled breath, with its levels increasing during airway inflammation. For this reason, analysis of the exhaled fraction of NO (FeNO) is used in both the diagnosis and the management of asthma.

Table 2-29 Comparison of Methods Used to Measure Functional Residual Capacity

Method/Description	Key Points
Helium (He) Dilution (Closed-Circuit Method)	
• At the end of a normal exhalation (FRC), the patient is connected to a spirometer containing 5–10% He, and then breathes normally. • CO_2 is chemically absorbed by soda lime while O_2 is added to keep a constant end-expiratory level (about 0.25 L/min). • The test continues until equilibration is reached (% He is constant for 2 minutes). • FRC is calculated based on initial and final % He, volume of He and O_2 added to the system, and system deadspace.	• The spirometer must be leak free and the He analyzer properly calibrated. • After the FRC is obtained, VC, IC, ERV, and IRV should be measured. • FRC may be underestimated in individuals with air trapping. • Hypercapnia or hypoxemia may occur if CO_2 is not removed or O_2 not added. • Test results should be repeatable (±500 mL in adults). • Test validity depends on the proper starting point (at FRC) and an absence of leaks (e.g., poor mouth seal, perforated eardrums, tracheostomies).
Nitrogen (N_2) Washout (Open-Circuit Method)	
• At the end of a normal exhalation (FRC), the patient is connected to a 100% O_2 reservoir. • Expired N_2 and expired volume are measured continuously. • The test continues for 7 minutes or until % N_2 falls below 1.0% (more time may be needed for patients with air trapping). • FRC is computed based on total expired volume and final % N_2.	• The system must be leak free and the N_2 analyzer properly calibrated. • Some patients cannot maintain a good mouth seal or cooperate adequately. • Ventilatory drive may be depressed in some patients who breathe 100% O_2. • An initial alveolar % N_2 of 80% is assumed if the patient has been breathing room air for at least 15 minutes. • After the FRC is obtained, VC, IC, ERV, and IRV should be measured. • A minimum of 15 minutes should elapse before the test is repeated. • Test results should be repeatable (±500 mL in adults). • Test validity depends on starting at FRC and an absence of leaks (increased % N_2 indicates a leak).
Body Box (Body Plethysmography)	
• Transducers measure chamber + mouth pressure, and flow. • A mouthpiece shutter occludes the airway at end-expiration. • The patient "pants" against the closed shutter (compressing and expanding gas in the thorax and the chamber). • Changes in chamber pressure are proportional to changes in alveolar gas volume. • The volume of gas in the thorax is computed according to Boyle's law: $P_1V_1 = P_2V_2$.	• Careful calibration of multiple transducers is required. • The test measures total thoracic gas volume (TGV), which may be greater than He dilution or N_2 washout FRC (due to "trapped gas" in cysts or bullae, as can occur in emphysema). • Plethysmographic TGV is usually measured together with airway resistance/conductance. • Claustrophobic patients may not tolerate the procedure. • Test validity requires proper panting (as evidenced by "closed" P-V loops) at about 1 cycle/sec with hands against the patient's cheeks to avoid "bowing." • TGV should be averaged from a minimum of three to five acceptable panting maneuvers. • After the FRC is obtained, VC, IC, ERV, and IRV should be measured.

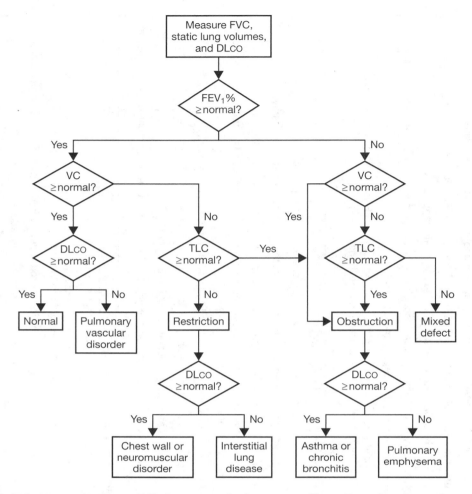

Figure 2-6 Interpretation of Pulmonary Laboratory Test Results. Less than normal is < 70% for the FEV$_1$% and < 80% predicted for the VC, TLC, and DLco.

Adapted from: Pellegrino R, Viegi G, Brusasco V, et al. Interpretative strategies for lung function tests. *Eur Respir J.* 2005;26:948–968.

Because many nondisease factors influence FeNO levels, you must instruct patients not to exercise, consume alcohol, smoke, or eat for at least 1 hour prior to testing. In addition, because both steroids and beta agonists alter FeNO levels, you should record all medications being taken by the patient. Last, because forced expiratory efforts decrease FeNO, you should conduct the analysis *before* spirometry.

The test requires that the patient inhale NO-free air for 2–3 seconds to TLC, then exhale steadily at a low flow (50 mL/sec) for or at least 6 seconds (more than 4 seconds for children), during which time the FeNO is measured by a calibrated analyzer. The requisite flow is achieved by having the patient exhale against a fixed resistance, with the measurement system using visual cues to keep this parameter within the targeted range. NO contamination from the nose (which has higher NO concentrations than air coming from the lungs) is prevented because the backpressure created by the system's expiratory flow resistance closes off the soft palate.

To ensure quality, at least three acceptable maneuvers should be obtained. **Figure 2-7** provides a sample graphic display of three such maneuvers during sampling of a patient with normal FeNO levels. The reported FeNO is the mean value of at least two plateau measurements whose FeNO levels fall within 10% of each other.

FeNO is measured by a rapidly responding and very sensitive analyzer in units of parts per billion (ppb). Note the consistent plateau levels of about 16 ppb occurring toward the end of each breath in Figure 2-7, indicating both acceptability and repeatability of the maneuvers.

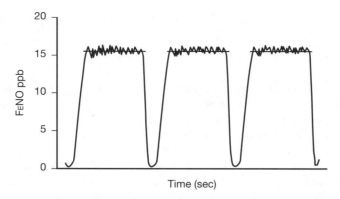

Figure 2-7 Example Display of FᴇNO from Normal Subject. Note the consistent plateau levels of about 16 ppb occurring toward the end of each breath, indicating both acceptability and repeatability of the maneuvers.

Courtesy of: Strategic Learning Associates, LLC, Little Silver, New Jersey.

Table 2-30 provides interpretive guidelines for FᴇNO measurements based on cutpoints recommended by American Thoracic Society. Like any laboratory measure, FᴇNO values should always be interpreted in conjunction with the patient's history, physical examination, and related diagnostic procedures, including pulmonary function tests.

Blood Gases and Related Measures

Obtaining and interpreting arterial and arterialized capillary blood samples, as well as related non-invasive measures, can be tested on this section of the NBRC exams. However, most questions on

Table 2-30 FᴇNO Cutpoints and Related Clinical Considerations for Adults and Children

	Low Cutpoint	**Intermediate Values**	**High Cutpoint**
Adult	< 25 ppb	25–50 ppb	> 50 ppb
Child	< 20 ppb	20–35 ppb	> 35 ppb
Eosinophilic inflammation?	Unlikely	Interpret based on clinical context	Likely
Response to steroids?	Unlikely	Interpret based on clinical context	Likely
Diagnostic considerations	Consider other causes of symptoms (e.g., CF, sinusitis, COPD, GERD, anxiety)	Be cautious; monitor FeNO trends	In symptomatic patients (not taking steroids), generally confirms diagnosis of asthma
Management considerations for asthmatics	• If symptoms persist, consider other diagnoses • In asymptomatic patients on inhaled steroids, indicates good compliance with treatment—consider decreasing the dose	• In symptomatic patients, may indicate persistent allergen exposure, inadequate inhaled steroid dose, or poor adherence • In asymptomatic patients, indicates adequate inhaled steroid dosing and good adherence	• May indicate poor treatment compliance, poor inhaler technique, inadequate inhaled steroid dose, or steroid resistance • Increased risk for exacerbation; inhaled steroid withdrawal may lead to relapse

Adapted from: Dweik RA, Boggs PB, Erzurum SC. An official ATS clinical practice guideline: interpretation of exhaled nitric oxide levels (FeNO) for clinical applications. *Am J Respir Crit Care Med.* 2011;184(5):602–615.

these measures require that you apply this information to patient care. For this reason, we cover these topics primarily in Chapter 11.

Apnea Monitoring

Apnea monitoring is used to warn caregivers of life-threatening cardiorespiratory events, particularly in hospitalized neonates being treated for recurrent apnea accompanied by bradycardia or O_2 desaturation. At-risk babies also may be discharged from the hospital with a prescription for home apnea monitoring, as will some older children and adults with conditions affecting the control of breathing (see Chapter 17 for details on home apnea monitoring).

Apnea monitors use two sensors placed on the chest wall to detect respiratory movements via changes in electrical impedance. Typically hospital monitors display a continuous waveform representing the cycle of chest motion, with the respiratory and heart rates also provided. *Although these systems can warn of adverse events, you should always confirm a patient's status by visual inspection.* Moreover, because impedance changes measure only chest wall movement and not airflow, simple apnea monitoring cannot be used to detect obstructive sleep apnea. Patients suspected of obstructive sleep apnea should undergo polysomnography.

Key points in performing apnea monitoring include the following:

- Set the low/high heart rate alarm limits (typically 80–210 for neonates; lower limits for older babies).
- Set the apnea time alarm limit (typically 15–20 seconds).
- For event recording:
  ○ Clear memory and set the desired option for waveform recording.
  ○ Set the event log limits for low/high heart rate and apnea time.
- Secure the sensors on the right and left sides of the chest, midway between the nipple line and the midaxillary line where the greatest chest motion is occurring (a sensor 'belt' facilitates placement).
- Connect the patient cable, turn the monitor on, and confirm a successful system check.
- Confirm that the monitor signals match the patient's heart and respiratory rate.

You can use an apnea monitor's event recording (chest motion, heart rate trend) to identify the following conditions:

- *Apnea:* the cessation of respiratory effort. Short (less than 10 seconds) periods of central apnea can be normal for all ages.
- *Pathologic apnea:* apnea occurring for longer than 20 seconds or associated with cyanosis, abrupt marked pallor, hypotonia, or bradycardia (< 80–100 beats/min in neonates).
- *Periodic breathing:* a breathing pattern characterized by three or more respiratory pauses of more than 3 seconds' duration with less than 20 seconds of respiration between pauses. Periodic breathing is not associated with cyanosis or changes in heart rate and can be a normal event.

To differentiate the various causes of altered respiratory rate, you compare the apnea monitor's respirations to the heart rate, as summarized in **Table 2-31**. Note that apnea monitoring cannot identify the cause of apnea (central versus obstructive) or by itself identify related symptoms (e.g., cyanosis, pallor, hypotonia, choking).

Table 2-31 Interpretation of Apnea Monitoring Signals

Respirations	Heart Rate	Likely Significance
Absent	Decreased	Pathologic apnea
Decreased	Increased	Hypoxemia*
Decreased/irregular	Unchanged	Periodic breathing
Increased	Increased	Motion/activity artifact
*Confirmed via simultaneous pulse oximetry.		

Overnight Pulse Oximetry

Overnight or *nocturnal* oximetry uses a recording pulse oximeter to log changes in Spo_2 and heart rate while the patient is sleeping. Overnight oximetry can help identify patients with sleep apnea–hypopnea syndrome (SAHS) and assess their response to therapy. In addition, overnight oximetry can determine whether serious desaturation occurs in certain COPD patients during sleep.

Key points in performing overnight oximetry include the following:

- Set up and verify equipment operation:
  - Set the device to trend monitoring and select the period (e.g., 8 hours).
  - If settable, adjust the capture rate to the shortest allowable (usually 2–6 seconds).
  - Confirm that there is sufficient memory to capture the data for the planned period.
  - If needed, turn the low alarm off and begin trend monitoring.
- Instruct and prepare the patient (remove artificial fingernails and nail polish).
- Attach the sensors and begin recording.
- Return in the morning to gather the data.

If overnight oximetry is conducted in the home:

- Provide simple step-by-step written instructions for the patient and family.
- Demonstrate proper setup and operation of the equipment on the patient.
- Require a return demonstration to verify its proper use.
- Provide a phone number where the patient can get help.

Upon completion of the procedure, you transfer the data to a computer for storage and analysis using the applicable data acquisition software.

Figure 2-8 provides a 5-hour segment of a typical overnight oximetry trend graph for a patient being assessed for SAHS. The graph includes both the Spo_2 and the pulse rate, as well as marks indicating potential periods of motion artifact (to help eliminate false-positive results). This graph shows several major desaturation periods, visible as "valleys" in the Spo_2 trend, associated with increases in heart rate. *A desaturation event occurs when the Spo_2 drops by 4% or more.* The average number of desaturation events per hour of sleep is the oxygen desaturation index (ODI). Oximetry software typically reports the total number of desaturation events and the ODI, along with the percentage of time that the Spo_2 was below a given level, most commonly 90%.

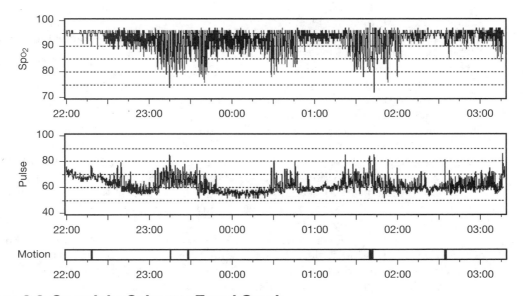

Figure 2-8 Overnight Oximetry Trend Graph.

Courtesy of: Sleep Solutions, Inc., Pasadena, Maryland.

In general, an ODI of 15 or more indicates the presence of SAHS. In these cases, a follow-up polysomnography exam is not needed to confirm the diagnosis or begin therapy, except as may be required to titrate CPAP treatment (described later in this chapter). Patients suspected of sleep-disordered breathing who exhibit fewer than 15 desaturation events per hour should undergo full polysomnography to diagnose SAHS and help determine its cause.

In COPD patients, decreases in arterial O_2 saturation may occur in the absence of apnea, hypopnea, or snoring. For this reason, the ODI is not as useful in assessing COPD patients' nocturnal desaturation. Instead, Medicare allows reimbursement for nocturnal O_2 therapy in the following circumstances:

- Nocturnal oximetry demonstrates a greater than 5% drop in Spo_2 or an Spo_2 less than 88%.
- The patient has signs or symptoms of hypoxemia (e.g., impaired cognitive process, insomnia).

These criteria are basically the same as for continuous long-term O_2 therapy (LTOT) in COPD (Sao_2 ≤ 88% or Pao_2 ≤ 55 torr on room air). When nocturnal desaturation is associated with pulmonary hypertension, daytime somnolence, or cardiac arrhythmias, continuous (as opposed to just night-time) O_2 therapy is indicated. For those patients already certified for continuous LTOT who also exhibit nocturnal desaturation, the liter flow can be titrated upward in 1 L/min increments until the nighttime Spo_2 consistently exceeds 88% and desaturation events cease.

Titration of CPAP or BiPAP During Sleep

Once a patient is diagnosed with SAHS, most physicians will order a CPAP/BiPAP titration study to assess the effectiveness of this therapy and tailor it to the patient's needs. Titration studies can be conducted via laboratory polysomnography or using an unattended auto-CPAP system.

Polysomnography Titration

Polysomnography titration of CPAP/BiPAP is indicated after a sleep study confirms the diagnosis of SAHS. Regardless of the approach taken, you should ensure that all patients undergoing CPAP/BiPAP titration should first receive appropriate instructions (with demonstration), be carefully fitted with a comfortable mask, and be given the time needed to get use to the device. Once this is accomplished, the titration procedure commences as follows:

- Start CPAP at 4 cm H_2O (use a higher pressure if the patient complains of "not getting enough air" or cannot fall asleep).
- Maintain each CPAP pressure level for an observation interval of at least 5 minutes.
- If *any* of the following events (defined in Chapter 1) occur during the interval, increase the CPAP level by at least 1 cm H_2O:
  - Two or more obstructive apneas
  - Three or more hypopneas
  - Five or more respiratory effort–related arousals (RERAs)
  - Three or more minutes of loud snoring
- Continue increasing the CPAP level until the obstructive events are abolished or controlled, or until you reach a maximum CPAP level of 20 cm H_2O.
- Quantify the control level using the respiratory disturbance index (RDI) (see Chapter 1) at the selected pressure during an observation interval of at least 15 minutes that includes a period of rapid eye movement (REM) sleep in the supine position. Control is classified as follows:
  - *Optimal*: the titrated CPAP level reduces the RDI to less than 5 and REM sleep is not continually interrupted by arousals
  - *Good*: the titrated CPAP level reduces the RDI to 10 or less (or by 50% if the baseline RDI was less than 15) and REM sleep is not continually interrupted by arousals
  - *Adequate*: at the titrated CPAP level, the RDI remains above 10 but is reduced 75% from baseline and REM sleep is not continually interrupted by spontaneous arousals
- If the patient cannot tolerate high CPAP pressures, *or* there are continued obstructive respiratory events at higher levels of CPAP (> 15 cm H_2O), *or* the patient exhibits periods of central sleep apnea during titration, consider a trial of BiPAP:

○ Start at EPAP = 4 cm H_2O and IPAP = 8 cm H_2O
○ Recommended minimum IPAP–EPAP differential = 4 cm H_2O
○ Recommended maximum IPAP–EPAP differential = 10 cm H_2O
○ Recommended maximum IPAP = 30 cm H_2O
○ Raise EPAP to abolish obstructive events
○ Raise IPAP to abolish hypopnea and snoring
○ If events persist at maximum tolerated IPAP, increase EPAP in 1 cm H_2O increments

Auto-CPAP Titration

Many modern CPAP units incorporate a mode in which pressure levels are automatically optimized to abolish or control obstructive events. Typically these units use sensors to monitor pressure, flow, and system leaks (see Chapter 4). Using these input data, a computer algorithm identifies the event and adjusts the pressure accordingly. For example, the algorithm may identify apnea as an 80% reduction in flow lasting at least 10 seconds. Based on a defined number of occurrences of this event, the device will begin a programmed step-up in CPAP pressure until the problem resolves or the preset maximum pressure is reached. **Figure 2-9** provides a trend graph of CPAP pressure and obstructive events over a 7-hour period that demonstrates how auto-CPAP functions.

6-Minute Walk Test

The 6-minute walk test (6MWT) measures the distance a patient can walk on a flat surface in 6 minutes. It evaluates how well the body responds to exertion and is used to determine overall functional capacity or changes in capacity due to therapy in patients with moderate to severe heart or lung disease. **Table 2-32** summarizes the indications for the 6MWT.

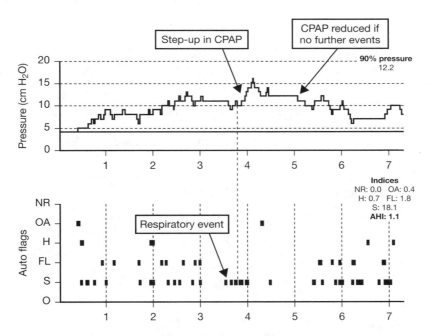

Figure 2-9 Trend Graph of Auto-CPAP (REMstar Auto). The occurrence of a respiratory event (snoring) 4 hours into sleep triggers a programmed step-up in CPAP pressure until the problem resolves, at which point the pressure is incrementally reduced if no additional events occur.

Abbreviations: NR, nonresponsive apnea/hypopnea; OA, obstructive apnea; H, hypopnea; FL, flow limitation; S, snore; AHI, apnea/hypopnea index (sum of OA + H).

Courtesy of: Philips Respironics, Murrysville, Pennsylvania.

Table 2-32 Indications for the 6-Minute Walk Test

Functional Status (Single Measurement)	Pre- and Post-treatment Comparisons
COPD	Lung transplantation
Cystic fibrosis	Lung resection
Heart failure	Lung volume reduction surgery
Peripheral vascular disease	Pulmonary rehabilitation
Fibromyalgia	COPD
Effects of aging	Pulmonary hypertension
	Heart failure

The 6MWT does not measure O_2 uptake, nor does it help identify either the cause of dyspnea or the factors limiting exercise tolerance. *If such information is needed, you should recommend a comprehensive cardiopulmonary exercise test.*

The 6MWT should *not* be performed on patients who have either had an MI or experienced unstable angina during the month prior to the test. Relative contraindications include a resting heart rate > 120 beats/min, a systolic blood pressure > 180 mm Hg, or a diastolic blood pressure > 100 mm Hg.

The American Thoracic Society has developed a standardized protocol for the 6MWT. The first consideration is the walking course itself, which must be 30 meters in length with a clearly set starting line and turnaround point, and with the distance marked in 3-meter increments. In terms of equipment, you will need a stopwatch, a movable chair, and a recording worksheet. **Figure 2-10** provides a 6MWT worksheet like that recommended by the ATS.

6-Minute Walk Test		**Walk #:**	**Date:**	
Patient Name:		**Patient ID:**		**Gender:** M F
Race/ Ethnicity:		**Height (cm):**	**Weight (kg):**	**Blood Pressure:**
Medications taken before the test (dose and time):				

Supplemental O_2 during the test?	No	Yes	Flow L/min:	Device:

Lap counter	1	2	3	4	5	6	7	8	9	10	11	12	13	14	15

	Start/baseline	**End of test**
Time		
Heart rate		
SpO_2		
Dyspnea (Borg scale)		
Fatigue (Borg scale)		

Stopped or paused before 6 minutes?	Yes	No	Reason:

Other symptoms at end of exercise:	☐ Angina ☐ Dizziness	☐ Hip or leg pain ☐ Diaphoresis	☐ Ashen appearance ☐ Other:

Number of laps:		x 60 m/lap	+ partial lap of	m	=	Total distance (6MWD)
Predicted 6MWD:	m	% Predicted (actual/predicted)		%		

Comments:
Interpretation:

Test administrator (name):	**Signature:**

Figure 2-10 American Thoracic Society Recommended Documentation Form for the 6-Minute Walk Test.

Adapted from: ATS statement: guidelines for the six-minute walk test. *Am J Respir Crit Care Med.* 2002;166:111–117.

You will also need a sphygmomanometer to measure blood pressure, as well as a visual Borg Scale to assess the patient's dyspnea and level of exertion. If used, a pulse oximeter must be lightweight and not have to be held by the patient while walking. Last, for potential emergencies, you must have immediate access to a source of oxygen, an automated electronic defibrillator (AED), and a telephone.

To prepare for the 6MWT, patients should wear comfortable clothing and walking shoes/sneakers, bring their usual walking aid (e.g., cane, walker), follow their usual medical regimen, and avoid vigorous exercise for 2 hours before testing. If a recent ECG is available, the results should be reviewed by a physician before testing. For patients with a history of stable angina on exercise, direct them to take their angina medication before the test and have rescue nitrates available. For patients on supplemental O_2, oxygen should be provided at the prescribed flow using the same portable system normally used.

The ATS-recommended 6MWT protocol is outlined in the accompanying box. You should immediately stop the test if the patient develops chest pain, severe dyspnea, leg cramps, staggering, diaphoresis, or a pale or ashen appearance. In these cases, sit the patient in a chair, retake the vital signs, administer O_2 as appropriate, and arrange for a physician assessment. Once you are sure the patient is stable, record the time stopped, distance walked, and the reason the patient could not continue.

ATS 6-Minute Walk Protocol

1. With the patient sitting at rest for at least 10 minutes, gather all needed data and measure/record vital signs.

2. Assemble all equipment (lap counter, stopwatch, colored tape, Borg Scale, recording worksheet).

3. If Sp_{O_2} is to be monitored, record the baseline value.

4. Have the patient stand and rate his or her baseline dyspnea and exertion levels using the Borg Scale.

5. Move to the starting point and set the stopwatch to zero.

6. Position the patient at the starting line and provide the requisite ATS-mandated demonstration and instructions.

7. Start the timer as soon as the patient starts to walk.

8. Remain at the starting line while you watch the patient and tally the completed "laps."

9. At the completion of each lap, make sure the patient sees you tallying the lap.

10. At the end of each minute, provide encouragement to the patient and specify the remaining time.

11. After exactly 6 minutes, firmly say "Stop," mark the stop point on the floor with tape, and have the patient sit down.

12. Repeat the Borg Scale assessment, being sure to remind the patient of the prior ratings. In addition, ask, "What, if anything, kept you from walking farther?"

13. If using a pulse oximeter, record the end-of-walk Sp_{O_2} and pulse rate.

14. Record the number of laps, additional distance covered in any partial lap, and the total distance walked (rounded to the nearest meter).

15. Congratulate the patient on a good effort.

Data from: American Thoracic Society. ATS statement: guidelines for the six-minute walk test. *Am J Respir Crit Care Med.* 2002;166: 111–117.

The outcome measure for the 6MWT is the 6-minute walking distance (6MWD). Prediction equations for the 6MWD exist, but are not very useful in assessing those with cardiopulmonary disease. In general, a 6MWD less than 500–600 meters can be used to screen for abnormal functional capacity. However, because the test is not diagnostic of any specific condition, patients who exhibit a low 6MWD should undergo further pulmonary and cardiac function testing. If you are using the 6MWT to assess treatment, you should expect at least a 10–20% *improvement* in the 6MWD to consider it effective.

Cardiopulmonary Exercise Testing

Cardiopulmonary exercise testing involves measurement of heart and lung function during progressive increases in workload, usually performed on a treadmill. The standard work unit used for exercise testing is the metabolic equivalent of task (MET): 1 MET = 3.5 mL O_2 consumption/kg of body weight, about equal to normal resting O_2 consumption per minute. MET levels are varied during exercise by altering treadmill speeds and inclinations. Most protocols increase exercise intensity by 1–2 METs at each step-up in workload.

Exercise testing is conducted under direct physician supervision in a cardiac, pulmonary, or exercise physiology lab. A fully stocked crash cart with defibrillator, O_2, suction, and airway equipment must be on hand, and all involved staff should be ACLS certified. General contraindications against exercise testing include acute MI, uncontrolled heart failure, unstable angina, significant cardiac dysrhythmias, acute pulmonary disorders, and severe hypertension.

Two types of exercise tests are commonly performed: the cardiac stress test and the comprehensive exercise capacity assessment. The classic cardiac "stress test" assesses the patient's 12-lead ECG, heart rate, and blood pressure, and is indicated for the following purposes:

- Diagnosing coronary artery disease (CAD)
- Evaluating risk and prognosis in patients with a history of CAD
- Assessing prognosis after MI
- Providing the basis for the rehabilitation prescription
- Evaluating the impact of medical treatment for heart disease

Data are continuously gathered at each increment in workload, and patient symptoms are monitored. ST-segment depression or elevation indicates myocardial ischemia and constitutes a positive test result.

The more comprehensive exercise capacity test employs a metabolic cart to measure ventilation parameters (tidal volume, respiratory rate) and gas exchange (O_2 consumption and CO_2 production) during the test protocol. This approach is used for the following purposes:

- Differentiating between cardiac and pulmonary limitations to exercise capacity
- Evaluating responses to treatments intended to increased exercise tolerance
- Determining appropriate exercise levels in rehabilitation programs
- Detecting exercise-induced bronchospasm
- Evaluating exercise capacity in heart transplant candidates
- Evaluating claimants for cardiopulmonary disability

The accompanying box outlines the elements commonly included in the comprehensive exercise capacity test procedure. In most cases, patients scheduled for an exercise test should be told to take their regular medications and avoid strenuous activity on the day of the test. In addition, you should instruct patients to avoid caffeine, smoking, or eating for at least 2 hours prior to the test and to wear loose, comfortable clothing and nonslip footwear suitable for walking, such as sneakers.

Basic Comprehensive Exercise Capacity Test Procedure (Treadmill) Procedure

1. Obtain the appropriate medical and medication history and PFT results; measure the patient's height and weight.
2. Place and secure the ECG leads, pulse oximetry probe, and sphygmomanometer cuff.
3. Obtain a baseline resting 12-lead ECG, SpO_2, and blood pressure (BP).
4. If ordered, obtain a baseline arterial blood sample (ABG/lactate level).
5. Instruct the patient in the operation of the treadmill.
6. Confirm leak-free fit of the breathing interface; have the patient breathe through system for 2–3 minutes, until stable.
7. Provide 2–3 minutes of unloaded warm-up activity (e.g., 1–2 mph, 0% grade).
8. Apply the prescribed protocol to increment the patient workload.

9. Measure BP, HR, SpO_2, Borg exertion rating, and symptoms (if any) toward end of each graded interval.

10. End the test when:

    a. VO_{2max} or maximum steady-state heart rate is achieved (stop at the end of that stage).

    b. The patient cannot continue due to exhaustion.

    c. An abnormal or hazardous response occurs.

11. If ordered, obtain an arterial sample immediately following test cessation.

12. Provide 2–3 minutes of unloaded cool-down activity (e.g., 1–2 mph, 0% grade).

13. Have the patient stop activity.

14. Continue to monitor blood pressure and heart rate until they return to baseline.

15. If assessing for exercise-induced bronchospasm, immediately obtain PFT measures.

Abnormal or hazardous responses that justify ending the test include wide swings in blood pressure; development of severe angina, dyspnea, or a serious arrhythmia; or the patient becoming dizzy, confused, or cyanotic.

Table 2-33 provides the common parameters measured during exercise capacity testing, including their typical values at peak capacity.

The primary measure used to evaluate exercise capacity is the VO_{2max}. Test results are normal if patients can attain their predicted VO_{2max} and a heat rate at or near their predicted maximum (HR_{max}) at peak exercise. Normal patients also have no difficulty increasing their ventilation in response to increased work intensity, and they can maintain normal SpO_2 levels at all levels of exercise.

In general, a patient has reduced exercise capacity if either the VO_{2max} is less than 15 mL/kg or a peak exercise level of at least 5 METs cannot be achieved. Reduced exercise capacity can be due to poor physical conditioning or the presence of a pulmonary or cardiovascular disorder. Low exercise capacity due to poor conditioning is evident when the patient has a low VO_{2max}, but a normal anaerobic threshold (> 40% of the VO_{2max}). Such patients also are prone to developing abnormally high heat rates at peak exercise capacity.

Patients whose exercise limitation is due mainly to a pulmonary disorder cannot increase their ventilation sufficiently to keep pace with increased metabolic demands. This limitation manifests itself as a reduction in breathing reserve. A normal individual has a breathing reserve of at least 30%, meaning that at peak exercise only 70% or less of the maximum voluntary ventilation (MVV) is being used, with the MVV estimated as $FEV_1 \times 40$. At peak exercise, a patient with a pulmonary disorder

Table 2-33 Measurements Made During Comprehensive Exercise Capacity Testing

Measurement	Definition	Typical Values at Peak Exercise Capacity
VO_{2max}	Maximum uptake of O_2 per minute at peak exercise capacity	Men: 35–90 mL/kg/min Women: 25–75 mL/kg/min
Anaerobic threshold	Exercise intensity beyond which progressive increases in blood lactate occur	> 40% VO_{2max}
HR_{max}	Maximum heart rate at peak exercise capacity	220 – age
Breathing reserve	Proportion of MVV that is unused after reaching maximum minute ventilation at peak exercise	> 30%
SpO_2	O_2 saturation (pulse oximetry)	> 88%
O_2 pulse	Oxygen consumption per heart beat at peak exercise capacity	Men: > 12 mL/beat Women: > 8 mL/beat
VO_2, oxygen consumption; HR, heart rate; MVV, maximum voluntary ventilation.		

may have little or no breathing reserve available. Moreover, it is not unusual for such patients to "desaturate" during exercise. A fall in SpO_2 with exercise is most common among those individuals with advanced COPD or interstitial lung disease who have marginal O_2 saturations at rest.

Patients whose exercise limitation is due mainly to a cardiovascular disorder typically have a reduced anaerobic threshold, low O_2 pulse, and higher than predicted heart rate at peak exercise capacity. The reduced O_2 pulse occurs because the diseased heart cannot increase stroke volume sufficiently to meet increased exercise demands.

If the test is being done to detect exercise-induced bronchospasm, look for at least a 20% drop in FEV_1 post exercise. If the test is being conducted to justify participation in a pulmonary rehabilitation program, the patient's Vo_{2max} should be less than 75% of predicted, with a breathing reserve of less than 30%.

Oxygen Titration with Exercise

According to the American Association for Respiratory Care (AARC), O_2 titration with exercise is indicated for the following purposes:

- Assessing the adequacy of arterial oxygenation during exercise in patients suspected of desaturation, especially those with pulmonary disease who complain of dyspnea on exertion or have a decreased $DLco$ and/or low Pao_2 at rest
- Determining the optimal amount of supplemental O_2 needed to treat desaturation previously documented to have to have occurred during exertion

Contraindications and patient preparation are basically the same as for cardiopulmonary stress testing, albeit with additional cautions against performing this test on patients with a resting SpO_2 of less than 85% on room air.

O_2 titration with exercise can be performed in PFT or exercise labs, pulmonary rehabilitation centers, clinics, and physicians' offices. Often this test is performed during exercise capacity testing and requires the same basic equipment, except for the metabolic cart. If a treadmill is not available, a step test or the 6MWT can be substituted. A cycle ergometer is not recommended for O_2 titration, because *patients' O_2 needs during exercise must be established while carrying the portable system they use or that is planned for use.* Heart rate monitoring via pulse oximeter is mandatory; ECG monitoring should be used if possible. Because pulse oximetry estimates arterial O_2 saturation, the AARC recommends that the SpO_2 be validated by arterial sampling and CO-oximetry. If a CO-oximeter is not available, measurement of the Pao_2 via standard blood gas analysis can suffice.

The basic procedure is depicted in **Figure 2-11**. After gathering relevant patient data, obtain a baseline Sao_2 on room air (or the patient's prescribed resting O_2 liter flow). If the Sao_2 is less than 85%, terminate the protocol and record the reason. For patients who continue with the test, have them begin walking and slowly increase their activity until it replicates the highest intensity they will likely perform in the home environment, usually equivalent to a 3 or 4 on the Borg rating of perceived exertion (Table 2-13). After having the patient maintain this activity level for at least 3 minutes, remeasure the Sao_2 (or SpO_2 if calibrated against the Sao_2).

If the patient's O_2 saturation at the peak activity level equals or exceeds 88%, the patient does not need any additional oxygen and the test can be terminated. If the patient's Sao_2 drops by 2% or more, or if the Sao_2 is less than 88% (Pao_2 ≤ 55 torr), increment the O_2 flow by 1 L/min (up to 6 L/min). After stabilization on the new O_2 flow for 3 minutes, reassess the Sao_2 while the patient continues to exercise. Repeat this procedure until the Sao_2 is at least 88% or the Pao_2 is greater than 55 torr. *To provide an extra margin of safety, the AARC recommends setting the target Sao_2 during titration to 93%.* The resulting liter flow should be the value prescribed by the ordering physician for use during applicable activities.

Hemodynamic Monitoring

Hemodynamic monitoring involves bedside measurements obtained from indwelling systemic arterial, central venous, or pulmonary artery catheters. These measures include both blood samples and vascular pressures and flows. **Table 2-34** outlines the key information that hemodynamic monitoring provides by sampling location.

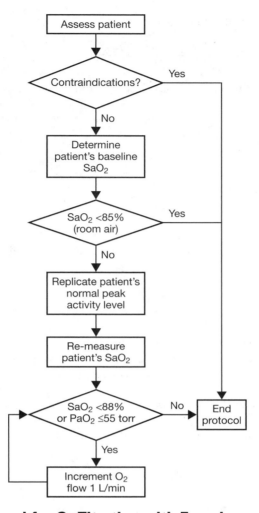

Figure 2-11 Basic Protocol for O₂ Titration with Exercise.
Courtesy of Strategic Learning Associates, LLC, Little Silver, New Jersey.

Table 2-34 Hemodynamic Monitoring Information by Sampling Location

| Location | Blood Collection | | Pressure Monitoring | |
	Sample	Reflects	Pressure(s)	Reflects
Systemic artery	Arterial blood	Pulmonary gas exchange (ABG)	Systemic arterial pressure	• LV afterload • Vascular tone • Blood volume
Central vein	Venous blood (unmixed)	Not useful for assessing gas exchange, but can be used instead of venipuncture for most lab tests	Central venous pressure (CVP)	• Fluid volume • Vascular tone • RV preload
Pulmonary artery (PA)	Mixed venous blood (balloon deflated)	Gas exchange at the tissues; can be used to compute cardiac output (Fick method)	Pulmonary artery pressure (PAP)	• RV afterload • Vascular tone • Blood volume
			Pulmonary artery wedge pressure (PAWP) (balloon inflated)	• LV preload
LV = left ventricle; RV = right ventricle.				

Performing Hemodynamic Assessments

In regard to hemodynamic monitoring procedures, the NBRC likely will focus on arterial line insertion; general aspects of indwelling catheter use, troubleshooting, and infection control; and the interpretation of the data obtained. Arterial lines insertion is covered in Chapter 11. Chapter 4 provides details on the use and troubleshooting of pressure-measuring devices. Here we focus on the specific aspects of indwelling catheter use, including troubleshooting and infection control. The following sections address interpretation of vascular pressure, blood sample, and flow data.

General considerations that apply to the proper use of indwelling catheters include the following:

- For accurate pressure measurements, you need to ensure that the transducer is at the same level as the pressure it measures; for CVP and PA pressures, this level is the patient's *phlebostatic axis* (i.e., the intersection of the fourth intercostal space with the midaxillary line).
- Both CVP and PAWP are affected by intrathoracic pressure changes during spontaneous and positive pressure breathing; to minimize this effect, make your measurements at end-expiration.
- Do not remove patients from PEEP/CPAP to measure CVP or PAWP. If PEEP is less than or equal to 10 cm H_2O, simply obtain the end-expiratory reading; if PEEP is greater than 10 cm H_2O, apply the following correction formula: corrected pressure = measured pressure – [0.5 × (PEEP/1.36)].
- To obtain a valid blood sample from an indwelling catheter, you first need to remove fluid from the "deadspace" of the system (i.e., by using a separate syringe or closed reservoir to aspirate the flush solution until whole blood appears); only then do you obtain the blood sample.
- When sampling mixed venous blood from a PA catheter, you must be sure the balloon is deflated and the sample withdrawn slowly (otherwise you may get arterialized blood).
- To avoid clot formation, after obtaining the blood sample, briefly flush the system.

Unfortunately, indwelling catheters are a common cause of bloodstream infections. See Chapter 5 for details on methods for avoiding bloodstream infections associated with indwelling vascular lines.

Interpreting Hemodynamic Pressures

The NBRC expects you to know the common reference ranges of vascular pressures and the causes of abnormal values, as outlined in **Table 2-35**. In general, pressures rise above normal due to increased cardiac activity (increased contractility and/or rate), hypervolemia, distal vasoconstriction, or flow obstruction. Pressures fall below normal due to decreased cardiac activity, hypovolemia, or distal vasodilation.

In critical care settings, vascular pressures are often measured and displayed continuously on a monitor at the bedside. **Figure 2-12** provides an example of a display of systemic arterial pressure, CVP, and the accompanying ECG, as well as an annotated single cycle depicting the key events.

Although most hemodynamic monitors compute mean vascular pressures, the NBRC often tests your ability to estimate these measures. You estimate both the systemic and pulmonary arterial mean pressures using the following formula:

Estimated mean pressure = diastolic + 1/3 (systolic – diastolic)

For example, the mean arterial pressure of a patient with a systolic value of 110 mm Hg and a diastolic value of 70 mm Hg would be calculated as follows:

Estimated mean pressure = 70 + 1/3 (110 – 70)
= 70 + 40/3 = 70 + 13.3
≈ 83 mm Hg

Table 2-35 Vascular Pressures: Reference Ranges and Causes of Abnormalities

Reference Ranges	Increased	Decreased
Systemic Arterial Pressure		
Systolic: < 120 mm Hg Diastolic: < 80 mm Hg Mean: 70–105 mm Hg	• Increased LV contractility (e.g., inotropes) • Vasoconstriction (e.g., alpha agonist) • Increased blood volume • Increased cardiac rate • Arteriosclerosis • Essential hypertension	• LV failure (e.g., MI, CHF) • Vasodilation (e.g., alpha blockers) • Hypovolemia • Decreased cardiac rate • Arrhythmias • Shock
Central Venous/Right Atrial Pressure		
2–6 mm Hg	• Increased venous return/hypervolemia • RV failure (e.g., cor pulmonale) • Tricuspid or pulmonary valve stenosis • Pulmonary hypertension • Hypoxemia (e.g., COPD) • Pulmonary embolism • Cardiac tamponade/constrictive pericarditis • Positive-pressure ventilation • Pneumothorax	• Vasodilation • Hypovolemia • Shock • Spontaneous inspiration
Pulmonary Artery Pressure		
Systolic: 15–30 mm Hg Diastolic: 8–15 mm Hg Mean: 9–18 mm Hg	• Increased RV contractility • Hypervolemia • Pulmonary hypertension • Hypoxemia (e.g., ARDS, COPD) • Pulmonary embolism • Left ventricular failure • Cardiac tamponade • Mitral stenosis • Vasoconstriction (e.g., vasopressors)	• RV failure • Vasodilation (e.g., NO, sildenafil) • Hypovolemia
Pulmonary Arterial Wedge Pressure		
6–12 mm Hg	• LV failure/cardiogenic shock • Hypervolemia • Cardiac tamponade/constrictive pericarditis • Mitral stenosis • Positive-pressure ventilation/PEEP • Pneumothorax	• Shock other than cardiogenic • Hypovolemia • Spontaneous inspiration

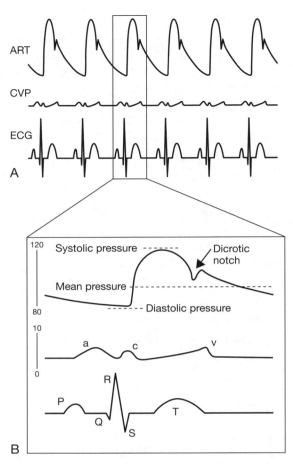

Figure 2-12 Monitor Display of Vascular Pressures and ECG. From top to bottom, view A displays the systemic arterial pressure (ART), CVP, and ECG at a normal sweep speed. View B extracts a single cycle run at a higher sweep speed. Note first the rapid rise in arterial pressure due to ventricular contraction, which immediately follows the ECG QRS complex. The peak and low points of the arterial waveform correspond to the systolic and diastolic pressures, respectively, with the dicrotic notch indicating aortic valve closure. The difference between the systolic and diastolic pressures equals the pulse pressure, normally about 40 mm Hg in the systemic circulation. Critical care monitors also often display the computed average or mean arterial pressure. Due to its lower pressure, the CVP waveform is displayed on a different pressure scale. At high scan speed (view B), three distinct waves can be visualized. The "a" wave corresponds to the rise in pressure with atrial contraction, which closely follows the P wave of the ECG. The "c" wave reflects ventricular contraction and bulging of the closed tricuspid valve back into the atrium. The "v" wave corresponds to the increase in pressure occurring as the right atrium refills.

Courtesy of: Strategic Learning Associates, LLC, Little Silver, New Jersey.

Interpreting Blood Flows and Resistances

Cardiac output (CO) is the total volume flow of blood per minute through the circulation. It is the simple product of the average stroke volume (SV) times the heart rate (HR) in beats per minute:

$$\text{CO (mL/min)} = \text{SV (mL/beat)} \times \text{HR (beats/min)}$$

Table 2-36 Commonly Measured Hemodynamic Parameters

Parameter	Formula	Normal Range
Cardiac output (CO)	N/A; Fick or thermal dilution value	4–8 L/min
Cardiac index (CI)	CI = CO (L/min) ÷ BSA	2.5–4.0 L/min/m²
Stroke volume (SV)	SV = CO (mL/min) ÷ HR	60–130 mL/beat
Stroke (SI)	SI = CI ÷ HR or SV/BSA	30–50 mL/m²
Systemic vascular resistance (SVR)	SVR = [(MAP – CVP) ÷ CO] × 80*	900–1400 dynes-sec/cm⁵ (15–20 Wood units)
Pulmonary vascular resistance (PVR)	PVR = [(MPAP – PAWP) ÷ CO] × 80*	110–250 dynes-sec/cm⁵ (< 2 Wood units)

BSA, body surface area (m²); HR, heart rate (beats/min); MAP, mean arterial pressure (mm Hg); CVP, central venous pressure (mm Hg); MPAP, mean pulmonary artery pressure (mm Hg); PAWP, pulmonary artery wedge pressure (mm Hg).
* The units used to measure vascular resistance (dynes-sec/cm⁵) are cgs units. The factor of 80 converts the traditional "Wood" units (mm Hg/L/min) to the corresponding cgs units.

Direct monitoring of stroke volume at the bedside is difficult. Instead, to measure CO at the bedside, we use flow data obtained via a PA catheter. Although the Fick method can be used, it has been replaced by the thermal dilution technique. Thermal dilution determines CO by measuring blood temperature changes occurring between two points on the PA catheter. The traditional method involves injecting a cool saline solution into the right atrial port of the catheter. A newer method that can provide continuously updated measurements without injections uses a catheter that heats the blood via a thermal filament. In either case, a computer measures the rate of temperature change, from which it calculates the CO.

Using one of these methods, measured adult CO typically varies between 4 and 8 L/min. This wide range is due to the fact that CO depends on body size—in particular, body surface area (BSA). For this reason, interpretation of CO must be adjusted for body surface area. We call this measure the cardiac index (CI) and compute it as follows:

$$CI = \frac{CO}{BSA}$$

where CI is the cardiac index in L/min/m² and BSA is the body surface area as estimated using the Dubois nomogram or its prediction equation.

Knowledge of CO, heart rate, CVP, mean arterial and pulmonary arterial pressures, and PAWP allows computation of several other hemodynamic parameters, as defined in **Table 2-36**.

The NBRC expects that you know the normal ranges for adult CO, CI, and SV and be able to compute a patient's CI and SV (given the requisite data). In addition, you should be able to interpret all the values in Table 2-36. See the accompanying box for a simple example.

Simple Hemodynamic Computations and Interpretation

Problem

Given a patient with a cardiac output of 4.0 L/min, heart rate of 100/min, and a body surface area of 2.0 m², compute his stroke volume and cardiac index.

Solution

Stroke volume

SV (mL) = CO (mL/min) ÷ HR
SV = 4000 ÷ 100 = 40 mL

Cardiac index

$$CI \ (L/min/m^2) = CO \div BSA$$
$$CI = 4.0 \div 2 = 2.0 \ L/min/m^2$$

Interpretation

The patient's stroke volume and cardiac index are both below normal. Decreased stroke volume is associated with decreased cardiac contractility (e.g., an MI) or increased afterload (e.g., vasoconstriction).

To interpret vascular resistance measures, you need to understand the concept involved. As with resistance to gas flow through a tube, vascular resistance represents a change in pressure per unit flow:

$$R = \frac{\Delta P}{\dot{V}}$$

where R is resistance, ΔP is the pressure difference across the tube, and $\dot{V}$ is the flow. In terms of vascular resistance, the "tubes" are the systemic and pulmonary circulations. In both circulations, the flow equals the cardiac output. For the systemic circulation, the pressure difference is that between the start (mean arterial pressure) and the end (CVP) of the system. Likewise, ΔP across the pulmonary circulation equals the starting mean PA pressure minus the ending left ventricular end-diastolic pressure (LVEDP), which is equivalent to the PAWP.

The causes of increased vascular resistance are complex. With the exception of those conditions causing hypervolemia or affecting cardiac contractility, essentially all the factors specified in Table 2-35 as increasing pressures in the systemic and pulmonary circulations are caused by increased vascular resistance—for example, hypertension (systemic or pulmonary), arteriosclerosis, hypoxemia (pulmonary circulation only), and vasopressor drugs. In addition, one of the body's responses to cardiogenic and hypovolemic shock (which both *decrease* systemic and pulmonary vascular pressures) is to increase vascular resistance by vasoconstriction.

Interpreting Blood Sample Data

In terms of obtaining blood for analysis, samples collected from an arterial line provides standard ABG data. *The blood obtained from the distal port of a PA catheter is mixed venous blood,* useful in assessing tissue oxygenation. When obtained concurrently, arterial and mixed venous samples can be used to compute cardiac output and physiologic shunt.

To assess tissue oxygenation, we need to know *how much oxygen is left over after the blood leaves the capillaries.* We call this measure the *mixed venous oxygen content,* or $C\bar{v}O_2$. With a normal Hb, PaO_2, and cardiac output, the $C\bar{v}O_2$ ranges between 14 and 16 mL/dL, equivalent to a $S\bar{v}O_2$ between 68% and 77% at a $P\bar{v}O_2$ of 38–42 torr.

The NBRC will often assess your understanding of mixed venous oxygen content as related to both tissue oxygen delivery *and* demand. Oxygen delivery is the product of arterial oxygen content times cardiac output ($CaO_2 \times CO$). For the body as a whole, O_2 demands equal O_2 consumption, or $\dot{V}O_2$. The relationship between O_2 delivery and demand is best understood using the following version of the Fick equation for cardiac output:

$$C\bar{v}O_2 = CaO_2 - \frac{\dot{V}O_2}{CO \times 10}$$

where $\dot{V}O_2$ equals the whole-body O_2 consumption in mL/min and CO equals the cardiac output in L/min.

Table 2-37 Conditions Associated with Changes in Mixed Venous O₂ Content (C$\bar{v}$o₂)

Low C$\bar{v}$o₂	
Decreased Oxygen Delivery[a]	**Increased Oxygen Demand**[a]
↓ Hb (e.g., anemia, hemorrhage)	Hyperthermia
↓ Pao₂, Sao₂ (e.g., hypoxemia, suctioning)	Trauma/burns
↓ CO (e.g., hypovolemia, shock, arrhythmias)	Shivering
	Seizures
High C$\bar{v}$o₂	
Increased Oxygen Delivery	**Decreased Oxygen Demand**
↑ CO	Hypothermia
Hyperoxemia (e.g., ↑ Fio₂, polycythemia)	Anesthesia
	Pharmacologic paralysis
	Cyanide poisoning[b]
	Sepsis[b]

[a] Oxygen delivery = CO × Cao₂; oxygen demand = whole-body $\dot{V}$o₂.
[b] In both cyanide poisoning and sepsis, C$\bar{v}$o₂ can be higher than normal, even if tissue hypoxia is present. For this reason, in patients with pathologic conditions that decrease O₂ demand, mixed venous lactate may be a better indicator of tissue oxygenation.

According to this formula, C$\bar{v}$o₂ will rise if either of the factors responsible for O₂ delivery increases—that is, with an increase in either arterial O₂ content or cardiac output. C$\bar{v}$o₂ also will rise if O₂ consumption decreases (all else being equal). In contrast, C$\bar{v}$o₂ will fall if either arterial O₂ content or cardiac output decreases or if O₂ consumption increases. **Table 2-37** demonstrates these relationships and summarizes the common clinical conditions associated with changes in C$\bar{v}$o₂.

In general, with a normal Hb level, *if the S$\bar{v}$o₂ is less than 50% or the P$\bar{v}$o₂ is less than 27 torr, the patient has impaired tissue oxygenation.* An S$\bar{v}$o₂ less than 30% (corresponding to a P$\bar{v}$o₂ of approximately 20 torr) can lead to unconsciousness and permanent organ damage.

Instead of using the C$\bar{v}$o₂ alone, many clinicians prefer to use the difference between the arterial and mixed venous oxygen content to assess tissue oxygenation. Normally, the C(a–$\bar{v}$)o₂ is less than 7.0 mL/dL. According to the Fick equation, C(a-$\bar{v}$)o₂ will increase if oxygen consumption increases or cardiac output decreases. In contrast, C(a-$\bar{v}$)o₂ decreases when oxygen consumption falls or cardiac output increases.

Concurrently obtained arterial and mixed venous samples also can be used to measure the physiologic shunt in the pulmonary circulation. Shunting occurs when venous blood bypasses ventilated alveoli and returns unchanged into the left (arterial) side of the circulation. Shunting *always* lowers Cao₂, in direct proportion to the amount of blood flow bypassing ventilated alveoli. Due to design "flaws" in the pulmonary and cardiac circulations, a small anatomic shunt (3–5%) is normal. Shunting above this level is abnormal.

The true physiologic shunt in the lungs is computed using the following equation:

$$\% \, shunt = \frac{Cc'o_2 - Cao_2}{Cc'o_2 - C\bar{v}o_2}$$

where Cc'o₂ equals the "ideal" pulmonary end-capillary oxygen content. To compute Cc'o₂, you must substitute the alveolar Po₂ (Pao₂) into the formula for calculating total O₂ content.

Fortunately, the NBRC is not likely to ask you to compute the true percent shunt. Instead, you will be expected to *estimate* the percent shunt based on the alveolar–arterial oxygen tension gradient, or P(A-a)O$_2$. Assuming a normal C(a-$\bar{\text{v}}$)O$_2$, one can estimate the percent shunt of a patient breathing 100% oxygen as follows:

$$\% \, shunt = \frac{\text{P(A}-\text{a})\text{o}_2 \times 0.003}{[\text{P(A}-\text{a})\text{o}_2 \times 0.003 + 5]}$$

where P(A-a)O$_2$ is the alveolar–arterial oxygen tension gradient and 5 is the normal C(a-$\bar{\text{v}}$)O$_2$ in mL/dL. Rather than perform this computation, you instead can apply the rule of thumb provided in the accompanying box.

Estimating the Percent Shunt [assumes Pao$_2$ > 100 torr and C(a-$\bar{\text{v}}$)o$_2$ = 5]

Rule of Thumb: Breathing 100% oxygen, every 100 torr P(A-a)o$_2$ equals about a 5% shunt.

Example: A patient breathing 100% O$_2$ has a P(A-a)o$_2$ of 300 torr. What is her approximate percent shunt?

Solution: 300/100 = 3

Approximate % shunt = 3 × 5 = 15%

Putting It All Together

In terms of basic hemodynamics, the NBRC often will ask a question or two that require you to integrate your knowledge of pressure, flow, and resistance parameters as related to common clinical conditions. **Table 2-38** outlines the typical hemodynamic changes you will see in selected critically ill patients. The accompanying box provides an example interpretation.

Table 2-38 Hemodynamic Changes in Common Clinical Conditions

Condition	SAP	CVP	CO	PAP	PAWP	PVR	SVR
Dehydration/hypovolemic shock	↓	↓	↓	↓	↓	↑	↑
LV failure/cardiogenic shock	↓	↑	↓	↑	↑	↑	↑
Septic shock	↓	↓	↑ (early)	↓	↓	↓	↓
Neurogenic shock	↓	↓	↓	↓	↓	↓	↓
Pulmonary hypertension	N	↑	N or ↓	↑	N	↑	N
Pulmonary embolism	↓	↑	↓	↑	N or ↓	↑	↑

N, normal; ↑, increased; ↓, decreased; SAP, systemic arterial pressure; CVP, central venous pressure; CO, cardiac output; PAP, pulmonary artery pressure; PAWP, pulmonary artery wedge pressure; PVR, pulmonary vascular resistance; SVR, systemic vascular resistance.

Example of a Hemodynamic Interpretation

Problem

Measurements taken via a pulmonary artery catheter on a patient with a decreased cardiac output and low arterial blood pressure indicate the following:

- Increased CVP
- Increased PAP
- Increased PAWP

Interpretation

The increased CVP and PAP could be due to LV failure/cardiogenic shock, pulmonary hypertension, or pulmonary embolism. However, the elevated PAWP is most consistent with LV failure/cardiogenic shock.

COMMON ERRORS TO AVOID

You can improve your score by avoiding these mistakes:

- Don't assume that all that wheezes is asthma; patients with congestive heart failure may also exhibit wheezing due to peribronchial edema.
- Don't assume that a lack of central cyanosis means satisfactory oxygenation; a patient with anemia can be severely hypoxemic without cyanosis.
- Never delay needed interventions for a newborn to assess Apgar scores.
- Do not use a numeric pain scale with young children or patients who are unable to express themselves.
- Do not attempt patient education until all major barriers to learning have been resolved.
- Do not use mechanical (vane-type) respirometers to measure forced vital capacity.
- Do not use peak expiratory flows alone to categorize a patient's pulmonary impairment.
- Never accept bedside spirometry results until you have three acceptable maneuvers.
- Do not recommend or use apnea monitoring to assess patients for obstructive apnea.
- Do not recommend or use the 6MWT to identify the *cause* of a patient's dyspnea or exercise intolerance.
- Avoid cardiopulmonary exercise testing in patients with uncontrolled heart failure or unstable angina.
- Do not use a cycle ergometer when titrating a patient's supplemental O_2 needs.
- Do not remove patients from PEEP/CPAP to measure CVP or PAWP.

SURE BETS

In some situations, you can always be sure of the right approach to a clinical problem or scenario:

- Always consider peripheral cyanosis, coolness of the extremities, and slow capillary refills as signs of circulatory failure.
- Always consider recommending airway clearance for patients whose sputum production exceeds 30 mL/day.
- Always think pulmonary edema when a patient has pink, frothy secretions.
- Always remember that the trachea and PMI shift *toward* areas of atelectasis and *away* from space-occupying lesions such as pneumothoraces and pleural effusions.
- If you detect crepitus, always consider the possibility of pneumothorax and warn the attending doctor.
- When you detect a pulse deficit, you can be sure there is a cardiac arrhythmia, such as atrial fibrillation.
- Recognize that only alert patients can cooperate and fully participate in their own care.
- Always consider a patient to be comatose if the Glasgow Coma Scale score is less than 8.
- Tachypnea, thoracic–abdominal dyssynchrony, and the use of accessory muscles always indicate increased work of breathing.
- Whenever in doubt regarding DNR status, always initiate emergency life support when needed.
- When reading an x-ray, always verify patient identification and film orientation.
- Always consider foreign body aspiration a possibility in children presenting with airway obstruction (and as justification for both chest and lateral neck x-rays).
- High breathing rates and low tidal volumes always increase deadspace ventilation per minute.
- To consider a change in an expiratory flow parameter to be clinically significant, expect at least a 12–15% improvement from baseline.
- The primary indicator of an abnormal cardiopulmonary exercise test is a low Vo_{2max}.
- For accurate vascular pressure measurements, ensure that the transducer is at the same level as the pressure it measures, typically the patient's phlebostatic axis.

PRE-TEST ANSWERS AND EXPLANATIONS

Following are this chapter's pre-test answers and explanations. Be sure to review each answer's explanation thoroughly to help you understand why it is correct. If the explanation is still unclear to you, review the chapter content.

2-1. **Correct answer: A.** Cor pulmonale. Cor pulmonale is right heart failure due to lung disease. Right heart failure occurs when chronic hypoxemia causes pulmonary vasoconstriction, which puts a strain on the right ventricle. Right heart failure also causes blood to back up in the venous system, including the neck veins.

2-2. **Correct answer: B.** Left upper lobe collapse. Volume loss in the upper lobe will pull the trachea *toward* the collapsed lung. In this case the trachea has shifted to the left, indicating that either volume loss has occurred on the left or a space-occupying lesion (tension pneumothorax, effusion, tumor) on the right is pushing the trachea to the left.

2-3. **Correct answer D.** Pneumothorax. A patient with a dull percussion note and bronchial breath sounds most likely has pulmonary infiltrates, atelectasis, or consolidation of the affected area. A pneumothorax normally results in a hyperresonant note.

2-4. **Correct answer: C.** Pneumonia. Bronchial breath sounds normally are heard only over the trachea. When heard over the lung periphery, consolidation (due to pneumonia) is present. Tissue consolidation enhances transmission of the turbulent flow sounds in the larger airways to the chest surface.

2-5. **Correct answer: A.** Left-sided pneumothorax. An acutely ill patient with dyspnea, hypotension, unilateral findings of reduced chest expansion, a hyperresonant percussion note, absence of breath sounds and tactile fremitus, and a tracheal shift most likely has a large pneumothorax on the affected side. If the pneumothorax is severe enough to disrupt cardiac function, blood pressure will also fall.

2-6. **Correct answer: B.** Severe hypoxemia. An abnormal sensorium (e.g., confusion or stupor) is often caused by inadequate cerebral oxygenation. In fact, whenever a critically ill patient exhibits this finding, assume that it is due to hypoxemia until proven otherwise.

2-7. **Correct answer: C.** Use a numeric pain scale. A numeric pain scale is *not* useful for young children or patients who cannot express themselves. To assess a young child's pain, get input from a family member. Without such information, you may have to rely on observing behaviors indicating pain, such as moaning, crying, or grimacing.

2-8. **Correct answer: B.** Orthopnea. Orthopnea is present when a patient has difficulty breathing when lying down. Most often this is due to either congestive heart failure or abdominal factors impairing diaphragm movement. Most patients learn that elevating the head with pillows can help alleviate orthopnea.

2-9. **Correct answer: B.** Chronic bronchitis. Chronic bronchitis is defined primarily by its symptoms: chronic cough and sputum production.

2-10. **Correct answer: A.** Recent weight gain. Any patient who (1) is significantly underweight, (2) has recently exhibited significant weight loss, (3) has poor dietary habits or inadequate food intake, or (4) is impoverished, isolated, or unable to prepare his or her own food is at high risk for malnutrition. Weight gain is not normally associated with malnutrition.

2-11. **Correct answer: D.** Occupational history. Of the items listed, occupational history is most important in the diagnosis of lung disease. Many lung diseases are associated with inhalation of dust or toxic chemicals in the work setting.

2-12. **Correct answer: B.** Immediately call a code and begin resuscitation efforts. If there is any doubt regarding a DNR order, start resuscitation. Formal or informal directives such as "slow code" or "code gray" bypass the patient's rights and generally are inappropriate.

2-13. **Correct answer: C.** Have her "teach" the information back to you. Teach-back is the best way to determine whether a patient has learned information. A return demonstration is appropriate for procedural skills, whereas discussion is the best method for assessing attitudinal change.

2-14. **Correct answer: C.** Right phrenic nerve paralysis. An elevated hemidiaphragm indicates either phrenic nerve paralysis on the affected side or hepatomegaly (generally right side only). Pleural effusions blunt the costophrenic angles, whereas hyperinflation tends to flatten the affected hemidiaphragm(s), as does tension pneumothorax.

2-15. **Correct answer: A.** Croup. Croup is the most likely problem. On an AP x-ray, croup is characterized by the "steeple sign"—that is, a narrowed and tapering airway below the larynx due to subglottic edema. Typically, the lateral neck x-ray in these patients is normal.

2-16. **Correct answer: D.** Bundle branch block. QRS complexes appear wider than normal (more than 0.12 second) in PVCs, bundle branch block, ventricular fibrillation, and hyperkalemia.

2-17. **Correct answer: B.** 8.00 L/min. Alveolar minute ventilation is $\dot{V}_E = f \times (V_T - V_D)$. In this case the deadspace is estimated at 1 mL/lb predicted body weight, or 150 mL. Substituting the patient's values in the equation, alveolar minute ventilation = $20 \times (550 - 150) = 8000$ mL/min, or 8.00 L/min.

2-18. **Correct answer: B.** The patient cannot sustain prolonged spontaneous ventilation. This patient has a tidal volume of 250 mL (8750 mL ÷ 35 breaths/min = 250 mL/breath) and a rapid shallow breathing index (RSBI) of 140 (35 ÷ 0.25 = 140). When the RSBI exceeds 105 early in a spontaneous breathing trial, the attempt is likely to fail.

2-19. **Correct answer: A**. Anterior–posterior (AP) view, improperly rotated. In the AP view, the medial borders of scapula are seen in the upper lung fields, ribs appear more horizontal, and the heart is more magnified. With proper alignment, the thoracic spine lines up with center of the sternum and is positioned equally between the medial ends of each clavicle.

2-20. **Correct answer: C.** A restrictive disorder. A patient with a decreased FVC, normal FEV_1, and increased $FEV_1\%$ is exhibiting the classic pattern of a restrictive pulmonary disorder—decreased volumes and normal (or increased) flows.

2-21. **Correct answer: C.** 3300 mL. The functional residual capacity (FRC) equals the sum of the residual volume and the expiratory reserve volume (FRC = RV + ERV). Rearranging this equation (to solve for RV) yields RV = FRC − ERV. In this case, RV = 4500 − 1200, or 3300 mL.

2-22. **Correct answer: C**. 2 and 3. In adults with a diagnosis of asthma who are complying with treatment, high NO values (> 35 ppb) indicate the need for higher steroid dosing or the addition of a beta agonist. If compliance cannot be confirmed, the problem likely is related to poor disease management or poor inhaler technique.

2-23. **Correct answer: A.** Hypoxemia. A decreased respiratory rate in combination with an increased heart rate in a neonate most likely indicates hypoxemia, which should be confirmed by pulse oximetry or an ABG.

2-24. **Correct answer: C.** 4% or more. Most sleep disorder specialists agree that a desaturation event represents a decrease in saturation of 4% or more. The total number of these desaturation events per hour is the oxygen desaturation index (ODI).

2-25. **Correct answer: B.** Patient B. When using the 6MWT to assess medical or surgical interventions, you should expect at least a 10–20% improvement in the 6MWD to consider the treatment effective. Only patient B has more than a 10% improvement in this measure [(200 − 150)/150 = 33% improvement].

2-26. **Correct answer: B.** Somewhat strong exertion (rating of 4). For O_2 titration during exercise, you have the patient initiate walking and slowly increase activity until it replicates the highest intensity likely achieved in the home environment, usually equivalent to a 3 to 4 on the Borg rating of perceived exertion.

2-27. **Correct answer: C.** Pulmonary artery. To assess gas exchange at the tissues, you need to assess blood *after it leaves the tissues*. For the body as a whole, you need *mixed venous blood*, which can be obtained only from the distal port of a pulmonary artery catheter.

2-28. **Correct answer: A.** Hypovolemia. A pulmonary artery wedge pressure (PAWP) of 20 mm Hg is higher than the normal pressure of 6–12 mm Hg. All of the causes listed except hypovolemia can increase PAWP. Hypovolemia tends to lower *all* vascular pressures.

2-29. **Correct answer: D.** Patient D. All patients with poor exercise capacity have a reduced Vo_{2max}. In addition, patients with a pulmonary limitation to exercise tend to have a normal anaerobic threshold (if it can be reached) but a decreased breathing reserve. Patients with a cardiovascular limitation to exercise typically have a reduced anaerobic threshold but normal breathing reserve. In the presence of a low Vo_{2max}, poor effort is revealed by a normal anaerobic threshold and breathing reserve.

2-30. **Correct answer: B.** Increase CPAP to 10 cm H_2O for 5 minutes and continue observation. You should increase the CPAP level by at least 1 cm H_2O during a titration observation interval (up to the maximum pressure, typically 20 cm H_2O) if any of the following events occur: 2 or more obstructive apneas, 3 or more hypopneas, 5 or more RERAs, 3 or more minutes of loud snoring.

POST-TEST

To confirm your mastery of this chapter's topical content, you should take the chapter post-test, available online at http://go.jblearning.com/respexamreview. A score of 80% or more indicates that you are adequately prepared for this section of the NBRC written exams. If you score less than 80%, you should continue to review the applicable chapter content. In addition, you may want to access and review the relevant Web links covering this chapter's content (courtesy of RTBoardReview. com), also online at the Jones & Bartlett Learning site.

CHAPTER 3

Recommend Procedures to Obtain Additional Data

Craig L. Scanlan

Other than providing therapy, your role as a respiratory therapist often will involve making recommendations to others to improve patient care. Making recommendations related to enhancing *therapeutic* outcomes is covered in Chapter 13. However, the NBRC also assesses your ability to recommend needed *diagnostic procedures* for your patients.

OBJECTIVES

In preparing for the shared NBRC exam content, you should demonstrate the knowledge needed to recommend:

1. Radiographic and other imaging studies
2. Diagnostic bronchoscopy
3. Sputum Gram stain, culture, and sensitivities
4. Bronchoalveolar lavage
5. Pulmonary function testing
6. Lung mechanics
7. Blood gas analysis, pulse oximetry, and transcutaneous monitoring
8. Capnography
9. Electrocardiogram
10. Hemodynamic monitoring
11. Sleep studies

In preparing for the RRT-specific NBRC exam content, you should demonstrate the knowledge needed to recommend:

12. Blood tests
13. Insertion of monitoring catheters
14. Thoracentesis

WHAT TO EXPECT ON THIS CATEGORY OF THE NBRC EXAMS

CRT exam: 4 questions; about 25% recall, 75% application
WRRT exam: 5 questions; about 20% recall, 20% application, and 60% analysis
CSE exam: indeterminate number of questions; however, exam I-C knowledge is a prerequisite to success on CSE Information Gathering sections

PRE-TEST

Carefully respond to each of the following questions. After completing the pre-test, compare your answers to those provided at the end of this chapter. Then thoroughly review each answer's explanation to help understand why it is correct.

3-1. A patient admitted to the emergency department is suspected of having suffered pulmonary injury due to inhalation of toxic fumes. To determine the location and extent of potential injury, you would recommend which of the following procedures?
  A. V/Q scan
  B. Chest x-ray
  C. Blood gas analysis
  D. Fiberoptic bronchoscopy

3-2. Your patient in the ICU is suspected of having developed a bacterial ventilator-associated pneumonia. Which of the following procedures would you recommend as best able to diagnose the cause of this problem?
  A. Sputum culture and sensitivity
  B. Chest x-ray
  C. Bronchoalveolar lavage
  D. CT scan

3-3. To estimate the metabolic rate of a patient receiving mechanical ventilation, which of the following would you recommend?
  A. Hemoximetry
  B. ABG analysis
  C. Capnography
  D. Maximum voluntary ventilation

3-4. To evaluate and follow the course of a patient with interstitial lung disease, which of the following pulmonary function testing procedures would you recommend?
  A. Diffusing capacity (DLco)
  B. He dilution FRC and TLC
  C. Forced expiratory volumes/flows
  D. Methacholine challenge test

3-5. Which of the following tests of lung mechanics would you recommend to detect the presence of auto-PEEP on a patient receiving ventilatory support?
  A. Pressure–volume loop
  B. Flow–volume loop
  C. Static compliance (inspiratory hold)
  D. Airway resistance (inspiratory hold)

3-6. The wife of a patient receiving postoperative incentive spirometry asks if this therapy will help get rid of his snoring, daytime sleepiness, and morning headaches. In communicating this information to the patient's surgeon, you would recommend which of the following diagnostic procedures?
  A. Lateral neck x-ray
  B. Arterial blood gas
  C. Polysomnography
  D. Diffusing capacity

3-7. To continuously monitor the adequacy of ventilation of a patient in the ICU being supported by mask BiPAP, you would recommend which of the following?
  A. Transcutaneous P_{CO_2}
  B. Pulse oximetry
  C. ABG analysis
  D. Capnography

3-8. As you are fitting him with a nonrebreathing mask, a 62-year-old patient in the emergency department complains of severe, crushing chest pain. Which of following tests would you recommend for this patient?
  1. Electrocardiogram (ECG)
  2. Ventilation–perfusion (V/Q) scan
  3. Cardiac biomarkers (e.g., troponin, CK)
  4. Bedside spirometry

  A. 1 and 3
  B. 1 and 2
  C. 2 and 3
  D. 1, 2, 3, and 4

3-9. To assess tissue oxygenation in a patient with ARDS, you would recommend which of the following?
  A. A CVP line
  B. A pulmonary artery catheter
  C. An arterial line
  D. Pulse oximetry

3-10. Which of the following would you recommend as the best method for diagnosing a patient suspected of having a pulmonary embolism?
 A. Prothrombin time
 B. CT angiography
 C. AP chest radiograph
 D. Capnography

3-11. A patient with tachycardia and tachypnea exhibits confusion and disorientation with evidence of tissue hypoxia but has a normal PaO_2 and SpO_2 breathing room air. Which of the following tests would you recommend to further assess this patient?
 1. Hemoglobin concentration
 2. Hematocrit level
 3. HbCO level

A. 3 only
B. 1 and 2
C. 2 and 3
D. 1, 2, and 3

3-12. A patient in respiratory distress has an upright AP chest x-ray in which the left costophrenic angle, left hemidiaphragm, and most of the lower third of the left lung field are obscured by a uniformly white area of increased density. Which of the following would you recommend at this time?
 A. Postural drainage and percussion
 B. A CPAP recruitment maneuver
 C. Intubation and mechanical ventilation
 D. A therapeutic thoracentesis

WHAT YOU NEED TO KNOW: ESSENTIAL CONTENT

Radiographic and Other Imaging Studies

Imaging studies that you may be expected to recommend include chest and lateral neck x-rays; computed tomography (CT), magnetic resonance imaging (MRI) and positron emission tomography (PET) scans; pulmonary angiography; ultrasound imaging; and V/Q scans. **Table 3-1** outlines the primary reasons for recommending these imaging studies for your patients.

Diagnostic Bronchoscopy

You should recommend diagnostic bronchoscopy in the following circumstances:

- Assessing lesions of unknown etiology that appear on a chest x-ray
- Evaluating recurrent atelectasis or pulmonary infiltrates
- Assessing the patency of the upper airway
- Investigating the source of hemoptysis
- Evaluating unexplained cough, localized wheeze, or stridor
- Following up on suspicious or positive sputum cytology results
- Obtaining lower respiratory tract secretions, cell washings, or biopsies for cytologic or microbiologic assessment
- Determining the location and extent of injury from toxic inhalation or aspiration
- Evaluating problems associated with artificial airways—for example, tube placement or tracheal damage
- Facilitating endotracheal tube insertion during difficult intubations
- Locating and clearing mucus plugs causing lobar or segmental atelectasis
- Removing abnormal endobronchial tissue or foreign bodies

According to the AARC, you should recommend *against* performing diagnostic bronchoscopy in patients who meet the following criteria:

- Cannot be adequately oxygenated during the procedure
- Have a bleeding disorder that cannot be corrected
- Have severe obstructive airway disease
- Are hemodynamically unstable

Table 3-1 Recommending Imaging Studies

Recommend to	Comments
Chest X-ray	
• Evaluate signs and symptoms of respiratory and cardiovascular disorders • Follow known chest disease processes to assess progression or improvement • Monitor patients receiving ventilatory support • Monitor patients after thoracic surgery • Assess surgical risk in patients with cardiac or respiratory symptoms • Confirm proper placement of ET tubes, CVP and PA catheters, and nasogastric (NG) and chest tubes • Comply with government requirements for chest radiography, as in occupational lung disease	Although performing a chest x-ray after thoracentesis is common practice, the American College of Radiology recommends it only if pneumothorax is suspected (e.g., if air rather than fluid is aspirated).
Neck X-ray	
• Help diagnose causes of stridor and respiratory distress • Detect the presence of aspirated foreign bodies • Detect retropharyngeal abscesses and hematomas	AP versus lateral neck films are taken to differentiate croup from epiglottitis; however, the classic AP-view "steeple sign" described for croup is not specific to that disorder and can be absent.
Thoracic CT	
• Evaluate abnormalities identified by chest x-ray (e.g., interstitial lung disease and pulmonary nodules) • Stage lung cancer • Detect tumor metastases to the lung • Detect mediastinal masses/nodes • Detect pulmonary embolism (CT angiography) • Detect and evaluate aortic aneurysm • Assess trauma to thoracic organs and structures	Patient cooperation is essential because the patient must remain motionless. Helical CT angiography is replacing V/Q scans as a test for pulmonary embolism.
Thoracic MRI	
• Evaluate the heart, major vessels, and lungs for pathology • Assess the chest wall and surrounding soft tissues for abnormalities • Evaluate posterior mediastinal masses • Detect and evaluate aortic aneurysm • Detect/assess mediastinal, vascular, and chest-wall metastasis of lung cancer • Stage lung cancer in patients who are allergic to radiographic contrast media	Patients must remain motionless. Thoracic MRI is contraindicated for patients with pacemakers, metallic surgical clips or heart valves, or infusion or chemotherapy pumps. Ventilatory support must be provided by a manual all plastic resuscitator or via a ventilator certified for MRI use. MRI is less accurate than CT for assessing lung parenchymal disease.
PET Scan	
• Differentiate malignant versus benign masses • Assess tumor metastases/response to therapy • Determine tumor biopsy site(s) • Detect and localize impaired blood flow to the myocardium	Often combined with CT scanning to enhance diagnostic accuracy. Most common use in pulmonary medicine is to diagnose, stage, and evaluate treatment of non–small-cell lung cancer.

Table 3-1 Recommending Imaging Studies (*continued*)

Recommend to	Comments
Pulmonary Angiography	
• Evaluate the pulmonary arteries for pulmonary embolism, stenosis, AV malformation, or aneurysm	Contraindicated in patients with bleeding abnormalities, extremely high blood pressure, or shock. *Being replaced by CT angiography.*
V/Q Scan	
• Detect and quantify the effects of a pulmonary embolism • Assess regional pulmonary blood flow in patients undergoing lung resection surgery	Patients must be able to cooperate during the test (breathe through a mouthpiece, hold breath for 10 seconds or more, and remain still during procedure).
Transthoracic Ultrasound	
• Detect free fluid in the thorax (e.g., pleural or pericardial effusion, hemithorax) • Detect pneumothorax • Detect mediastinal masses • Detect pulmonary atelectasis or consolidation • Assess the pleural surfaces for pleuritis or granulomatous processes • Assess thoracic wall lesions and rib masses • Assess trauma to the diaphragm, heart, and large thoracic vessels, as well as bone fractures • Guide thoracentesis and percutaneous needle biopsies	Generally ineffective in imaging tissues or organs through aerated lung tissue or pneumothorax.

Bronchoalveolar Lavage

Bronchoalveolar lavage (BAL) involves the instillation and removal of sterile normal saline solution into a lung segment via the suction channel of a fiberoptic bronchoscope. The withdrawn fluid then undergoes chemical, cytologic, and/or microbiologic assessment. According to the American Thoracic Society, BAL is indicated in patients with nonresolving pneumonias, unexplained lung infiltrates (interstitial or alveolar), or suspected alveolar hemorrhage. BAL also is a key tool for diagnosing bacterial ventilator-associated pneumonia (VAP) and can be helpful in confirming a diagnosis of various lung cancers. The only major contraindication to BAL is a predisposition for bleeding.

Sputum Gram Stain, Culture, and Sensitivity

You should recommend a sputum Gram stain and culture and sensitivity (C&S) on any patient suspected of having a respiratory tract infection and for whom focused antibiotic therapy might be needed. By identifying whether the organisms are primarily Gram positive or Gram negative, the stain can be used to guide initial antibiotic therapy. Sputum C&S determines the susceptibility of any infectious organisms present to *specific* antibiotics and, therefore, can help the doctor choose the most appropriate drug(s) for the patient. Because organism identification by culturing can require 2 days or longer, this method is being replaced by more rapid techniques such as antibody and DNA testing.

Blood Tests (RRT-Specific Content)

Blood test results can provide important information regarding a patient's status. **Table 3-2** lists some of the most common lab tests you may want to recommend based on selected patient scenarios commonly seen on the NBRC exams.

Table 3-2 Recommending Blood Tests

Patient Scenario	Recommended Test(s)
Patients with evidence of tissue hypoxia but normal Pao_2 and Spo_2	• Hemoglobin and hematocrit to determine O_2 carrying capacity • Hemoximetry to assess for actual Sao_2 and abnormal saturation (e.g., HbCO, metHb)
Postoperative patients with low-grade fever	• White blood cell count with differential to rule out possible bacterial pneumonia • Blood cultures (for sepsis)
Postoperative patients with sudden dyspnea, hemoptysis, chest pain, or tachycardia (signs of pulmonary embolism)	• D-Dimer • ischemia-modified albumin (IMA)
Patients with fluid balance disturbance	• Electrolytes to assess possible causes of fluid imbalance • Hematocrit to assess for hemodilution or concentration
Patients with decreased or absent urine output over time	• Urinalysis for specific gravity, pH • Electrolytes • BUN and creatinine to assess for possible renal disease/failure • Glomerular filtration rate (GFR)
Patients with chest pain due to suspected myocardial infarction or ischemia	• Cardiac biomarkers (CK, CK-MB, troponin I) to assess for cardiac muscle damage • Electrolytes
Patients with suspected hepatitis, history of alcohol or drug abuse	• Liver enzymes to asses liver function • Selected drug screening panels
Patients with acid-based disturbances	• ABG (pH, Pco_2, HCO_3, BE) • Electrolytes
Patients with PVCs or cardiac dysrhythmias without previous history of cardiac disease	• Electrolytes (especially potassium and calcium)
Patients on anticoagulation therapy or uncontrolled bleeding	• CBC and WBC differential • Prothrombin time (PT) • International Normalized Ratio (INR) • Activated partial thromboplastin time (APTT)

Pulmonary Function Tests

Pulmonary function testing ranges from simple bedside assessment of peak flows to complex computerized lab studies. **Table 3-3** outlines the primary reasons why you would recommend each of these tests for your patients.

Lung Mechanics

The term "lung mechanics" refers to the physical properties of the lungs and thorax—specifically the elastic and frictional forces opposing ventilation. Elastic resistance to ventilation is measured as *compliance* of the lungs, thorax, and lungs/thorax combined. Frictional opposition to ventilation is measured as *airway resistance*. How you measure these properties on mechanically ventilated patients is discussed in Chapter 11. Here we focus on *why* you would recommend measuring lung mechanics.

Table 3-3 Recommending Common Pulmonary Function Tests

Specific Test	Recommend to
Peak expiratory flow rate (PEFR)	• Monitor airway tone of patients with asthma over time (via diary) • Assess changes in airway tone in response to bronchodilator therapy
Bedside spirometry	• Screen for lung dysfunction suggested by history and physical indicators or other abnormal diagnostic tests • Assess changes in lung function in response to treatment • Assess the risk for surgical procedures known to affect lung function
Pre-/post-bronchodilator spirometry (bedside or lab)	• Confirm need for bronchodilator therapy • Individualize the patient's medication dose • Determine patient status during acute and long-term drug therapy • Determine if a change in dose, frequency, or medication is needed
Laboratory spirometry (FVC volumes and flows)	• Quantify the severity and prognosis associated with lung disease • Follow up on bedside spirometry results that are not definitive (e.g., restrictive conditions) • Assess the potential pulmonary effects of environmental or occupational exposures • Monitor for adverse reactions to drugs with known pulmonary toxicity • Assess the degree of pulmonary impairment for rehabilitation or disability claims
Maximum voluntary ventilation (MVV)	• Assess the integrated function of the airways, lungs, thoracic cage, and respiratory muscles • Evaluate preoperative pulmonary function • Predict breathing reserve for exercise testing • Evaluate respiratory disability
Functional residual capacity (FRC) and total lung capacity (TLC)	• Evaluate the degree of hyperinflation in obstructive abnormalities • Determine the volume of gas trapped in cysts or bullae (by comparing it to body box measurement of thoracic gas volume)
Carbon monoxide diffusing capacity (DL$_{CO}$)	• Evaluate/follow the course of interstitial lung diseases such as pulmonary fibrosis and pneumoconiosis • Evaluate/follow course of emphysema and cystic fibrosis • Differentiate among chronic bronchitis, emphysema, and asthma in patients with obstructive patterns • Quantify the degree of pulmonary impairment for disability claims • Evaluate cardiovascular disorders affecting diffusion or pulmonary blood flow • Evaluate the pulmonary effects of systemic diseases such as rheumatoid arthritis and lupus • Evaluate the effects of drugs known to cause pulmonary damage, such as amiodarone and bleomycin • Help predict arterial desaturation during exercise in patients with lung disease

(continues)

Table 3-3 Recommending Common Pulmonary Function Tests (*continued*)

Specific Test	Recommend to
Bronchial provocation (e.g., methacholine challenge test)	• Exclude a diagnosis of airway hyperreactivity • Evaluate occupational asthma • Assess the severity of airway hyperresponsiveness • Determine the relative risk of developing asthma • Assess response to therapeutic interventions
Exhaled nitric oxide (FeNO)	• Establish the correct diagnosis of airway hyperreactivity/asthma • Predict the response to and titrate corticosteroids in patients with asthma • Monitor asthma medication adherence
Airway resistance (body plethysmography)	• Evaluate airway responsiveness to provocation • Identify the specific type and severity of obstructive lung disease • Localize the primary site of flow limitation

The four most common measures of lung mechanics obtained for mechanically ventilated patients are static compliance, airway resistance, the pressure–volume curve, and the flow–volume curve. Most often, static compliance and airway resistance are computed using the end-inspiratory occlusion method (inspiratory hold). Pressure–volume and flow–volume curves are generated by the ventilator's sensors and can be continuously displayed on a graphics screen. **Table 3-4** summarizes when you should recommend each of these measures of lung mechanics for patients receiving ventilatory support.

Blood Gas Analysis, Pulse Oximetry, and Transcutaneous Monitoring

No aspect of bedside assessment is more important in respiratory care than the monitoring and evaluation of oxygenation, ventilation, and acid–base status. These processes are best assessed

Table 3-4 Recommending Measures of Lung Mechanics

Measure	Recommend to
Static compliance	• Regularly monitor patients during patient–ventilator system checks • Detect trends in patients subject to rapid changes in lung distensibility (e.g., ARDS, pulmonary edema)
Airway resistance	• Regularly monitor patients during patient–ventilator system checks • Detect trends in patients subject to rapid changes in airway caliber (e.g., asthma)
Pressure–volume curve	• Detect trends in patients subject to rapid changes in compliance (e.g., ARDS, pulmonary edema [slope of curve]) • Detect trends in patients subject to rapid changes in airway resistance (e.g., asthma [width of curve]) • Detect suspected overinflation ("beaking" appearance) • Determine optimum PEEP levels (just above lower inflection point)
Flow–volume curve	• Assess response to bronchodilator therapy (changes in peak expiratory flow and slope of expiratory flow curve) • Detect auto-PEEP (expiratory flow does not return to baseline before start of next breath)

by measuring relevant blood parameters, either invasively (by arterial sampling) or noninvasively through the skin or in the expired air.

Oxygenation of arterial blood can be assessed by blood gas analysis (ABG), hemoximetry, pulse oximetry, and transcutaneous P_{O_2} monitoring (mainly in infants and children). Ventilation can be assessed by ABGs, transcutaneous monitoring of P_{CO_2}, or capnography (discussed here in a separate section). Full assessment of acid–base status requires an ABG. **Table 3-5** outlines the key indications for these various measurements.

Regarding these methods, ABG analysis is always the gold standard against which all other measures are compared. *If the goal is the most accurate evaluation of oxygenation, ventilation, and acid-base status, always recommend ABG analysis.*

The only real limitations of ABG analysis are that (1) it does not measure actual Hb content or saturation and (2) it does not reveal the presence of abnormal hemoglobins, such as carboxy-hemoglobin (HbCO). *If you need accurate measures of any of these parameters, you must use or recommend hemoximetry (CO-oximetry).* The most common patient scenario in which you should recommend hemoximetry is smoke inhalation/CO poisoning. In addition, you should recommend hemoximetry when you need to calibrate pulse oximetry reading (Sp_{O_2}) against the actual arterial saturation.

Often called the "fifth vital sign," pulse oximetry is the most widely used measure of blood oxygenation. However, *pulse oximetry should never be substituted for ABG analysis or hemoximetry when the clinical situation demands accurate assessment of oxygenation.* You also should recommend *against* pulse oximetry in patients with poor peripheral perfusion and when there is a need to monitor for hyperoxemia, as when protecting a premature infant against retinopathy of prematurity.

Traditionally, transcutaneous P_{O_2} and P_{CO_2} monitoring has been limited to infants and small children. However, the Ptc_{CO_2} can be measured reliably in hemodynamically stable adults, making it a good choice for continuous monitoring of ventilation when capnography is impractical—for example, during noninvasive ventilation. However, the setup time required for transcutaneous monitors means that this approach should never be recommended in emergencies.

Table 3-5 Indications for Various Invasive and Noninvasive Blood Measurement

Method	Indications
Blood gas analysis	• Evaluate ventilation (Pa_{CO_2}), acid–base (pH, Pa_{CO_2}, and HCO_3), and oxygenation (Pa_{O_2}) status • Assess the patient's response to therapy or diagnostic tests (e.g., O_2 therapy, exercise testing) • Monitor severity and progression of a documented disease process
Hemoximetry (CO-oximetry)	• Determine actual blood oxyhemoglobin saturation (Sa_{O_2}) • Measure abnormal Hb levels (HbCO, metHb, and sulfhemoglobin)
Pulse oximetry (Sp_{O_2})	• Monitor the adequacy of Sp_{O_2} • Quantify the response of Sp_{O_2} to therapeutic or diagnostic interventions • Screen for functional shunts in babies with congenital heart disease • Comply with regulations or recommendations by authoritative groups (e.g., anesthesia monitoring)
Transcutaneous monitoring (Ptc_{O_2}, Ptc_{CO_2})	• Continuously monitor the adequacy of arterial oxygenation and/or ventilation • Continuously monitor for excessive arterial oxygenation (hyperoxemia) • Quantify real-time changes in ventilation and oxygenation during diagnostic or therapeutic interventions • Screen for functional shunts in babies with congenital heart disease

Capnography

You should recommend capnography for the following purposes:

- Noninvasively monitoring the effectiveness (P_{ETCO_2}) and efficiency (P_{aCO_2}-P_{ETCO_2}) of ventilation, usually during mechanical ventilation
- Monitoring the severity of pulmonary disease and assess the response to therapies intended to lower physiologic deadspace and/or better match ventilation to perfusion (V/Q)
- Confirming and monitor correct placement of an ET tube after intubation
- Optimizing chest compressions, and detecting return of spontaneous circulation (ROSC) during CPR
- Measuring CO_2 production (to assess metabolic rate)
- Providing graphic data to help evaluate the ventilator–patient interface

The utility of capnography during CPR is based on the fact that P_{ETCO_2} correlates well with cardiac output. Absent blood flow to the lungs, P_{ETCO_2} levels remain low. With good blood flow to the lungs—either due to chest compressions or due to restoration of cardiac function— P_{ETCO_2} levels rise.

Regarding graphic evaluation of the ventilator–patient interface, end-tidal CO_2 trend analysis can indicate potential hyperventilation/hypoventilation, which should be confirmed by ABG analysis. Analysis of the shape of the capnogram also can be helpful in identifying conditions such as circuit rebreathing and disconnection. Chapter 6 addresses the setup and calibration of capnographs, while Chapter 11 reviews the interpretation of capnography data in more detail.

Electrocardiography

You should recommend obtaining a 12-lead electrocardiogram to meet the following needs:

- Screening for heart disease (e.g., CAD, left ventricular hypertrophy)
- Ruling out heart disease in surgical patients
- Evaluating patients with chest pain
- Following the progression of patients with CAD
- Evaluating heart rhythm disorders (using rhythm strips)

A 12-lead ECG also can be used to assess the effect of metabolic disorders associated with electrolyte disturbances—in particular, calcium and potassium imbalances.

Hemodynamic Monitoring

Hemodynamic monitoring ranges from simple and safe noninvasive methods, such as auscultatory blood pressure measurement, to complex and hazardous invasive techniques, such as pulmonary artery catheterization. In general, the more critically ill the patient, the greater the need for invasive hemodynamic monitoring.

Noninvasive Blood Pressure Measurement

As a component of the vital signs, blood pressure should be measured noninvasively and regularly for all patients. The frequency of measurement varies according to the patient's cardiovascular stability. Automated noninvasive bedside systems allow measurement intervals as short as every 5 minutes.

Invasive Hemodynamic Monitoring (RRT-Specific Content)

Although the decision to insert an indwelling catheter is a medical one, you need to be aware of the circumstances in which your patients could benefit from hemodynamic monitoring. Likewise, given the many complications associated with indwelling lines, you must be familiar with the contraindications. This knowledge is particularly important for arterial lines ("A-lines"), which are often recommended, inserted, and removed by RTs. **Table 3-6** summarizes the key indications and contraindications for indwelling catheters by location.

Table 3-6 Indications and Contraindications for Indwelling Catheters

Indications	Contraindications
Systemic Arterial Monitoring	
• To continuously monitor arterial pressure in unstable/hypotensive patients or those receiving vasoactive drugs • To obtain frequent ABGs for patients in respiratory failure or receiving mechanical ventilation	• Inadequate collateral arterial circulation (as confirmed by Allen test) • Evidence of infection or peripheral vascular disease in the selected limb • Severe bleeding disorder • Presence of a surgical/dialysis shunt in the selected arm (consider the contralateral limb)
Central Venous Monitoring	
• To monitor CVP/right ventricular function in unstable or hypotensive patients • To provide volume resuscitation • To infuse drugs that can cause peripheral phlebitis (certain vasopressors and chemotherapeutic agents) • To provide a route for total parenteral nutrition • To perform plasmapheresis or hemodialysis • To introduce transvenous pacing wires • To provide venous access in patients with poor peripheral veins	• Evidence of infection at the insertion site • Abnormalities at insertion site (vascular injury, prior surgery, rib/clavicle fractures, chest wall deformity) • Suspected injury to the superior vena cava • Severe bleeding disorder (Note: The subclavian vein cannot be compressed to stop bleeding.) • Presence of intravascular pacemaker or vena cava filter • Severe obesity (a technical difficulty) • Bullous lung disease (high risk of pneumothorax)
Pulmonary Artery Monitoring	
• To identify the cause of various shock states • To identify the cause of pulmonary edema • To diagnose pulmonary hypertension • To diagnose valvular disease, intracardiac shunts, cardiac tamponade, and pulmonary embolus • To monitor and manage complicated MI • To assess the hemodynamic response to therapies • To manage multiple organ failure • To manage hemodynamic instability after cardiac surgery • To optimize fluid and inotropic therapy • To measure tissue oxygenation and cardiac output • To perform atrial and ventricular pacing	• Certain dysrhythmias (Wolff-Parkinson-White syndrome, LBBB) • Tricuspid or pulmonary valve endocarditis, stenosis, or mechanical prosthesis • Right heart mass (thrombus and/or tumor) • Infection at the insertion site • The presence of an RV assist device, transvenous pacemaker, or defibrillator • Severe bleeding disorder

Sleep Studies

Sleep studies that respiratory therapists might recommend include overnight pulse oximetry and polysomnography.

Overnight Oximetry

You should recommend overnight oximetry for the following purposes:

- Helping identify patients with obstructive sleep apnea–hypopnea syndrome (SAHS)
- Helping assess SAHS patients' response to therapy, such as CPAP
- Identifying whether serious desaturation occurs in COPD patients during sleep

Laboratory polysomnography (which includes oximetry) is the gold standard for diagnosing SAHS. However, polysomnography is expensive and not available to all patients with suspected sleep-disordered breathing. In comparison, overnight oximetry is readily available, is inexpensive, and can be performed in the patient's home.

In regard to screening those individuals with COPD, it is well known that some of these patients experience large drops in arterial O_2 saturation during sleep. This nocturnal desaturation generally can be predicted from daytime saturation levels and is probably due to hypoventilation occurring during REM sleep. When screening COPD patients for nocturnal desaturation, the focus should be on those with hypercapnia, erythrocytosis, or evidence of pulmonary hypertension.

Polysomnography

You should recommend polysomnography for patients who exhibit signs or symptoms associated with sleep-disordered breathing, such as daytime somnolence and fatigue, morning headaches, pulmonary hypertension, and polycythemia. According to the AARC, polysomnography is specifically indicated in patients with the following conditions:

- COPD with awake $Pao_2 > 55$ torr, and whose condition includes pulmonary hypertension, right heart failure, polycythemia, or excessive daytime sleepiness
- Chest wall or neuromuscular restrictive disorders, and whose condition includes chronic hypoventilation, polycythemia, pulmonary hypertension, disturbed sleep, morning headaches, daytime somnolence, or fatigue
- Disorders of respiratory control with chronic hypoventilation (daytime $Paco_2 > 45$ torr) or whose illness is complicated by pulmonary hypertension, polycythemia, disturbed sleep, morning headaches, daytime somnolence, or fatigue
- Excessive daytime sleepiness or sleep maintenance insomnia
- Snoring associated with observed apneas and/or excessive daytime sleepiness

Polysomnography is also indicated to help diagnose certain neurologic and movement disorders, such as restless leg syndrome and nocturnal seizures, as well as parasomnias like sleepwalking. In addition, polysomnography is used to assess the adequacy of sleep-related interventions, including titrating CPAP in patients with obstructive SAHS and determining BiPAP levels for patients with central sleep apneas or respiratory insufficiency due to chronic neuromuscular disorders, such as amyotrophic lateral sclerosis.

Thoracentesis (RRT-Specific Content)

Thoracentesis is a physician-performed procedure involving withdrawal of fluid from the pleural space for either diagnostic or therapeutic purposes. You would recommend a *diagnostic* thoracentesis to help determine the cause of the accumulated fluids (e.g., transudative versus exudative) or to obtain cell samples to assess for certain malignancies. You would recommend a *therapeutic* thoracentesis for any patient with an effusion large enough to cause respiratory distress. Details on assisting physicians with this special procedure are provided in Chapter 16.

COMMON ERRORS TO AVOID

You can improve your score by avoiding these mistakes:

- Never recommend diagnostic bronchoscopy in patients who are hemodynamically unstable or who cannot be adequately oxygenated during the procedure due to severe hypoxemia.
- Never let pulse oximetry data substitute for ABG analysis or hemoximetry when the clinical situation demands accurate assessment of blood oxygenation.

- Never use pulse oximetry to detect hyperoxemia (abnormally high Pa_{O_2}).
- Never recommend or insert a radial arterial line when the Allen test indicates inadequate collateral circulation on that side.

SURE BETS

In some situations, you can always be sure of the right approach to a clinical problem or scenario:

- You should always recommend a sputum Gram stain and culture and sensitivity for any patient suspected of having a respiratory tract infection.
- To determine if a change in the dose or frequency of an aerosolized bronchodilator is needed, always recommend pre-/post-bronchodilator spirometry.
- To assess the presence and severity of restrictive abnormalities, always recommend both TLC/FRC measurement and the diffusing capacity test (DLco).
- If the goal is the most accurate evaluation of oxygenation, ventilation, and acid–base status, always recommend obtaining and analyzing an arterial blood sample (ABG).
- Always recommend CO-oximetry for patients suspected of suffering smoke inhalation.
- Always recommend polysomnography for patients who complain of or exhibit signs or symptoms associated with sleep-disordered breathing, such as daytime somnolence and fatigue.
- Always recommend a therapeutic thoracentesis for any patient with a confirmed large pleural effusion causing signs or symptoms of respiratory distress.

PRE-TEST ANSWERS AND EXPLANATIONS

Following are this chapter's pre-test answers and explanations. Be sure to review each answer's explanation thoroughly to help you understand why it is correct. If the explanation is still unclear to you, review the chapter content.

3-1. **Correct answer: D.** Fiberoptic bronchoscopy. Injury from toxic inhalation or aspiration can affect the airways. In these patients, the location and extent of injury is best determined initially using fiberoptic bronchoscopy.

3-2. **Correct answer: C.** Bronchoalveolar lavage (BAL). A sputum culture and sensitivity could help diagnose this problem. However, BAL is the best tool available to diagnose ventilator-associated pneumonia (VAP) and, therefore, is the better choice for this patient.

3-3. **Correct answer: C.** Capnography. Capnography is used primarily to noninvasively monitor the effectiveness (PET_{CO_2}) and efficiency (Pa_{CO_2}-PET_{CO_2}) of ventilation, usually during mechanical ventilation. Most capnographs also can compute the accumulated CO_2 volume over time. CO_2 production per minute is one measure of metabolic activity, with the other being O_2 consumption.

3-4. **Correct answer: A.** Diffusing capacity (DLco). The primary indication for the DLco test is to evaluate interstitial lung diseases such as pulmonary fibrosis and pneumoconiosis. In addition, the DLco test can help differentiate among the various patterns of airway obstruction (emphysema patients typically have a low DLco). The DLco test also can help predict arterial desaturation during exercise in patients with lung disease.

3-5. **Correct answer: B.** Flow–volume loop. Of the tests listed, only the flow–volume loop would help detect the presence of auto-PEEP on a patient receiving ventilatory support. On the flow–volume loop of a patient with auto-PEEP, the expiratory flow does not return to baseline before the start of the next breath.

3-6. **Correct answer: C.** Polysomnography. You should recommend polysomnography for patients who complain of or exhibit signs or symptoms associated with sleep-disordered breathing (e.g., daytime somnolence and fatigue, morning headaches, pulmonary hypertension, and polycythemia).

3-7. **Correct answer: A.** Transcutaneous P_{CO_2} analysis. Although traditionally used only with infants and children, the transcutaneous P_{CO_2} is an accurate measure of ventilation in stable adults and, therefore, is a good choice for continuous monitoring of ventilation when capnography is impractical (e.g., during noninvasive ventilation).

3-8. **Correct answer: A.** 1 and 3. An ECG is indicated in evaluating patients with chest pain, and cardiac biomarkers such as troponin I and CK can help diagnose an acute myocardial infarction.

3-9. **Correct answer: B.** A pulmonary artery catheter. To assess tissue oxygenation, we need to know how much oxygen is *left over* after the blood leaves the capillaries (mixed venous oxygen content or $C\bar{v}_{O_2}$). This measure can be obtained only from the distal port of a pulmonary artery catheter.

3-10. **Correct answer: B.** CT angiography. Although standard pulmonary angiography and V/Q scans are still used to detect pulmonary embolism (PE), CT angiography is replacing these methods as the best tool for diagnosing PE.

3-11. **Correct answer: D**. 1, 2, and 3. Hemoglobin and hematocrit levels should be obtained to determine the O_2 carrying capacity of the blood, and hemoximetry performed to measure actual Sa_{O_2} and the presence of any dyshemoglobins such as HbCO or metHb.

3-12. **Correct answer: D**. A therapeutic thoracentesis. The x-ray description is consistent with a large pleural effusion. Recommend a therapeutic thoracentesis for patients with large effusions causing respiratory distress.

POST-TEST

To confirm your mastery of this chapter's topical content, you should take the chapter post-test, available online at http://go.jblearning.com/respexamreview. A score of 80% or higher indicates that you are adequately prepared for this section of the NBRC written exams. If you score less than 80%, you should continue to review the applicable chapter content. In addition, you may want to access and review the relevant Web links covering this chapter's content (courtesy of RTBoardReview. com), also online at the Jones & Bartlett Learning site.

CHAPTER 4

Manipulate Equipment by Order or Protocol

Craig L. Scanlan

Manipulate Equipment by Order or Protocol represents the single largest section of the NBRC CRT exam and also is one of the most difficult topics for candidates. Consistent with the topic's importance, this chapter is the most comprehensive in the text. For each category of equipment, we present guidelines on selecting, using, and troubleshooting the applicable devices. This information will not only help you answer questions in this category, but also help you achieve high scores on other sections of the NBRC exams that have equipment-related questions. For this reason, we recommend returning here whenever you need to clarify how to properly use equipment.

OBJECTIVES

In preparing for the shared NBRC exam content, you should demonstrate the knowledge needed to select, use, and troubleshoot the following equipment:

1. Gas cylinders, reducing valves, flowmeters, and O_2 blenders
2. Oxygen administration devices
3. Humidifiers, nebulizers, and mist tents
4. Aerosol drug-delivery systems
5. Incentive breathing devices
6. Percussors and vibrators (covered in Chapter 9)
7. Positive expiratory pressure and vibratory devices (covered in Chapter 9)
8. Resuscitation devices
9. Artificial airways
10. Ventilators, CPAP devices, and breathing circuits
11. Vacuum systems, suction, and pleural drainage devices
12. Manometers
13. CO, He, O_2, and specialty gas analyzers
14. Bedside pulmonary function devices
15. ECG monitors and 12-lead ECG machines
16. Point-of-care blood gas analyzers
17. Noninvasive oximetry monitoring devices
18. Bronchoscopes

In preparing for the RRT-specific NBRC exam content, you should demonstrate the knowledge needed to select, use, and troubleshoot the following additional equipment:

19. Portable oxygen systems (covered in Chapter 17)
20. Incubators/isolettes
21. He/O_2-delivery systems
22. High-frequency chest wall oscillators (covered in Chapter 9)
23. High-frequency ventilators
24. Hemodynamic monitoring devices

WHAT TO EXPECT ON THIS CATEGORY OF THE NBRC EXAMS

CRT exam: 22 questions; about 20% recall, 50% application, and 30% analysis
WRRT exam: 12 questions; about 15% recall, 15% application, and 70% analysis
CSE exam: indeterminate number of questions; however, exam II-A knowledge can appear in both the CSE Information Gathering and Decision-Making sections

PRE-TEST

Carefully respond to each of the following questions. After completing the pre-test, compare your answers to those provided at the end of this chapter. Then thoroughly review each answer's explanation to help understand why it is correct.

4-1. You measure an oxygen concentration of 55% being delivered by an air-entrainment mask set to deliver 31% oxygen. Which of the following actions is most appropriate?
  A. Add an aerosol collar to the mask
  B. Decrease the oxygen input flow
  C. Check the entrainment ports
  D. Increase the oxygen input flow

4-2. Which of the following is the approximate total output flow delivered from a 35% air-entrainment mask operating at 8 L/min?
  A. 12 L/min
  B. 48 L/min
  C. 52 L/min
  D. 72 L/min

4-3. You observe that the reservoir bag on a patient receiving O_2 at 10 L/min does not deflate at all when the patient inspires. What should you do *first?*
  A. Tell the patient to breathe more deeply
  B. Decrease the O_2 flow to 6 L/min
  C. Check the mask for a snug fit
  D. Remove mask valve flaps

4-4. Which of the following is the most probable cause of insufficient mist in a croup tent?
  A. Decreased temperature within the canopy
  B. Insufficient cooling of the gas
  C. Inadequate size of the tent
  D. A clogged nebulizer capillary tube

4-5. A physician specifies in her respiratory orders the following objective for a patient with an artificial airway: "to overcome the patient's humidity deficit." Which of the following devices should you select for this patient?

  A. Small-volume jet nebulizer
  B. Large-reservoir heated jet nebulizer
  C. Unheated passover humidifier
  D. Vibrating mesh nebulizer

4-6. To ensure proper function of a radiant warmer applied to a low-birth-weight infant in NICU, what would you do?
  A. Set the temperature control to servo mode and target 32°C
  B. Place and secure the temperature probe on an extremity (hand or foot)
  C. Use a reflective material to cover the temperature probe
  D. Set the controller low-temperature alarm for 30°C

4-7. While a patient is being ventilated with a bag-valve resuscitator, the bag fills rapidly and collapses on minimal pressure, although little chest movement by the patient is noted. The cause of the problem may be which of the following?
  A. Absence of the inlet valve
  B. Excessive oxygen flow
  C. Plugged endotracheal (ET) tube
  D. Plugged inlet valve

4-8. An intubated adult patient with severe expiratory airway obstruction requires ventilatory support. Which of the following factors is most important in selecting a ventilator for this patient?
  A. Ability to compensate for airway interface leaks
  B. Variable flow control and adjustable I:E ratios
  C. Ability to run on 12-volt DC (battery) power
  D. Certification for use during MRI procedures

4-9. Which type of circuit tubing is required for high-frequency oscillation ventilation?
- **A.** Wide-diameter, high-compliance tubing
- **B.** Narrow-diameter, high-compliance tubing
- **C.** Wide-diameter, low-compliance tubing
- **D.** Narrow-diameter, low-compliance tubing

4-10. To provide a low to moderate concentration of oxygen to a patient receiving noninvasive nasal bilevel ventilation via a device that uses a turbine or blower to generate pressure, what should you do?
- **A.** Connect the device to a 50-psi O_2 outlet
- **B.** Apply a nasal cannula to the patient under the mask
- **C.** Bleed supplemental O_2 from a flowmeter into the circuit
- **D.** Add a reservoir bag to the device's breathing circuit

4-11. Which of the following alarm conditions indicates a potential system leak when delivering volume control mechanical ventilation.
- **A.** High volume + low pressure
- **B.** Low volume + high pressure
- **C.** High volume + high pressure
- **D.** Low volume + low pressure

4-12. A patient with a chronic neuromuscular condition requires nocturnal positive-pressure ventilation over the long term. Which of the following airways should you recommend for this patient?
- **A.** Oral ET tube
- **B.** Fenestrated tracheostomy tube
- **C.** Laryngeal mask airway
- **D.** Standard tracheostomy tube

4-13. An infant is receiving 50% O_2 via an isolette's built-in O_2 controller. A doctor orders the FIO_2 increased to 0.65. What is the most appropriate action at this time?
- **A.** Provide additional O_2 to the infant via the "blow-by" method
- **B.** Recommend intubation and initiate mechanical ventilation
- **C.** Provide additional O_2 to the infant via a simple mask
- **D.** Setup an O_2 blender/heated humidifier oxyhood system

4-14. Prior to intubation in an emergency, injection of air into the pilot line of the endotracheal (ET) tube fails to inflate the cuff. What should you do?
- **A.** Check the cuff for leaks
- **B.** Check the valve on the pilot line
- **C.** Replace the ET tube
- **D.** Inspect the pilot line for patency

4-15. Resistance is encountered while suctioning a teenage child through a size 6-mm ID ET tube with a 14-Fr catheter. Which of the following is the most appropriate action for you to take?
- **A.** Lubricate the catheter
- **B.** Use a 10-Fr catheter
- **C.** Turn the patient's head
- **D.** Instill normal saline solution

4-16. All of the following could cause suctioning to stop suddenly during tracheobronchial aspiration *except*:
- **A.** Disconnected tubing
- **B.** Clearance of secretions
- **C.** A full suction reservoir
- **D.** A mucus plug in the catheter

4-17. The emergency room doctor orders administration of 70% He/30% O_2 to a spontaneously breathing patient suffering an acute exacerbation of asthma. Which of the following systems would be appropriate for delivery of this mixture?
1. Tightly fitted nonrebreathing mask @ 12 L/min
2. Large-volume nebulizer @ 100% with aerosol mask
3. High-flow nasal cannula @ 40 L/min
- **A.** 1 only
- **B.** 1, 2, or 3
- **C.** 3 only
- **D.** 1 or 3

4-18. After attaching a yoke connector to an E-size cylinder and opening the cylinder valve, you notice a leak at the gas outlet. Which of the following are possible causes for this leak?
1. The gas outlet bushing is missing or damaged
2. Pin-indexed safety system (PISS) pins are missing
3. The yoke hand screw is not tight enough
- **A.** 1 and 2
- **B.** 2 and 3

C. 1 and 3
D. 1, 2, and 3

4-19. While obtaining an arterial sample for analysis using a point-of-care analyzer, you should do all of the following *except*:
A. Analyze the sample within 3 minutes
B. Place the sample in an ice slush
C. Thoroughly mix the sample
D. Prevent sample exposure to air

4-20. An alert 55-year-old patient who two days earlier had abdominal surgery has coarse crackles and rhonchi on the left side, a respiratory rate of 13 breaths/min, and an SpO_2 of 96% on nasal cannula at 2 L/min. The surgeon is concerned that the patient may be developing atelectasis. Which of the following approaches should you select to manage this patient?
A. Intermittent positive-pressure breathing
B. Incentive spirometry with directed coughing
C. Incentive spirometry alone
D. Aerosolized bronchodilator therapy

4-21. A home care patient receiving long-term low-flow O_2 via standard nasal cannula and a pulse dose/demand flow system calls and reports that the device is not working. After confirming a good O_2 source, tight fittings, and the proper device settings, which instruction would you give to the patient?
A. Switch to a backup supply of continuous O_2 at 2 to 3 times the demand flow setting
B. Remove the standard nasal cannula and switch to a reservoir nasal cannula
C. Switch to a backup supply of continuous O_2 at one-third to one-half the demand flow setting
D. Call the home care company to request delivery of a replacement unit

4-22. Which of the following valves in a typical high-frequency oscillation ventilator (HFOV) is used to regulate the mean airway pressure?
A. Limit valve
B. Flush valve
C. Dump valve
D. Control valve

4-23. You can use a fluid column pressure manometer for all of the following purposes *except*:
A. To measure atmospheric pressure
B. To measure static pressures
C. To calibrate other manometers
D. To measure rapid pressure changes

4-24. You need to measure the forced vital capacity (FVC) of an adult patient at the bedside. Which of the following devices should you select to make this measurement?
A. A portable electronic spirometer
B. Strain-gauge pressure transducer
C. Mechanical turbine-type respirometer
D. Water-sealed bell spirometer

4-25. Upon inspection of a portable spirometer's FVC curve obtained on an adult outpatient, you determine that the back-extrapolated volume is excessive. Prior to repeating the maneuver, which of the following instructions should you provide to the patient?
A. "Don't hesitate"
B. "Blast out faster"
C. "Blow out longer"
D. "Breathe deeper"

4-26. After setting up a 12-lead ECG on a patient, you note a noisy and unstable signal. All of the following would help to resolve this problem *except*:
A. Verifying that the leads are connected properly
B. Checking the ECG main lead cable for damage
C. Turning off filtering of extraneous electrical activity
D. Confirming that the patient is staying motionless

4-27. To spot check a patient's oxygen saturation at the bedside, you should select which of the following devices?
A. Oxygen analyzer
B. Hemoximeter
C. Transcutaneous monitor
D. Pulse oximeter

4-28. A neonatal intensive care unit (NICU) nurse calls you to check an infant on a transcutaneous Po_2/Pco_2 monitor due to a rapid rise in $Ptco_2$ and concurrent fall in $Ptcco_2$ below 10 torr. What is the most likely cause of this problem?

A. The presence of peripheral vasoconstriction

B. A defective sensor or sensor membrane

C. Interference due to bright ambient lighting

D. Air leakage around the sensor's fixation ring

4-29. A 2-year-old child is admitted to the emergency department with severe asthmatic symptoms. The attending physician orders a bronchodilator that is available in both solution and MDI preparations.

Which of the following is the best delivery system for this drug to this patient?

A. Breath-actuated MDI with mask

B. Small-volume nebulizer (SVN) with mouthpiece

C. MDI with holding chamber and a mask

D. SVN using the "blow by" technique

4-30. You are assisting a nurse in ICU measure a patient's central venous pressure (CVP) with a strain-gauge pressure transducer. You note that the pressure transducer is positioned well above the middle of the patient's lateral chest wall. What effect, if any, would this have on the CVP measurement?

A. It would not affect the measurement

B. It would underestimate the CVP

C. It would cause damping of the signal

D. It would overestimate the CVP

WHAT YOU NEED TO KNOW: ESSENTIAL CONTENT

Gas Cylinders, Reducing Valves, Flowmeters, and O_2 Blenders

In hospitals, O_2 and air are supplied to the bedside via piping at the standard pressure of 50 psi for direct application to equipment, such as ventilators and O_2 blenders. To control flow to a patient, attach a *flowmeter* to the 50-psi outlet, using the appropriate DISS connector.

High-pressure gas cylinders may be required in areas lacking piped gas, in the home or some extended-care facilities, and during patient transport. In addition, all specialized gases (He, NO, CO, and CO_2) are provided in cylinders. Because cylinders' pressures are much higher than 50 psi, they cannot be connected directly to equipment. Instead, you must use a *pressure-reducing valve*. For equipment requiring 50 psi, select a *preset* pressure-reducing valve. *Adjustable* pressure-reducing valves are used only in conjunction with a Bourdon flow gauge. **Table 4-1** provides guidelines for selecting gas-delivery equipment.

Table 4-1 Guidelines for Selecting Gas-Delivery Equipment

Purpose	Setting	Needed Equipment
To provide 50-psi unrestricted flow to ventilators or blenders	Piped source available (most hospital units)	• None; connect directly to piped gas source at 50 psi
	Piped source not available	• Large gas cylinder (H or K) with preset (50-psi) pressure-reducing valve • For air, piston air compressor with reservoir
To deliver a controlled flow of gas to a patient or equipment	Piped source available (most hospital units)	• Connect calibrated Thorpe tube flowmeter to piped gas source at 50 psi
	Piped source not available	• Gas cylinder with reducing valve and flowmeter—cylinder size selected based on portability needs and planned duration of usage • For air, portable diaphragm compressor
	Ambulatory or home care setting	• Liquid O_2 system (with portable unit) • O_2 concentrator (stationary or portable)

If portability is the first consideration, select either a small cylinder (A through E), a portable liquid O_2 system, or a portable O_2 concentrator. Note that small cylinders use a post-type valve stem with pin-indexed holes (PISS) for attaching reducing valves or regulators.

When using cylinders for transport, you'll want a flowmeter that is *unaffected by gravity*—either a Bourdon gauge or a variable orifice regulator like the Praxair Grab 'n Go™ or Western Medica's Oxytote™. If the patient is being transported for an MRI study, you must either use iron-free equipment (e.g., aluminum cylinders and carts and brass and/or aluminum regulators) or provide an O_2-delivery tubing extension long enough to keep sensitive equipment out of the exam room.

If there is no need for portability or the duration of use exceeds an hour, you should select a large cylinder (G, H, or K). Large cylinders use threaded outlets for connecting reducing valves or regulators. In general, these cylinders store at least 10 times more gas than their smaller counterparts.

Cylinders, Reducing Valves, and Regulators

Once you have selected the appropriate cylinder and attachments, apply the following guidelines for assembly and use, including transport:

1. Before transporting a cylinder to its point of use:
   a. Check that the label and cylinder color match (if in doubt, do not use it).
   b. For large cylinders, make sure the protective cap is in place.
2. Transport large cylinders chained to a wheeled cart; place small cylinders in the gurney/wheelchair holder or on the mattress.
3. Properly secure the cylinder at the point of use.
4. Always "crack" the cylinder valve to clear dust or debris.
5. Attach the needed reducing valve or regulator and ensure leak-free connection.
6. Connect the needed equipment to reducing valve/regulator outlet (DISS connection).
7. Slowly open the cylinder valve, and record pressure compute flow duration.
8. Before disconnecting equipment, close the cylinder valve and release pressure from any attached devices.

Most problems with cylinders and regulators involve leakage at the valve stem or in the regulator. If a leak occurs when the cylinder valve is opened:

1. Tighten the connection between the regulator and cylinder valve and regulator and any attached equipment.
2. If a PISS connection, recheck for missing or extra washers.
3. If the regulator is leaking, replace it.

If gas does not flow from the cylinder regulator, first check the pressure gauge for adequate pressure/contents. If the gauge indicates cylinder pressure, you should replace the regulator.

Air Compressors

Although medical-quality air can be provided via cylinders, air compressors are the preferred source. Air may be piped to the bedside from large-volume compressors or delivered via portable units at the point of care. Only large-volume compressors with reservoirs can meet the unrestricted flow needs of equipment such as ventilators. Small portable compressors generally are limited to powering devices such as small-volume nebulizers.

If a compressor fails to operate when the switch is turned on, check the electrical outlet for power and the unit's fuse or circuit breaker. If an operating compressor's output appears inadequate:

1. Check the inlet filter for obstruction.
2. Check the tubing and connected equipment for obstruction.
3. Check the tubing and connections for leaks.

Oxygen Blenders

Select an O_2 blender when you need to deliver a range of precise O_2 concentrations to either equipment or a patient. All blenders require unrestricted air and O_2 source gas at standard line pressure (50 psi). Most blenders output 50 psi at the set $O_2\%$, which can be applied directly to power equipment or meter flow going to the patient. To set up a standard O_2 blender:

1. Connect 50-psi hoses from the air and O_2 sources to the respective blender inlets.
2. Check/confirm the pressure alarms by separately disconnecting each gas source; if either alarm fails, replace the device.
3. Verify 100% and 21% O_2 settings with an oxygen analyzer.
4. Set the blender to the prescribed $O_2\%$.
5. Attach the required delivery device.
6. Verify the prescribed $O_2\%$ using an O_2 analyzer.

If a blender pressure alarm sounds when both gas sources are attached:

1. Verify that both gas sources are at the required inlet pressures (usually $\geq$ 35 psig).
2. Check for leaks between the gas source and the blender.
3. If these check out, replace the blender.

Most O_2 *blenders do not monitor the actual* $O_2\%$. If you observe a large discrepancy between the blender setting and the measured $O_2\%$, first recheck the air and O_2 hoses to make sure that they have not accidently been switched (requires illegal "cheater" adaptors). If this is not the case, and you confirm the $O_2\%$ discrepancy, replace the blender.

Portable O_2 Systems (RRT-Specific Content)

Because they are used primarily in the ambulatory and home care settings, portable O_2 systems (liquid O_2 and concentrators) are discussed in Chapter 17, Pulmonary Rehabilitation and Home Care.

Oxygen Administration Devices

You should select or recommend O_2 therapy in the following situations:

- Documented hypoxemia (Pao_2 < 60 torr or Sao_2 < 90% on room air)
- Signs of hypoxemia (e.g., dyspnea, tachypnea, tachycardia, cyanosis, confusion)
- Severe trauma
- Acute myocardial infarction
- Short-term therapy or surgical intervention (e.g., postanesthesia recovery)

Most O_2 modalities are disposable single-use devices categorized as being either low- or high-flow systems. **Table 4-2** summarizes these devices, their flow settings, Fio_2 ranges, advantages, disadvantages, and best use. The following guidelines apply to their assembly and use:

- If assembly is required, carefully follow the manufacturer's recommended procedure.
- Use a simple bubble humidifier for low-flow systems set to deliver more than 4 L/min.
- Make sure all threaded components are properly seated and tightened and all tubing connections snug.
- With heated humidifiers or any nebulizers, use large-bore corrugated tubing to avoid blockage by condensate.

Table 4-2 Common Oxygen Administration Devices

Device	Flow	F_{IO_2}	Advantages	Disadvantages	Best Use
			Low Flow		
Standard nasal cannula	¼–8 L/min (adults) ≤ 2 L/min (infants)	22–45%	• Can be used on adults, children, and infants • Easy to apply • Disposable • Low cost • Well tolerated	• Unstable, easily dislodged • High flows uncomfortable • Can cause dryness/bleeding • Polyps, deviated septum may block flow	• Stable patient needing low F_{IO_2} • Home care patient requiring long-term therapy
Simple mask	5–10 L/min	35–50%	• Can be used on adults, children, and infants • Quick, easy to apply • Disposable • Low cost	• Uncomfortable • Must be removed for eating • Prevents radiant heat loss • Blocks vomitus in unconscious patients	• Emergencies • Short-term therapy requiring moderate F_{IO_2}
Partial rebreathing mask	6–10 L/min (prevent bag collapse)	40–70%	• Same as for simple mask • Moderate to high F_{IO_2}s	• Same as for simple mask • Potential suffocation hazard	• Emergencies • Short-term therapy requiring moderate to high F_{IO_2}s
Nonrebreathing mask	Minimum 10 L/min (prevent bag collapse)	60–80%	• Same as for simple mask • High F_{IO_2}s	• Same as for simple mask • Potential suffocation hazard	• Emergencies • Short-term therapy requiring high F_{IO_2}s • Heliox therapy

High Flow

		Advantages	Disadvantages	Indications
Air-entrainment mask	Varies; output should be ≥ 40 L/min to ensure FiO_2	• Easy to apply • Disposable • Inexpensive • Stable • Precise FiO_2s	• Limited to adult use • Uncomfortable • Noisy • Must be removed for eating • $FiO_2 \geq 0.35$ not ensured • FiO_2 varies with back-pressure	• Unstable patient requiring precise, low FiO_2
Air-entrainment nebulizer	10–15 L/min input; output should be > 60 L/min to ensure FiO_2	• Provides temperature control and extra humidity	• $FiO_2 < 28\%$ or ≥ 0.35 not ensured • FiO_2 varies with back-pressure • High infection risk	• Patients with artificial airways requiring low to moderate FiO_2s via T-tube or tracheal mask • Post extubation (aerosol mask)
High-flow nasal cannula	1–40 L/min adults; 1–20 L/min children; 1–8 L/min infants	• Easy to apply • Stable, precise FiO_2s • Provides gas at BTPS without condensation • Meets/exceeds nonrebreather performance • Decreases anatomic deadspace (CO_2 washout)	• Requires special (proprietary) cannulas and humidification system • Can create occult CPAP • Potential electrical risks • Some units associated with contamination/infection	• As an alternative to a nonrebreather mask for patients needing moderate to high FiO_2, including those with claustrophobia or facial burns • Patients with hypothermia requiring O_2 • Patients requiring heliox or NO therapy

BTPS: body temperature, pressure saturated (37° C and 100% relative humidity)
Adapted from: Wilkins RL, Stoller JK, Scanlan CL. *Egan's fundamentals of respiratory care* (8th ed.). St. Louis, MO: Mosby; 2003.

Table 4-3 Factors Affecting the F$_{IO_2}$ of Low-Flow Oxygen Systems

Less Air Dilution/Higher F$_{IO_2}$	More Air Dilution/Lower F$_{IO_2}$
Device Related	
Higher O_2 input	Lower O_2 input
Reservoir present (masks)	Reservoir absent (cannula)
Leak present (masks)	Leak absent (masks)
Valves present (masks)	Valves absent (masks)
Patient Related	
Lower inspiratory flow	Higher inspiratory flow
Lower tidal volume	Higher tidal volume
Slower rate of breathing	Faster rate of breathing
Smaller minute volume	Larger minute volume

Low-Flow Devices

Low-flow devices include standard nasal cannulas and masks. These devices deliver O_2 at *flows less than the patient's inspiratory flow*, so that the O_2 is always diluted with some room air. Masks overcome some of this air dilution by providing an O_2 reservoir. **Table 4-3** summarizes factors affecting the amount of air dilution and the F$_{IO_2}$ in low-flow systems.

Note that the low-flow F$_{IO_2}$ ranges in Table 4-2 are estimates only. *For adults receiving nasal O_2, each L/min of O_2 raises the F$_{IO_2}$ by approximately 4%.* For example, a patient on a nasal cannula at 2 L/min would have an estimated F$_{IO_2}$ of about 29% (21 + 8). However, because low-flow system F$_{IO_2}$s vary, you should always evaluate the patient's response to therapy, as described in Chapter 11.

Special consideration is required for patients receiving continuous low-flow O_2 therapy outside the hospital (refer to Chapter 17). For these patients, the goal is to make the most efficient use of the available O_2 and extend the time available for portable O_2 use. Both goals are accomplished using *oxygen-conserving devices.*

Oxygen-conserving devices overcome the inefficiency of standard nasal cannulas, which typically waste one-half to two-thirds of the delivered O_2. This waste can be either by using either a reservoir cannula or a pulse dose/demand flow system. Compared with standard nasal cannulas, these devices can reduce O_2 usage by 50–75%. For an ambulatory patient carrying a full D cylinder, that difference would extend the available usage time from approximately 1.5 hours to 5 hours.

Reservoir cannulas store O_2 during exhalation and release it during inhalation. Unfortunately, many ambulatory care patients object to the appearance of these devices and fail to use them. For this reason, reservoir cannulas have generally been replaced by pulse dose/demand flow systems.

Pulse dose/demand flow systems use a sensor to detect inspiration and trigger a valve to deliver O_2 only during that phase of breathing. Unfortunately, these devices have different setting and adjustment protocols. For this reason, when switching patients from a nasal cannula to a demand flow system, *you should start them out at one-half the original flow and then adjust the flow to achieve the desired SpO_2.* This should be done both at rest and under the exertion levels that the patient will commonly encounter.

To ensure continuity of therapy, patients using pulse dose/demand flow systems who suspect a problem with their unit should *immediately switch to a backup supply of continuous O_2 via nasal cannula at the equivalent flow* (2–3 times that of the conserving device). More in depth troubleshooting guidelines for demand flow O_2-delivery systems are provided in **Table 4-4**.

High-Flow Devices

High-flow devices deliver O_2 at *flows exceeding the patient's inspiratory flow*, thereby generally ensuring a stable F$_{IO_2}$. Most high-flow systems use air entrainment, by which source O_2 driven through a high-velocity jet draws in air through surrounding ports, mixing it with the O_2. Bigger ports and smaller jets cause more air dilution, lower O_2 concentrations, and higher total flows, while smaller ports and bigger jets cause less air dilution and higher O_2 concentrations, but lower total flows.

Table 4-4 Troubleshooting Common Problems with Demand Flow O$_2$-Delivery Systems

Problem	Possible Causes	Remedies
Low-battery light flashes	Batteries are low	• Replace old batteries with new batteries
Alarm stays on	Batteries are low	• Replace old batteries with new batteries
	No inspiration is sensed	• Turn unit off, then back on to reset the alarm • Check all cannula and tube connections to ensure they are tight and not kinked or otherwise obstructed • Adjust the cannula to ensure a comfortable fit, then initiate inspiration
Hissing sound coming from inside the device	Pressure from oxygen regulator is too high	• Reduce pressure to the recommended level
No oxygen is delivered	Leaks in delivery system	• Check all cannula and tubing connections to ensure they are tight
	Kinks in delivery tubing	• Check all tubing to ensure there are no kinks, bends, obstructions, or objects putting pressure on the tube
	Oxygen source is off (concentrator) or empty (LOX reservoir or gas cylinder)	• Turn concentrator on, fill/refill LOX reservoir, replace gas cylinder
Oxygen is delivered continuously	Selector knob is set to continuous flow	• Check the selector to ensure it is set to pulse mode
	Unit is in bypass mode due to failure to sense inspiration	• Turn the unit off, then back on to reset the alarm • Check all cannula and tube connections to ensure they are tight and not kinked or otherwise obstructed • Adjust the cannula to ensure a comfortable fit, then initiate inspiration

Air-entrainment devices mix air and O$_2$ at specific ratios. **Table 4-5** provides the approximate air-to-O$_2$ ratios for common O$_2$ concentrations delivered by these systems, as well as their total output flows for an input of 10 L/min. *Changing the O$_2$ input of an air-entrainment device does not alter the air/O$_2$ ratio or delivered O$_2$%, only the total output flow.*

Table 4-5 Air-to-O$_2$ Ratios and Total Flow Output of Air-Entrainment Devices

O$_2$ Percent	Air-to-O$_2$ Ratio	Total Ratio Parts	Total Flow* at 10 L/min O$_2$ Input
80	0.3:1	1.3	13
70	0.6:1	1.6	16
60	1:1	2	20
50	1.7:1	2.7	27
40	3:1	4	40
35	5:1	6	60
31	7:1	8	80
28	10:1	11	110
24	25:1	26	260
*Total flow (air + oxygen) = O$_2$ input flow (L/min) × total ratio parts.			

Because entrainment devices dilute oxygen with air, they always provide less than 100% O_2. Moreover, *the higher the delivered O_2% from an entrainment device, the lower its total output low* (Table 4-5). For example, at the 60% setting, an entrainment device with a 10 L/min O_2 input produces only 20 L/min total output flow, which may not be sufficient to meet some patients' inspiratory flow demands. In this case, additional air dilution would occur and the FIO_2 would become variable. You can observe this problem on some patients receiving O_2 therapy via an air-entrainment nebulizer when the mist disappears from the mask or T-tube port(s) during inspiration, indicating air dilution. In this situation, what is labeled as a high-flow system becomes a low-flow system, delivering a variable FIO_2.

Because patients' inspiratory flows vary greatly, *the best way to ensure a stable FIO_2 is to provide a total flow of at least 40 L/min.* As indicated in Table 4-5, for an input flow of 10 L/min, this occurs only at or below the 40% O_2 settings. Total output flow can be boosted somewhat by increasing the O_2 input flow, although this flow is limited by the back-pressure created at the jet, typically to 12–15 L/min.

An alternative high-flow approach that does not depend on air entrainment is the *high-flow nasal cannula*. This device typically includes a blender to mix air and O_2, a high-flow flowmeter, a heated humidification system, an O_2 sensor, and a heated delivery system to prevent condensation. By providing warm, humidified gas to the airway, a high-flow nasal cannula overcomes the discomfort experienced with high flows delivered via a standard cannula. The higher flows (up to 40 L/min in adults) minimize air dilution, yielding moderate to high FIO_2s. As an added benefit, high-flow nasal cannulas increase the efficiency of ventilation by "washing out" CO_2 from the upper airway deadspace. **Table 4-6** provides the approximate FIO_2s that high-flow nasal cannulas can provide to adults at various flows.

Because high-flow cannula humidifiers employ sensors and alarm indicators like those used with ventilator humidifiers, troubleshooting these devices is also similar. Note that a low-temperature alarm often occurs temporarily when the water reservoir is changed. A persistent high-temperature warning is more serious and generally requires that the device be discontinued or replaced. *If no replacement is available, you should substitute an O_2 modality that matches the high-flow system's FIO_2 as closely as possible—for example, a nonrebreathing mask if delivering a high FIO_2.* Additional serious alarms requiring your immediate attention are those signaling an out-of-range O_2%, failure of the gas supply, or empty water reservoir.

O_2 Therapy Enclosures

O_2 enclosures constitute a separate category of O_2-delivery systems. Generally you use O_2 enclosures only with infants and children. **Table 4-7** provides a summary of these devices, including their flow settings, advantages, disadvantages, and best use.

Infant Environmental Control via Isolette or Warmer (RRT-Specific Content)

Environmental control of both temperature and humidity is indicated for any newborn infant whose gestational age is less than 32 weeks or whose birth weight is less than 1500 g. Because it provides control of both temperature and humidity, the isolette is the preferred environmental control system for these infants. In contrast, if the infant requires frequent handling or is attached to multiple support systems (e.g., ventilator, IV lines, hemodynamic monitors), a semi-open radiant warmer can be used, with supplemental O_2 provided via oxyhood. To reduce insensible water loss, most infants in

Table 4-6 Approximate Adult FIO_2 Provided by High-Flow Nasal Cannulas

Flow (100% O_2)	Approximate FIO_2
10 L/min	60%
15 L/min	80%
20 L/min	90%
30 L/min	95%

Table 4-7 Oxygen Therapy Enclosure Systems

Device	Flow	FIo₂ Range	Advantages	Disadvantages	Best Use
Oxyhood	≥ 7 L/min	21–100%	Full range of FIo₂s	• Difficult to clean, disinfect	For infants requiring supplemental oxygen
Isolette	8–15 L/min	40–50%	Provides temperature control	• Expensive, cumbersome • Unstable FIo₂ (leaks) • Difficult to clean, disinfect • Limits patient mobility • Fire hazard	For infants requiring supplemental oxygen and precise thermal regulation
Tent/croupette	12–15 L/min	40–50%	Provides concurrent aerosol therapy	• Expensive, cumbersome • Unstable FIo₂ (leaks) • Requires cooling • Difficult to clean, disinfect • Limits patient mobility • Fire hazard	For toddlers or small children requiring low to moderate FIo₂s and bland aerosol

Adapted from: Wilkins RL, Stoller JK, Scanlan CL. *Egan's fundamentals of respiratory care* (8th ed.). St. Louis, MO: Mosby; 2003.

radiant warmers are wrapped in a Saran blanket, which minimizes evaporation from the body surface. The accompanying box specifies key elements in setting up a newborn infant in an isolette or radiant warmer.

Setting Up a Newborn Infant in an Isolette or Radiant Warmer

- Prewarm the unit to 35°C or the infant's neutral thermal environment temperature (NTE).
- If using an isolette, attach and fill the humidity reservoir with sterile water.
- Set the F_{IO_2} to the prescribed level via the isolette servo-controller or oxyhood blender.
- Set the isolette humidity to the prescribed level or 70–80% to start (if condensation occurs, reduce in 2–5% increments until the problem resolves).
- Place the infant in the unit after warm-up is complete.
- Place and secure the temperature probe on the infant's upper abdomen (use a reflective cover with a radiant warmer).
- Set the high/low alarms for temperature (± 1°C above/below the servo setting), humidity, and F_{IO_2}.
- Set the temperature control to servo mode and the target temperature to 36.5°C.
- Assess temperature stability after 15 minutes.
- Recheck the infant's axillary temperature every 15 to 30 minutes until it is within normal limits.
- Monitor for heat loss during procedures; keep the isolette portholes closed whenever possible.
- When phototherapy is in use, monitor for temperature changes and adjust as needed.
- Reposition the temperature probe every 24 hours and as needed.

O_2 Device Selection

In general, sicker patients require higher and more stable F_{IO_2}s, whereas less acutely ill patients usually can be managed with lower, less exact F_{IO_2}s. **Table 4-8** provides guidance in selecting an O_2-delivery system based on these factors.

A high-flow cannula (at 1–8 L/min) can be used as an alternative to an oxyhood in infants requiring controlled O_2 therapy. Besides controlling the F_{IO_2}, high-flow cannulas also may produce variable amounts of CPAP, which can benefit some neonates. CPAP pressures created with high-flow cannulas vary directly with the flow and inversely with the amount of nasal leakage, generally ranging from 2 to 6 cm H_2O.

Table 4-8 Selecting an Oxygen Administration Device Based on Desired F_{IO_2} and Stability

Desired O₂%	Needed Stability in Delivered O₂%	
	Stable/Fixed	**Variable**
Low (< 35%)	• Air-entrainment mask • Air-entrainment nebulizer • High-flow cannula	• Standard nasal cannula • Tent/croupettes (child) • Isolette (infant)
Moderate (35–60%)	• Air-entrainment nebulizer • High-flow cannula	• Simple mask • Isolette (infant) • Tent/croupettes (child)
High (> 60%)	• Multiple air-entrainment nebulizers in parallel • Oxyhood (infant) • High-flow cannula	• Partial rebreathing mask • Nonrebreathing mask

Adapted from: Wilkins RL, Stoller JK, Scanlan CL. *Egan's fundamentals of respiratory care* (8th ed.) St. Louis, MO: Mosby; 2003.

Most small children needing a low to moderate F_{IO_2} can accept a standard nasal cannula, to be used in conjunction with a *calibrated low-flow flowmeter*. If the child cannot tolerate a cannula, you may need to recommend using an O_2 tent/croupette. Providing high F_{IO_2}s to small children can be difficult, because they often do not tolerate masks. If they can tolerate a cannula, consider using a high-flow cannula system at 5–20 L/min to provide the high F_{IO_2}.

Table 4-9 applies these concepts to the selection of specific O_2 systems in a variety of common clinical scenarios you are likely to see on NBRC exams.

O_2 Device Troubleshooting

All O_2-delivery systems should be checked at least once per day. More frequent checks with an O_2 analyzer should be performed in systems susceptible to fluctuations in F_{IO_2} or when applied to unstable patients, those with ET or tracheal tubes, or those requiring high F_{IO_2}s.

Table 4-10 summarizes the most common problems with low-flow O_2-therapy devices, along with their causes and potential solutions.

Table 4-11 summarizes the most common problems with high-flow O_2 therapy devices, along with their causes and potential solutions. Note that obstructing an entrainment device's output flow *decreases* air entrainment, resulting in a higher delivered O_2 concentration but a lower overall flow, with an unpredictable effect on the patient.

The primary problems with O_2 therapy enclosures are (1) inability to maintain the desired F_{IO_2} and (2) temperature regulation. If an enclosure's O_2 level is lower than expected, check for and correct any major leaks and ensure that the flow is sufficient to maintain the desired O_2%. If an infant or child must be removed from an O_2 enclosure for a procedure, provide an equivalent O_2% via an alternative device, such as a simple mask.

Overheating of infants in enclosures can cause dehydration, while underheating can cause cold stress, increased O_2 consumption, and apnea. To ensure a neutral thermal environment in an oxyhood, you should use a servo-controlled heated humidifier with appropriate temperature alarms. Because tents and croupettes impair radiant heat loss, these devices must be cooled, usually via

Table 4-9 Example O_2 Device Selection Scenarios

Patient Scenario	Recommended O_2-Delivery System
A stable adult medical patient needing a low to moderate F_{IO_2}	Nasal cannula, 1–6 L/min
A patient admitted to the emergency department with chest pain and a suspected MI	Nonrebreathing mask, > 10 L/min *or* high-flow nasal cannula ($\geq$ 20 L/min)
A patient just extubated from ventilatory support on 30% O_2	Air-entrainment nebulizer and aerosol mask
An unstable COPD patient requiring a precise low F_{IO_2}	Air-entrainment mask, 24% or 28%
A postoperative patient with an ET tube requiring a moderate F_{IO_2}	Air-entrainment nebulizer and T-tube with open reservoir *or* high-flow nasal cannula ($\leq$ 20 L/min)
A stable postoperative patient with a tracheostomy tube needing low F_{IO_2}	Air-entrainment nebulizer, 30–35%, and tracheostomy collar
An ICU patient with a high minute volume needing high F_{IO_2} (intact upper airway)	Two air-entrainment nebulizers in parallel with aerosol mask *or* high-flow nasal cannula ($\geq$ 30 L/min)
A stable 2-year-old child needing a low F_{IO_2}	Nasal cannula ¼–2 L/min with calibrated low-flow flowmeter
An infant requiring short-term supplemental O_2	Simple O_2 mask
An infant requiring high F_{IO_2} and temperature control	Oxyhood with servo-controlled heated humidification system *or* high-flow nasal cannula (1–8 L/min)
A small child requiring moderate F_{IO_2} and bland aerosol	Croup tent with supplemental O_2

Table 4-10 Troubleshooting Common Problems with Low-Flow O$_2$ Therapy Devices

Problem/Clue	Cause(s)	Solution
Nasal Cannulas		
No gas flow can be felt coming from the cannula	Flowmeter not on	Adjust flowmeter as needed
	System leak	Check connections
	Humidifier down tube is obstructed	Repair or replace device
Humidifier pop-off sounding	Obstruction distal to humidifier	Find and correct obstruction
	Flow set too high	Lower flow
	Obstructed naris	Use alternative O$_2$ appliance
Patient complains of soreness over lip or ears	Irritation/inflammation due to appliance straps/loops	Loosen straps
		Place cotton balls at pressure points
		Use an alternative device
Masks		
Patient constantly removes mask	Claustrophobia	Use an alternative device
	Confusion	Restrain or sedate patient
No gas flow detected	Flowmeter not on	Adjust flowmeter as needed
	System leak	Check connections
Humidifier pop-off sounding	Obstruction distal to humidifier	Find and correct obstruction
	High input flow	Omit humidifier (short term)
	Jammed inspiratory valve	Repair or replace mask
Reservoir bag collapses when the patient inhales	Inadequate flow	Increase flow
Reservoir bag remains inflated during inhalation	Large mask leak	Correct leak
	Inspiratory valve jammed/reversed	Repair or replace mask
Patient develops erythema over face or ears	Irritation/inflammation due to appliance or straps	Reposition mask/straps
		Place cotton balls over ear pressure points
		Provide skin care

a thermostatically controlled refrigeration system. Temperatures within such enclosures should be continually monitored and adjusted for patient comfort.

Of course, all O$_2$-therapy devices present a fire hazard, with O$_2$ enclosures being the most dangerous. To minimize the risk of fire, you must keep all electrical equipment out of the enclosure.

He/O$_2$-Delivery Systems (RRT-Specific Content)

Due to their reduced density, mixtures of helium with oxygen (heliox) can help decrease the work of breathing, especially in patients with large airway obstruction. Tanks of 100% helium are available, but require a blending system to mix the helium with O$_2$. However, were the O$_2$ source to fail in such systems, the patient could receive 100% He and quickly suffer from anoxia. For this reason, most centers use premixed cylinders in one of three common combinations: 80% He/20% O$_2$, 70% He/30% O$_2$, or 60% He/40% O$_2$. *To ensure patient safety, always use helium combined with at least 20% O$_2$.*

If the gas mixture is delivered by flowmeter, you must either use a device calibrated for the specified He% or apply a correction factor (1.8 for 80/20, 1.6 for 70/30, and 1.4 for 60/40). For example, for every 10 L/min of indicated flow on an O$_2$ flowmeter delivering an 80% He/20% O$_2$ mixture, the actual heliox flow is 18 L/min (10 L/min × 1.8).

Table 4-11 Troubleshooting Common Problems with High-Flow O_2 Therapy Devices

Problem/Clue	Cause(s)	Solution
Air-Entrainment Masks		
Patient's Sao_2 lower than expected	Inadequate total flow	• Increase input flow • Check for/correct any flow obstructions
	Inadequate O_2 concentration	• Switch to device capable of higher Fio_2
Patient complains of dryness	Inadequate water vapor content	• Use aerosol collar plus an air-driven nebulizer to increase humidification
Air-Entrainment Nebulizers		
Patient's Sao_2 lower than expected	Inadequate total flow (only for high O_2% settings, such as > 35–40%)	• Maximize input flow • Add open reservoir to expiratory side of T-tube • Connect multiple nebulizers together in parallel • Provide inspiratory reservoir with one-way expiratory valve • Set nebulizer to low O_2% and bleed in extra O_2 • Use a specialized high-flow/high O_2% generator
Delivered O_2% higher than set or expected	Obstruction to flow in circuit	• Drain tubing condensate • Check/correct kinking or other outlet obstructions

For spontaneously breathing patients, heliox generally is delivered via a tight-fitting nonrebreathing mask at a flow sufficient to meet the patient's inspiratory demands. Alternatively, you can deliver heliox using a high-flow cannula. Heliox mixtures also can be delivered to mechanically ventilated patients—both those with cuffed artificial airways and via the noninvasive route. Heliox, however, can alter ventilator performance. For this reason, only ventilators approved by the FDA for delivering heliox should be used. Even with approved ventilators, you may need to add special modules or use conversion factors to adjust settings.

Irrespective of the delivery method, all patients receiving helium–oxygen mixtures should be closely monitored, and an O_2 analyzer with active alarms should always be used to continuously measure the Fio_2 of the mixture provided to the patient. Details on providing/modifying heliox therapy are provided in Chapter 12.

Humidifiers, Nebulizers, and Mist Tents

A *humidifier* adds molecular water to gas via evaporation from a water surface. A *nebulizer* generates and disperses small particles of liquid into the air as aerosol. If the liquid is water or normal saline (bland aerosol therapy), such aerosols add water content to the inspired gas.

Humidifiers and Humidification

Three primary types of humidifiers are used: bubble humidifiers, passover humidifiers, and heat and moisture exchangers (HMEs). A bubble humidifier disperses small bubbles of gas through a water reservoir. A passover humidifier sends gas either directly over the water surface or over a wick or membrane. Both types of devices are considered *active humidifiers* and may incorporate heating elements and reservoir feed systems.

Many NBRC exam candidates have difficulty with questions related to humidifier output and condensation. The following are the key facts and concepts that you need to know to address exam questions about humidification systems:

- All modern humidifiers saturate the gas passing through them—that is, they achieve 100% relative humidity.
- The actual water vapor content (absolute humidity) delivered to the patient depends on two factors:
  - The humidifier's temperature (the higher the temperature, the greater the absolute humidity)
  - Whether the gas leaving the humidifier warms, cools, or remains at the same temperature
- Condensation in the delivery system occurs only if the gas cools on its way to the patient.

Figure 4-1 demonstrates these concepts in three delivery systems using (A) an unheated humidifier, (B) a heated humidifier, and (C) a heated humidifier with heated wires in the delivery circuit. Due to evaporative cooling, the unheated humidifier operates *below* room temperature (10°C). Although the gas leaving is 100% saturated, it has low water vapor content (about 10 mg/L). As it passes through the tubing, the surrounding room temperature *warms* the gas to 20°C. This increases the capacity of the gas to hold water vapor, but not its content. As a result, *no condensation occurs, and the relative humidity decreases* (to about 54%). Although this is adequate for patients receiving medical gases via the upper airway, it is not sufficient for patients with artificial tracheal airways.

For these patients, the simple solution is to add heat, which raises the water vapor content delivered to the patient (example B in Figure 4-1). However, now the gas leaving the humidifier will be *cooled* by the surrounding room temperature. To offset this cooling and achieve BTPS conditions at the patient's airway (100% relative humidity at 37°C), we must set the humidifier's temperature higher than 37°C—in this example, 45°C. *As this hot, saturated gas transverses the cooler circuit, significant condensation occurs*. If not removed, this condensate can block the tubing or be aspirated by the patient.

To prevent condensation when using heated humidifiers, we need to prevent cooling, normally by placing heated wires in the circuit. As shown in example C in Figure 4-1, the humidifier temperature can then be set to the desired airway temperature (generally 34–41°C). *As long as the heated wires maintain this temperature throughout the circuit, condensation will not occur, and the patient will receive the gas at or near BTPS conditions.*

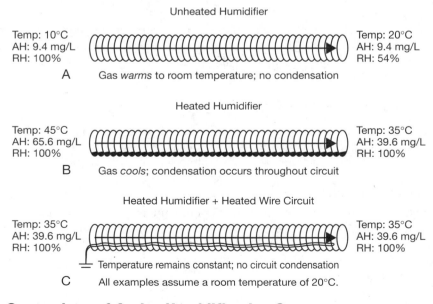

Unheated Humidifier

Temp: 10°C
AH: 9.4 mg/L
RH: 100%

Temp: 20°C
AH: 9.4 mg/L
RH: 54%

A   Gas *warms* to room temperature; no condensation

Heated Humidifier

Temp: 45°C
AH: 65.6 mg/L
RH: 100%

Temp: 35°C
AH: 39.6 mg/L
RH: 100%

B   Gas *cools*; condensation occurs throughout circuit

Heated Humidifier + Heated Wire Circuit

Temp: 35°C
AH: 39.6 mg/L
RH: 100%

Temp: 35°C
AH: 39.6 mg/L
RH: 100%

Temperature remains constant; no circuit condensation

C   All examples assume a room temperature of 20°C.

Figure 4-1 Comparison of Active Humidification Systems.

A simpler and less expensive solution to the problem of rain-out in ventilator circuits is to use a heat and moisture exchanger. Like the nose, HMEs capture a portion of the patient's expired water vapor via condensation and humidify the inspired gas via evaporation of this condensate. Because they require no heating or reservoir systems, HMEs are called *passive humidifiers*. However, because HMEs require *bidirectional flow* for proper function, their use is generally limited to humidifying gas in ventilator circuits. Details on humidification during mechanical ventilation are provided in Chapter 8.

Nebulizers

Devices used to generate bland aerosols include large-volume jet nebulizers and ultrasonic nebulizers. **Table 4-12** compares and contrasts these devices in terms of operating principles and best use.

Specialized high-output jet nebulizers are available to deliver bland aerosols into mist tents. Typically these devices generate higher flows and water outputs than those designed for application to the airway. Because heat buildup in enclosures is a problem, these systems always run cool (never heated).

Assembly and Use of Humidifiers and Nebulizers

Humidifiers and nebulizers either come preassembled or require minimal assembly. The following guidelines should help avoid most problems:

- Should any assembly be required, carefully follow the manufacturer's procedure.
- During any assembly, prevent contamination by avoiding contact with internal parts.
- If the device does not come prefilled, fill its reservoir with sterile H_2O.
- Use a compensated Thorpe-tube flowmeter to ensure accurate flows with jet nebulizers.
- Make sure all threaded components are properly seated and tightened.
- To help prevent obstruction from condensate when using a heated humidifier or nebulizer, use large-bore corrugated delivery tubing.
- Make sure that all tubing connections are snug.

Table 4-12 Operating Principles and Best Uses for Jet and Ultrasonic Nebulizers

Jet Nebulizers	Ultrasonic Nebulizers
Key Operating Principles	
• Produce aerosols via shearing of water into particles at a high-velocity gas jet	• Produce small (1–3μm), high-density aerosols using high-frequency sound waves
• Typically incorporate baffles to remove large particles from the suspension	• Need a separate source of carrier gas
• The low pressure at the gas jet can be used to entrain air, providing for increased flow and variable F_{IO_2}	• Sound-wave amplitude determines aerosol output (mg/min)
• Heating the water reservoir will increase total water output	• Aerosol density (mg/L) based on the ratio of amplitude to gas flow—the greater the amplitude and the lower the gas flow, the higher the density
Best Use	
• Patients with tracheal airways requiring long-term supplemental humidification	• Short-term application to patients with thick or inspissated secretions
• Short-term application to patients with upper airway edema (e.g., croup, post extubation) and to help thin secretions	• Single-treatment application for sputum induction—may use hypertonic saline
• Single-treatment application for sputum induction—may use hypertonic saline	

Troubleshooting Humidifiers and Nebulizers

Table 4-13 summarizes problems commonly encountered with humidification devices, along with their causes and potential solutions. **Table 4-14** provides similar information for nebulizers used to deliver bland aerosols.

Aerosol Drug-Delivery Systems

You use aerosol drug-delivery systems to administer medications to patients via the inhalation route. The common aerosolized drugs are covered in Chapter 10. Here we focus on the selection, use, and troubleshooting of aerosol drug-delivery devices, including small-volume nebulizers (SVNs), metered-dose inhalers (MDIs), dry-powder inhalers (DPIs) and electronic nebulizers—that is, compact ultrasonic nebulizers (USNs) and vibrating mesh nebulizers (VMNs). **Table 4-15** compares the advantages and disadvantages of these devices.

Table 4-13 Troubleshooting Common Problems with Active Humidifiers

Problem/Clue	Cause(s)	Solution
Bubble Humidifier		
No gas flow coming from the cannula	Flowmeter not on	• Adjust flowmeter
	System leak*	• Check connections
Humidifier pop-off sounding	Obstruction distal to humidifier	• Find/correct obstruction
	Flow is set too high	• Use an alternative device
	Obstructed naris	• Use an alternative device
Heated Humidifier		
Intermittent flow or "bubbling" in tubing circuit	Water vapor condensation	• Drain condensate (away from patient)
		• Place water traps in the circuit
		• Employ a heated-wire circuit
Airway temperature too high	Temperature set too high	• Reset to 34–41°C
	Abrupt decrease in flow	• Ensure proper flow
	Temperature probe not in circuit	• Insert temperature probe in the circuit
	Unit warmed up without flow through circuit	• Let temperature equilibrate with flow before application
	Unit failure	• Replace unit
Airway temperature too low	Unit not plugged in	• Plug unit into wall outlet
	Circuit breaker activated	• Reset circuit breaker
	Temperature set too low	• Reset to 34–41°C
	Cool water added to reservoir	• System will readjust
	Abrupt increase in flow	• Ensure proper flow
	Reservoir low or empty	• Refill/replenish reservoir
	Unit failure	• Replace unit
Loss of pressure (during positive-pressure ventilation)	Leak in unit or connections	• Check/tighten connections
		• Replace unit

*You can also use the humidifier pop-off to test an O_2 system for leaks. If you obstruct the system at or near the patient interface and the pop-off sounds, the system is leak free; failure of the pop-off indicates a leak.

Table 4-14 Troubleshooting Common Problems with Bland Aerosol Delivery Systems

Problem/Clue	Cause(s)	Solution
Large-Volume Jet Nebulizer		
Inadequate mist output	Inadequate input flow	• Increase input flow
	Siphon tube obstruction	• Repair or replace unit
	Jet orifice misalignment	• Repair or replace unit
Aerosol mist disappears during inspiration (T-tube or mask)	Inadequate flow	• Maximize input flow • Add open reservoir to expiratory side of T-tube • Connect multiple nebulizers together in parallel
Airway temperature too high or too low	Heat setting incorrect	• Adjust to ensure 34–41°C at airway
	Malfunctioning heater	• Repair or replace unit
Ultrasonic Nebulizer		
No "geyser" produced in nebulizer chamber	Unit not on or connected to line power	• Connect unit to line power and turn on
	Circuit breaker tripped	• Reset circuit breaker
	Amplitude set too low	• Increase amplitude/output
	Inadequate fluid level	• Ensure adequate fluid level
Misting in chamber but no aerosol delivered	Inadequate flow through chamber	• Increase flow through chamber
Aerosol density too high/low	Incorrect amplitude or flow setting	• Increase density by lowering flow and/or increasing amplitude • Decrease density by increasing flow and/or lowering amplitude
Patient's Spo$_2$ lower than desired	Lack of supplemental O$_2$	• Provide supplemental O$_2$ flow, adjust to provide desired Spo$_2$

Selection

Figure 4-2 outlines a general algorithm for selecting an aerosol drug delivery system for spontaneously breathing patients. As indicated in this figure, your first must determine the available formulations for the prescribed drug. Given that some drugs are available only in a single formulation (such as DPI only), your choice in these cases will be limited to that system. For example, Advair (fluticasone propionate and salmeterol) is available only in a DPI formulation, and both Cayston® (aztronam—an antibiotic used to treat *Pseudomonas aeruginosa* infection) and Ventavis (iloprost—a prostaglandin used to treat pulmonary hypertension) are approved for administration only via specific electronic (vibrating mesh) nebulizers. Given the cost and complexity of electronic nebulizers, their use generally is limited to administering formulations that require them and for delivery of these drugs to patients receiving mechanical ventilation. Details on aerosol drug delivery to patients via mechanical ventilation circuits are provided in the later section "Ventilators, CPAP Devices, and Breathing Circuits."

If multiple formulations of a medication are available, you should assess the patient to determine the best delivery system. In general, SVN administration should be reserved for acutely ill adults who cannot use either a DPI or an MDI. Most infants and small children should receive

Table 4-15 Advantages and Disadvantages of Aerosol Drug-Delivery Systems

Advantages	Disadvantages
MDI	
• Convenient	• Patient activation/coordination required
• Low cost	• High percentage of pharyngeal deposition
• Portable	• Has potential for abuse
• No drug preparation required	• Difficult to deliver high doses
• Difficult to contaminate	• Not all medications formulated for MDI delivery
MDI with Valve Holding Chamber or Spacer	
• Less patient coordination required	• More complex for some patients
• Less pharyngeal deposition	• More expensive than MDI alone
• No drug preparation	• Less portable than MDI alone
	• Not all drugs formulated for MDI delivery
DPI	
• Less patient coordination required	• Requires high inspiratory flow
• Breath activated	• Some units are single dose
• Breath hold not required	• Can result in pharyngeal deposition
• Can provide accurate dose counts	• Not all medications formulated for DPI delivery
	• Difficult to deliver high doses
	• Cannot be used for drug delivery during mechanical ventilation
SVN (Jet Nebulizer)	
• Less patient coordination required	• Wasteful (large residual volume)
• Can provide high doses/continuous therapy	• Drug preparation required
• Nebulizes both solutions and suspensions	• Contamination possible if not cleaned carefully
• Inexpensive/disposable	• Not all medications formulated for SVN delivery
	• Pressurized gas source required
	• Long treatment times
Electronic Drug Nebulizers (Compact Ultrasonic and Vibrating Mesh Devices)	
• Create a fine-particle mist that is ideal for lower respiratory tract delivery	• Expensive
• Do not require propellants/compressor system	• Prone to electrical or mechanical failure; requires backup
• Small residual volume/less waste	• Batteries need to be replaced/recharged periodically
• Small, silent, and portable	• Patients need training in device assembly/disassembly
• Can aerosolize small volumes, eliminating need for diluent (may require dose reduction)	• Aerosol production can be position dependent
• Adds no flow/volume to ventilator circuit	• Vibrating mesh plates require regular cleaning and have limited life span/require replacement
• Fast nebulization rate/shorter duration of treatments	• Ultrasonic not recommended for aerosolizing suspensions and transducer heat can degrade some drugs

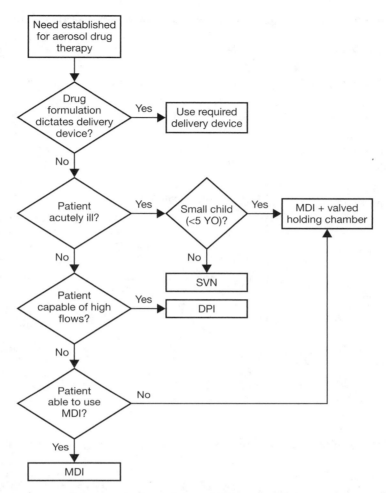

Figure 4-2 Basic Selection of Aerosol Drug-Delivery Devices for Spontaneously Breathing Patients. In many cases, the drug formulation will dictate the choice. Otherwise, assessment of the patient's acuity, age, inspiratory flows, and ability to properly use an MDI will determine the best device to use on a patient. If several different devices qualify, patient preference should be the deciding factor.

aerosolized drugs via an MDI with a holding chamber and mask (an SVN is an alternative if tolerated). If an adult who is not acutely ill has difficulty properly coordinating MDI actuation with breathing, you should consider adding a holding chamber. A breath-actuated MDI is an alternative for such patients. Patients prescribed steroids by MDI should use either a spacer or a holding chamber to minimize pharyngeal deposition. DPIs are ideal for maintenance therapy in outpatient adults, larger children, and adolescents who can generate sufficient inspiratory flow to carry the powder into the lungs.

Assembly and Use

With the exception of the electronic nebulizers, most aerosol delivery devices come preassembled. **Table 4-16** highlights what you need to do when assembling and checking the operation of MDIs, DPIs, and SVNs. Electronic nebulizers should be assembled, disassembled, and cleaned strictly according to the manufacturer's specifications.

Aerosol drug delivery is both patient and device dependent. **Table 4-17** outlines the optimal technique and key therapeutic issues involved in spontaneously breathing patients' use of the common aerosol delivery devices.

Table 4-16 Assembly and Operational Check of Aerosol Delivery Devices

Small-Volume Nebulizer	Metered-Dose Inhaler	Dry-Powder Inhaler
• Select a mask or mouthpiece (use a mask if patient cannot use a mouthpiece)	• Check the expiration date; discard if expired	• Check the expiration date; discard if expired
• Connect the SVN to mask or T-tube	• Inspect the canister outlet and boot for any dirt or foreign objects	• Confirm sufficient remaining doses (if multidose system)
• If using a T-tube, connect mouthpiece and reservoir tube	• If needed, rinse the canister outlet and boot in warm, running water; air dry	• Inspect outlet for dirt or caked powder—use dry cloth or small brush to wipe away; *never use water*
• Connect gas-delivery tubing to nebulizer input	• Warm the canister in your hand, then shake vigorously	• Remove any mouthpiece cap
• Connect gas-delivery tubing to flowmeter/compressor	• Fit the canister firmly in its boot, and remove the boot cap	• Load the dose of medicine (usually by moving a lever or twisting a knob until it clicks)
• Aseptically place drug and diluent in SVN reservoir (4 mL fill volume is ideal)	• If the canister is new or has not been used in a while, test spray it into the air	• Keep mouthpiece in horizontal position to avoid loss of drug
• Turn flowmeter/compressor on and set to recommended flow/pressure	• Confirm proper patient technique	• Confirm proper patient technique
• Confirm adequate aerosol production	• After administration, disassemble apparatus and recap mouthpiece	• After administration, recap mouthpiece and store at room temperature in a dry place
• After administration, rinse SVN with sterile water, blow dry with gas source, and store aseptically in plastic bag		

Table 4-17 Optimal Technique and Therapeutic Issues in Using Aerosol Delivery Devices

Optimal Technique	Therapeutic Issues
Metered-Dose Inhaler for Beta₂ Agonists, Steroids, Cromolyn Sodium, and Anticholinergics	
• Patient should open mouth wide and keep tongue down	• Young children and the elderly may have difficulty coordinating inhalation with device actuation
• Actuate during 3- to 5-sec deep inhalation, followed by 10-sec breath hold	• Patients may incorrectly stop inhalation at actuation
• Holding MDI 2 inches away from open mouth may enhance lung deposition	• To reduce the amount of drug swallowed and absorbed systemically, patients should rinse the mouth with water
• Use closed-mouth method only if (1) patient cannot use open-mouth technique, (2) a spacer is not available, and (3) the drug is not a steroid	
Spacer or Valved Holding Chamber (VHC) for Use with MDIs	
• Slow (30 L/min or 3–5 sec) deep inhalation, followed by 10-sec breath hold immediately following actuation	• Indicated for patients having difficulty properly using an MDI
• Actuate only once into the spacer/VHC per inhalation	• Simple spacers still require coordinated actuation; VHCs are preferred
• Face mask (if used) should fit snugly and allow 3–5 breaths/actuation	• A face mask allows MDIs to be used with small children but reduces lung deposition by 50%
• Rinse plastic VHCs once a month in water with diluted dishwashing detergent and let air dry	• Because spacers and VHCs decrease oropharyngeal deposition, they can help reduce the risk of topical side effects such as thrush
	• Use antistatic VHCs or rinse plastic nonantistatic VHCs with dilute household detergents to enhance efficacy and delivery to the lungs

Table 4-17 Optimal Technique and Therapeutic Issues in Using Aerosol Delivery Devices (*continued*)

Optimal Technique	Therapeutic Issues
Breath-Actuated MDI for Beta₂ Agonists	
• Maintain a tight seal around the mouthpiece and slightly more rapid inhalation than with a standard MDI, followed by a 10-sec breath hold	• Useful for patients who cannot coordinate inhalation with actuation, such as the elderly • Patients may incorrectly stop inhalation at actuation • Cannot be used with spacers or VHCs
Dry-Powder Inhaler for Beta₂ Agonists, Steroids, and Anticholinergics	
• Do not use with a spacer or VHC • Lips must be tightly sealed around the mouthpiece to avoid loss of drug • After loading, most DPIs must be held horizontal to avoid loss of drug • Requires rapid (60 L/min or 1–2 sec), deep inhalation • Patient must exhale to room (not back into device) • Children younger than 4 years may not generate sufficient flow to use this device	• Dose is lost if patient exhales into the device after loading • Exhaling into device may cause clogging due to moisture caking and powder residue • Rapid inhalation increases deposition in large airways • To reduce amount of drug absorbed systemically, patient should rinse mouth with water • The device should never be washed or rinsed in water • Between uses, the device should always be stored with the cap on in a dry place
Small-Volume Nebulizer for Beta₂ Agonists, Steroids, Cromolyn Sodium, and Anticholinergics	
• Slow tidal breathing with occasional deep breaths • Use a tightly fitting face mask for those patients who are unable to use a mouthpiece • Avoid using the "blow-by" technique (i.e., holding the mask or open tube near the infant's nose and mouth)	• Less dependent on the patient's coordination and cooperation • As effective as MDI + VHC for bronchodilators delivery to patients with mild to moderate exacerbations of asthma • Method of choice for cromolyn in young children • More expensive and time consuming than other methods • Output depends on device, fill volume, and driving gas flow • Use of a face mask reduces lung deposition by 50% • Bacterial infections can occur if the SVN is not cleaned properly

Troubleshooting

Most problems with MDIs and DPIs involve poor patient technique. With SVNs, the most common problem is inadequate aerosol production. **Table 4-18** summarizes the problems you are likely to encounter with aerosol delivery devices and their solutions.

Table 4-19 outlines the problems commonly encountered with electronic mesh nebulizers, including their causes and potential solutions. Note that the most common problem is clogging of the mesh plate with residual drug, which is easily corrected by cleaning the device according to the manufacturer's protocol.

Table 4-18 Troubleshooting Aerosol Delivery Devices

Metered-Dose Inhaler	Dry-Powder Inhaler	Small-Volume Nebulizer

• Poor patient response: check and correct patient technique
 	
• Empty canister (floats horizontally in water): replace with new canister
 	
• Cold canister: hand warm
 	
• Loose fitting in boot: reset
 	
• Failure to detach cap: remove
 	
• Obstructed outflow: remove foreign material or clean canister outlet and boot
	• Poor patient response: check and correct patient technique
	
	• Powder residue in outlet: clean with a dry cloth or small brush; make sure device is always stored with cap on in a dry place
	
	• Patient observes powder in air during use: confirm proper technique, especially DPI position (horizontal), tight lip seal, and exhalation to room (not back into device)
		• Inadequate aerosol production caused by:
		
		  ○ Inadequate pressure/flow: make sure the source gas is turned on and properly set (6-8 L/min)
		
		  ○ Leaks in delivery system: confirm that all connections are tight
		
		  ○ Inadequate fill volume: fill SVN to 4-5 mL
		
		  ○ Nebulizer malpositioned: reposition vertically
		
		  ○ Obstructed jet: replace SVN

Table 4-19 Troubleshooting Electronic Mesh Nebulizers

Problem	Cause	Solution
No visible aerosol when using batteries	Batteries inserted incorrectly	Insert batteries properly, being sure to match (+) and (−) poles
	Batteries low in charge (power warning)	Replace/recharge batteries or use AC power
	Cable from power unit to nebulizer not properly connected	Make sure that the cable is properly connected
	Mesh plate clogged with residual drug	Clean the device as per manufacturer's protocol
No visible aerosol when using AC power	AC power unit not correctly plugged into a working outlet	Insert the plug into a working outlet and verify that the power light is lit
	Cable from power unit to nebulizer not properly connected	Make sure that the cable is properly connected
	Mesh plate clogged with residual drug	Clean device as per manufacturer's protocol
No visible aerosol when power source is properly functioning	No solution in the medication reservoir	Fill reservoir with prescribed solution
	Mesh plate clogged with residual drug	Clean device as per manufacturer's protocol
	Nebulizer position preventing proper solution contact with mesh plate	Position unit according to manufacturer's specifications
Weak nebulization/ longer than expected treatment time	Mesh plate clogged with residual drug	Clean device as per manufacturer's protocol
	Batteries low in charge (power warning)	Replace/recharge batteries or use AC power
	Nebulizer unit has reached end of life span	Nebulizer unit may need to be replaced
Medication left over in unit after treatment	Batteries low in charge (power warning)	Replace/recharge batteries or use AC power
	Mesh plate clogged with residual drug	Clean device as per manufacturer's protocol
	Nebulizer unit has reached end of life span	Nebulizer unit may need to be replaced

Incentive Breathing Devices

Incentive spirometry (IS) involves the use of devices to assist patients in performing a sustained maximal inspiration—that is, a slow, deep breath followed by a breath hold. When used *together with* deep breathing exercises, directed coughing, early ambulation, and appropriate analgesia, IS may help lower the incidence of postoperative pulmonary complications, including atelectasis. The primary contraindication against IS is inability of the patient to perform the maneuver, with the primary hazard being hyperventilation.

Incentive spirometers are disposable devices that typically monitor flow, with some providing a volume accumulator. For adults, select a device that can accumulate at least 2500 mL, with lesser volumes being used for children. A high/low flow scale can help patients maintain the desired slow flow, while the volume accumulator can help estimate inspired volumes, which are needed for goal setting. For units lacking a volume accumulator, you estimate the volume by multiplying the flow times the inspiratory time. For example, if the patient sustains a flow of 700 mL/sec for 3 seconds, then the inspired volume would be 700 mL/sec × 3 sec = 2100 mL. Because most units come preassembled, you need only check for loose parts, proper tubing/valve connections, and free movement of the flow and volume indicators (by turning the unit upside down).

Given that IS normally is self-administered, good preliminary instruction is critical. Details on the use of IS are provided in Chapter 8. Following are some key points to consider when incentive breathing is ordered for a patient:

- Always use IS in conjunction with deep breathing exercises, directed coughing, early ambulation, and appropriate analgesia.
- Ideally, surgical patients should be provided with instructions and practice *preoperatively*.
- Instruction should establish reasonable goals, emphasize the value of breath holding, stress the need for frequent use (6–10 times/hour), and point out how to avoid hyperventilation by allowing recovery time between breaths.
- Patients who cannot follow instructions cannot benefit from IS; consider IPPB or IPV for these patients.
- If you need to accurately measure inspired volumes, attach a respirometer with a high-efficiency particulate air (HEPA) filter to the IS device.

After preliminary patient instruction and confirmation of proper technique, you should arrange for periodic patient visits to assess and adjust volume goals and provide additional instruction as needed.

Incentive breathing devices are simple and generally trouble free. Loose connections and improper positioning or functioning of one-way valves are the most common and easily correctable problems. If simple corrective action does not fix the problem, replace the unit.

Mechanical Devices Used to Aid Airway Clearance

A number of mechanical devices are used in conjunction with bronchial hygiene methods to aid patients in secretions clearance. These units include mechanical percussors and vibrators, oscillators, and positive expiratory pressure (PEP) devices. Because these devices all are used to aid airway clearance, they are covered in Chapter 9.

Resuscitation Devices

Resuscitation devices provide ventilation and oxygenation in emergency situations and during short patient transport. Three resuscitation devices are in widespread use: (1) self-inflating manual resuscitators (bag-valve-mask systems [BVMs]); (2) gas-powered resuscitators; and (3) mouth-to-valve mask resuscitators.

Resuscitation Device Selection

The following guidelines apply to the selection of resuscitation devices:

- BVMs are the standard and should be your first choice; select the correct size for the patient.
- Use a mouth-to-valve mask resuscitator to ventilate adults when a BVM is not available or fails.
- Consider a gas-powered resuscitator only for adults being ventilated via mask, and use only a manually triggered, flow-limited device.

Always select the appropriate BVM with the correct stroke volume and mask size. Typically, manufacturers provide four sizes: adult (≤ 800 mL), pediatric (≤ 500 mL), infant (≤ 300 mL), and neonatal (≤ 100 mL). Some pediatric, infant, and neonatal models provide a pressure relief valve to help avoid gastric insufflation and barotrauma.

A gas-powered resuscitator may be considered if the healthcare provider's small hand size or fatigue prevents adequate ventilation with a BVM. Note that malfunction or misuse of these devices can cause severe patient injury. To avoid such complications, select a unit that limits flow to 40 L/min and keeps pressures below 60 cm H_2O. Be sure to trigger the device manually during CPR; automatic triggering can generate high PEEP levels and impede venous return during chest compressions.

Resuscitation Device Assembly and Use

Most BVMs are disposable and need minimal assembly. Key considerations in their use include the following:

- Use an O_2 reservoir with a volume at least equal to the bag stroke volume.
- Connect the BVM to an O_2 flowmeter set to the maximum level allowed by the manufacturer; however, *never delay ventilation to obtain oxygen.*
- If the patient is not intubated, attach an appropriate-size mask to the standard connector.
- If needed, attach a PEEP valve to the expiratory port and adjust it to the desired level.
- For children and infants, monitor airway pressures via a manometer.
- Always test the device for proper function before application (see the discussion of troubleshooting).
- To ensure the highest possible F_{IO_2}, manually provide for slow refilling of the bag (if time permits).

Most mouth-to-valve mask resuscitators come preassembled. If not, assemble the device per the manufacturer's instructions. If the mask has an O_2 supply port, attach it to an O_2 source. *Never delay ventilation to obtain oxygen.*

Resuscitation Device Troubleshooting

Before applying a resuscitator to a patient, check it for proper function. For BVMs, follow these two simple steps:

1. Occlude the patient connector, and then squeeze the bag. If the bag has a pressure relief valve, it should pop off. If the bag does not have a relief valve, it should not be possible to compress the bag.
2. Squeeze the bag, and then occlude the patient connection. The bag should reinflate via the inlet valve, and any attached O_2 reservoir bag should deflate.

Failure of the first test indicates that either the nonrebreathing valve or the bag inlet valve is missing or leaking. Failure of the second test indicates that the bag inlet valve is jammed or positioned incorrectly. *If the BVM fails either test, replace it.* If no replacement is available, use a mouth-to-valve mask resuscitator or initiate mouth-to-mouth ventilation.

During BVM use, apply the following troubleshooting guidelines:

- If the valve jams open, check the input flow. If this flow is excessive, reduce it to the recommended maximum. If this step does not correct the problem, replace the device.
- If secretions or vomitus accumulate and jam the valve, replace the device.
- If a pressure pop-off continually activates, squeeze the bag more slowly. If this fails to lower airway pressure, consider potential causes (e.g., pneumothorax, endobronchial intubation) before overriding it.

As with BVMs, always check the function of a mouth-to-valve mask resuscitator's valve before use. If you can inhale through the device's one-way valve, the device is either misassembled or malfunctioning. Try quickly reversing the valve. If that does not work, replace the device. If no replacement is available, initiate mouth-to-mouth ventilation.

Artificial Airways

An artificial airway is required when the patient's natural airway can no longer perform its proper functions. Conditions requiring these devices include airway compromise, respiratory failure/need for ventilatory support, and the need to protect the lower airway.

Table 4-20 outlines the basic indications, key factors in selection and use, and troubleshooting considerations associated with the airways you will encounter most frequently.

In addition to these devices, you may encounter four other specialized tracheal airway devices: (1) fenestrated tracheostomy tubes, (2) "speaking" tracheostomy tubes, (3) speaking valves, and (4) tracheostomy buttons. **Table 4-21** outlines the basic indications, key factors in selection and use, and troubleshooting considerations associated with these devices.

Ventilators, CPAP Devices, and Breathing Circuits

Selection

Four key questions dictate choice of a ventilator device:

1. Which patient variables apply?
2. Where will the device be used and for how long?
3. How will the device be used?
4. Which added capabilities are needed or desired?

Table 4-22 provides common answers to these key questions and guidance on recommending the type of ventilator you should select for each circumstance.

Ventilators and CPAP Device Assembly and Use

Most ventilators and CPAP devices require little or no assembly. However, before applying a ventilator to a patient, you need to select and assemble the appropriate breathing circuit *and* confirm its operation. Ventilator and operational verification procedures are described in Chapter 6. Here we focus on the breathing circuit.

All ventilators and CPAP devices use an external circuit to move gas to and from the patient. Most adult circuits use large-bore corrugated tubing. Standard pediatric and neonatal ventilators use smaller-diameter, low-compliance tubing to minimize compressed volume loss. Most high-frequency oscillator ventilators also use smaller-diameter, low-compliance tubing, which is needed to ensure proper transmission of the pressure pulses going to and from the patient. All disposable circuits should come labeled with a compliance factor. This factor is used by computerized ventilators to compensate for compressed volume loss.

In addition, breathing circuits usually include either an active or a passive humidification system and can provide bacterial filtration and monitoring functions. Often the circuit also provides the mechanism to create PEEP/CPAP. Last, specialized oral or nasal interfaces may be incorporated into circuits designed for CPAP or noninvasive positive pressure ventilation (NPPV).

Table 4-20 Indications, Selection, Use, and Troubleshooting of Selected Artificial Airways

Indications	Selection and Use	Troubleshooting
Oropharyngeal Airways		

1. To prevent tongue from obstructing the upper airway during bag-mask ventilation
2. As a "bite block" in intubated patients
3. Generally contraindicated in conscious patients
	• Proper sizing: measure from the corner of the mouth to the angle of the jaw
	• Proper positioning: airway should curve over and extend past the base of the tongue
		• If airway obstruction due to the tongue is not relieved:
		  ○ Remove the airway, reinsert
		  ○ Recheck the size of the airway
		• If patient gags or retches, remove the device and maintain airway by positioning the head/neck; consider a nasopharyngeal airway as an alternative

Nasopharyngeal Airways		

1. To prevent upper airway obstruction when an oropharyngeal airway cannot be placed
2. To minimize trauma associated with repetitive suctioning via the nasal route
3. Contraindicated for infants and small children
	• Proper sizing: for an average-size female, select a #6 (24 Fr); for an average-size male, select a #7 (28 Fr)
	• When lubricated, the airway should fit through the inferior meatus without force
	• If too large, it can cause mucosal trauma, gagging, vomiting, and gastric distension
	• Always insert with the beveled side pointed toward the centerline
	• Use a safety pin to ensure that the airway does not slip into the nose
		• If you cannot pass the airway:
		  ○ Be sure the airway is lubricated
		  ○ Try the other nare
		  ○ Try a smaller airway
		• If a suction catheter will not pass:
		  ○ Lubricate the catheter
		  ○ Consider a larger airway

Endotracheal Tubes		

1. To establish and protect the airway against aspiration in emergency situations or with unconscious patients
2. To provide short-term positive-pressure ventilation (< 7 days)
3. To bypass an upper airway obstruction (may require tracheotomy)
	• Proper sizing is critical
	• Inflate cuff to confirm integrity before intubating; deflate fully and lubricate before insertion
	• Typical adult insertion length from tip to incisors: 19–21 cm for females and 21–23 cm for males
	• Always check position by breath sounds + CO_2 analysis; confirm with x-ray
	• See Chapter 8 for intubation procedure and Chapter 16 for assisting with intubation
		• Tube position (breath sounds)
		  ○ If breath sounds are not equal bilaterally, deflate cuff, withdraw tube 1–2 cm (adults), reinflate cuff, recheck
		  ○ If breath sounds are not heard or the stomach distends, remove tube and reintubate
		• Leaks
		  ○ If large leak occurs, reinflate cuff, recheck for leaks
		  ○ If leak persists, check pilot balloon, inflation line, and valve for leaks (bypass by inserting a small-gauge needle with three-way stopcock into the pilot line)
		  ○ If the inflation line system is leak free, cuff is likely blown; reintubate
		• Obstruction—follow the obstruction algorithm provided in Chapter 8

Laryngeal Mask Airways (LMAs)

Indications	Notes	Troubleshooting
1. As an alternative to ET intubation for emergency ventilatory support and airway control in or out of the hospital 2. To provide ventilatory support and/or airway control for patients who are difficult to intubate (high Mallampati classification) 3. Contraindicated in patients at high risk of aspiration	• Proper sizing is critical (infant/small child, 1–1.5; child, 2–3; adolescent/small adult, 3–4; adult, 4–6) • Prior to insertion, fully deflate mask cuff and lubricate mask rim and posterior surface • After proper positioning, inflate mask and confirm effective ventilation; do not exceed maximum volume	• If you need maximum inflation volume to seal, consider a larger mask • Malposition of the airway can cause obstruction or leaks—reposition the patient's head, readjust tube position, or adjust cuff inflation volume • A fiber-optic scope can confirm proper placement

Esophageal–Tracheal Combination Tubes

Indications	Notes	Troubleshooting
1. As an alternative to ET intubation for emergency ventilatory support and airway control in or out of the hospital 2. To provide ventilatory support and/or airway control for patients who are difficult to intubate due to trauma, bleeding, vomiting, or other factors obscuring the vocal cords 3. Available only for adults; contraindicated in patients with esophageal disease	• Proper sizing: 41 Fr for patients more than 5 ft tall; 37 Fr for smaller patients • Leak-test cuffs and then deflate before insertion • Insert until two black marks at the proximal end of tube are between upper incisors • Inflate distal white cuff (15 mL) and ventilate first through connector #2; good breath sounds confirm tracheal placement • If gurgling is heard over the epigastrium while ventilating via distal connector, tube is in esophagus; inflate proximal blue cuff (50–75 mL) and ventilate through connector #1	• If you cannot ventilate through either connector, tube may be inserted too far (proximal cuff obstructs glottis); to rectify, withdraw 2–3 cm at a time while ventilating through connector #1 until breath sounds are heard over lungs • Confirm tube placement via capnography

Tracheostomy Tubes

Indications	Notes	Troubleshooting

1. To provide long-term positive-pressure ventilation (> 7 days)
2. To bypass upper airway obstruction (when oral or nasal intubation is not feasible)
3. For patients needing a permanent artificial airway
	• Proper sizing is critical (see Chapter 8)
	• Inflate cuff to confirm integrity before intubating; deflate fully and lubricate before insertion
	• Confirm placement via x-ray
	• Be sure to secure neckplate/flange to avoid extubation; change disposable ties as needed for comfort and cleanliness
	• Make sure that a correctly sized spare inner cannula is kept at the bedside
	• See Chapters 8 and 16 for guidance on changing tracheostomy tubes and providing tracheostomy care
		• Leaks
		  ○ If large leak occurs, reinflate cuff, recheck for leaks
		  ○ If leak persists, check pilot balloon, inflation line, and valve for leaks (bypass by inserting a small-gauge needle with three-way stop cock into the pilot line)
		  ○ If the inflation line system is leak free, the cuff likely is blown; reintubate
		• Obstruction—follow the obstruction algorithm provided in Chapter 8

Table 4-21 Indications, Selection, Use, and Troubleshooting of Specialty Tracheal Airway Devices

Indications	Selection and Use	Troubleshooting
Fenestrated Tracheostomy Tubes		
1. To facilitate weaning from a tracheostomy tube 2. To support patients needing intermittent (e.g., nocturnal) ventilatory support	• Sized the same as regular tracheostomy tubes (see Chapter 8) • Proper placement confirmed by fiberoptic bronchoscopy • Outer cannula has fenestration (opening) above cuff • Removal of inner cannula opens the fenestration • Plugging tube after cuff deflation allows normal upper airway function • Remove plug to suction • To provide positive pressure or protect lower airway, reinsert inner cannula and reinflate cuff	• *Never plug tube with the cuff inflated (attach a warning tag to the plug)* • If respiratory distress occurs when tube is plugged, make sure cuff is deflated • If deflation of cuff does not relieve distress, tube may be improperly positioned; carefully reposition
"Speaking" Tracheostomy Tubes		
1. To allow patients with needing a tracheostomy tube to vocalize, even when receiving mechanical ventilation 2. For patients not needing a cuff for airway protection, consider a speaking valve instead	• Sized the same as tracheostomy tubes (see Chapter 8) • Include a separate small line that adds gas flow (4–6 L/min) to an outlet above the cuff, allowing patient vocalization • A "Y" connector controls when flow is applied • Cuff must be inflated for vocalization	• Leaks and obstructions are managed the same as a regular tracheostomy tube • Separately label gas supply and cuff lines to avoid mix-up (connecting cuff line to a flow-meter will burst cuff)
Tracheostomy Buttons		
1. To maintain an open stoma after tracheostomy tube removal 2. To facilitate weaning from a tracheostomy tube 3. To provide long-term access for suctioning of the lower airway	• Consists of a short cannula flanged at both ends • Exact insertion length controlled using spacers • Proper placement confirmed by fiberoptic bronchoscopy • A cap seals the button and forces the patient to use upper airway • Some buttons provide an adaptor for positive-pressure ventilation	• Regularly pass a suction catheter through button to ensure patency • If respiratory distress occurs, the tube may be protruding too far into trachea; reposition by changing number of spacers
Speaking Valves		
1. To allow patients with tracheostomy tubes/buttons and good protective reflexes to vocalize, swallow, and cough normally 2. Contraindicated for unconscious patients or for use with HMEs	• One-way valve allows inspiration through tube but blocks expiration • *When used with tracheostomy tubes, cuff must be fully deflated* • Always suction through tube and above cuff before attaching • To provide O_2, use a tracheostomy collar or an O_2 adaptor • If used with ventilator, select time- or volume-cycled mode and adjust alarms (expiration will not occur through breathing circuit)	• If patient experiences distress with valve and cuff deflated, likely causes are upper airway obstruction, secretion problems, or too-large tracheostomy tube; *remove valve immediately* • To prevent sticking due to dried secretions, valve should be cleaned daily in soapy water, rinsed, and air dried • Should not be worn during sleep because valve could become clogged and cause obstruction

Table 4-22 Selecting a Ventilator

Question	Answer	Recommended Device
Which patient variables apply?	Patient is an infant or small child	Ventilator certified for use on specific age group
	Patient has or needs an artificial tracheal airway	Standard multipurpose ICU ventilator; if artificial tracheal airway not needed, select a noninvasive positive-pressure ventilator
	Patient has severe expiratory airflow obstruction	Ventilator with variable flow control and adjustable I:E ratios
	Patient has hypoxemic respiratory failure only, adequate ventilation	Ventilator capable of high levels of PEEP and/or airway pressure release ventilation (APRV); if refractory hypoxemia, consider high-frequency oscillation ventilator
	Patient is candidate for weaning	Ventilator capable of SIMV, CPAP, pressure support, bilevel ventilation with capability to monitor spontaneous breathing parameters
Where will the device be used and for how long?	In the acute care setting	Standard multipurpose, pneumatically powered microprocessor-controlled ICU ventilator capable of volume or pressure control
	Home or long-term care setting	Electrically powered ventilator with volume-control A/C or SIMV
	For short-term transport	BVM or simple pneumatically powered transport ventilator (for long-term transport, consider an electrically powered ventilator capable of running on 12-volt DC)
	During MRI procedures	Pneumatically powered, pneumatically or fluidically controlled ventilator certified for MRI use
How will the device be used?	On critically ill/unstable patients	Standard multipurpose microprocessor-controlled ICU ventilator with graphics display
	On stable home or long-term care patients	A ventilator with vent-inoperative, high-pressure, and disconnect alarms
Which additional capabilities are needed or desired?	Advanced alarm and monitoring functions	Standard multipurpose microprocessor-controlled ICU ventilator with graphics display
	Data analysis/storage and programmability	Standard multipurpose microprocessor-controlled ICU ventilator with graphics display

Two general types of breathing circuits are used: (1) the dual-limb or "wye" circuit and (2) the single-limb circuit. Single-limb circuits may include a true expiratory valve or a leakage-type exhaust port. **Table 4-23** summarizes the appropriate use of these different breathing circuits. Due to their unique design, most high-frequency oscillators use more complex and proprietary breathing circuits (discussed subsequently).

Table 4-23 Appropriate Use of Common Ventilator/CPAP Circuits

Circuit Type	Appropriate Use
Dual-limb "wye" circuit	Most critical ventilators
	Continuous-flow CPAP circuit
Single-limb circuit with expiratory valve	Transport and home care ventilators
Single-limb circuit with leakage-type exhaust port	Noninvasive positive-pressure ventilators

Dual-Limb Circuits

Figure 4-3 shows a typical dual-limb "wye" circuit, the type most commonly used with critical care ventilators. It includes three basic components that together resemble the letter "Y": (1) an inspiratory limb that delivers fresh gas from the ventilator to the patient, (2) a standard 15-mm patient connector/swivel adapter, and (3) an expiratory limb that directs expired gas to the ventilator's expiratory valve or PEEP/CPAP valve. Additional components may include plug connectors for the heated wires, a pressure-sensing line, and ports for temperature probes.

Most critical care ventilators incorporate an *internal* electromechanical expiratory valve that closes when the machine triggers to inspiration and opens to allow exhalation. When linked to a pressure transducer and an electronic circuit, this valve also can regulate PEEP/CPAP by preventing expiration below a specific pressure baseline. Alternatively, when a dual-limb breathing circuit is used to provide continuous-flow CPAP, the expiratory limb is connected to a separate PEEP/CPAP valve, such as an underwater column or spring-loaded disk. In this case, you adjust the PEEP/CPAP level either by varying the depth of the water column (each centimeter = 1 cm H_2O PEEP/CPAP) or by adjusting the disk spring tension.

The mechanical deadspace or rebreathed volume in dual-limb circuits is that between the patient connector/swivel adapter (located at the "tail" of the wye) and the patient's airway. *Any tubing or device (such as an HME) added distal to this point will increase mechanical deadspace.*

Single-Limb Circuits

There are two types of single-limb circuits: (1) those with built-in expiratory valves and (2) those with leakage-type exhaust ports. **Figure 4-4** depicts a single-limb breathing circuit with a built-in expiratory valve, which is used with most transport and home care ventilators. These circuits have a separate pneumatic line running from the ventilator to the expiratory valve. When pressurized, the expiratory valve blocks gas outflow during inspiration. At the beginning of expiration, this valve depressurizes and allows expired gases to escape. By maintaining a set level of pressure throughout expiration, the expiratory valve also can provide CPAP/PEEP. The expiratory valve also may incorporate a port for the collection or monitoring of expired gases. *The mechanical deadspace in these circuits is that between the built-in expiratory valve and patient's airway.*

Figure 4-5 shows a single-limb circuit with a leakage-type exhaust port, as used with most NPPV ventilators. These circuits are very simple, consisting of a single section of large-bore tubing and an open exhaust port, usually in the form of either a small orifice or a set of slotted vent holes. The continuous flow that noninvasive ventilators provide forces expired gas out this exhaust port during exhalation. Combined with the leakage common to all NPPV interfaces, this simple setup prevents rebreathing of most expired gas, thereby minimizing mechanical deadspace. When provided, PEEP/CPAP is created by the continuous regulation of pressure and system flow/leakage via the ventilator's demand valve.

As indicated in Figure 4-5, a single-limb circuit with a leakage-type exhaust port also includes a pressure-monitoring line. This line connects the ventilator's pressure sensor to the main tubing at or near the exhaust port. *Proper connection of this pressure line is essential to ensure proper ventilator function.*

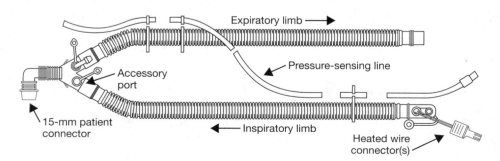

Figure 4-3 Typical Dual-Limb Heated Wire Ventilator Circuit.

Courtesy of: Strategic Learning Associates, LLC, Little Silver, New Jersey.

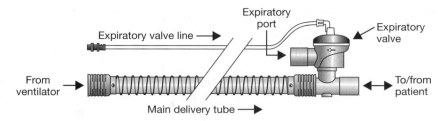

Figure 4-4 Single-Limb Breathing Circuit with Built-In Expiratory Valve.

Courtesy of Strategic Learning Associates, LLC, Little Silver, New Jersey.

Because many NPPV ventilators use a simple air blower to generate pressure, circuit modification may be needed to provide supplemental O_2. Typically this is done by placing a small-bore tubing adapter at either the patient interface or the machine outlet. After connecting this adapter to a flowmeter via small-bore tubing, you bleed O_2 into the circuit until the desired level is confirmed by O_2 analysis. Note that high O_2 flows can interfere with the proper triggering or cycling of some NPPV ventilators. For this reason, you should always follow the manufacturer's recommendations when considering how best to increase the F_{IO_2} of these devices.

High-Frequency Oscillation Ventilation Circuits (RRT-Specific Content)

Although several high-frequency oscillation ventilation (HFOV) devices are available, the CareFusion (Sensormedics) 3100A (for infants and children weighing less than 35 kg) and 3100B (for patients weighing more than 35 kg) models are the mostly commonly used for this mode of support. Details on the indications and application of HFOV are provided in Chapter 10. Here we focus on the HFOV circuit.

Figure 4-6 depicts the breathing circuit assembly of the CareFusion (Sensormedics) 3100B device. The basic configuration is similar to a simple "wye" circuit, with a continuous flow of heated, humidified gas (the "bias flow") provided to the patient via separate inspiratory and expiratory limbs. Gas in the patient circuit is oscillated via an electrically driven diaphragm at a selectable frequency between 3 and 15 cycles per second (Hz). Mean airway pressure is controlled by a pneumatic valve (the *control valve*) that provides variable resistance to outflow of gas from the circuit. Unique to this circuit are two additional pneumatic valves, both designed to ensure patient safety. The *limit valve* opens when the airway pressure meets or exceeds the ventilator's maximum pressure alarm setting. The *dump valve* activates when either the airway pressure rises above 60 cm H_2O or falls below 5 cm H_2O. When activated, this valve opens the entire circuit to ambient air, allowing the patient to breathe spontaneously at normal atmospheric pressure. As with many standard ventilator circuits, a pressure sensing port line is incorporated into the circuit as well as two temperature probe ports. Last, a water trap with stopcock is connected to the diaphragm for collection and removal of circuit condensate.

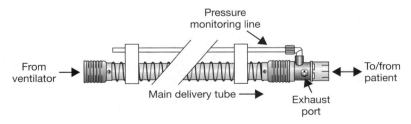

Figure 4-5 Single-Limb Circuit with a Leakage-Type Exhaust Port as Used with Common NPPV Ventilators.

Courtesy of: Strategic Learning Associates, LLC, Little Silver, New Jersey.

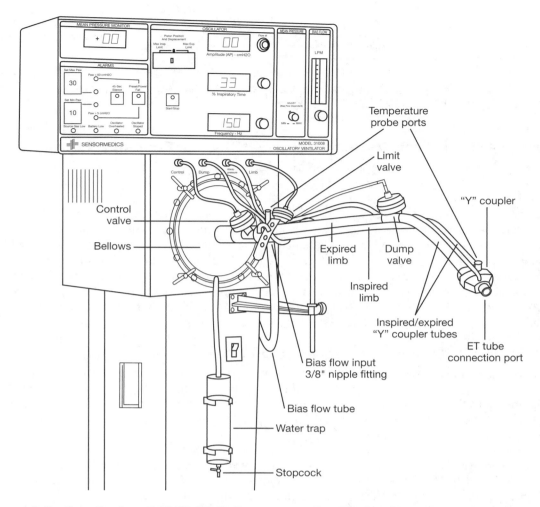

Figure 4-6 CareFusion 3100B High-Frequency Oscillation Ventilator Circuit.

Courtesy of: CareFusion Corporation.

NPPV Interfaces

NPPV circuits also include a patient interface. **Figure 4-7** depicts the three most common NPPV interfaces: the oronasal mask, the nasal mask, and nasal pillows. Oral mouthpieces/lip seals are used as well, primarily in the long-term care and home settings. In the acute care setting, the lower leakage associated with oronasal masks may make them the best choice for short-term treatment

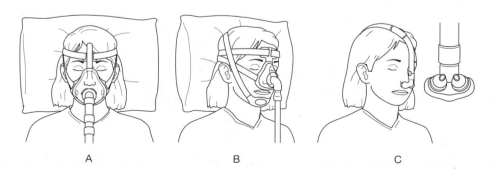

Figure 4-7 Common Noninvasive Positive-Pressure Ventilation Patient Interfaces. (A) Oronasal mask. (B) Nasal mask. (C) Nasal pillows.

of hypoxemic respiratory failure. However, for patients with hypercapnic respiratory failure, nasal appliances are preferred due to their lesser deadspace. Oral devices have proved successful in managing patients with chronic hypercapnic respiratory failure in need of intermittent support, such as those with progressive neuromuscular diseases.

Ultimately, the best interface is the one that the patient prefers and uses. Ideally, you should have several different interfaces available for the patient to try and use sizing tools to help customize the fit. Whichever device is selected, it must be positioned and secured well enough to prevent major leakage, yet remain loose enough to avoid discomfort or pressure sores. To avoid tissue damage during long-term usage, you may need to consider special cushioning materials or alternative devices.

Circuit Assembly

Proper circuit assembly involves connecting all components to the proper ventilator outlets and inlets and checking to confirm that all connections are tight and leak free. Generally, you connect the inspiratory limb to either a HEPA filter at the ventilator's gas outlet or to the outlet side of a heated humidifier. By trapping particles that are larger than 0.3 µm, HEPA filters help protect patients from bacterial contamination. Because condensation impairs performance, *HEPA filters must be positioned upstream of active humidifiers*. To prevent airborne cross-contamination, some ventilators also have an expiratory HEPA filter, *which must be heated to prevent blockage from condensation*.

Because the Sensormedics HFOV circuit is more complex, the three valve lines and pressure sensing port line are color coded. To prevent disconnection, all lines attach to their valves/ports using a Luer lock mechanism. Care should be taken not to crimp or perforate any of the lines, as this can cause ventilator malfunction. In addition, to avoid inadvertent circuit disconnection due to oscillatory forces and prevent condensate from reaching the patient's airway, the circuit must be properly supported and angled down to the diaphragm as per manufacturer recommendations. Last, prior to each patient use and whenever control valves are replaced, the circuit must be calibrated (see the "Circuit Testing/Calibration" section).

All patients needing ventilatory support via a tracheal airway require properly humidified gas, provided via either an active heated humidifier or a passive HME. To prevent condensate generated by heated humidifiers from obstructing flow, water traps can be placed at low points in the circuit. If a heated-wire circuit is used, the connector(s) must be plugged into the low-voltage outlets on the humidifier. *If an HME is used, it must be placed to ensure bidirectional flow, where it will always add some deadspace*. Details on humidification during invasive ventilatory support are provided in Chapter 10.

Circuit Testing/Calibration

After connection to a ventilator, all standard circuits should be tested for leaks. On a microprocessor-controlled ventilator, the leak test typically is conducted during the device's setup program. To run a manual leak test, trigger the ventilator to deliver a small volume (200–300 mL for adult ventilators) at low flow into a circuit that is occluded at the patient connector. If the resulting pressure readily exceeds the ventilator's pressure limit or can be held at a static level during an inspiratory pause, no leakage is present. If a leak is apparent, recheck all connections and repeat the test. If a repeat test also fails, replace the circuit.

The Sensormedics HFOV circuit requires calibration before application to a patient, using the following procedure:

1. Insert stopper at patient circuit wye.
2. Turn on source gas, set *Bias Flow* to 20 L/min and set the *Max Pressure* alarm to 59 cm H$_2$O.
3. Set *Mean Pressure Adjust* control to Max (full clockwise).
4. Push in and hold RESET button while observing the Mean Pressure digital readout (Battery Low LED will light when RESET button is pressed).
5. Adjust the *Patient Circuit Calibration* screw on the right side of the control package to achieve a pressure of 39 to 43 cm H$_2$O; do not overturn. If the specified pressure cannot be achieved, *locate the leak*.
6. Release the RESET button; the Battery Low LED should turn off.

Incorporating Aerosol Drug-Delivery Systems in Ventilator Circuits

Depending on the drug, available equipment, and protocol, you will use a small-volume jet nebulizer (SVN), metered-dose inhaler (MDI), or an electronic (ultrasonic or mesh) nebulizer to deliver aerosolized drugs to patients on ventilators. The following guidelines apply when incorporating aerosol drug-delivery systems in ventilator circuits:

1. If in use, remove HME before aerosol therapy begins (traps aerosol particles).
2. Bypass/disable active humidifier during drug delivery (dry gas improves lung deposition).
3. Use an *expiratory* HEPA filter to prevent drug residue from entering the ventilator.
4. Use an in-line spacer with MDIs.
5. In dual-limb circuits, place aerosol system in the *inspiratory* limb, 15–30 cm (6–12 in.) from the wye connector; in single-limb circuits, place it between patient and exhalation port.
6. Use manual (MDI) or automated means (SVNs or electronic nebulizers) to synchronize aerosol generation with the start of inspiration (for SVNs, synchronized flow from ventilator must meet manufacturer's specifications).
7. If continuous flow is used with an SVN, adjust ventilator volume or pressure limit to compensate (*need not be done with MDIs or electronic nebulizers*).
8. Upon completion of the treatment, remove nebulizer from circuit, reconnect humidifier or HME, and return ventilator settings and alarms to previous values.

PEEP/CPAP Valves

Most ventilators provide PEEP/CPAP via either an electromechanical valve type or a pressurized balloon/diaphragm. You do not normally select a PEEP/CPAP valve, as these devices are built into either the ventilator or its circuit. The exception is the underwater column-PEEP/CPAP valve, which can be used with any ventilator or circuit that separates out the patient's expired gases. Spring-loaded disk PEEP/CPAP valves also may be added to bag-valve-mask units to provide the desired elevation in airway pressure.

Troubleshooting Ventilator Circuits and Interfaces

Quality-control procedures can prevent or minimize most common problems with ventilators and their circuits. When problems do occur, they can be due to the ventilator, its circuit, or the patient. Because you must always attend to patient needs first, *when any major problem is suspected, immediately remove the patient from the ventilator and provide appropriate support using a manual resuscitator connected to an O_2 source*. If this action resolves the problem, you know that the ventilator or circuit was the cause, and can have others troubleshoot the system while you continue to support the patient.

Chapters 11 and 12 describe how you should respond to alarms and changes in the status of patients receiving mechanical ventilation. Here we focus on troubleshooting the ventilator circuit and related equipment.

The most common problems encountered with ventilator circuits include leaks, obstructions, expiratory/PEEP valve problems, humidification and temperature regulation problems, and infection/cross-contamination. Specific to NPPV are problems with the patient interface.

Leaks, Obstructions, and Expiratory/PEEP Valve Problems

Table 4-24 summarizes common circuit-leak, obstruction, and expiratory/PEEP valve problems that you may encounter, along with their relevant symptoms/clues and potential solutions.

Circuit leaks are among the most common problems causing loss of ventilator volume and pressure. However, ventilator malfunction can have the same effect. To distinguish a circuit leak from a ventilator malfunction, run a circuit leak test. If the leak test is negative, then the ventilator may not be delivering the preset volume. To determine whether a ventilator is delivering the preset volume, compare the volume setting to that measured *at the ventilator outlet* using a calibrated respirometer.

Circuit obstructions always are associated with low-volume and high-pressure alarms. Expiratory obstruction is the more serious of the two conditions, as it can result in rebreathing,

Table 4-24 Troubleshooting Common Ventilator Circuit Problems

Problem	Clue	Solution
Leaks	Low-volume + low-pressure alarm	• Check/correct loose circuit connections
Inspiratory obstructions (e.g., kinks, condensate, HME blockage)	Low-volume + high-pressure alarm	• Find/correct obstruction • Drain condensate • Replace HME
Expiratory obstructions (e.g., kinks, condensate, blocked exhalation port [patient, bedding])	Low-volume + high-pressure alarm	• Find/correct obstruction • Drain condensate • Prevent expiratory port blockage
Expiratory/PEEP valve malfunction	Open or leaking: • Low-volume alarm • Low-PEEP/CPAP alarm Obstructed/sticking: • High-pressure alarm • High-PEEP/CPAP • Expiratory flow impeded	Single-limb circuits: • Check expiratory valve line • Replace circuit Double-limb circuit with internal expiratory valve: • Replace ventilator

asphyxia, or barotrauma. The most dangerous type of expiratory obstruction occurs when the exhalation port on single-limb circuits becomes obstructed. To avoid this problem, you must prevent patients from grasping the circuit, and make sure that nothing obstructs the exhalation port, such as bedding.

Humidification and Temperature-Regulation Problems

To avoid humidification or temperature-regulation problems on mechanically ventilated patients with artificial airways, you must ensure that gas delivered to the patient's airway is carrying *at least* 30 mg/L water vapor. Most HMEs meet this standard, as long as the minute ventilation is not excessive and there are no expiratory leaks. Heated humidifiers also easily meet this requirement, typically delivering gas saturated with water vapor (100% relative humidity) to the airway at temperatures between 34°C and 41°C. However, because few humidification systems measure humidity levels, it is difficult to verify that these conditions are being met. *To ensure adequate humidification, always confirm that a few drops of condensation remain at or near the patient connection.*

Heated-wire systems pose a few additional problems, especially if the wire temperature is controlled separately from the humidifier. If the wires heat the gas in the circuit above the humidifier temperature, then the relative humidity of the gas decreases as it flows to the patient, which can dry secretions and cause mucus plugging. However, if the heating is insufficient to maintain temperatures equal to the humidifier outlet, then cooling and tubing condensation will occur.

Last, when heated-wire circuits deliver gas to infants under radiant warmers or in incubators, two temperature zones are created—that of the room and that of the incubator or warmer. This situation "confuses" the servo-control mechanism. To avoid this problem in radiant warmers, cover the temperature probe at the wye with a light reflective shield, which will minimize spurious radiant warming. If the infant is in an incubator, the position of the probe/wires varies according to the set temperature:

- If the incubator temperature is set to less than 32°C, the temperature probe should be placed at the circuit wye.
- If the incubator temperature is set to greater than 32°C, the temperature probe and heater wire portion of the circuit should be placed just *outside* the incubator, with an unheated extension delivering the gas into the enclosure.

Infection and Cross-Contamination

In heated humidification systems that do not use heated wires, the condensate is a potential source of nosocomial infection. Methods that can help minimize nosocomial infections associated with ventilator circuits include the following:

- Using HMEs or heated-wire circuits to eliminate condensate (not applicable to all patients)
- Changing circuits only when visibly soiled or malfunctioning
- Avoiding unnecessary disconnections—for example, for suctioning (consider an in-line/ closed suction system)
- Avoiding excessive condensate in the circuit and accidental drainage into the patient's airway
- Avoiding contamination during circuit disconnection or disposal of condensate

NPPV Interface Problems

NPPV patient interfaces are the last major area of ventilator circuit troubleshooting. **Table 4-25** summarizes the most common problems with these interfaces and their potential solutions.

Vacuum/Suction Systems

Airway suctioning is indicated for the following purposes:

- Removing accumulated pulmonary secretions
- Obtaining a sputum specimen
- Maintaining the patency of an artificial airway
- Stimulating a cough in patients who are unable to cough effectively

Table 4-25 Common Problems with Noninvasive Positive-Pressure Ventilation Interface

Interface	Problems	Remedy
Nasal masks	Mouth leakage	Use chin strap (see Figure 4-7)
	Discomfort	Refit, adjust strap tension, change mask type
	Nasal bridge redness, pressure sores	Reduce strap tension, use forehead spacer, use nasal pillows, use artificial skin
	Skin rash	Use steroid cream, switch mask type
Oronasal masks	Rebreathing	Use non-rebreathing (plateau) exhalation valve
	Impedes speech/eating	Permit periodic removal if tolerated
	Claustrophobia	Choose a clear mask with minimal bulk
	Aspiration	Exclude patients who cannot protect their airway; use nasogastric tubes for nausea/abdominal distension
Nasal pillows	Mouth leakage	Use chin strap
	Discomfort	Ensure proper fit, adjust strap tension, change mask type
	External nares redness, pressure sores	Clean/replace or use different-size pillows; reduce strap tension; temporarily use nasal mask
Oral devices	Dry mouth, throat, lips	Provide supplemental humidification; apply oral lubricant/ saliva replacement
	Numb lips	Extend the distance between lips and flange
	Gum discomfort	Try a smaller seal
	Device falls out at night	Tighten the holder/use a larger seal
	Nasal leak	Consider nose plugs
	Sore jaw	Discourage biting down on appliance; device should "float" in mouth
	Excessive salivation	Usually temporary/resolves after initial use

Table 4-26 Selection of Suctioning Devices

Question	Considerations	Recommendations
Where to suction	Oral cavity/nasal passages (newborn)	Choose bulb suction
	Oropharynx	Choose Yankauer tip
	Trachea	Select standard suction catheter
	Bronchus (right or left)	Use a Coude (curved) tip catheter
	Nasal route (frequent)	Consider nasopharyngeal airway
Patient size/age	Catheter diameter	Varies; apply formula
	Catheter length	Limit depth to just beyond the ET/tracheostomy tube tip
Patient condition	Meconium aspiration	Use meconium aspirator connected to ET tube
	Ventilator/PEEP	Use in-line/closed suction system
	Leakage aspiration	Consider continuous aspiration system
Goals	Airway clearance	Use standard systems
	Sputum collection	Use sputum collection (Lukens) trap

All suction equipment includes three components: (1) a negative pressure or vacuum source, (2) a collection system, and (3) a suction device for removing secretions or other fluids.

Negative pressure is provided by either a portable suction pump or a central piped vacuum wall outlet. You use portable suction pumps where wall vacuum outlets are unavailable, as in some ambulatory clinics, for patient transport, and in the home. Most portable suction pumps are electrically powered, by either line current or battery. Hand-powered portable suction pumps are available as well. You should select a battery- or hand-powered unit for transporting patients who may need suctioning.

Wall vacuum outlets are attached to a central piping system that connects to a powerful suction pump. To adjust the negative pressure, you use a regulator that attaches to a DISS suction outlet. Suction regulators can provide either continuous or intermittent vacuum. Use continuous vacuum for airway suctioning; intermittent suction is used mainly for gastrointestinal and surgical drainage.

Table 4-26 outlines the key considerations in selecting suction equipment and specifies the appropriate device given the circumstances.

Suction systems incorporate either a trap or float valve in the collection bottle to prevent aspiration of fluids into the suction pump or regulator. Before suctioning, always *confirm that the collection bottle is not full and the valve is not closed.* In addition, you should ensure that all tubing connections are tight, as any leaks will impair suction ability. Then turn the suction on, either by using the on/off switch on electrical units or by adjusting the wall regulator. To set the suction level, crimp the tubing coming from the collection bottle while adjusting the vacuum control and observing the negative pressure gauge.

Negative pressure should be set to the lowest level needed to readily remove the patient's secretions and flush them out of the tubing with water.

Table 4-27 provides guidelines for setting the initial negative pressure levels for suctioning adults, children, and infants using portable and wall suction systems.

Table 4-27 Guidelines for Initial Negative Pressure Levels

Patient Group	Portable Suction Pump	Wall Regulator
Adults	−12 to −15 in. Hg	−100 to −120 mm Hg
Children	−7 to −12 in. Hg	−80 to −100 mm Hg
Infants	−5 to −7 in. Hg	−60 to −80 mm Hg

After adjusting the vacuum pressure, connect the selected suction device to the system and implement the procedure. Chapter 9 provides details on procedures used to remove bronchopulmonary secretions, including suctioning. Following are a few additional equipment considerations:

- Any device used to suction the lower airways should initially be sterile.
- The external diameter of suction catheters should occlude less than 50% of the airway lumen in children and adults, and less than 70% in infants.
- To minimize contamination, hypoxemia, and potential lung derecruitment in patients receiving invasive ventilatory support, use a in-line/closed suction catheter system.
- To help prevent hypoxemia, pre- and post-oxygenate adult and pediatric patients by providing 100% O_2 for at least 30–60 seconds either manually (for spontaneously breathing patients) or via the ventilator; for neonates, increase the F_{IO_2} to 10% above baseline.
- Patients at high risk for hypoxemia during suctioning should by monitored by pulse oximeter.
- To help minimize trauma to the nasal mucosa in patients requiring frequent nasotracheal suctioning, use a nasopharyngeal airway.
- Suction catheters should be inserted only to just beyond the tip of the tracheal airway (*shallow suctioning*), a distance equal to the tube plus adapter length.
- Upon completion of closed suctioning, fully retract the catheter until the tip is visible in the sleeve, turn off the suction source, and lock the suction control valve in the off position.

Most problems with suction systems are identified through the preprocedural equipment check. If when crimping the tubing coming from the collection bottle you get inadequate suction, perform the following steps to correct the problem:

1. Make sure that the vacuum source is on.
   a. For a portable electrical pump, confirm that it has electrical power and that it is switched on (if the pump still does not run, check the fuse/circuit breaker).
   b. For wall units, make sure that the regulator provides continuous vacuum, that it is properly fitted to the vacuum outlet, and that its control switch is set to on.
2. Check for/correct leaks.
   a. Check all tubing connections for a tight fit.
   b. Check the seal between any bottles or traps with screw-on lids.
3. Check for/correct obstructions.
   a. Check all tubing for kinks or compression (e.g., bed wheels).
   b. Check whether any float valve is blocking the suction source.

If a leak appears due to the suction device itself (e.g., Yankauer tip, catheter) and cannot easily be corrected, replace the device.

Other than leaks, in-line/closed suction catheter systems are associated with two other problems: tracheal tube displacement and partial tube obstruction. To avoid tube displacement with these systems, *firmly grasp the airway connector when advancing or withdrawing the catheter*. To prevent partial tube obstruction, be sure to fully retract the catheter upon completing the procedure.

Pleural Drainage Systems

Pleural drainage systems remove free air and/or fluid from the pleural space via a chest tube. As depicted in **Figure 4-8**, all standard pleural drainage systems have three key components:

1. A one-way seal to prevent air from returning to the pleural space
2. A suction control for adjusting the negative pressure applied to the chest tube
3. A collection chamber for gathering fluid aspirated through the chest tube

Traditional pleural drainage systems like that shown in Figure 4-8 use a "wet" seal and suction control. Some newer units employ a dry seal and suction control. Here we focus on use of the traditional "wet" systems.

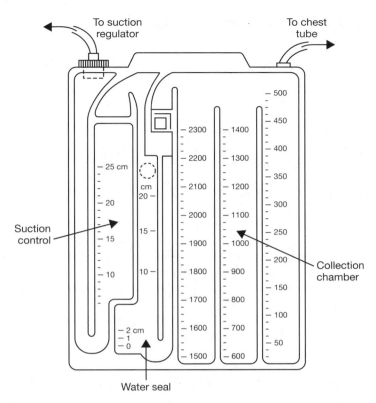

Figure 4-8 Traditional "Wet" Three-Chamber Pleural Drainage System.

Courtesy of: Strategic Learning Associates, LLC, Little Silver, New Jersey.

To assemble a pleural drainage system for evacuation of pleural air or fluid:

1. Aseptically open the package, being sure not to touch any tube connectors or internal surfaces.
2. Position the system *below the patient's chest level*, usually by hanging it on the bed frame.
3. Fill the water seal chamber with sterile water to the desired level, (usually 2 cm).
4. Fill the suction control chamber with sterile water to the desired level, usually 20 cm; make sure the vent is unobstructed.
5. Connect the collection chamber tubing to the chest tube, avoiding kinks or loops.
6. Connect the suction chamber tubing to the suction outlet.
7. Apply negative pressure until bubbling appears in the suction control chamber.
8. Ensure that the water seal chamber level rises and falls with patient breathing or ventilator cycle.

Once a pleural drainage system is operating, you should monitor the fluid levels regularly to ensure proper function:

1. If the water seal chamber level is less than 2 cm, refill it.
2. If the suction control chamber level is less than the prescribed suction level, refill it.
3. If the pleural fluid collection chamber fills, replace the unit with a new one.

If you need to transport the patient, make sure the system remains below the patient's chest level and *do not* clamp the chest tube. This will maintain the water seal and prevent any air from getting into the pleural space.

If there is no bubbling in the suction control chamber:

1. Check the suction control regulator to confirm that it is on.
2. Check the suction chamber tubing for connection leaks or obstructions/kinking; correct any problems.
3. Check the atmospheric vent to ensure that it is open and not obstructed.

If there is continuous bubbling in the water seal chamber, there is a leak either at the patient *or* in the drainage system. If the patient has a bronchopleural fistula and is receiving positive pressure, some air leakage is normal. Otherwise, you need to determine the source of the leak and correct it. To determine the source of the leak, briefly pinch the chest tube near its insertion point into the patient. If bubbling in the water seal chamber stops, the leak is at the insertion point or in the patient; if not, the leak is between the patient and the collection system.

1. For an insertion point or patient leak, immediately contact the physician. Patient leaks usually are due to either an outwardly displaced chest tube or an open insertion wound; use a sterile petroleum jelly gauze pad to temporarily stop insertion point leaks.
2. For a collection system leak, check and tighten all tubing connections, apply tape to temporarily seal any tears or holes, and prepare a new drainage unit.

If the water level in the water seal chamber does not fluctuate with breathing, the drainage system is obstructed. In these cases:

1. Check the collection chamber tubing for kinks or dependent loops; correct any problems if present.
2. "Milk" the tubing connected to the chest tube by compressing and releasing it along its length *toward* the collection chamber (do this regularly to prevent clotting or obstruction).
3. If milking the tubing fails to restore pressure fluctuations in the water seal chamber:
   a. Check the patient for signs of pneumothorax.
   b. Immediately notify the physician of the problem.

Should the patient exhibit clear signs or symptoms of pneumothorax, be sure to immediately notify the physician and obtain both a thoracentesis kit and a tube thoracotomy tray.

Manometers

A manometer measures pressure. Three pressure-measuring devices are commonly used in respiratory care: fluid columns, aneroid manometers, and electronic pressure transducers. **Table 4-28** describes each of these devices, along with their common applications and usage considerations.

With fluid columns, the measured pressure equals the height of the column, with the units based on the column scale and fluid. For example, when using a mercury barometer, the pressure is equivalent to the height of the mercury column in millimeters (mm Hg). Likewise, for a saline-filled CVP manometer, the pressure equals the height of the water column in centimeters (cm H_2O). The U-tube fluid manometer represents a special case (**Figure 4-9**). These devices are typically used as a calibration standard for mechanical manometers or electronic pressure transducers. As shown in Figure 4-9, you read the pressure as the *difference in height* between the two liquid levels.

The following key pointers provide guidance on selecting a pressure measurement device for specific tasks:

- To measure atmospheric pressure when calibrating a blood gas analyzer, use a barometer.
- To intermittently measure low pressures (MIP/NIF, cuff pressures), use an aneroid manometer calibrated in the units being reported.
- To continuously measure rapidly changing pressures, use a calibrated electronic pressure transducer.

Table 4-28 Types of Manometers and Their Clinical Applications

Device Description	Common Applications	Considerations
Fluid Columns		
Measure pressure as the height of a column of fluid with known density (i.e., water or mercury)	• To measure atmospheric pressure (barometer) • To measure static/slowing changing pressures (e.g., CVP) • To measure systolic/diastolic blood pressures (occlusion method) • To calibrate other pressure-measuring devices	• Most accurate measure of static pressures • Not suited for measuring rapidly changing pressures • Accuracy depends on position (must be vertical) • Can be messy/hazardous (mercury)
Aneroid (Liquid-Free) Manometers		
Measure pressure in a flexible chamber; changes in chamber size activate a geared pointer, which provides a scale reading analogous to pressure	• To measure blood pressures (occlusion method) • To measure airway pressure (e.g., ventilator pressures or MIP/MEP) • To measure tracheal tube cuff pressures • To measure gas cylinder pressures • To measure suction vacuum pressures	• Avoid the mess/hazards with fluid columns • Can display rapidly changing pressures • Not useful if measurements need to be stored or analyzed • Require calibration to ensure accuracy
Electronic Pressure Transducers		
Typical design ("strain gauge") measures electrical current changes that vary with its expansion and contraction of a flexible metal diaphragm	• To continuously measure rapidly changing pressures such as those in the blood vessels, at the airway or in a body plethysmograph	• Best for measuring rapidly changing pressures, including graphics display • Output can be digitized and stored for computer analysis • Require physical *and* electrical calibration

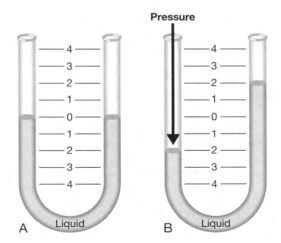

Figure 4-9 U-Tube Manometer. (A) At zero pressure relative to the atmosphere, the liquid levels on the two sides of the U-tube are equal. (B) When pressure is applied to one side of the manometer, the liquid is displaced. You read the pressure as the difference in height between the two levels. In this example, the difference in height is +2 − (−2) = 4 units.

- If pressure data need to be stored or analyzed, use an electronic pressure transducer and computer system.
- To calibrate either an aneroid manometer or electronic pressure transducer, use a U-tube fluid column.

To obtain accurate pressure measurements, the device you use must be properly calibrated. First, if the device measures pressure *relative* to atmospheric, it should read zero when open to ambient air. If not, either reset the device to zero or replace it. Second, the device must accurately measure the pressures that it will encounter. To do so requires *calibration*. To calibrate a simple aneroid manometer, you compare its readings to either a fluid column or a precision lab instrument designed for calibration verification. Calibrating electronic transducers is a more complicated process usually performed by biomedical engineers.

Accurate pressure measurements also require a leak-free system. When you assemble any pressure measurement system, you need to check and confirm that all connections are tight.

O_2, He, CO, and Specialty Gas Analyzers

Most RTs are skilled in monitoring F_{IO_2}s using portable O_2 analyzers. Details on the use and trouble-shooting of these devices are provided in Chapter 6. However, the NBRC also expects that RTs be familiar with other specialty gas analyzers. **Table 4-29** outlines the method employed, use, performance standards, and calibration considerations for all gas analyzers that you may encounter in practice.

The key consideration in selecting a gas analyzer is the response time. If real-time analysis is needed during breathing, the analyzer response time must be less than 500 msec. Also noted in Table 4-29 is the recommendation that essentially all gas analyzers undergo a two-point calibration before each use.

Bedside Pulmonary Function Devices

Devices used to measure pulmonary function at the bedside include mechanical "vane-type" respirometers and portable electronic spirometers. Use a mechanical respirometer to measure tidal volume, minute volume, inspiratory capacity, or slow vital capacity. Use a portable spirometer to obtain measures of forced expiratory volumes/flows.

Mechanical Respirometers

Mechanical respirometers, such as the Wright or Haloscale, measure gas volume via a rotating vane, with a gear mechanism translating these rotations into movement of indicator hands on a watch-like dial. An on/off switch unlocks and locks the gear mechanism, while a reset button zeros the indicator hands. *Measurements made with these devices are unidirectional, always being from device inlet to outlet.*

Mechanical respirometers generally are accurate to within 2% of their recommended flow range. Like any turbine system, however, these devices tend to over-read at high flows and under-read at low flows. Moreover, these devices are easily damaged by flows outside their recommended range. *For this reason, they should never be used to measure forced flows or volumes.*

Before each use, you should check the respirometer for proper function. To do so:

1. Inspect the device's inlet and outlet to make sure they are clean and dry.
2. Check the foil vane—if it is bent or damaged, send the device for repair.
3. Check for proper function by resetting the indicators to zero, turning the unit on, and then:
    a. Cupping the device in the palm of your hand, with the inlet unobstructed
    b. Gently blowing toward the device's inlet (the indicators should rotate smoothly)
4. Check the on/off control while the indicators are rotating.
5. Press the reset button to return the indicators to zero.

Table 4-29 Therapy and Diagnostic Gas Analysis

Gas	Analysis Method(s)	Usage	Performance Standards and Calibration Considerations

O_2	• Paramagnetic
	• Electrochemical:
	  ○ Galvanic cell
	  ○ Polarographic
	• ZrO_2
		• Bedside FIO_2 monitoring
		• Metabolic analysis ($\dot{V}O_2$)
			• For bedside monitoring (primarily Galvanic cell or polarographic sensors):
			  ○ Accuracy: ± 2% for bedside monitoring
			  ○ Response time: 90% of scale range in ≤ 20 sec
			• For metabolic analysis (primarily ZrO_2 sensors):
			  ○ Accuracy: 1.0%
			  ○ Precision: 0.01%
			  ○ Response time: < 100 msec
			• Two-point calibration (21% and 100%) should be done just prior to each test

N_2	• Emission spectroscopy
	• Mass spectrometry
		• FRC determination (nitrogen washout)	• For real-time (breath) analysis:
			  ○ Accuracy: ± 0.2% over the entire range N_2% (0–80%)
			  ○ 95% response time: 30–60 msec to a 10% step change in N_2%
			• Two-point calibration (100% O_2 and room air) should be done just prior to each test
			• Linearity should be checked every 6 months with a 40% N_2 calibration gas mixture

He	• Thermal-conductivity	• FRC determination (helium dilution)
		• Single-breath DLCO (as tracer gas)
			• For FRC or DLCO:
			  ○ Measurement range: 0–10%
			  ○ Resolution: 0.01%
			  ○ 95% response time: 15 sec to a 2% step change in He%
			  ○ Stability: ± 0.5% full scale, confirmed weekly (drift ≤ 0.02% in 10 min)
			• Two-point calibration (zero and full scale) should be done just prior to each test
			• CO_2 and water must be removed before the sample is analyzed—CO_2 first (because its absorption creates water vapor), followed by removal of water vapor

(continues)

Table 4-29 Therapy and Diagnostic Gas Analysis (*continued*)

Gas	Analysis Method(s)	Usage	Performance Standards and Calibration Considerations
CO	• Infrared absorption • Electrochemical	• Single-breath DLco • Assessment of smoking status	• Accuracy is less important than linearity and stability (DLco is based on relative changes in CO%) • Linearity: within ± 0.5% from zero to full span (checked every 3 months) • Stability: ± 0.001% absolute CO% • Two-point calibration (zero and full scale) should be done just prior to each test

NO, NO$_2$	• Chemiluminescence
	• Electrochemical
		• Nitric oxide therapy
		• Monitoring airway inflammation (expired NO)
			• For nitric oxide:
			  ○ Resolution: 1 ppm
			  ○ Accuracy between 1 and 20 ppm: ± (0.5 ppm + 20% actual concentration)
			  ○ Accuracy above 20 ppm: ± (0.5 ppm + 10% actual concentration)
			  ○ Response time for breath-by-breath analysis: < 500 msec
			  ○ Response time for monitor/alarm of 0–90% rise time: ≤ 30 sec
			  ○ Drift: < 1% of full scale/24 hours
			• For NO$_2$:
			  ○ Accuracy: ± 20% of the actual %, or 0.5 ppm, whichever is greater
			  ○ Daily 1-point automated "zero" calibration (room air) while on patient
			  ○ Monthly two-point high range using 45 ppm NO/10 ppm NO$_2$ calibrating gases

Once you confirm proper function, you should set up the device for expired volume measurements, as depicted in **Figure 4-10**. As assembled, this setup can be attached directly to an ET or tracheostomy tube. To connect to a patient with a normal intact airway, use a mask or mouthpiece with nose clips.

To use a respirometer to obtain expired volume measurements:

1. Instruct the patient in the desired maneuver (slow vital capacity, minute volume).
2. Attach the equipment to the patient on the *exhalation side of the one-way valve*.
3. Move the on/off switch to the on position during patient *inhalation*.
4. Have the patient perform the desired maneuver (timed for minute volume).
5. When the maneuver is completed, move the on/off switch to the off position.
6. Record the desired measures (for minute volume, compute $V_T = \dot{V}_E \div f$).
7. For multiple measures on the same patient, store the valve/filter assembly in a clean bag at the bedside.

If a properly functioning device fails to operate, you should recheck the position of the on/off switch and make sure the respirometer is properly positioned with respect to the valve assembly (Figure 4-10).

Portable Electronic Spirometers

Portable electronic spirometers combine a flow sensor with a computer module. The computer module stores reference equations, provides input keys to specify patient data and select test options, converts the flow signal into volume, and outputs data via a screen and/or printer. The flow sensor may either sense flow directly (e.g., using a hot wire or Doppler technology) or by measuring the "back-pressure" created as gas flows through a restriction. **Figure 4-11** depicts a spirometer pneumotachometer that quantifies flow by measuring pressure differences across a resistive element.

In selecting a portable spirometer, you should make sure that it meets the following criteria:

- Meets ATS standards for diagnostic spirometry:
    - Volume range 0.5–8.0 L with accuracy of ± 3% or 0.05 L, whichever is greater
    - Flow range ± 14 L/sec with accuracy of ± 5% or 0.20 L/sec, whichever is greater

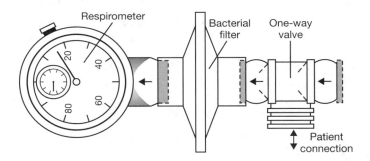

Figure 4-10 Basic Equipment Setup of Wright Respirometer for Bedside Volume Measures. A one-way breathing valve separates the patient's inspiratory and expiratory volumes. A HEPA filter protects the patient and respirometer from contamination. Replacement of the valve and filter allows the respirometer to be used on multiple patients (if the respirometer becomes contaminated, gas sterilize and properly aerate it). Here the respirometer is positioned to measure expiratory volumes (its normal use), with its inlet attached to the expiratory side of the breathing valve. To measure inspiratory volumes, you would reverse this positioning by attaching the filter and the respirometer's *outlet* to the inspiratory side of the valve.

Adapted from: Kacmarek RM, Foley K, Cheever P, Romagnoli D. Determination of ventilatory reserve in mechanically ventilated patients: a comparison of techniques. *Respir Care.* 1991;36:1085–1092.

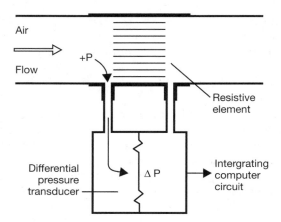

Figure 4-11 Differential Pressure (Fleisch) Pneumotachometer. Air flowing through a resistive element (parallel tubes) creates a pressure difference across the element, directly proportional to flow. These pressure changes are measured by a pressure transducer that sends its output signal to a computerized circuit, which converts the flow signal to volume via electronic integration. For continuous use, the pneumotachometer typically is heated to maintain a constant temperature and prevent condensation.

Adapted from: Sullivan WJ, Peters GM, Enright PL. Pneumotachography: theory and clinical application. *Respir Care.* 1984;29:736–749.

- Allows selection of common adult/child reference equations (e.g., NHANES III, Polgar)
- Adjusts normal values for gender, height, age, and ethnicity
- Provides automated validity checks on the maneuver:
  - Back-extrapolated volume
  - Time to peak expiratory flow
  - End-of-test volume
- Provides appropriate corrective prompts based on maneuver validity checks
- Stores and allows comparison of multiple/repeat test results on patients
- Prints both tabular data and applicable graphs (FEV versus time; flow versus volume)

Proper use of portable spirometers involves (1) regular calibration and (2) a procedure that provides valid results. Calibration of PFT equipment is covered in Chapter 6. Here we focus on proper application of the procedure.

Unlike many physiologic measurements, forced expiratory measures are very dependent on the patient correctly performing the procedure. Key procedural elements required to ensure accurate and reproducible results when performing bedside spirometry are outlined in Chapter 2. The most common technique-related problems include the following:

- Incomplete inhalation (less than inspiratory capacity)
- Inadequate expiratory force
- Breathing during maneuver
- Leakage (poor lip seal/exhalation through the nose)
- Too slow a start to forced exhalation
- Stopping exhalation before all gas is expelled
- Coughing during the maneuver

Devices that incorporate automated validity checks can detect many of these errors. To detect and correct these problems, the National Lung Health Education Program (NLHEP) recommends several validity checks and corrective prompts, as specified in **Table 4-30**. If the spirometer does not provide automated checks, you will need to detect these errors by carefully observing the patient during the maneuver and examining the graphic results. Chapter 6 provides details on how to detect patient-related errors affecting the validity of spirometry measurements.

Table 4-30 NLHEP Recommended Validity Checks and Corrective Prompts for Portable Spirometers

Problem Observed on Validity Check	Corrective Prompts
Back-extrapolated volume > 150 mL	"Don't hesitate"
Time to peak expiratory flow > 120 msec[a]	"Blast out faster"
Forced expiratory time < 6.0 sec and end-of-test volume[b] > 100 mL	"Blow out longer"
Repeat FEV_6 values do not match within 150 mL	"Take a deeper breath"
[a]More than 160 msec for school-age children and adolescents. [b]End-of-test volume = change in exhaled volume during the last 0.5 sec of the maneuver.	

When used and maintained according to the manufacturer's instructions, portable spirometers are generally trouble free. As outlined in **Table 4-31**, malfunctions that do occur usually involve power source problems, computer software or hardware errors, incorrect calibration, or misassembly or damage to the sensor.

ECG Monitors

Bedside monitors typically provide a continuous display of multiple patient parameters, which can include the ECG, respirations, blood pressure, SpO_2, and expired CO_2. Because bedside ECG monitors help warn of abnormal changes in heart rate or rhythm and can provide data essential in arrhythmia management, their continuous use is considered a standard of care for critically ill patients. For the same reason, portable (battery-powered) patient monitors should be selected for critically ill patients requiring intrahospital or interhospital transport.

Bedside ECG monitors use a three-lead system to acquire the ECG signal, with lead placement as depicted in **Figure 4-12**. You generally need only clean the skin site with an alcohol swab before placing the disposable self-adhesive electrodes. In some cases, to get good contact you may need to shave away body hair or gently abrade the underlying skin.

Once all three electrodes are positioned, you select among leads I, II, or III using a selector on the monitor. Limb lead II is the most common monitoring lead, because it normally produces the largest positive R wave (important because the R-R interval is used to compute the ECG heart rate). After obtaining a satisfactory signal, you should set the low and high rate alarms, typically at 50 and 120 to start. As with ventilator alarms, you want to avoid setting the high/low rates too close to the patient's actual rate, as this will cause frequent false alarms.

On ECG monitors that include both ECG rate and pulse oximeter rate displays, the two measures can often be different—with one setting off an alarm and one indicating normal. A discrepancy like this indicates either (1) pulseless electrical activity (ECG acceptable, but low or no pulse oximeter rate), or (2) an error in one of the monitored parameters. In these cases, check both the ECG leads *and* the pulse oximetry sensor for proper position and good contact.

12-Lead ECG Machines

Modern 12-lead ECG machines provide computerized data acquisition and storage. ECG data are obtained using 10 sensors or leads, which provide 12 separate electrical views of the heart's electrical activity. Once obtained, the 12-lead ECG can be stored in the computer's memory, printed as a "hard copy" for reading, or electronically sent to a remote location for interpretation. Clinicians use the data obtained from a 12-lead ECG to assess rhythm disturbances, determine the heart's electrical axis, and identify the site and extent of myocardial ischemia or damage (see Chapter 2).

If they are to provide accurate data, ECG machines must be calibrated regularly. Typically, calibration is performed by the biomedical engineering department using an ECG simulator. Simulator calibration also allows testing of the machine's self-diagnostics and alarm/warning systems, including the ability to sense a poor signal or a missing lead.

Table 4-31 Troubleshooting Common Problems with Portable Spirometers

Problem/Clue	Cause(s)	Solution(s)
Device does not turn on	Device lacks electrical power	• If AC powered, confirm connection to working line power outlet • If battery powered, check/replace batteries
Device turns on, but does not complete or fails the power-on self-test (POST)	Failure of boot/start-up program or central processing unit (CPU) failure	• Record error message • Turn device off, wait 20 seconds, then turn it back on • Replace device if continued boot failure
Sensor will not zero	Sensor is moving during zeroing	• Place sensor on tabletop and repeat
Device fails volume calibration (± 3%)	Incorrect temperature or pressure/altitude input	• Recalibrate device, being sure to enter proper temperature and pressure/altitude
	Loose connections or leaks in spirometer system	• Tighten connections and correct leaks
	Flow sensor misassembled or damaged	• Reassemble or replace flow sensor
	Flow sensor obstructed with foreign matter	• Clean or replace flow sensor
Test begins/volume accumulates before patient exhales	Sensor and/or tubing is not stationary at the start of test	• Have the patient hold the sensor assembly steady until prompted to begin
Flow measures appear to be reversed (differential pressure sensors only)	Flow sensor inlet and outlet pressure tubing connections reversed	• Check/correct and confirm proper tubing connections
Device does not sense beginning of exhalation	Sensor pressure tubing not connected	• Check/correct and confirm proper tubing connections
	Flow sensor misassembled or damaged	• Reassemble or replace flow sensor
Falsely high or low volume or flow readings suspected	Device out of calibration	• Recalibrate device, being sure to enter proper temperature and pressure/altitude
	Incorrect temperature or pressure/altitude input	• Recalibrate device, being sure to enter proper temperature and pressure/altitude
	Flow sensor misassembled or damaged	• Reassemble or replace flow sensor
	Leaks in patient or spirometer system (low readings only)	• Correct leaks • Use nose clips • Ensure proper lip seal
	Teeth, lips, or tongue obstructing mouthpiece (low readings only)	• Correct patient technique
Falsely high or low percent normal computations suspected	Incorrect patient data entry (e.g., age, height, gender)	• Verify/re-enter correct patient data

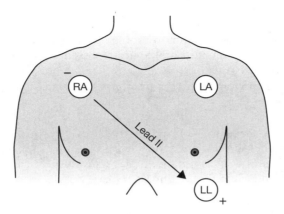

Figure 4-12 ECG Monitor Lead Placement. Place the RA/white electrode below the right clavicle, the LA/black electrode below the left clavicle, and the LL/red electrode just below the left pectoral muscle. When set to lead II, the RA electrode is the negative pole, the LL electrode is the positive pole, and the LA electrode serves as the ground lead. Due to the electrical axis of the normal heart, this configuration usually produces the largest positive R wave.

Figure 4-13 shows the proper lead placement for obtaining a 12-lead ECG. Note that there are only 10 actual leads to place, not 12. One (the right leg) does not really count, as it is just a ground lead. The difference is the three augmented limb leads (aVR, aVL, and aVF), which use the RA, LA, and LL electrodes to obtain their data.

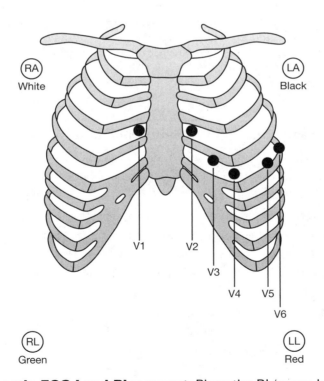

Figure 4-13 Diagnostic ECG Lead Placement. Place the RL/green lead on the right leg, the LL/red lead on the left leg, the RA/white lead on right arm, and the LA/black lead on the left arm. Then place the six chest leads as follows: V1—fourth intercostal space, right sternal border; V2—fourth intercostal space, left sternal border; V3—between V2 and V4; V4—fifth intercostal space, midclavicular line; V5—fifth intercostal space, anterior axillary line; and V6—fifth intercostal space, midaxillary line.

Once all sensors are positioned properly, you should verify a good-quality, artifact-free ECG signal. Most units automatically detect common problems and will not begin recording until a good signal is obtained. The two most common problems are absent or "noisy" signals. Failure to obtain a signal usually is due to a loose, missing, or defective lead. A noisy ECG signal may be caused by a poor electrical connection, motion artifact, or improper filtering of extraneous electrical activity. In either case, you should follow these steps:

1. Verify that the ECG snaps and connectors are clean and corrosion free.
2. Verify that the lead electrodes are connected properly to the patient.
3. Verify that the electrode gel is not dry; replace any suspect electrodes.
4. Check the ECG main cable for continuity; replace it if damaged.
5. Confirm that the patient is motionless; if necessary, support the patient's limbs.
6. Verify that the device's filter settings (if available) are properly set.

Point-of-Care Blood Gas Analyzers

Point-of-care testing (POCT) is indicated for patients in urgent need of assessment for whom central laboratory processing would delay needed therapy. Typically, patients who might need POCT include those receiving care in the emergency department, critical care units, and operating rooms.

Most POCT instruments measure patient blood samples using disposable analysis cartridges specifically designed for each desired battery of tests. The most common POCT tests done by respiratory therapists are for arterial blood gases (ABGs) and combined panels that include ABG measures plus other selected parameters important in managing critically ill patients.

If POCT is ordered for ABG analysis, in addition to the POCT analyzer you will need an ABG kit and the appropriate analysis cartridge. Which analysis cartridge you select depends on the tests being ordered. Typically, the simple ABG cartridge provides measures of pH, Po_2, and Pco_2, with calculated values for HCO_3, BE, total CO_2, and O_2 saturation. A variety of combined panel tests provide these measures plus selected electrolyte concentrations, the anion gap, the hematocrit, hemoglobin content, glucose levels, blood lactate, and/or the blood urea nitrogen (BUN).

Key elements in using a common POCT unit (Abbott Laboratories I-STAT) for blood analysis are outlined in the accompanying box. Other devices may employ slightly different procedures.

Key Procedural Elements in Using the Abbott Laboratories I-STAT POCT Instrument

- Turn the analyzer on.
- From the menu provided, specify the cartridge type/test panel to be performed.
- Scan or enter the operator and patient IDs.
- Carefully remove the cartridge from its pouch; avoid touching any contact pads.
- Obtain the sample as usual and analyze it within 3 minutes (do *not* place it in ice).
- Mix the sample thoroughly and dispense it into the cartridge well to the fill mark.
- Close the sample well cover, insert the cartridge into its port, and confirm placement.
- Enter any requested information—for example, type of sample, F_{IO_2}, patient temperature.
- View the results shown on the analyzer's display screen.
- Remove the cartridge when indicated by the analyzer.
- Turn analyzer off and place in the downloader/recharger.

POCT analyzers are highly reliable devices. Because calibration occurs with each cartridge test, minimal user intervention is needed. **Table 4-32** summarizes the few problems that you may encounter in using a POCT analyzer, along with their causes and potential solutions.

Table 4-32 Troubleshooting Common Problems with POCT Analyzers

Problem/Clue	Cause	Solution
Analyzer does not turn on	Batteries discharged or dead	Confirm that the batteries are properly charged; if you cannot properly charge the batteries, replace them.
Analyzer turns on but fails to display proper start-up information	Software start-up/boot error	Reboot the analyzer (turn it off, wait 10–20 seconds, turn it on); replace the device if the second start-up fails.
Calibration error message	A problem with the sample, calibrating solutions, sensors, or device's electrical or mechanical functions	Follow the error message guidance and report findings (may be a numeric error code referenced in user's manual); repeat the analysis using a fresh sample and new cartridge.
Failed electrical simulator test	A problem with the device's electrical functions	Report findings and replace the device.
Flagged results	Results outside the analyzer's reportable ranges	Send the sample to the central lab for analysis.
Results rejected based on quality control criteria	A problem with the sample, calibrating solutions, sensors, or device's electrical or mechanical functions	Repeat the analysis using a fresh sample and new cartridge. If sample integrity is not in question, results that are not rejected should be reported as usual. If results are rejected twice, send the sample to the central lab.

Note that you may obtain POCT results outside the device's critical range, such as a pH less than 7.20 or greater than 7.60. Such readings are *not* the same as flagged or "outside reportable range" results and should be treated as potentially valid data. To validate measures falling outside a device's critical range, repeat the analysis using a fresh sample and new cartridge. Some protocols require out-of-range results be repeated in the central lab. *Either way, never wait for repeat results if the findings are life threatening or coincide with a deteriorating clinical picture.* For example, if the POCT result indicates a Po_2 less than 40 torr and the patient exhibits signs of hypoxemia, increase the Fio_2 while awaiting the repeat test results.

Noninvasive Oximetry Monitoring Devices

The noninvasive oximetry monitoring devices you should be most familiar with include pulse oximeters and transcutaneous monitors. You select a pulse oximeter to spot check, monitor, or obtain trend data on a patient's oxygen saturation (Spo_2). You select a transcutaneous monitor to provide continuous estimates of arterial blood gases (Po_2 and Pco_2). Details on assessing and interpreting noninvasive oximetry data are provided in Chapter 11.

Pulse Oximeters

Although pulse oximeters vary widely in design, the steps involved in their setup and assembly are similar. **Table 4-33** outlines the basic steps, including key considerations for obtaining good saturation data.

For monitoring critically ill patients, pulse oximetry readings should be compared to a simultaneous measure of actual arterial O_2 saturation, as measured by laboratory oximetry. You can then use the difference between the Sao_2 and Spo_2 to "calibrate" the pulse oximetry reading.

The most common problem with pulse oximeters is an unstable or poor-quality signal. In these cases, you should take the following steps:

- Recheck the site and clean it along with the probe (if a multiuse probe) with alcohol.
- Reposition the probe to ensure that the transmitted light is directly opposite the detector.

Table 4-33 Key Considerations in the Setup of Pulse Oximeters

Setup Steps	Key Considerations
1. If AC powered, connect the power cord to an appropriate power source.	• Most oximeters use a battery to provide power if an AC outlet is unavailable.
2. Connect the appropriate probe to the oximeter.	• There are special probes for infants and children. • Proper probe size is essential for accurate readings.
3. Turn the power on.	• Most oximeters perform a power-on self-test before reading the SpO_2. • Always verify that the unit has passed the POST.
4. Attach the probe to the patient.	• For continuous monitoring, use a disposable probe attached with adhesive or Velcro strips. • For spot checks, a nondisposable, multipatient probe is satisfactory. • Always disinfect a multiuse probe with alcohol before use. • Overly tight oximeter probes may cause inaccurate readings or skin damage.
5. Verify a good signal.	• If displayed, observe the waveform to verify a good pulse signal. • Alternatively, use the oximeter's rate LED to verify a good signal. • Always validate the oximeter's rate against an ECG monitor or palpated pulse.
6. For continuous monitoring, set the alarm limits.	• Set the low alarm according to institutional protocol, usually between 92% and 94%.
7. For overnight oximetry, set the devices for trend recording.	• Select the planned period (e.g., 8 hours, 12 hours). • Adjust the capture rate/response time to the fastest allowable value (usually 2–6 seconds). • Confirm sufficient memory is available to record for the specified period/capture rate. • If needed or appropriate, turn alarms off.

- Remove any fingernail polish or "fake" nails (in emergencies, rotate the probe 90°).
- Try a different site, particularly if the probe has been in place for several hours.
- Replace the probe (if disposable) or try a different type of probe.
- If poor peripheral perfusion affects signal quality, consider using an ear sensor or a forehead reflectance sensor.

If an oximeter displays an error message indicating that the probe is off or disconnected, check the probe's connection to the oximeter and determine whether it is malpositioned. Reconnect or reposition the probe as needed. Last, if bright ambient light appears to be interfering with the reading, shield or cover the probe or reposition it to an unaffected area.

Transcutaneous Monitors

Transcutaneous blood gas monitoring provides continuous, noninvasive estimates of arterial PO_2 and PCO_2 via a sensor placed on the skin. The sensor includes PO_2 and PCO_2 electrodes like those in laboratory ABG analyzers, along with a heating element. The heating element "arterializes" the blood by dilating the underlying capillary bed and increasing its blood flow. Oxygen and CO_2 diffuse from the capillaries through the skin and into the sensor's contact gel, where their pressures are measured by the electrodes. These pressures are referred to as transcutaneous (tc) partial pressures (i.e., $Ptco_2$ and $Ptcco_2$).

Common indications for transcutaneous blood gas monitoring are listed in Chapter 3. Transcutaneous monitoring also may be used in children or adults to continuously assess the adequacy of ventilation (via the $Ptcco_2$) when capnography is not available or technically difficult (as during noninvasive ventilation).

You should avoid using a transcutaneous monitor on patients with poor skin integrity or those with an adhesive allergy. Because accurate $Ptco_2$ and $Ptcco_2$ values generally require good perfusion, you should not use these devices on patients in shock or with poor peripheral circulation. Lengthy setup and stabilization time (10–20 minutes) also makes transcutaneous monitoring a poor choice in emergency situations.

Although transcutaneous monitors vary in design, the following key setup and assembly steps are common across devices:

1. Membrane the sensor and calibrate the device as per the manufacturer's instructions.
2. Adjust the temperature to the desired level (usually 42–45°C).
3. Choose a site that has good superficial circulation (e.g., the side of chest, the abdomen, inner thigh) and clean it with alcohol.
4. Apply the adhesive fixation ring to the sensor (some protocols apply the ring to the skin).
5. Apply the contact gel to the sensor face and inside the fixation ring; *avoid air bubbles.*
6. Apply the sensor to the selected site; make sure the edges are sealed, with the sensor lying flat on the skin.
7. Allow 10–20 minutes for the reading to stabilize.
8. To avoid burns/skin damage, change the sensor site frequently (every 2–6 hours, depending on the sensor temperature and manufacturer's recommendation).

Like lab ABG analyzers, transcutaneous Po_2/Pco_2 monitors require two-point calibration using precision gas mixtures. Most manufacturers provide a calibration system with their monitors, and a semi-automated software routine prompts you through the steps. Failure to calibrate is usually due to a leaking membrane or excessive trapped air under the membrane. In both cases, the calibrating Pco_2 values and the high Po_2 measure will be lower than expected. If a transcutaneous monitor fails to calibrate, you should re-membrane the sensor.

To validate transcutaneous readings, the $Ptco_2$ and $Ptcco_2$ should be compared with a concurrently obtained ABG. *For an infant with an anatomic shunt, both the transcutaneous and arterial values must be obtained on the same side.* If the transcutaneous and arterial values differ significantly, poor peripheral circulation is the likely cause. If the patient has good peripheral circulation but the two readings still differ, try an alternative sensor site. If an alternative sensor site does not provide valid data, re-membrane and recalibrate the sensor. If the two values still differ significantly, consider another mode of monitoring, such as pulse oximetry or serial ABGs.

Aside from difficulty validating the $Ptco_2$ and $Ptcco_2$ against a patient's arterial values, the most common problem with transcutaneous monitoring is air leaking around the adhesive ring. Air leaks always cause a dramatic fall in $Ptcco_2$. If the leak is large, the $Ptco_2$ and $Ptcco_2$ values will mimic those of room air ($Po_2 \approx 150$ torr; $Pco_2 \approx 0$ torr). In these cases, reapply the sensor using a new adhesive ring.

Hemodynamic Monitoring Devices (RRT-Specific Content)

The use of indwelling vascular catheter systems and interpretation of the hemodynamic data they provide are discussed in Chapters 2, 11, and 16. Here we focus on the problems you can encounter in using hemodynamic monitoring devices. **Table 4-34** outlines the most frequent problems to expect and how to solve them.

As noted in Table 4-34, any partial obstruction in the measurement system, such as that caused by air bubbles or small clots, can "dampen" the pressure signal (i.e., reduce its amplitude). **Figure 4-14** portrays damping of a pulmonary artery pressure waveform and its correction by flushing the line.

Table 4-34 Troubleshooting Vascular Lines

Problem/Causes	Solution
Unexpectedly High or Low Venous/PA Pressure Readings	
Change in transducer reference level	Position transducer at phlebostatic axis (midchest)
Damped Pressure Waveform	
Catheter tip against vessel wall	Pull back, rotate, or reposition catheter while observing pressure waveform
Partial occlusion of catheter tip by clot	Aspirate clot with syringe and flush with heparinized saline
Clot in stopcock or transducer	Disconnect and flush stopcock and transducer; if no improvement, change stopcock and transducer
Air bubbles in transducer or connector tubing	Disconnect transducer and flush out air bubbles
Absent Waveform/No Pressure Reading	
Catheter occluded	Aspirate blood from line
Catheter out of vessel	Notify doctor and prepare to replace line
Stopcock off to patient	Position stopcock correctly
Loose connection	Tighten loose connection
Transducer not connected to monitor	Check and tighten cable connection
Monitor set to zero, calibrate, or off	Make sure monitor set to proper function/display
Incorrect scale selection	Select appropriate scale (arterial = high; venous = low)
Signal Artifact	
Patient movement	Wait until patient is quiet before taking a reading
Electrical interference	Make sure electrical equipment is connected and grounded correctly
Catheter fling	Notify doctor to reposition catheter

Also as noted in Table 4-34, when measuring "right-sided" vascular pressures (e.g., CVP or PA), changes in the transducer level can affect the accuracy of the reading. To obtain accurate readings, you must ensure that the base of the fluid column or pressure transducer is positioned at a level equal to the point of measurement, the right atrium (the *phlebostatic axis*). Otherwise, the system will behave like a U-tube manometer, overestimating pressures if placed too low and underestimating pressures if placed too high. Note that any change in the patient's position will have the same effect and require releveling the system.

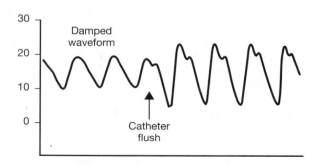

Figure 4-14 Damping of Pulmonary Artery Pressure Measurement Due to Partial Obstruction of the Fluid Line (Due to Bubbles and/or Small Clots). Flushing the catheter eliminates the damping and restores the normal pulse-pressure waveform.

Courtesy of: Strategic Learning Associates, LLC, Little Silver, New Jersey.

Bronchoscopes

As discussed in Chapter 16, therapists may assist physicians with bronchoscopy. Key equipment involved includes the bronchoscope itself, its light source, its suction and biopsy valves, assorted bronchoscopic instruments (e.g., brushes, forceps, aspiration needles), an oral insertion guide/bite block, specimen-collection devices, a regulated vacuum source and suction supplies, syringes, pulse oximeter, O_2-delivery equipment, and a BVM resuscitator. Troubleshooting of these accessory devices is covered separately in other sections of this chapter. Here we focus on the care of the bronchoscope during use and its subsequent cleaning, disinfection, and storage.

A fiberoptic bronchoscope is a very delicate instrument. Its outer sheath, filaments in the viewing channel, and objective (distal) lens are very easily damaged. In addition, the working channel lining can easily be ruptured by rigid or sharp instruments. When damage occurs to the fiberoptic filaments, numerous black dots begin appearing in the eyepiece. Damage to the working channel can allow fluid invasion of the scope, causing a foggy image. The possibility of fluid invasion is confirmed by leak testing the scope during cleaning and disinfection.

To avoid damage to the scope, you must ensure proper handling of the device. Key points in this regard follow:

- Avoid letting the distal end strike any hard surface (damages the distal objective lens).
- Avoid forced angulation of the insertion tube (damages the fiberoptic filaments).
- Avoid direct axial twisting of the insertion tube (damages the fiberoptic filaments).
- Use only instruments with external diameters properly sized for the working channel.
- Keep the proximal portion of scope as straight as possible during insertion.
- Avoid use of force when inserting instruments into the working channel.
- Avoid using petroleum-based lubricants for insertion (damage the scope's outer sheath).
- Always replace (do not repair) bronchoscope instruments.
- Always use a bite block whenever the tube is inserted via the mouth or oral ET tube.

In addition, to avoid endobronchial ignition or fire during Nd-YAG laser bronchoscopy, you should ensure that the F_{IO_2} is kept below 0.40 (if possible) and that alcohol is *not* used to clear the laser tip. Moreover, the physician should make sure that the laser tip is at least 5 mm away from scope outlet and as far away from the ET tube as possible when fired.

If during bronchoscopy suction appears inadequate, first check the vacuum regulator setting and all connections to the scope. If the problem persists, remove and clean or replace the scope's suction valve.

Because fiberoptic bronchoscopes are a proven source for the spread of infection, you must properly clean, disinfect, and store this equipment after completion of the procedure. The accompanying box outlines the key elements involved in processing bronchoscopes after use.

Processing of Bronchoscopes After Use

Cleaning

1. While still at the bedside, flush water or saline through the scope's working channel for 20 seconds.

2. To avoid drying of organic material, immediately transport the scope in a sealed contaminated equipment bag to a processing area.

3. Mechanically clean (e.g., by ultrasonic technology) all reusable accessory instruments and send them for autoclaving.

4. Remove all disposable parts, cap and seal all light/electrical connectors, and place the scope in a cleaning basin.

5. Following the manufacturer's protocol, perform a leak test on the scope (get it repaired if it fails the test).

6. Add enzymatic cleaner to the water and soak the scope for 5 minutes.

7. Using the enzymatic solution, wipe external surfaces with wet gauze and flush the suction channel.

(continues)

Processing of Bronchoscopes After Use (*continued*)

8. Insert an appropriate-size cleaning brush through the working channel and brush all ports until no more visible debris is being removed.

9. Flush the channel again to remove all loosened material.

10. Drain the enzymatic solution from the basin.

11. Rinse all internal and external surfaces with water to prepare the scope for disinfection.

High-Level Disinfection

1. Place the bronchoscope in either an automatic endoscope reprocessor (AER) or a basin used for manual disinfection.

2. Use only FDA-cleared disinfectants that are compatible with the scope; confirm proper disinfectant concentration with each process.

3. Fully immerse the scope in the disinfectant, exposing all surfaces for the proper time (20 minutes or longer for glutaraldehyde); if manually disinfecting the scope, fill the working channel with the disinfectant using a syringe.

Postprocessing

1. After proper immersion time, rinse the scope and its working channel with either sterile or filtered tap water according to the recommendations of the disinfectant supplier.

2. Dry the working channel with 70% alcohol, purged with compressed air.

3. Remove the watertight caps from the scope and hang it vertically in a storage cabinet without attaching any valve.

4. Document the disinfection process (patient ID, date of the procedure, bronchoscopist, model and the serial number of the scope, and the date of reprocessing).

Adapted from: Mehta AC, Prakash UB, Garland R, et al. Consensus statement: prevention of flexible bronchoscopy-associated infection. *Chest.* 2005;128:1742–1755.

COMMON ERRORS TO AVOID

You can improve your score by avoiding these mistakes:

- Never use a Thorpe tube to meter O_2 during patient transport; instead, use a gravity-independent device such as a Bourdon gauge.
- Avoid selecting or using an air-entrainment device when a patient needs a high FIO_2; use a nonrebreathing mask or high-flow cannula instead.
- Never use helium unless it is combined with at least 20% O_2.
- Never heat the gas used to deliver bland aerosols into pediatric mist tents; these systems must always run cool.
- Never use a gas-powered resuscitator on an infant or child.
- Avoid regular changing of ventilator circuits; change them only when absolutely necessary.
- Avoid using oronasal (full-face) masks for noninvasive ventilation of patients with hypercapnic respiratory failure.
- Avoid using oropharyngeal airways in conscious patients.
- Never plug a fenestrated tracheostomy tube with the cuff inflated.
- Never clamp a patient's chest tube during transport; the one-way seal must be maintained.
- Never use a mechanical vane-type respirometer to measure forced expiratory volumes; use a portable electronic spirometer instead.
- Never accept an adult's FEV maneuver that lasts for less than 6 seconds.
- Avoid using transcutaneous O_2/CO_2 monitors in emergency situations or on patients in shock or with poor peripheral circulation.
- Never wash or rinse a dry-powder inhaler in water.
- Never forcefully bend or twist the insertion tube portion of a fiberoptic bronchoscope.
- Avoid using petroleum-based lubricants for bronchoscope insertion.

SURE BETS

In some situations, you can always be sure of the right approach to a clinical problem or scenario:

- Always evaluate the patient's *actual response* to O_2 therapy (e.g., via the SpO_2), not just the FIO_2.
- Always deliver the highest possible FIO_2 (via nonrebreathing mask or high-flow cannula) to patients in emergency settings suspected of being hypoxemic.
- Always have home care patients who experience problems with an O_2-conserving device switch to a nasal cannula at an equivalent liter flow (2–3 times the conserving device rate).
- Always ensure a neutral thermal environment when delivering O_2 to infants.
- To avoid overinflation, always select a manual resuscitator with the correct stroke volume and mask size.
- Whenever a major problem occurs during mechanical ventilation, always remove the patient from the ventilator and provide support using a manual resuscitator connected to an O_2 source.
- Always treat a combined low-volume and high-pressure alarm condition during mechanical ventilation as signaling an obstruction.
- To ensure adequate active humidification in a ventilator circuit, always confirm that a few drops of condensation remain at or near the patient connector.
- If using an active humidification system in a ventilator circuit, always ensure that the inspiratory HEPA filter is positioned proximal to or upstream from the humidifier.
- When providing aerosol drug therapy through a ventilator circuit, always remove the HME before the procedure and replace it afterward.
- Always perform the required breathing circuit testing/calibration before applying a ventilator to a patient.
- Check the position of an endotracheal tube by breath sounds and (if available) capnometry—but always *confirm* this position with a chest x-ray.
- To positively identify the contents of a medical gas cylinder, always read the cylinder label.
- Always verify the prescribed O_2% provided by a blender using a calibrated O_2 analyzer.
- Before using any computerized electronic device, always verify that it passes its power-on self-test (POST).
- Always send flagged point-of-care test results to the central laboratory for analysis.
- Always check a pulse oximeter's displayed rate against an ECG monitor or count the actual pulse rate.
- When measuring right-sided heart pressures (e.g., CVP, PA, PAWP), always position the manometer or pressure transducer at the level of the right atrium (the phlebostatic axis).
- Always use a bite block when inserting a fiberoptic bronchoscope via the mouth or through an oral ET tube.

PRE-TEST ANSWERS AND EXPLANATIONS

Following are this chapter's pre-test answers and explanations. Be sure to review each answer's explanation thoroughly to help you understand why it is correct. If the explanation is still unclear to you, review the chapter contents.

4-1. **Correct answer: C.** Check the entrainment ports. Because air-entrainment devices mix air and O_2 at a constant ratio, an alteration in the delivered O_2% can result only from a change in the mixing ratio. Most commonly, this occurs with port obstruction, which will decrease air entrainment and raise the delivered O_2%.

4-2. **Correct answer: B.** 48 L/min. Total output flow = sum of the ratio parts × input flow. A 35% air-entrainment mask mixes air an oxygen at a fixed 5:1 ratio; thus $(5 + 1) \times 8 = 48$ L/min.

4-3. **Correct answer: C.** Check the mask for a snug fit. If a nonrebreathing mask bag does not deflate when the patient inspires, either the flow is higher than needed, there are large leaks, or the inspiratory valve is jammed. The most common cause is leakage, which is easily corrected by snugly fitting the mask to the patient's face.

4-4. **Correct answer: D.** A clogged nebulizer capillary tube. Because most croup tents use large-volume jet nebulizers, insufficient mist indicates nebulizer malfunction. The most common cause of malfunction is clogging of the capillary tube that feeds liquid water to the jet.

4-5. **Correct answer: B.** Large-reservoir heated jet nebulizer. The large-reservoir air-entrainment jet nebulizer is the primary gas-powered aerosol generator used to provide humidification to the respiratory tract of spontaneously breathing patients.

4-6. **Correct answer: C.** Use a reflective material to cover the temperature probe. To ensure proper function of a radiant warmer applied to a low-birth-weight infant in the NICU, you would set the temperature control to servo mode and a target temperature of 36.5°C, place and secure the temperature probe on the infant's upper abdomen, use a reflective material to cover the temperature probe, and set the controller's high/low-temperature alarms ± 1°C above/below the targeted servo setting.

4-7. **Correct answer: A.** Absence of the inlet valve. If a bag-valve resuscitator fills rapidly but collapses on minimal pressure and delivers little volume, the likely problem is a missing, torn, or malpositioned inlet valve. In this case, when you squeeze the bag, gas escapes out the inlet port instead of going to the patient. Had the bag been checked before use, a replacement could have been secured.

4-8. **Correct answer: B.** Variable flow control and adjustable I:E ratios. Of the functions listed, the most important ventilator capability for an intubated adult patient with severe expiratory airway obstruction would be variable flow control and adjustable I:E ratios. This will allow clinicians to make sure the expiratory time is sufficiently long to prevent air trapping/auto-PEEP.

4-9. **Correct answer: D.** Narrow-diameter, low-compliance tubing. To ensure proper transmission of the pressure pulses going to and from the patient, most high-frequency oscillator ventilators use narrow-diameter, low-compliance tubing.

4-10. **Correct answer: C.** Bleed supplemental O_2 from a flowmeter into the circuit. Most NPPV ventilators use a simple air blower to generate pressure. To provide supplemental O_2 with these devices, you bleed O_2 into the circuit until you achieve the desired FiO_2. Because high supplemental O_2 flows can affect NPPV ventilator function, always follow the manufacturer's recommendations when considering how best to increase the FiO_2 of these devices.

4-11. **Correct answer: D.** Low volume + low pressure. When delivering volume control ventilation, potential system leaks are indicated by a low-volume and low-pressure alarm condition. In such cases you should quickly check for and correct any loose circuit connections.

4-12. **Correct answer: B.** Fenestrated tracheostomy tube. A fenestrated tracheostomy tube is the best choice to support patients needing intermittent (e.g., nocturnal) ventilatory support. For positive-pressure ventilation, the inner cannula is inserted to close the fenestration and the cuff inflated to provide a seal. When the patient is not on the ventilator, the inner cannula is removed (to open the fenestration), the cuff is deflated, and the tube is plugged. This allows normal use of the upper airway.

4-13. **Correct answer: D.** Set up an O_2 blender/heated humidifier oxyhood system. Isolettes provide control over the FiO_2 up to approximately 0.60 (60% O_2). However, the need for frequent access/opening of the isolette ports makes it difficult to maintain a stable FiO_2, especially at the higher levels. For this reason, a blender/oxyhood system is the best way to ensure a stable FiO_2 for an infant in an isolette.

4-14. **Correct answer: C.** Replace the ET tube. A cuff that fails to inflate when injected with air has a large leak. The faulty ET tube should be replaced and the new tube tested in the same manner.

4-15. **Correct answer: B.** Use a 10-Fr catheter. The catheter is too large for the ET tube. The outside diameter of a suction catheter should be no more than about 50% as large as the inside diameter (ID) of the artificial airway (70% in infants). To quickly estimate the correct catheter size, multiply the ID of the tracheal tube by 2 and select the next smallest catheter. In this example, to suction a patient with a 6.0-mm tube, $2 \times 6 = 12$. The next smallest catheter = 10 Fr.

4-16. **Correct answer: B.** Clearance of secretions. Conditions that could cause suctioning to stop suddenly include (1) disconnected tubing (leak/loss of vacuum), (2) a full suction reservoir (ball-valve shutoff), and (3) plugging of the catheter. Normal clearance of secretions would not cause loss of suction pressure.

4-17. **Correct answer: D.** 1 or 3. For spontaneously breathing patients, heliox generally is delivered via a tight-fitting nonrebreathing mask at a flow sufficient to meet or exceed the patient's inspiratory demands. Alternatively, you can deliver heliox using a high-flow cannula.

4-18. **Correct answer: C.** 1 and 3 only. If the yoke connectors for cylinders A–E are not properly tightened, a leak could result. In addition, the small receiving nipple on the yoke normally is sealed to the gas outlet with a washer. A missing or damaged washer could also cause a leak. Missing PISS pins would not cause a leak.

4-19. **Correct answer: B.** Place the sample in an ice slush. The procedure used for point-of-care blood gas analysis is similar to that used when preparing a sample for central lab analysis. The exceptions are that (1) the sample should be analyzed within 3 minutes, and (2) the sample should *not* be placed in ice.

4-20. **Correct answer: B.** Incentive spirometry with directed coughing. Incentive spirometry is a good choice for treating suspected or confirmed atelectasis in an alert patient who does not have evidence of bronchospasm. It should never be used alone, however, but always in combination with a bronchial hygiene protocol, to include directed coughing.

4-21. **Correct answer: A.** Switch to a backup supply of continuous O_2 at 2 to 3 times the demand flow setting. To ensure continuity of therapy, patients using pulse dose/demand flow systems who report a problem with their unit should immediately switch to a backup supply of continuous O_2 via nasal cannula at the equivalent flow (2 to 3 times the rate of the conserving device).

4-22. **Correct answer: D.** Control valve. Mean airway pressure in a HFOV typically is regulated by a pneumatic valve (the control valve) that provides variable resistance to outflow of gas from the circuit. Unique to this circuit are two additional pneumatic valves, both designed to ensure patient safety. The limit valve opens when the airway pressure meets or exceeds the ventilator's maximum pressure alarm setting. The dump valve activates when either the airway pressure rises above 60 cm H_2O or falls below 5 cm H_2O.

4-23. **Correct answer: D.** To measure rapid pressure changes. Fluid column pressure manometers are used to measure static or slowing changing pressures and to calibrate other pressure measuring devices. They are not suited for measuring rapidly changing pressures.

4-24. **Correct answer: A.** A portable electronic spirometer. If you need to measure a patient's forced vital capacity or related measures (e.g., peak flow, FEV_t) at the bedside, you should choose a portable electronic spirometer. Because they can be damaged by high flows, mechanical turbine-type devices like the Wright model should not be used to measure forced inspiratory or expiratory volumes.

4-25. **Correct answer: A.** "Don't hesitate." In adults, a back-extrapolated volume greater than 150 mL indicates patient hesitation at the beginning of the breath, which will invalidate test results. In these cases, you need to make sure the patient does not hesitate when beginning the forced exhalation.

4-26. **Correct answer: C.** Turning off filtering of extraneous electrical activity. The two most common problems in obtaining a good 12-lead ECG recording are absent or "noisy" signals. In either case you should check and confirm that (1) the main lead cable is undamaged, (2) the ECG electrodes are connected properly to the patient, (3) the electrode gel is not dry, (4) the patient is motionless, and (5) the device's filters are properly set to eliminate extraneous electrical activity.

4-27. **Correct answer: D.** Pulse oximeter. If you need to spot check or monitor a patient's oxygen saturation, you should select a pulse oximeter. Select a laboratory hemoximeter to obtain precise measures of both normal and abnormal Hb saturations. A transcutaneous monitor would be your best choice to continuously and noninvasively monitor arterial blood gases (P_{O_2} and P_{CO_2}), particularly in infants.

4-28. **Correct answer: D.** Air leakage around the sensor's fixation ring. The most common problem with transcutaneous monitoring is leakage around the adhesive fixation ring. Air leaks always cause a fall in P_{tcCO_2}. If the leak is large, the P_{tcO_2} and P_{tcCO_2} will mimic those in room air ($P_{O_2} \approx 150$ torr; $P_{CO_2} \approx 0$ torr). In these cases, reapply the sensor using a new fixation ring.

4-29. **Correct answer: C.** MDI with holding chamber and a mask. Most infants and small children should receive aerosolized drugs via an MDI with a valved holding chamber and a mask. If tolerated by the patient, an SVN with a mask could be considered as an alternative. Avoid using the "blow-by" technique with small-volume nebulizers.

4-30. **Correct answer: B.** It would underestimate the CVP. When measuring right-sided vascular pressure such as CVP, you must ensure that the base of the fluid column or pressure transducer is positioned at the level of the right atrium (the phlebostatic axis). Otherwise, the system will behave like a U-tube manometer and overestimate pressures if placed too low, or underestimate pressures if placed too high.

POST-TEST

To confirm your mastery of this chapter's topical content, you should take the chapter post-test, available online at http://go.jblearning.com/respexamreview. A score of 80% or more indicates that you are adequately prepared for this section of the NBRC written exams. If you score less than 80%, you should continue to review the applicable chapter content. In addition, you may want to access and review the relevant Web links covering this chapter's content (courtesy of RTBoardReview. com), also online at the Jones & Bartlett Learning site.

CHAPTER 5

Ensure Infection Control

Craig L. Scanlan

Infection control is a minor topic on NBRC exams, but it is a big part of your job. Most students and clinicians know the basics, such as hand hygiene and isolation procedures. However, the NBRC exams include some areas of infection control with which you may not be as familiar, such as equipment disinfection. Moreover, protocols recently have been developed in an effort to decrease the incidence of ventilator-associated pneumonia (VAP) and central line–associated bloodstream infections, as well as to combat the spread of atypical viral infections. For these reasons, you should spend a reasonable portion of your prep time on this topic, with an emphasis on those areas with which you are least familiar.

OBJECTIVES

In preparing for the shared NBRC exam content, you should demonstrate the knowledge needed to:

1. Ensure cleanliness of equipment by
   a. Selecting or determining the appropriate agent and technique for disinfection and/or sterilization
   b. Performing procedures for disinfection and/or sterilization
   c. Monitoring the effectiveness of sterilization procedures
2. Ensure proper handling of biohazardous materials
3. Adhere to infection control policies and procedures
4. Adhere to the ventilator-associated pneumonia protocol
5. Implement infectious disease protocols, such as that for avian flu/severe acute respiratory syndrome (SARS)

WHAT TO EXPECT ON THIS CATEGORY OF THE NBRC EXAMS

CRT exam: 3 questions; about 66% application and 33% analysis
WRRT exam: 2 questions; all analysis
CSE exam: indeterminate number of questions; however, exam II-B knowledge can be tested on CSE Decision-Making sections

PRE-TEST

Carefully respond to each of the following questions. After completing the pre-test, compare your answers to those provided at the end of this chapter. Then thoroughly review each answer's explanation to help understand why it is correct.

5-1. What is the first step in processing reusable equipment?
  A. Pasteurization
  B. Cleaning
  C. Disinfection
  D. Sterilization

5-2. The label of a disinfectant indicates that it does *not* inactivate or kill either *Mycobacterium tuberculosis* or bacterial spores. Which class of disinfectant is this?
  A. Surface active
  B. Low level
  C. Intermediate level
  D. High level

5-3. A patient with pneumonia has her noninvasive ventilatory support discontinued. Which of the following should be used to disinfect the device's nondisposable breathing circuit before it is placed back into service?
   A. Pasteurization
   B. Isopropyl alcohol
   C. Acetic acid
   D. Hydrogen peroxide

5-4. For patients receiving bronchodilator therapy via small-volume nebulizer (SVN), which of the following precautions would be beneficial in preventing nosocomial infection?
   1. Use a different SVN for each patient
   2. Change the nebulizer and tubing every 24 hours
   3. Perform thorough hand washing prior to each therapy session
   A. 1 only
   B. 2 only
   C. 1 and 3
   D. 1, 2, and 3

5-5. A business woman returning from a country experiencing an outbreak of an atypical virus infection initially complained of flu-like symptoms, which after hospital admission have worsened into a severe pneumonia. Which of the following infection control precautions would you recommend for this patient?
   1. Airborne precautions
   2. Contact precautions
   3. Droplet precautions
   A. 1 and 2
   B. 1, 2, and 3
   C. 1 and 3
   D. 2 and 3 only

5-6. All of the following help minimize the risk of contamination during suctioning *except*:
   A. Using a fresh sterile single-use catheter on each patient
   B. Using only sterile fluid to remove secretions from the catheter
   C. Minimizing suction time to 10-15 seconds
   D. Performing proper hand washing and gloving before suctioning

5-7. If sterilization is not feasible, which of the following are acceptable alternatives for processing a specialized reusable plastic airway?
   1. Exposure to a high-level chemical disinfectant
   2. Surface disinfection with 70% ethyl alcohol
   3. Pasteurization at 63°C for 30 minutes
   A. 1 and 2
   B. 2 and 3
   C. 1 and 3
   D. 1, 2, and 3

5-8. Which of the following *violates* CDC recommendations regarding infection control when inserting a vascular line?
   A. Performing vigorous hand hygiene before insertion
   B. Using sterile barrier precautions, including drapes
   C. Scrubbing the insertion site with hydrogen peroxide
   D. Covering the site with a sterile transparent dressing

5-9. Cultures taken from a respirometer that has been used in the surgical intensive care unit to monitor several patients indicate that it is contaminated. What is the most practical way to prevent cross-contamination?
   A. Provide a new respirometer for each patient
   B. Sterilize the respirometer after each use
   C. Replace the respirometer with a water-sealed spirometer
   D. Use a disposable HEPA filter and one-way valve for each patient

5-10. All of the following will reduce the incidence of ventilator-acquired pneumonia (VAP) for your patients *except*:
   A. Elevating the head of the bed at least 30°
   B. Implementing daily spontaneous breathing trials
   C. Continuously aspirating subglottic secretions
   D. Changing ventilator circuits every 48 hours

WHAT YOU NEED TO KNOW: ESSENTIAL CONTENT

Key Terms and Definitions

Basic to your understanding of infection control are some key terms and definitions, summarized in **Table 5-1**.

Ensure Equipment Cleanliness

Most of the key information on the processing and maintenance of equipment and devices derives from guidelines developed by the Centers for Disease Control and Prevention (CDC).

Selecting Appropriate Methods to Ensure Equipment Cleanliness

To help you select the best method to ensure equipment cleanliness, the CDC defines three levels of infection risk, as delineated in **Table 5-2**. Note that some of the same liquid chemical solutions (e.g., glutaraldehyde [Cidex] and ortho-phthalaldehyde [OPA]) can be used to either sterilize or provide high-level disinfection of equipment and are commonly used for heat-sensitive items. The differences in level of activity of these solutions reflect time and temperature variables. For example, high-level disinfection with glutaraldehyde (Cidex) can be achieved in 20 minutes at room temperature, but true sterilization requires a full 10 hours.

Table 5-1 Key Terms Used in Infection Control

Term	Meaning
Antiseptic	A chemical that kills microorganisms on living skin or mucous membranes
Bacteriostatic	A descriptive term for chemical agents that inhibit the growth of bacteria but do not necessarily kill them
Cleaning	The physical removal of foreign material (e.g., dirt or organic material), usually with water, detergents, and mechanical action (washing); cleaning generally removes rather than kills microorganisms
Decontamination	The removal of disease-producing microorganisms to leave an item safe for further handling
Disinfection	A general term for the inactivation of disease-producing microorganisms on inanimate objects, usually specified by level
Disinfection, high-level	The destruction of vegetative bacteria, mycobacteria, fungi, and viruses, but not necessarily bacterial spores; some high-level disinfectants can sterilize given adequate contact time
Disinfection, intermediate-level	The destruction of vegetative bacteria, mycobacteria, most viruses and fungi, but not resistant bacterial spores
Disinfection, low-level	The destruction of most vegetative bacteria, some fungi, and some viruses (e.g., hepatitis B/C, HIV), but not mycobacteria or bacterial spores; low-level disinfectants are typically used to clean environmental surfaces
Germicides	Chemical agents capable of killing microorganisms; *bactericidal*, *virucidal*, *fungicidal*, and *sporicidal* are related terms for chemicals capable of killing these specific categories of microorganisms
Sanitation	A process that reduces microorganisms on environmental surfaces to minimize any infectious hazard (e.g., on furniture, floors)
Sterilization	The destruction of all forms of microbial life including bacteria, viruses, spores, and fungi

Table 5-2 Infection Risk Categories of Equipment

Description	Example	Processing
Critical Items		
Devices introduced into the bloodstream or other parts of the body	• Surgical devices • Intravascular catheters • Implants • Heart–lung bypass components • Dialysis components • Bronchoscope forceps/brushes	Sterilization For heat-tolerant items: • Steam under pressure (autoclaving) For heat-sensitive items: • Gas or ionized vapor (ethylene oxide, hydrogen peroxide) • Immersion in a liquid chemical sterilant (e.g., glutaraldehyde, ortho-phthalaldehyde)
Semicritical Items		
Devices that contact intact mucous membranes	• Endoscopes/bronchoscopes • Oral, nasal, and tracheal airways • Ventilator circuits/humidifiers • PFT mouthpieces/tubing • Nebulizers • Laryngoscope blades • Nondisposable resuscitation bags • Pressure, gas, or temperature probes	Sterilization or high-level disinfection via either: • Immersion in a liquid high-level disinfectant (e.g., glutaraldehyde, ortho-phthalaldehyde) • Pasteurization (immersion in hot water at > 158°F [70°C] for 30 minutes)
Noncritical Items		
Devices that touch only intact skin or do not contact the patient	• Face masks (external) • Blood pressure cuffs • Ventilators	Detergent washing or exposure to low- or intermediate-level disinfection

Disinfecting, Sterilizing, and Maintaining Equipment

The CDC recommends the following general measures for sterilization or disinfection and maintenance of equipment and devices:

1. Disassemble and thoroughly clean all equipment before sterilization or disinfection.
2. Consider all reusable breathing circuit components (e.g., tubing, valves, nebulizers, humidifiers) to be semicritical items.
3. Whenever possible, use steam sterilization (autoclaving) or high-level disinfection for reprocessing semicritical equipment not sensitive to heat and moisture.
4. Use low-temperature sterilization methods (gas, vapor, plasma, or liquid sterilant) for equipment that is heat sensitive. After disinfection, protect these items with appropriate rinsing, drying, and packaging, taking care not to recontaminate them.
5. When rinsing reusable semicritical equipment after immersion in a liquid disinfectant, use sterile water. If this is not feasible, rinse the device with filtered water or tap water, and then rinse with isopropyl alcohol and dry with forced air or in a drying cabinet.
6. Avoid reprocessing equipment designed for single use only.

Regarding sterilization, disinfection, and maintenance of *specific* respiratory care equipment and devices, the CDC recommends the following:

- Ventilators
  - Do not routinely sterilize or disinfect the internal machinery of ventilators.
  - Do not routinely change in-use ventilator circuits, attached humidifiers/HMEs, or closed-suction systems; change only if they are visibly soiled or malfunctioning.
  - Sterilize or high-level disinfect nondisposable circuit volume/flow-measuring devices, O_2 sensors, and thermometers between patients.
  - Periodically drain and discard any collected circuit condensate using gloves; avoid letting the condensate drain toward the patient; decontaminate hands when done.
  - Use sterile water to fill humidifiers.
  - Do not place bacterial filters distal to humidifier reservoirs.
- Oxygen "wall" humidifiers
  - Follow the manufacturer's instructions for use of O_2 humidifiers.
  - Change any in-use humidifier tubing and/or the cannula or mask when it malfunctions or becomes visibly contaminated.
- Large-volume nebulizers (e.g., those used with aerosol masks, T-tubes)
  - Whenever possible, use prefilled, sterile disposable nebulizers.
  - If nebulizers are not prefilled, fill reservoirs with sterile water before use and discard the old water before refilling.
  - Do not drain condensate back into reservoir or allow it to flow into airway.
  - Do not handle the internal parts of large-volume nebulizers; replace them if malfunctioning.
  - Replace large-volume nebulizers with sterile or high-level–disinfected units every 24 hours.
- Small-volume drug nebulizers (SVNs)
  - Use only sterile fluid for nebulization; dispense fluids aseptically.
  - Whenever possible, use single-dose medications. If multidose vials are used, follow the manufacturer's instructions for handling.
  - Between treatments on the same patient, SVNs should be cleaned, rinsed with sterile water, and dried.
- Room-air humidifiers
  - Do not use large-volume room-air humidifiers that create aerosols unless they can be sterilized or high-level disinfected at least daily and filled only with sterile water.
- Bag-valve resuscitators
  - Between their uses on different patients, sterilize or high-level disinfect reusable bag-valve resuscitators.
- Suctioning equipment
  - When using an open-suction system, use a sterile single-use catheter for each incident.
  - Use only sterile fluid to remove secretions from the suction catheter.
  - Change the suction collection tubing (up to the canister) between patients.
  - Change the suction collection canisters between patients (except in short-term care units).
- Pulmonary function testing (PFT) equipment (includes American Thoracic Society recommendations)
  - There is no need to routinely sterilize or disinfect the internal workings of closed-circuit spirometers. Instead, the mouthpiece and HEPA filter should be changed between patients.
  - If any reusable components show breath condensation, they should undergo high-level disinfection or sterilization between patients.
  - When using open-circuit devices through which the patient only exhales, disinfect or change only those elements through which rebreathing occurs.

- Use separate disposable valves and HEPA filters to isolate nondisposable bedside PFT equipment (e.g., respirometers, peak flow meters, flow sensors) from each patient tested. If they cannot be isolated from the patient or circuit, these items must be sterilized or undergo high-level disinfection between uses.
- To protect yourself from infection, testing always should be conducted using standard precautions.
- Airborne precautions should be used when there is potential for exposure to infectious agents transmitted by that route, such as tuberculosis.
- Hands always should be washed between patients and immediately after direct handling of used circuit components, whether reusable or disposable.

Monitoring the Effectiveness of Sterilization Procedures

Mechanical, chemical, and biological techniques can be used to assess the effectiveness of sterilization procedures, and generally are used together. **Table 5-3** summarizes these monitoring methods.

Properly Handle Biohazardous Materials

Biohazardous materials include both noninfectious and infectious agents. The materials of most importance to RTs are infectious items such as isolation or contaminated wastes, blood and blood products, and contaminated sharps. Key CDC recommendations for the handling of infectious waste are summarized here:

- Separate infectious and noninfectious wastes at the point of generation; manage isolation wastes using the same methods as for medical wastes from other patient areas.
- Discard and contain all solid infectious wastes except sharps at their point of origin in clearly identifiable leak-proof and tear/puncture-resistant containers marked with the biological hazards symbol.
- Prevent biohazard bags from coming into contact with sharp objects; if a biohazard bag gets contaminated or punctured, double-bag it.
- To properly handle contaminated sharps:
  - Never recap used needles, handle them using both hands, or point a needle toward any part of the body; rather, use either a one-handed "scoop" technique or a mechanical device for holding the needle sheath.

Table 5-3 Methods to Monitor Sterilization Procedures

Description	Comments
Mechanical Methods	
Assess the cycle time, temperature, and pressure of sterilization equipment.	Correct readings do not ensure sterilization, but incorrect readings might indicate a problem.
Chemical Indicators	
A chemical reaction causes the indicator color to change when the proper sterilizer conditions (e.g., the correct temperature or gas concentration) are achieved.	Indicator changes are visible after processing and, therefore, can provide immediate warning as to potential problems. If an indicator does not change color as expected, the affected item(s) should not be used.
Biological Indicators	
Assess whether sterilization actually kills bacterial spores impregnated on paper strips that are exposed to growth media and incubated after processing. Biological indicators should be included in every cycle that contains critical items; otherwise, they should be used at least once a week for each sterilizer.	Best method for verifying sterilization; the incubation period requires holding equipment until negative results are confirmed. If mechanical and chemical monitoring indicate proper processing but culture is positive for growth, recall critical items only.

- Do not remove used needles from disposable syringes by hand, and do not bend, break, or otherwise manipulate used needles by hand.
- Place all used sharps in an impervious, rigid, puncture-resistant container made for this purpose.
- Most liquid wastes (e.g., blood, suction fluids) can be either inactivated using state-approved treatment technologies or carefully poured down a utility sink drain or toilet. Liquid wastes should be placed in capped or tightly stoppered bottles for transport.
- When transporting waste or sharp containers, place them within a rigid container lined with plastic bags.
- After each use, disinfect carts and recyclable containers used to transport waste. Single-use containers should be destroyed as part of the treatment process.
- Should a spill of blood or body fluids occur:
  - Use gloves and other personal protective equipment appropriate for the task.
  - If the spill contains large amounts of blood or body fluids, clean the visible matter with absorbent material and discard it as infectious waste.
  - Swab the area with cloth or paper towels wetted with an EPA-registered hospital disinfectant labeled "tuberculocidal" or with a registered germicide active against HIV or hepatitis B virus; then allow the surface to dry.
  - If an EPA-registered disinfectant is not available, use household bleach (1:100 dilution) to decontaminate nonporous surfaces after cleaning; if there is a large volume of blood or body fluid, use a more concentrated bleach solution (1:10).

Because medical wastes generally are no more infective than wastes coming from the home, their special treatment is not always practical or necessary. For this reason, the CDC now recommends that waste handling and disposal be based on the relative risk of disease transmission, in accordance with local and state regulations. Final disposition of infectious wastes usually involves treatment by either sterilization or incineration, with the solid waste products being buried in a sanitary landfill and liquid or ground-up waste being discharged into a sanitary sewer system.

Adhere to Infection Control Policies and Procedures

CDC Standard Precautions

Standard precautions are based on the assumption that every patient might have an infection that could be transmitted to others. **Table 5-4** specifies the CDC's recommendations for standard precautions.

Given that most hospital-acquired infections occur due to contact between patients and healthcare workers, good hand hygiene is the most important way to help prevent transmission of infections. Good hand hygiene also is incorporated into the respiratory hygiene/cough etiquette guideline, which applies to patients, visitors, *and* healthcare workers. When caring for patients with signs or symptoms of a respiratory infection, you should wear a mask and maintain good hand hygiene. If you have a respiratory infection, you should avoid direct patient contact, especially with any high-risk patients. If this is not possible, then you should wear a mask while providing care.

Which personal protective equipment (PPE) you use in a particular situation depends on the transmission category under which your patient is receiving care (discussed in the next section). In general, PPE should be applied and removed in the following sequence:

Order of Applying PPE

1. Hair and foot coverings
2. Gown
3. Mask
4. Goggles or face shield
5. Gloves

Order of Removing PPE

1. Hair and foot coverings
2. Goggles or face shield
3. Mask
4. Gloves (remove by pulling gloves down from the wrist and turning them inside out)
5. Gown (remove from the inside out)

Table 5-4 CDC Standard Precautions Recommendations

Component	Recommendations
Hand hygiene	• Perform after touching blood, body fluids, secretions, excretions, or contaminated items • Perform immediately after removing gloves • Perform between patient contacts
Gloves	• Use for touching blood, body fluids, secretions, excretions, or contaminated items • Use for touching mucous membranes and nonintact skin
Gown	• Use during procedures and patient-care activities when contact of clothing/exposed skin with blood/body fluids, secretions, or excretions is anticipated
Mask, eye protection (goggles, face shield)[a]	• Use during procedures and patient-care activities likely to generate splashes or sprays of blood, body fluids, or secretions, especially suctioning and endotracheal intubation
Soiled patient-care equipment	• Handle in a manner that prevents transfer of microorganisms to others and to the environment • Wear gloves if equipment is visibly contaminated • Perform hand hygiene after handling
Needles and other sharps	• Do not recap, bend, break, or hand-manipulate used needles • If recapping is required, use a one-handed scoop technique • Use safety features when available • Place used sharps in puncture-resistant container
Patient resuscitation	• Use a mouthpiece, bag-valve resuscitator, or other ventilation device to prevent contact with the patient's mouth and oral secretions
Patient placement	• Use a single-patient room if the patient is at increased risk of transmission, is likely to contaminate the environment, does not maintain appropriate hygiene, or is at increased risk of acquiring infection or developing adverse outcome following infection
Respiratory hygiene/cough etiquette	Patients/visitors who are sneezing or coughing should be instructed to: • Cover the mouth/nose when sneezing/coughing • Use tissues and dispose of them in a no-touch receptacle • Observe hand hygiene after soiling of hands with respiratory secretions • In common waiting areas, wear a surgical mask if tolerated or maintain spatial separation of more than 3 feet if possible

[a]During aerosol-generating procedures on patients with infections likely to be transmitted via the airborne route (e.g., TB, SARS), wear a fit-tested N95 or higher respirator in addition to gloves, gown, and face/eye protection.

Transmission-Based Precautions

Transmission-based precautions represent additional measures designed to prevent infection by microorganisms that are transmitted via particular routes. *Transmission-based precautions are always used in combination with standard precautions.* These extra precautions address three routes of transmission:

- *Contact transmission*: the spread of microorganisms by direct or indirect contact with the patient or the patient's environment, including contaminated equipment
- *Droplet transmission*: the spread of microorganisms in the air via large droplets (larger than 5 μm)
- *Airborne transmission*: the spread of microorganisms in the air via small droplet nuclei (5 μm or smaller)

Most NBRC candidates understand that equipment can be a vehicle for contact transmission between patients and that aerosol therapy devices can spread microorganisms via either the droplet or airborne routes. However, the difference between these routes is not always well understood. Because large droplets fall out of suspension quickly, they travel only short distances. Thus *droplet transmission requires close contact*, generally 3 feet or less. In contrast, the smaller droplets generated when talking, coughing, or sneezing and during procedures such as suctioning are very stable and can travel over long distances, such as between rooms. **Table 5-5** summarizes the CDC's precautions designed to thwart each of these types of transmission, including the most common infections to which they apply.

Table 5-5 CDC Transmission-Based Precautions Recommendations

Applicable Infections (Examples)	Precautions
Contact Precautions	
Gastrointestinal infections (including diarrhea of unknown origin and suspected or confirmed *C. difficile* infections), wound and skin infections, multidrug-resistant infection or colonization (e.g., MRSA, SARS)	• Apply standard precautions • Place the patient in a private room • Wear clean gloves and gown when entering the room • Change gloves after contact with any infectious material • Remove gloves and gown before leaving the room; wash hands immediately with alcohol-based rub
Droplet Precautions	
Bacterial meningitis, whooping cough (*Bordetella pertussis*), influenza, mumps, rubella, diphtheria, Group A *Streptococcus pneumoniae* infections, SARS, and epiglottitis (due to *Haemophilus influenzae*)	• Apply standard precautions • Place the patient in a private room (special air handling and ventilation are not needed; the door can stay open) • Wear a surgical mask when within 3 feet of the patient • Use eye/face protection for an aerosol-generating procedure or contact with respiratory secretions • Patients transported outside their rooms should wear a mask and follow respiratory hygiene/cough etiquette
Airborne Precautions	
TB, measles (rubeola), chickenpox (varicella-zoster), *Aspergillus* infections, SARS, smallpox (variola)	• Apply standard precautions • Place the patient in a private negative-pressure airborne infection isolation room (AIIR) with the door closed • Wear a fit-tested,* NIOSH-certified N95 respirator when entering the room • Use eye/face protection for an aerosol-generating procedure or contact with respiratory secretions • Nonimmune healthcare workers should avoid caring for patients with vaccine-preventable airborne diseases (e.g., measles, chickenpox, smallpox) • If airborne precautions cannot be implemented, place the patient in a private room with the door closed; mask the patient • Patients transported outside their rooms should wear a mask and follow respiratory hygiene/cough etiquette

*In addition to being fit-tested for a respirator, you need to perform a user-seal check each time you use this device (according to the manufacturer's specifications).

CDC Central Line Bundle

Indwelling vascular lines—especially those terminating close to the heart or in one of the great vessels—are a major cause of bloodstream infections. Because such infections are associated with high patient morbidity and mortality, the CDC has established an evidence-based central line bundle to help prevent them. Although the primary focus is on central lines, application of this bundle to peripheral arterial lines should also help reduce infections associated with those catheters. The accompanying box summarizes the key recommendations included in the central line bundle.

Key Elements in CDC Central Line Bundle

Follow Proper Insertion Practices

- Perform vigorous hand hygiene before insertion.
- Adhere to aseptic technique.
- Choose the best site to minimize infections/mechanical complications.
  - Avoid the femoral site in adults.
  - For CVP and PA catheters, use subclavian (not jugular) access.
  - Avoid brachial sites for arterial lines in children.
- Use sterile barrier precautions (i.e., mask, cap, gown, sterile gloves, and sterile drape).
- Scrub the skin area for 30 seconds with chlorhexidine 2% in 70% isopropyl alcohol.
- After insertion, cover the site with sterile gauze or a sterile transparent dressing.

Handle and Maintain Lines Appropriately

- Comply with hand hygiene requirements.
- Swab access ports with chlorhexidine, povidone-iodine, or alcohol, and access them only with sterile devices.
- Replace dressings that are wet, soiled, or dislodged.
- Perform dressing changes under aseptic technique using sterile gloves.

Review of Status

- Perform daily audits to assess whether the line is still needed.
- Do *not* routinely replace catheters to minimize infection.
- Promptly remove unnecessary lines.

Adhere to the Ventilator-Associated Pneumonia Protocol

Ventilator-associated pneumonia (VAP) is pneumonia occurring in patients who have received mechanical ventilation for more than 48 hours. It is a leading cause of death among patients with hospital-acquired infections. Among those who survive, VAP increases ventilator days and prolongs both ICU and overall hospital length of stay. To decrease the incidence of this problem, the CDC recommends a set of preventive strategies called the "VAP bundle." The key components in the VAP bundle are as follows:

- Elevating the head of the bed by 30-45° (unless contraindicated)
- Implementing daily "sedation vacations" and spontaneous breathing trials
- Providing peptic ulcer disease prophylaxis (using sucralfate rather than H_2 antagonists)
- Providing daily oral care with chlorhexidine

VAP is associated with gastric reflux aspiration. Elevating the head of the bed helps prevent gastric aspiration, as does ulcer disease prophylaxis. Elevating the head of the bed also improves the distribution of ventilation and the efficiency of diaphragmatic action, which may help prevent atelectasis.

Daily cessation of sedatives can shorten the duration of mechanical ventilation. In conjunction with this sedation vacation, patients should undergo daily spontaneous breathing trials to help wean them from ventilatory support (see Chapters 10, 12, and 13 for details on weaning). In general, the sooner a patient can be extubated, the lower the risk for VAP. Of course, one needs to be on guard for accidental (self-) extubation when stopping sedatives. To minimize this risk, ensure that the patient is adequately supervised and that appropriate hand or arm restraints are used.

Other strategies potentially helpful in preventing VAP include general infection control procedures, airway management techniques, equipment maintenance, and oral care.

In terms of *general infection control* procedures, you should always implement both standard precautions *and* any needed transmission-based precautions for patients receiving ventilatory support. This must include rigorous hand hygiene before and after contact with a patient's mucous membranes, respiratory secretions, or related equipment (e.g., ventilator circuit, suction apparatus, ET tube).

Airway management techniques that can help decrease the incidence of VAP include the following:

- Avoid intubation whenever possible (*use noninvasive ventilation instead*).
- If intubation is necessary, use the oral route (nasal intubation is associated with sinus infection).
- Maintain tube cuff pressures in the 20–25 cm H_2O range; *avoid using the minimal leak technique.*
- Aspirate subglottic secretions using tracheal tubes having a suction lumen above the cuff.
- Use only sterile water or saline to flush suction catheters.
- Use an inline or "closed" suction catheter system to avoid breaking the ventilator circuit.

Regarding use of inline suction catheters—even though the supporting evidence is not strong—the AARC recommends that they be incorporated into VAP prevention protocols. This approach is consistent with the "closed circuit" concept—that is, the less frequently the ventilator circuit is opened or "broken," the less likely infection will occur.

Also consistent with the closed-circuit concept are specific *equipment maintenance* strategies. To that end, both the CDC and the AARC recommend *against* routine changing of ventilator circuits. Instead, you should change the circuit only when it is visibly soiled or malfunctioning. In terms of humidification, the incidence of VAP does not appear to differ between patients receiving active (heated humidifier) versus passive (HME) support. However, when using heated humidification, the CDC recommends that you regularly drain collected condensate *away from the patient* and properly discard it, ideally without breaking the circuit. If using HMEs, you should place them vertically above the tracheal tube and change them only when they are visibly soiled.

Oral care is the last strategy potentially helpful in preventing VAP. Good oral care involves (1) regularly assessing the oral cavity for hydration, lesions, or infections; (2) rotating the oral ET tube position at least every 24 hours; (3) providing frequent chlorhexidine rinses and teeth brushing; and (4) applying mouth moisturizer and/or lip balm after oral care.

Implement Specific Infectious Disease Protocols

Over the past decade, several new viral infections have emerged and raised concerns in the healthcare community. These infections can be difficult to diagnose and treat and have the potential to cause serious widespread epidemics, called *pandemics*. Examples include avian or bird influenza (an influenza A virus) and severe acute respiratory syndrome (SARS). Although the SARS epidemic ended in 2004, variants of that virus causing pulmonary infection have appeared as recently as 2013, and avian flu cases continue to be reported worldwide.

Typically these emerging viruses initially produce symptoms similar to those of ordinary influenza. However, they tend to be much more virulent and can quickly progress to an acute and life-threatening pneumonia and ARDS. For these reasons, all patients who present to a healthcare setting with flu-like symptoms should follow the previously described respiratory hygiene and cough etiquette protocol *and* be questioned regarding their recent travel history and contact with other sick individuals. If a patient is suspected of or confirmed as having an atypical influenza-like infection, the CDC currently recommends implementing a protocol that presumes *multiple routes of transmission*—that is, spread via both contact and through the air. Key elements in this combined contact and airborne protocol (based on the avian flu and SARS experience) include the following:

- Standard precautions:
  - Pay careful attention to hand hygiene before and after all patient contact or contact with items potentially contaminated with respiratory secretions.
- Contact precautions:
  - Use dedicated equipment such as stethoscopes, disposable blood pressure cuffs, and thermometers.
  - Designate "clean" and "dirty" areas for isolation materials.
  - Maintain a stock of clean patient care and PPE supplies outside the patient's room.
  - Don gloves, gown, and respiratory protection before entering the room.
  - Wear eye protection when within 3 feet of the patient or if splash or spray of respiratory secretions or other body fluids is likely.
  - Avoid unnecessary touching of surfaces and objects or the face with contaminated gloves.
  - Locate dirty receptacles close to the point of use and separate them from the clean supplies.
  - Carefully remove PPE in a manner that prevents contamination of clothing and skin.
- Airborne precautions:
  - Place the patient in an airborne infection isolation room (AIIR).
  - If an AIIR is unavailable, use portable HEPA filtration.
  - Use a fit-tested, NIOSH-approved N-95 respirator when entering the room.
  - Discard disposable respirators upon leaving the patient room or area.

In general, these precautions should be continued for 14 days after onset of symptoms or until laboratory testing indicates that the patient is not infected with the suspected virus. Depending on the known or suspected contagiousness of the infection, additional protocol elements may include the following:

- Patient transport:
  - Limit patient transport outside the AIIR to medically essential purposes; whenever possible, use portable equipment to perform procedures in the patient's room.
  - If transport is required, have the patient wear a surgical mask, put on a clean patient gown, and perform hand hygiene before leaving the room.
  - Use less-traveled hallways and elevators to limit contact between the patient and others.
- Visitors:
  - Limit visits to persons who are essential for the patient's emotional well-being and care.
  - Visitors who have been in contact with the patient are a possible source of infection and should be screened for the suspected infection and instructed on using PPE and other precautions.
- Medical waste:
  - Contain and dispose of contaminated medical waste and sharps according to facility-specific procedures and/or local or state regulations.
  - Wear disposable gloves when handling waste and perform hand hygiene after removing gloves.
- Patient-care equipment:
  - Follow standard practices for handling and reprocessing used patient-care equipment.
  - Wear gloves when handling and transporting used patient-care equipment.
  - Wipe equipment with an EPA-approved hospital disinfectant before removing it from the patient's room.

- Aerosol-generating procedures (e.g., aerosol drug delivery, sputum induction, bronchoscopy, suctioning, intubation, and noninvasive and high-frequency oscillatory ventilation):
  - Perform only those aerosol-generating procedures that are medically necessary and with only the needed personnel present.
  - PPE for aerosol-generating procedures should cover the torso, arms, and hands as well as the eyes, nose, and mouth. Consider a surgical hood with an N-95 respirator that fully cover the head, neck, and face; for the highest level of protection, use a powered air-purifying respirator (PAPR).
  - Perform aerosol-generating procedures in an AIIR; keep the doors closed and minimize entry and exit during the procedure.
  - Consider sedation during intubation and bronchoscopy to minimize coughing.
  - Use HEPA filtration on the expiratory limb of mechanical ventilators.

COMMON ERRORS TO AVOID

You can improve your score by avoiding these mistakes:

- Don't pasteurize or immerse any electrically powered equipment in liquid disinfectants; use gas sterilization instead.
- Don't confuse sterilization (which kills all microorganisms, including bacterial spores) with high-level disinfection (which kills all microorganisms *except* bacterial spores).
- Don't select steam autoclaving for any heat-sensitive items needing sterilization.
- Never drain tubing condensate back into humidifier or nebulizer reservoirs.
- Don't routinely change ventilator circuits; instead, change these components only if they are visibly soiled or malfunctioning.
- Don't recap, bend, break, or otherwise manipulate used needles with your hands.
- Don't routinely replace indwelling catheters to prevent infection.
- Avoid using the brachial site for arterial lines in children.
- Don't intubate a patient in respiratory failure if noninvasive ventilation will suffice.
- Avoid touching surfaces, objects, and your face with contaminated gloves.

SURE BETS

In some situations, you can always be sure of the right approach to a clinical problem or scenario:

- Always disassemble and inspect nondisposable equipment before cleaning it.
- Always ensure that all equipment that has been cleaned via washing is dried properly before further processing.
- Always ensure that all nondisposable critical items (i.e., devices introduced into the blood stream or other parts of the body) are sterilized before reuse.
- Always treat any nondisposable equipment that comes in contact with a patient's airway as semicritical and in need of either high-level disinfection or pasteurization before reuse.
- Always recognize that among respiratory therapy equipment, nebulizers and aerosol generators pose the greatest infection risk.
- Always use sterile solutions to fill nebulizers and aerosol generators.
- Always use low-resistance HEPA filters to isolate bedside and laboratory pulmonary function equipment from the patient.
- Always scrub vascular line ports with chlorhexidine, povidone-iodine, or alcohol before accessing them.
- Always wear a mask and maintain good hand hygiene when examining or caring for patients with signs and symptoms of a respiratory infection.
- Always perform a user-seal check each time you use an N-95 respirator for airborne precautions.

PRE-TEST ANSWERS AND EXPLANATIONS

Following are this chapter's pre-test answers and explanations. Be sure to review each answer's explanation thoroughly to help you understand why it is correct. If the explanation is still unclear to you, review the chapter content.

5-1. **Correct answer: B.** Cleaning. The first step in equipment processing is cleaning. Equipment is cleaned by removing dirt and organic material from its surfaces, usually by washing. If equipment is improperly cleaned, subsequent processing efforts may be ineffective.

5-2. **Correct answer: B.** Low level. A low-level disinfectant inactivates most bacteria, some viruses, and fungi, but cannot destroy resistant microorganisms such as *Mycobacterium tuberculosis* or bacterial spores.

5-3. **Correct answer: A.** Pasteurization. Reusable breathing circuits are semicritical items. Reusable semicritical equipment should be sterilized or undergo high-level disinfection. Of the available options, only pasteurization meets this standard.

5-4. **Correct answer: D.** 1, 2, and 3. To minimize the likelihood of infection in patients receiving bronchodilator therapy via SVN, you should (1) use a different SVN for each patient, (2) change the SVN and tubing every 24 hours, and (3) perform thorough hand washing prior to therapy. It is also recommended that the nebulizer *not* be rinsed with tap water, but rather be rinsed with sterile water and blown dry between uses.

5-5. **Correct answer: B.** 1, 2, and 3. If an atypical virus infection causing severe pneumonia is either suspected or confirmed, the patient should be managed using a combination of standard, contact, and strict airborne precautions.

5-6. **Correct answer: C.** Minimizing suction time to 10-15 seconds. To decrease the risk of contamination during suctioning, you should use a fresh sterile single-use catheter on each patient and use only sterile water or saline to clear the catheter. In addition, both the suction collection tubing and collection canister should be changed between patients, except in short-term care units (where only the collection tubing should be changed). Minimizing suction time decreases the likelihood of hypoxemia, but does not reduce the risk of infection.

5-7. **Correct answer: C.** 1 and 3. Because it directly comes in contact with mucous membranes, a reusable airway is a semicritical item. If sterilization of a semicritical item is not feasible, the alternatives are high-level disinfection and pasteurization.

5-8. **Correct answer: C.** Scrubbing the insertion site with hydrogen peroxide. When inserting an indwelling vascular line, you should (1) perform vigorous hand hygiene before insertion; (2) use sterile barrier precautions, including a drape over the site; (3) scrub the insertion area for 30 seconds with chlorhexidine; and (4) after insertion of the line, cover the site with sterile gauze or a sterile transparent dressing.

5-9. **Correct answer: D.** Use a disposable HEPA filter and one-way valve for each patient. The best way to prevent the contamination of a Wright respirometer used on different patients is to use a one-way valving system, preferably with a HEPA filter. This ensures that patients only breathe out through the device, thereby preventing cross-contamination.

5-10. **Correct answer: D.** Changing ventilator circuits every 48 hours. The VAP bundle includes elevating the head of the bed, implementing daily "sedation vacations" and spontaneous breathing trials, providing peptic ulcer prophylaxis, and applying rigorous oral care. Related airway management strategies include (1) avoiding intubation if possible; (2) intubating via the oral route; (3) maintaining proper cuff pressures; (4) aspirating subglottic secretions; (5) using only sterile fluids to flush suction catheters, and (6) using closed-suction catheters. *Ventilator circuits should be changed only when visibly soiled or malfunctioning.*

POST-TEST

To confirm your mastery of this chapter's topical content, you should take the chapter post-test, available online at http://go.jblearning.com/respexamreview. A score of 80% or more indicates that you are adequately prepared for this section of the NBRC written exams. If you score less than 80%, you should continue to review the applicable chapter content. In addition, you may want to access and review the relevant Web links covering this chapter's content (courtesy of RTBoardReview.com), also online at the Jones & Bartlett Learning site.

Perform Quality Control Procedures

CHAPTER 6

Craig L. Scanlan
(previous version co-authored with John A. Rutkowski)

The quality of care you provide depends in part on the proper performance of the equipment you use. Quality control (QC) processes help ensure that the devices you use perform as expected. For diagnostic equipment, QC processes ensure accurate measurements. For therapeutic equipment, QC processes ensure proper device function and patient safety. Unfortunately, unless you work in the blood gas or pulmonary function testing (PFT) lab, or collaborate directly with your biomedical engineering department, you likely do not regularly engage in QC activities. The NBRC, however, expects exam candidates to know the basics of QC as applied to the common devices used in respiratory care. For this reason, you should plan on spending a reasonable portion of your exam preparation on this topic.

OBJECTIVES

In preparing for the shared NBRC exam content, you should demonstrate the knowledge needed to:

1. Perform quality control procedures for:
   a. Blood gas analyzers and hemoximeters
   b. Point-of-care analyzers
   c. Pulmonary function equipment
   d. Mechanical ventilators
   e. Oxygen and specialty gas analyzers
   f. Noninvasive monitors
   g. Gas metering devices
2. Record and monitor QC data using accepted statistical methods

WHAT TO EXPECT ON THIS CATEGORY OF THE NBRC EXAMS

CRT exam: 4 questions; about 25% recall and 75% application
WRRT exam: 2 questions; 100% analysis
CSE exam: indeterminate number of questions; however, exam II-C knowledge can appear in both CSE Information Gathering and Decision-Making sections

PRE-TEST

Carefully respond to each of the following questions. After completing the pre-test, compare your answers to those provided at the end of this chapter. Then thoroughly review each answer's explanation to help understand why it is correct.

6-1. To avoid the preanalytical errors that are associated with air contamination of a blood gas sample, all of the following are appropriate *except*:
A. Removing all of the air bubbles
B. Mixing only after removing air
C. Capping the syringe quickly
D. Using a short-bevel needle

6-2. What is the best way to avoid arterial blood gas analysis errors associated with blood metabolism?
A. Analyze the sample immediately
B. Place the sample in an ice slush
C. Keep the sample at body temperature
D. Use dry (lithium) heparin

6-3. Inspection of a blood gas analyzer's QC data set reveals a single PaO_2 value (among 10) as being +2.8 SD from the mean. Which of the following is the *least* likely cause of this observation?
- **A.** Sample contamination
- **B.** Failure of the PO_2 electrode
- **C.** Statistical probability
- **D.** Improper sample handling

6-4. Under ideal conditions, electrochemical oxygen analyzers have an accuracy of:
- **A.** ±1%
- **B.** ±2%
- **C.** ±3%
- **D.** ±4%

6-5. Which of the following hemoximeter measurements are affected by air contamination?
- **A.** COHb levels
- **B.** Met Hb levels
- **C.** HbO_2 levels
- **D.** Total Hb levels

6-6. Which of the following devices would you select to assess the output accuracy of a Bourdon gauge regulator used for O_2 transport?
- **A.** Mercury manometer
- **B.** Clark electrode
- **C.** Paramagnetic oxygen analyzer
- **D.** Precision flowmeter

6-7. To periodically confirm the validity of blood gas analyzer results, which procedure would you perform?
- **A.** External statistical quality control
- **B.** Instrument performance validation
- **C.** Regular preventive maintenance
- **D.** Control media calibration verification

6-8. According to ATS recommendations, diagnostic spirometers should be calibrated to within:
- **A.** ± 1.5 cm H2O/L/sec resistance
- **B.** ± 3% or 50 mL, whichever is greater, using a 3-liter syringe
- **C.** ± 5% or 100 mL, whichever is greater, using a 3-liter syringe
- **D.** ± 10% or 500 mL, whichever is greater, using a 5-liter syringe

6-9. How often should ventilators be tested to verify their performance?
- **A.** Daily
- **B.** Between patient uses
- **C.** Once a week
- **D.** Once a year

6-10. A fuel cell oxygen analyzer is reading 18% when exposed to ambient air. What should the initial corrective action be?
- **A.** Calibrate the sensor
- **B.** Check the batteries
- **C.** Replace the fuel cell
- **D.** Replace the display

WHAT YOU NEED TO KNOW: ESSENTIAL CONTENT

Key Terms and Definitions

Basic to your understanding of QC are some key terms and definitions, summarized in **Table 6-1**.

Laboratory Blood Gas and Hemoximetry Analyzers

Most of the QC specifications for laboratory testing are based on governmental guidelines promulgated by the Centers for Medicare and Medicaid Services (CMS) and implemented through the Clinical Laboratory Improvement Act (CLIA) program. As with most laboratory tests, QC processes for blood gas and hemoximetry analyses focus on eliminating errors in sample collection and handling (the preanalytical phase), sample measurement (the analytical phase), and results reporting, interpretation, and application (the postanalytical phase). Here we focus primarily on QC during the preanalytical and analytical phases of blood gas and hemoximetry.

Preanalytical Phase

The preanalytical phase involves all sample collection and handling procedures conducted prior to actual analysis. For this reason, you must be proficient with the techniques involved in obtaining blood samples from various sites (see Chapter 11 for details). Also important is your strict adherence

Table 6-1 Key Terms Used in Quality Control

Term	Meaning
Accuracy	The degree to which a measurement reading coincides with its true value
Analyte	A substance undergoing analysis or measurement
Analytical errors	Results errors due to mistakes made during measurement and analysis
Bias	Systematic inaccuracy—that is, consistently high or low variation from a measure's true value
Calibration	Testing and adjusting an analyzer to provide a known relationship between its measurements and the level or quantity of the substances being analyzed
Calibration verification	Measurement of control media to confirm that the calibration of the analyzer has remained stable throughout the lab's reportable range
Coefficient of variation (CV)	Standard deviation as a percentage of the mean; useful in gauging precision
Control charts	A record of the measurements of standard samples by an analyzer, which is used for statistical evaluation of analyzer performance; also referred to as Levy-Jennings charts
Drift	The difference in a given measurement's value between successive analyzer calibrations
Gain	The ratio of the output/response signal of an analyzer to its input signal (the true value) over a range of measurements; equivalent to the calibration slope
Linearity	The change in error over an analyzer's measurement range; the amount of deviation from ideal "straight-line" performance
Mean	The arithmetic average of a group of measurements
Postanalytical errors	Results errors due to mistakes made in data handling, results reporting, or interpretation
Preanalytical errors	Results errors due to mistakes in collection, handling, or storage of samples prior to analysis
Precision	The reproducibility or repeatability of an analyzer's results for the same analyte over multiple measurements
Reportable range	The range of values over which a laboratory can verify the accuracy of the measurements
Standard deviation	A statistical measure indicating the variability of a set of measurements
Statistical QC	The application of statistical analysis and other procedures to detect problems that could invalidate patient results

to infection control procedures (see Chapter 5). In addition, to avoid interpretation errors, you always must document the patient's FIO_2, the O_2 delivery device, the mode of ventilation, and the results of any related assessments made at the time of sampling.

The most common preanalytical errors affecting blood gas and hemoximetry measurements are air contamination, venous admixture, and continued blood metabolism. As indicated in **Table 6-2**, these errors can yield invalid measurements, which can result in incorrect decisions and potential patient harm. To avoid these problems, you always must strive to ensure that the samples you obtain are free of these common errors.

Analytical Phase

The analytical phase of blood gas and hemoximetry measurement involves three key elements: (1) analyzer calibration and calibration verification, (2) actual sample testing, and (3) ongoing review of QC and proficiency testing results.

Table 6-2 Common Preanalytical Errors in pH/Blood Gas Analysis and Hemoximetry

Error	Effect	Recognition	Avoidance
Air contamination	• Decreases P_{CO_2} • Increases pH • Variable effect on $P_{O_2}/HbO_2\%$*	• Visible bubbles • Results not consistent with patient's condition	• Expel bubbles • Do not mix samples with air bubbles • Cap syringes; seal capillary tubes quickly
Venous admixture	• Increases P_{CO_2} • Decreases pH • Decreases $P_{O_2}/HbO_2\%$	• No pulsations as syringe fills • Results not consistent with the patient's condition	• Do not aspirate sample • Avoid brachial/femoral sites • Use short-bevel needles
Continued metabolism	• Increases P_{CO_2} • Decreases pH • Decreases $P_{O_2}/HbO_2\%$	• Time lag between collection and analysis of sample • Results not consistent with patient's condition	• Analyze within 30 minutes (3 minutes for capillary tube samples) • If anticipated storage time exceeds 30 minutes, place sample in ice slurry

*If the patient's actual Pa_{O_2} is > 150 torr, air contamination will lower the P_{O_2} and $HbO_2\%$; if the actual Pa_{O_2} is < 150 torr, it will raise the measured values

Analyzer Calibration and Calibration Verification

During calibration, the response of an analyzer is compared and adjusted to a known standard. The standards used to calibrate blood gas analyzers are precision gases and buffer solutions with known values for pH, P_{CO_2}, and P_{O_2}. Similarly, hemoximeter calibration involves measurement of standard solutions with known values for total Hb, HbO_2, carboxyhemoglobin (COHb), and methemoglobin (MetHb).

As depicted in **Figure 6-1**, calibration involves adjusting the analyzer to ensure that its response is accurate and linear—in other words, to ensure that the measured value (response) equals the known value. In this example, the precalibrated response of the analyzer is linear, but positively biased. For example, at a known value of 0, the analyzer response is 20; and at a known

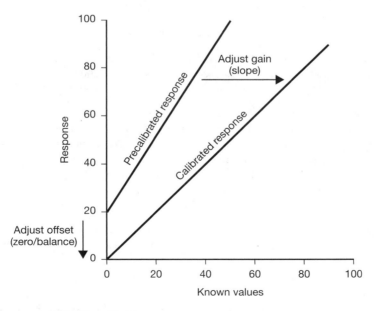

Figure 6-1 Instrument Calibration.

Courtesy of: Strategic Learning Associates, LLC, Little Silver, New Jersey.

Table 6-3 Typical Calibration Ranges for Blood Gas Analyzers

	Calibration Range
pH	6.840–7.384
Po_2	80–150 mm Hg
Pco_2	40–80 mm Hg

value of 40, the response is about 80—both clearly inaccurate. Calibration requires adjusting both the offset ("balancing" or "zeroing" the analyzer) and the gain or slope of the instrument. Only after these two adjustments are made can we say that the analyzer is properly calibrated—that the instrument response will accurately reflect the known value(s).

The method depicted in Figure 6-1 requires a "two-point calibration," in which two different known values are used. **Table 6-3** provides the typical ranges used for two-point calibration of blood gas analyzers. Only by performing a two-point calibration can you properly adjust both the offset and the gain (slope) of the analyzer and ensure an unbiased and linear response.

Single or one-point calibration also can be performed. However, when you measure only one known value, the slope or gain of the instrument remains in question, with measurement errors possible for values above or below the single confirmed point.

Modern analyzers include automated calibration routines. However, to ensure that the analyzers you use are providing valid measurements, you must perform *calibration verification*. Calibration verification involves analysis of prepared *control media*. Control media are analytes that are independently certified to provide a known measurement value when tested. Typically, calibration verification involves analysis of at least *three* different levels of control media spanning the full range of expected results and is conducted at least daily. In addition, calibration verification should be conducted after any instrument maintenance and whenever a question arises regarding instrument performance.

For blood gas analyzer calibration verification, commercial control media generally suffice. *However, both the AARC and the Clinical and Laboratory Standards Institute recommend tonometry as the best reference standard for assessing Po_2 and Pco_2 measurements.* Tonometry involves exposing and equilibrating liquid media (blood/control solution) to a reference gas with known partial pressures.

Sample Testing

Testing must be performed by individuals who meet the competency requirements for the procedure, as documented at least annually. Testing also must follow the protocol recommended by the instrument manufacturer. If you are responsible for performing the analysis, you always must take the following steps:

- Confirm that the specimen was properly labeled and stored prior to analysis.
- Assess the sample for any obvious preanalytical errors (e.g., air bubbles or clots).
- Confirm that the applicable calibration procedures were completed prior to analysis.
- Analyze the sample within an acceptable period of time.
- Mix the sample thoroughly and then discard a drop or two of blood from the syringe.
- Ensure that the sample is properly aspirated/injected into the analyzer.

Whenever you report the results of any test you conduct, you also should provide a brief statement addressing test quality, including any problems encountered with the specimen or its measurement.

Review of QC and Proficiency Testing Results

Comprehensive QC involves recording and continuously monitoring data using accepted statistical methods. To do so, you plot the results of control media analyses on graphs, with a separate chart constructed for each level of control and each analyte reported. The most common plotting format used for statistical QC is the Levy-Jennings chart. As depicted in **Figure 6-2**, a Levy-Jennings chart

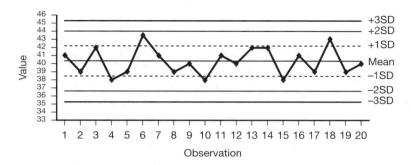

Figure 6-2 Levy-Jennings Chart for Pco₂ Control Value of 40 Torr Showing Analyzer in Control.

Courtesy of: Strategic Learning Associates, LLC, Little Silver, New Jersey.

plots individual values for control media over multiple measurements and compares these values with the mean and standard deviation (SD) of the data. Typically, bounding limits are set to within ±2 SD. Control measurements that consistently fall within these limits indicate that the analyzer is "in control" and ready for patient measurement. For example, Figure 6-2 depicts *normal variation* in the measurement of a Pco₂ control value standardized to 40 torr (mm Hg). This variation is considered normal because it consistently falls within the ±2 SD limits.

Control measurements that fall outside the bounding limits indicate *analytical error*. **Figure 6-3** depicts this situation, with the third to last observation falling well outside the ±2 SD bounding limit (actually greater than 3 SD from the mean). Single aberrant values like these are relatively common and are due to *random errors* of measurement that occur with any instrument. As long as subsequent measures are within the control limits, no remedial action is needed. In contrast, frequent random errors like this one would indicate a lack of precision—that is, poor repeatability of measurement. Any instrument that demonstrates poor repeatability over time is "out of control." In such cases, you would need to identify the problem, take corrective action, and confirm that the analyzer is back in control prior to reporting any patient results.

Figure 6-4 demonstrates a different type of error, called *systematic error* or *bias*. Note that beginning with observation 13 there is an upward trend in the reported values for the 40-torr Pco₂

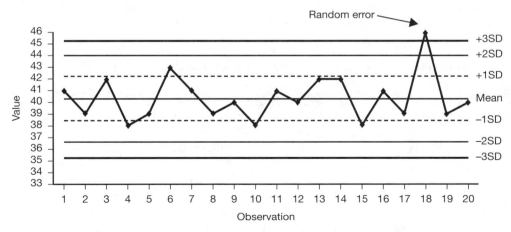

Figure 6-3 Levy-Jennings Chart for Pco₂ Control Value of 40 Torr Showing a Single Random Error. As long as subsequent measures are in control, no remedial action is needed.

Courtesy of: Strategic Learning Associates, LLC, Little Silver, New Jersey.

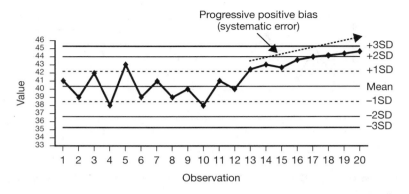

Figure 6-4 Levy-Jennings Chart for Pco$_2$ Control Value of 40 Torr Showing Developing Positive Bias Error. Bias errors usually indicate faulty procedure or component failure. No patient samples should be analyzed until the problem is found and corrected.

Courtesy of: Strategic Learning Associates, LLC, Little Silver, New Jersey.

control. Over time, this particular trend shifts the mean above the control value, causing a positive measurement bias. Generally bias errors are more serious than random errors, indicating either an incorrect procedure or instrument failure. As with recurrent random errors, whenever instrument bias is identified, no patient samples should be analyzed until the problem is corrected.

Table 6-4 compares and contrasts the common causes and corrective actions for these two types of analytic errors.

Supplementing "in-house" QC procedures is a process called *proficiency testing*. Under proficiency testing requirements, laboratories receive unknown samples from an outside agency on a regular schedule. These samples are analyzed and the results reported back to the sending agency. The agency then compares the results against its own and those of other laboratories using similar instrumentation. Discrepancies must be addressed and remediated for any lab to maintain CLIA certification, which is a prerequisite for Medicare/Medicaid reimbursement.

Point-of-Care Analyzers

As described in Chapter 4, point-of-care testing (POCT) involves the collection, measurement, and reporting of selected lab tests at or near the site of patient care, rather than via a central lab. Instruments used for POCT vary substantially. The most common POCT tests that you are likely to

Table 6-4 Comparison of Instrument Analytical Errors and Their Correction

Type of Error	Contributing Factors	Corrective Actions
Random errors	• Statistical probability • Contamination of sample • Improper handling of sample	• Reanalyze control sample after performing a two-point calibration • If repeat QC analysis is in control, no further action is needed • If repeat QC analysis is out of control, continue corrective actions according to manufacturer's recommendations
Bias errors	• Contaminated buffer solutions • Incorrect gas concentrations • Component degradation/failure • Incorrect procedure	• Troubleshoot suspected problem(s) • Repair or replace faulty components • Corrective action(s) continue until an acceptable two-point calibration is achieved and QC sample values are within ±2 SD of the mean

perform are for arterial blood gases (ABGs) or combined panels that include ABG measures plus other selected values essential in managing critically ill patients.

As with central lab measurements, POCT QC requires those personnel who perform the tests have documented competency with the equipment and procedures. In addition, *all POCT results must be auditable.* This means that the test results must be traceable to the patient tested, the instrument and its operator, the date and time of the test, and the process used. As with centralized lab testing, instrument maintenance records must be kept as well.

In terms of calibration, most POCT analyzers use self-contained disposable cartridges for each analysis. Typically, these cartridges include solutions that provide automated calibration prior to sample analysis. Other POCT analyzers employ a computer chip for calibration. When these devices fail to calibrate, analysis usually stops. For cartridge-based instruments, the first step in such cases is to rerun the test with a new cartridge. If a second attempt fails, you should remove the device from service and either obtain a replacement or send the sample to the central lab.

Most facilities also require that results obtained via POCT analysis regularly be compared with those provided by a calibrated bench-top analyzer. This is done by performing simultaneous analysis of the sample on both instruments ("inter-instrumental comparison"). Based on accumulated data and statistical rules, one can then determine if the POCT results meet the same standards for accuracy and precision as required for regular lab testing. In addition, most facilities use proficiency testing to help further ensure the quality of their POCT programs.

Pulmonary Function Test Equipment

As with analysis of blood specimens, erroneous PFT results can lead to inappropriate clinical decisions. For these reasons, an effective quality assurance program is required to make certain that PFT data are both accurate and reproducible. An effective PFT quality assurance program must include at least the following elements:

- Proper technician training and review
- Accurate spirometry equipment
- Daily spirometer checks
- Individual maneuver validity checks
- Monthly spirometry quality reports
- Documentation of equipment maintenance

Proper training and annual competency reviews of PFT technicians are key components of any quality process, as is ongoing documentation of both QC testing and equipment maintenance. Here we focus on ensuring the accuracy of the equipment and obtaining valid results.

Accuracy of PFT Equipment

To ensure the accuracy of PFT equipment, you need to confirm volume and flow values, check volume and flow linearity, assess system leakage, and validate time measurements. **Table 6-5** summarizes the QC tests used to confirm these measurements, as recommended by the American Thoracic Society (ATS) and the European Respiratory Society.

If using a volumetric spirometer (bell or bellows systems), you should check it daily for leaks (*before* the volume calibration check) and after any needed cleaning/reassembly activity. To do so, follow these steps:

1. Inject approximately 3 L of room air into the spirometer.
2. Occlude the breathing circuit at the patient interface.
3. Use the manufacturer's recommended method to pressurize the system to 3 cm H_2O.
4. Observe for any change in volume over 1 minute.

Depending on the device, a weight, spring, or rubber band is used to pressurize the system. When pressurized, the system should lose no more than 10 mL per minute. Larger losses indicate a leak, which must be corrected before patient testing. Common sources of leaks include loose connections, cracked tubing, and missing or damaged seals.

Table 6-5 PFT Equipment Quality Control

Test	Minimum Interval	Action
Leaks	Daily	3 cm H$_2$O constant pressure for 1 minute (< 10 mL)
Volume	Daily	Calibration check with a 3-L syringe check
Volume linearity	Quarterly	1-L increments with a calibrating syringe over the entire volume range
Flow linearity	Weekly	Test at least three different flow ranges
Time	Quarterly	Mechanical recorder check with a stopwatch
Software	New versions	Log the installation date and perform a test using a known subject, i.e. a "biological control"

Source: Miller MR, Hankinson J, Brusasco V, et al. Standardisation of spirometry. *Eur Respir J.* 2005:26;319–338. Reproduced with permission from the European Respiratory Society. This book has not been reviewed by the European Respiratory Society prior to its release; therefore, the European Respiratory Society may not be responsible for any errors, omissions, or inaccuracies, or for any consequences arising there from, in the content.

Volume calibration requires a large-volume (3.0 L) calibration syringe. The ATS volume accuracy standard for diagnostic spirometers is ± 3% or ± 50 mL, whichever is larger. On computerized systems, you may need to enter the ambient temperature and altitude or barometric pressure prior to calibration. You also may need to make sure that the BTPS (body temperature pressure, saturated) correction is *deactivated*; otherwise, the calibrating volume will be approximately 10% higher than actual. If the device uses an electronic transducer to measure flow, you also need to zero it before volume or flow calibration. **Figure 6-5** depicts a normal volume calibration graph, showing a percent error computation that falls within the ATS accuracy standard for a 3.0 L calibrating syringe (between 2.91 and 3.09 L).

If you obtain a low volume (less than 2.91 L), first repeat the leak check. If you obtain a high volume (more than 3.09 L), recheck the volume/flow zeroing, make sure that BTPS correction is off, and confirm that the temperatures of the syringe and spirometer are the same. Do not proceed with patient testing unless you can (1) identify the cause of the inaccurate reading and (2) obtain

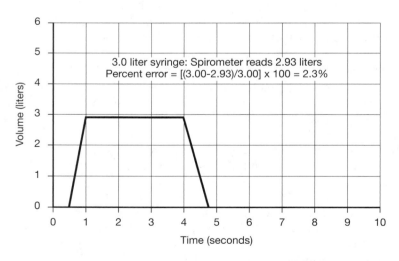

3.0 liter syringe: Spirometer reads 2.93 liters
Percent error = [(3.00-2.93)/3.00] x 100 = 2.3%

Figure 6-5 Plot of Volume Calibration of a Spirometer Showing the Percent Error Computation Falling Within the ± 3% Range of Accuracy Specified by the American Thoracic Society.

Source: National Institute for Occupational Safety and Health. *NIOSH spirometry training guide—unit three. The quality assurance program.* Publication No. 2004-154c. Atlanta, GA: Centers for Disease Control and Prevention; 2003.

an accurate volume calibration upon repeat measurement. The "gold standard" for flow calibration is a computer-controlled air pump that generates standard expiratory waveforms. Using this device, the recommended accuracy standard is ±5% of the reading or ±0.2 L/sec, whichever is greater. An acceptable alternative for flow calibration is to inject the full volume from the 3.0 L syringe into the spirometer using three different time intervals—for example, 0.5 second (about 6 L/sec), 6 seconds (about 0.5 L/sec), and somewhere in between. Volume linearity is confirmed if the recorded volume deviates by no more than 100 mL from the 3.0 L target volume. In addition, any deviations from the target volume should be unrelated to the flow (a rough index of flow linearity). Computerized spirometers typically include prompted routines to guide you through this process and maintain the appropriate time interval or flow.

You should record the leak test and volume and flow calibration results daily on a QC log. If repeated checks reveal inaccuracies for which you cannot identify any mechanical cause, you will need to recalibrate the device.

Obtaining Valid Test Results

Because forced expiratory maneuvers are technique dependent, obtaining accurate data depends on (1) proper patient instruction and coaching and (2) recognition and correction of patient performance errors. *Your goal is to obtain at least three error-free maneuvers that meet basic acceptability standards*. A forced vital capacity (FVC) maneuver meets acceptability standards if it is free of the following common errors:

- A slow or a false start to the maneuver (back-extrapolated volume ≥ 5% of FVC or 150 mL)
- Coughing during the maneuver
- Breathing during the maneuver
- Variable effort (e.g., prematurely ending exhalation)
- Exhalation time less than 6 seconds

Although many computerized spirometers automatically check the acceptability of each maneuver according to these criteria, the NBRC expects that you can recognize these problems via inspection of the FVC graph. **Table 6-6** depicts the most common validity errors you will encounter when measuring a patient's FVC.

After ensuring acceptability, you need to confirm the reproducibility of the patient's efforts. Efforts are reproducible *if the two largest values for <u>both</u> the FVC and the FEV_1 are within 0.150 L (150 mL) of each other*. If the effort fails to meet both criteria, you must continue testing until either both are met or the patient cannot continue.

Mechanical Ventilators

Ventilator QC involves a procedure called *operational verification*. Operational verification of non-computerized ventilators is performed manually following the manufacturer's recommendations. Most microprocessor-based ventilators include semi-automated self-test programs for operational verification.

Manual Ventilator Operational Verification

Table 6-7 outlines the basic manual operational verification procedure for noncomputerized ventilators, adapted from recommendations disseminated by the Emergency Care Research Institute.

Operational Verification of Computerized Ventilators

Most computer-controlled ventilators perform two types of operational verifications: a power-on self-test (POST) and an extended self-test (EST). Both of these QC procedures should be performed according to the manufacturer's recommendations.

A POST generally tests microprocessor function, zeros the sensors, and performs some basic checks related to patient functions, such as leak tests. *You should always confirm a successful POST before applying a ventilator to a patient and whenever you change the circuit.*

Table 6-6 Common Validity Errors Occurring During Measurement of Forced Vital Capacity

FVC Curve Indicating a Validity Error	Description of the Problem
A	Too slow a start to forced exhalation (back-extrapolated volume ≥ 5% of FVC or 150 mL). The graph reveals a characteristic S-shaped pattern in which the slope (flow) starts out low, then increases markedly toward the middle of the maneuver, finally plateauing toward the end. A normal FVC trace would have the greatest slope early in the breath.
B	Coughing during the maneuver. This graph shows an abrupt pause about a third of the way through the effort, followed by a short inspiratory effort preceding the cough and then an irregular pattern of exhalation. A normal FVC trace would be smooth throughout.
C	Breathing during the maneuver. This graph shows an extra breath as a short plateau occurring about a third of the way through the effort; in these cases, the measured volume may overestimate the actual FVC. A normal FVC curve consists of a single breath with a smooth and uninterrupted trace throughout.
D	Stopping expiration before all gas is exhaled. The graph reveals a normal and smooth high slope (high flow) early on; however, the curve ends abruptly in a plateau. In a normal FVC curve, the slope decreases progressively after the initial blast, smoothly transitioning to a plateau representing the true end-of-test volume.

Table 6-7 Manual Operational Verification of Noncomputerized Ventilators

Component or Function	Operational Verification Procedure (*Ventilator Not in Use*)
Battery test/power loss alarm	With the unit turned on, disconnect and then reconnect the power source. The machine's battery backup and disconnect alarms should function appropriately.
FIO$_2$/O$_2$ analyzer	See the "Gas Analyzers" section in this chapter.
Audible and visual alarms	Gas supply: disconnect the high pressure O$_2$ supply hose and, separately, the air hose (if used). The appropriate alarm(s) should result. Reconnect the hoses.
	Low-pressure, low-exhaled-volume, disconnect alarms: connect the ventilator to a test lung and set a stable minute volume; momentarily disconnect the circuit to check for the appropriate activation of all alarms.
	Apnea alarm: connect the ventilator to a test lung with the SMIV rate = 2/min and trigger the ventilator 8–12 times, then cease triggering to confirm appropriate activation of the alarm.
	High-pressure alarm: momentarily occlude the circuit to check for the appropriate activation of all audible and visual alarms.
	Inverse I:E ratio alarm: momentarily adjust the peak flow to create an inverse-ratio condition and confirm appropriate activation of the alarm.
Proximal airway pressure display	Connect the ventilator to a test lung and momentarily disconnect the pressure line or inspiratory limb of the circuit; the pressure display should read zero (±1 cm H$_2$O). Set the PEEP level to 10 cm H$_2$O and trigger several breaths; the pressure display should rise and then return to the appropriate baseline (±1 cm H$_2$O) at the end of each breath.
PEEP control	Connect the ventilator to a test lung, set a PEEP level of 5 cm H$_2$O, and trigger several breaths; the pressure display should rise and then return to 5 cm H$_2$O (±1 cm H$_2$O) at the end of each breath. Repeat at PEEP = 10 and PEEP = 15 cm H$_2$O.
Leak tests	*Occlusion method*: occlude the patient connection, set the pressure limit to its maximum and the peak flow to its minimum, and initiate a 200–300 mL breath (adult ventilators). The pressure limit should reach its maximum, and the high pressure alarm should activate.
	Plateau pressure method: set the inspiratory pause to 2 seconds or longer. When the ventilator triggers, observe the plateau pressure; a drop of 10% or more during the pause indicates a leak.
Modes	Use a test lung to verify proper operation of all ventilator modes.
Ventilator rate (and rate display)	Count the number of breaths delivered during a convenient interval, timed using a clock or a watch with a second hand. The measured rate should be within 1 breath per minute of the rate setting and rate display.
Delivered volume	Set the ventilator to a specific volume, connect a respirometer to the ventilator outlet, and trigger the ventilator; all measurements should be within ±5% of the setting.
Volume display	Connect a test lung to the circuit, cycle the machine, and compare the measured exhaled tidal volume and minute volume to their respective settings.
Sensitivity	Put the ventilator into an assist mode. Squeeze and release the test lung; an inspiration should result when the airway pressure or flow drops to the set sensitivity level.
Filters	Ensure that a high-efficiency particulate-air (HEPA) filter is present on the main inspiratory line.

Adapted from: Emergency Care Research Institute. Minimum requirements for ventilator testing. *Health Devices.* 1998;27(9–10):363–364.

Typically, an EST includes the a POST, followed by a series of more comprehensive function checks. *You should perform an EST between each application of a ventilator on different patients.* Extended self-testing of ventilators also should be documented in writing, with all records maintained as part of the QC program. Any ventilator that fails self-testing should be taken out of service for repair and replaced with one that has successfully completed operational verification.

Gas Analyzers

Oxygen Analyzers

Most O_2 analyzers use either a Clark electrode (the polarographic type) or a galvanic fuel cell to measure the P_{O_2}. Both types generally are accurate to within 2% of the actual concentration. Polarographic analyzers require external power to maintain the chemical reaction at the electrode. Galvanic cells do not require external power. However, both types require external power for alarm functions.

O_2 analyzer calibration involves four key steps:

1. Expose the sensor to a source of 100% O_2.
2. After the reading stabilizes, adjust the analyzer to 100%.
3. Remove the sensor from the 100% O_2 source
4. After restabilization, confirm a reading of 21% (± 2%).

Table 6-8 summarizes the common causes of O_2 analyzer calibration problems and measurement errors and outlines how to correct them.

Other Gas Analyzers

In addition to O_2 analysis, you may use specialty gas analyzers to measure N_2, He, CO, and NO/NO_2 concentrations in the PFT lab or at the bedside. See Chapter 4 for details on the analysis of these gases, as well as the applicable performance standards and calibration methods.

Table 6-8 Troubleshooting Polarographic and Fuel Cell O$_2$ Analyzers

Problem	Possible Cause	Suggested Solutions
Cannot calibrate to 21% O_2	• Probe not exposed to room air • Bad probe (electrode or cell) • Water condensation on probe membrane	• Ensure probe is exposed to room air • Recharge/replace probe • Dry probe membrane
Cannot calibrate to 100% O_2	• Low battery • Probe not exposed to 100% O_2 • Bad probe (electrode or cell) • Water condensation on probe membrane	• Replace battery • Ensure probe is exposed to 100% O_2 • Recharge/replace probe • Dry probe membrane
Measured %O_2 differs from expected value	• Low battery • Analyzer not calibrated • O_2 delivery device malfunction • Bad probe (electrode or cell)	• Replace battery • Calibrate analyzer • Confirm delivery device function • Recharge or replace probe
Analyzer reads 0% O_2	• Low battery • Probe not plugged into analyzer • Dead battery • Dead probe	• Replace battery • Plug probe into analyzer • Replace battery • Recharge or replace probe

Adapted from: Branson RD, Hess D, Chatburn RL. *Respiratory care equipment* (2nd ed.). Philadelphia: Lippincott; 1998.

Noninvasive Monitors

Pulse Oximeters

Pulse oximeters measures *relative* light intensities, as opposed to absolute values. For this reason, they do not require "true value" calibration, as previously described for blood gas analyzers. Instead, the following simple operational verification procedure is sufficient:

1. Connect the device to a normal person.
2. Compare the pulse reading with the actual pulse measured manually.
3. Check and confirm an Spo_2 reading of 97–100%.
4. Confirm loss of signal detection by removing the device.

An incorrect pulse rate, Spo_2 below 97%, or failure to detect loss of signal indicates a malfunctioning oximeter that should be taken out of service. **Table 6-9** identifies other common problems with oximeters and their solutions.

Transcutaneous Pco_2/Po_2 Monitors

The selection, use, calibration, and troubleshooting of transcutaneous Pco_2/Po_2 monitors is covered in Chapter 4. Noteworthy is the fact that this technology has continuously improved over the past several decades, making these systems easier and more reliable to use. In particular, sensors are smaller, require less frequent changing/calibration (twice a day) and membrane replacement (at least every 2 weeks), operate at lower temperatures (42°C), and can achieve capillary arterialization in as little as 3 minutes.

Capnometers/Capnographs

A capnometer measures exhaled CO_2 concentrations. A capnograph is a capnometer that graphically displays the expired CO_2 concentrations breath by breath. Chapter 11 provides details on the use of these devices. Here we focus on the procedures used to ensure the quality of data provided by capnographs.

To obtain accurate CO_2 measurements with a capnograph, you must properly set up the device, calibrate it, and maintain it while in use. Setup should follow the manufacturer's recommendations.

Table 6-9 Common Operational Problems with Oximeters and Their Solutions

Problem	Solution
The oximeter continues to "search" but cannot find a pulse or there is a pulse displayed but no Spo_2	• Readjust the sensor or apply it to a new site with better perfusion. • Check and confirm that the detector "windows" are clean. Make sure the sensor is plugged into the monitor. • Check the sensor for damage and replace if needed.
The heart rate and Spo_2 readings fluctuate rapidly	• Usually due to motion artifact (resolved when patient stops moving). • Use an oximeter with Masimo signal extraction technology (SET).
The oximeter reading seems to be inaccurate	• Check whether the oximeter pulse rate is the same as that determined by a cardiac monitor; if different, the sensor may need to be adjusted or replaced. • Check and confirm that the sensor is shielded from bright light.
The Spo_2 differs from that provided in a blood gas report	• Remember an ABG Sao_2 value usually is a computed rather than measured value; it is better to compare the Spo_2 to a hemoximeter's Sao_2 reading. • Use the difference between the Sao_2 and Spo_2 to "calibrate" the oximeter.

The setup, calibration, and maintenance procedures vary depending on whether the capnograph uses mainstream or sidestream technology.

Capnographs that employ mainstream sensors are used primarily for intubated patients, with the sensor placed at the airway connection. *Placement distal to the airway can result in inaccurate measurements due to rebreathing.* To prevent condensation from affecting the reading, most mainstream sensors are heated. For this reason, you must provide the recommended warm-up time. Accurate readings also require the proper-size sensor for the patient. Mainstream sensors can be applied to nonintubated patients using a mask or mouthpiece; however, accurate readings in such patients require supplemental O_2 flows of 6 L/min to prevent rebreathing due to the added mechanical deadspace.

Capnographs using sidestream technology can be applied to intubated patients, but are most useful for monitoring nonintubated patients. Newer low-flow sidestream capnographs that employ disposable nasal sampling cannulas can be used with infants, children, and adults. The primary problem with sidestream systems is occlusion of the sampling tubing with condensate. Manufacturers may address this problem by using water traps, moisture-absorbing filters, and/or water-absorbing Nafion tubing. Obstruction also can occur if the tube becomes kinked. Use of the recommended condensate prevention methods and proper tube placement can help avoid occlusion of sidestream sampling systems.

Most capnographs automatically zero themselves at start-up and during regular use by aspirating air through a CO_2 scrubber. As with ABG analyzer calibration, this one-point method adjusts only the offset (baseline drift) and does not properly correct instrument gain—a step that is required for accurate CO_2 readings. To assess and adjust instrument gain, you need to measure a known CO_2%. Most capnographs use a precision gas mixture of 5% CO_2 for this "high" calibration, equivalent to a P_{CO_2} of 38 mm Hg at sea level (ATPD = ambient pressure and temperature, dry). The most often cited standard for capnograph calibration is ±0.3%, or a range of 4.7–5.3% (36–40 mm Hg). Because aspiration through the sampling tube creates a pressure difference that can affect measurement, sidestream capnograph calibration must be performed using the same setup used on the patient.

Also, as with ABG gas analyzers, to *verify* calibration you need to confirm accuracy at *three levels* of measurement, usually by adding a "high" precision gas with 10% CO_2 (P_{CO_2} = 76 mm Hg) to the analysis. Because capnographs are calibrated under ATPD conditions but measure CO_2 under BTPS conditions, the calibration routine must account for the difference in values.

Instead of using precision gases for calibration, some mainstream capnographs employ filters to simulate the infrared absorption of various CO_2 concentrations. Alternatively, some devices store initial calibration results in memory and use this information to automatically adjust analyzer offset and gain with each use, or with a change in the sensor.

Gas Delivery and Metering Devices

A key responsibility for all RTs is the safe and effective delivery of medical gases. For this reason, you must be familiar with a wide variety of delivery devices and supply systems. Chapter 4 provides details on the selection and application of these devices. Here we emphasize standards and procedures to ensure safe and accurate delivery of medical gases.

Various nongovernmental agencies publish standards for the safe use and maintenance of the diverse systems employed to deliver medical gases to the patient. Based on these standards, the following general quality assurance recommendations apply:

- Medical gas distribution systems require alarms to monitor the operating supply, reserve supply, and line pressures. Two separate monitoring locations are required to ensure continuous surveillance. Critical care areas should have their own monitoring system with audible and visual alarms for pressure changes greater than 20% from normal.
- Periodic testing and inspection of piping systems should be done and recorded. These procedures should include assessment of station outlets for insertion, locking of the gas connector, gas leakage, wear, and damage.
- Indexed safety connections to prevent inadvertent delivery of the wrong gas should never be circumvented.

- If gas cylinders are used, rules and regulation for cylinder safety promulgated by CGA must be followed.
- If portable air compressors are used, the manufacturer's recommendations for preventive maintenance must be followed.
- Medical gas regulators and flowmeters require periodic preventive maintenance to ensure proper function. Whenever a device appears damaged or its function is questioned, it should be checked for accuracy using a precision (calibrated) flowmeter.

COMMON ERRORS TO AVOID

You can improve your score by avoiding these mistakes:

- Never aspirate an arterial blood gas sample or mix it if it contains air bubbles.
- Do not use any gas analyzer that cannot be calibrated at two points in the range of expected results.
- Never use a blood gas analyzer for reporting patient values if the QC results indicate it is out of control.
- Never proceed with pulmonary function testing if the spirometer has an uncorrected leak.
- Never apply a ventilator to a patient if it has failed its operational verification check.
- Never circumvent medical gas connection safety systems (e.g., PISS, DISS).

SURE BETS

In some situations, you can always be sure of the right approach to a clinical problem or scenario:

- Always perform a two-point calibration prior to using any gas analyzer or monitor.
- Always use tonometry if the accuracy of a blood gas analyzer's P_{O_2} and P_{CO_2} measurements is in doubt.
- Always document the patient's F_{IO_2}, the O_2 delivery device, the mode of ventilation, and the results of any related assessments made when obtaining a blood sample for analysis.
- Always perform leak testing on volumetric spirometers before volume calibration.
- Always perform an operational verification test prior to using a mechanical ventilator on any patient.
- Always include a statement about test quality in the final report of every pulmonary function test.
- Always include assessment of technician competency in any testing quality assurance program.

PRE-TEST ANSWERS AND EXPLANATIONS

Following are this chapter's pre-test answers and explanations. Be sure to review each answer's explanation thoroughly to help you understand why it is correct. If the explanation is still unclear to you, review the chapter content.

6-1. **Correct answer: D.** Using a short-bevel needle. To avoid preanalytical errors associated with air contamination of a blood gas sample, you should fully remove any air bubbles, cap the syringe quickly, and mix the sample only after all air has been removed.

6-2. **Correct answer: A.** Analyze the sample immediately. ABG errors caused by blood metabolism are time and temperature dependent. It is important to analyze all ABG samples within 30 minutes of procurement. If this is not possible, place the sample in an ice slurry and analyze it as soon as possible.

6-3. **Correct answer: B.** Failure of the P_{O_2} electrode. A single deviant control measurement represents a random error. Random errors can occur due to chance (statistical probability), or they may be caused by improper handling or contamination of the sample. A faulty electrode typically would cause measurement bias (multiple systematic high or low measurements).

6-4. **Correct answer: B.** ±2%. Two types of electrochemical O_2 analyzers are commonly used: the polarographic (Clark) electrode and the galvanic fuel cell. Both types generally are accurate to within 2% of the actual concentration.

6-5. **Correct answer: C.** HbO_2 levels. HbO_2 values for samples contaminated with air bubbles should be questioned. COHb, MetHb, SHb, and total Hb levels are unaffected by air contamination. Additionally, inadequate mixing prior to analysis will result in erroneous total Hb measurements.

6-6. **Correct answer: D.** Precision flowmeter. To assess the output or flow accuracy of a Bourdon gauge regulator used for O_2 transport, you would use a precision (calibrated) flowmeter.

6-7. **Correct answer: D.** Control media calibration verification. To periodically confirm the validity of a blood gas analyzer, you perform calibration verification using control media. Calibration verification requires analysis of at least three materials with known values (controls) spanning the range of results expected for clinical samples. At least one control should be analyzed every shift. All three levels of the control media should be analyzed at least once per day.

6-8. **Correct answer: B.** 3% or 50 mL, whichever is greater, using a 3-liter syringe (ATS recommendation).

6-9. **Correct answer: B.** Between patient uses. A complete ventilator operational verification procedure should be performed between each patient use. These procedures should follow the manufacturer's recommendations and be recorded in departmental QC logs.

6-10. **Correct answer: A.** Calibrate the sensor. If a galvanic cell O_2 analyzer reads 18% when exposed to ambient air, it should first be recalibrated to 20.9%. Replace the sensor only if an analyzer fails to calibrate at 21% and 100% oxygen.

POST-TEST

To confirm your mastery of this chapter's topical content, you should take the chapter post-test, available online at http://go.jblearning.com/respexamreview. A score of 80% or more indicates that you are adequately prepared for this section of the NBRC written exams. If you score less than 80%, you should continue to review the applicable chapter content. In addition, you may want to access and review the relevant Web links covering this chapter's content (courtesy of RTBoardReview. com), also online at the Jones & Bartlett Learning site.

CHAPTER 7

Maintain Records and Communicate Information

Craig Scanlan
(previous version co-authored with Louis M. Sinopoli)

Maintaining accurate records and properly communicating information is an essential part of your job. Improper record keeping can affect hospital income and licensure and accreditation status. More importantly, improper record keeping and poor communication can harm patients. It is for these reasons that the NBRC assesses your record keeping and communication skills. These skills require you to apply a variety of rules and standards while paying close attention to detail. Areas you need to emphasize include charting rules and standards, communication and coordination of patient care, and patient education.

OBJECTIVES

In preparing for the shared NBRC exam content, you should demonstrate the knowledge needed to:

1. Accept and verify patient care orders
2. Record therapy and results using conventional terminology
3. Communicate information regarding a patient's status to appropriate members of the healthcare team
4. Apply computer technology to support patient safety and document patient management
5. Communicate results of therapy and modify therapy according to protocol(s)
6. Explain planned therapy and goals to the patient in understandable terms
7. Educate the patient and family concerning health management smoking cessation

WHAT TO EXPECT ON THIS CATEGORY OF THE NBRC EXAMS

CRT exam: 5 questions; about 40% recall and 60% application
WRRT exam: 4 questions; 25% application and 75% analysis
CSE exam: indeterminate number of questions; however, exam III-A knowledge can appear in both CSE Information Gathering and Decision-Making sections

PRE-TEST

Carefully respond to each of the following questions. After completing the pre-test, compare your answers to those provided at the end of this chapter. Then thoroughly review each answer's explanation to help understand why it is correct.

7-1. On checking a ventilator patient's progress notes, you see that the attending physician's treatment plan includes starting spontaneous breathing trials. Your most appropriate action is to do which of the following?

A. Begin a spontaneous breathing trial immediately
B. Wait until after the patient's sedation is discontinued
C. Check to verify that a valid physician's order is present
D. Review the plan changes with the patient's nurse

7-2. After completing a ventilator check, you note that you incorrectly computed the patient's compliance in a prior entry. Which of the following is the most appropriate course of action?

A. Inform the medical director of the error

B. Erase the error and write over it with the correction

C. Copy the entire ventilator sheet over to correct the error

D. Line out the error, write the word "error," and correct and initial it

7-3. When must you contact the ordering physician when implementing a respiratory care treatment protocol?

A. After your initial assessment of the patient

B. Whenever a change in therapy is needed

C. Prior to providing the initial therapy

D. Whenever a limit or boundary rule takes effect

7-4. A prescription for an aerosolized drug for a patient under your care is complete except for the actual drug dosage. Which of the following is the appropriate action to take in this case?

A. Use the standard dosage listed in the package insert

B. Ask your medical director to rewrite the prescription

C. Contact the ordering physician for clarification

D. Postpone the therapy until the following day

7-5. The best way to routinely communicate a patient's clinical status to the appropriate members of the healthcare team is by reporting information:

A. To the respiratory therapy supervisor

B. To the next shift of respiratory therapy staff

C. In the respiratory therapy department records

D. In the patient's chart

7-6. If while giving therapy you note an adverse change in the patient's condition, you should:

1. Notify the nurse who is responsible for the patient

2. Contact the physician if a change in therapy seems warranted

3. Record the patient's reactions in the chart

A. 2 only

B. 1 and 3 only

C. 2 and 3 only

D. 1, 2, and 3

7-7. Midway through an aerosol drug treatment via intermittent positive-pressure breathing (IPPB), a patient complains of dizziness and tingling in her fingers. After stopping the therapy, adjusting the equipment to correct the problem, and then completing the treatment, you should record which of the following in the chart?

1. Medication used during the treatment

2. The patient's vital signs before and after the treatment

3. The nature of the problem and the way in which it was corrected

A. 1 and 2 only

B. 1 and 3 only

C. 2 and 3 only

D. 1, 2, and 3

7-8. When assessing a patient after a treatment, you note a significant deterioration in vital signs. What is the most appropriate action in this case?

A. Call for the institution's rapid response team

B. Report the findings to the next shift of the respiratory therapy staff

C. Chart the findings as an unexpected response to therapy

D. Orally communicate the findings to the patient's physician

7-9. A patient asks you if there are any over-the-counter (OTC) medications available to help her quit smoking. Which of the following would you suggest she discuss with her doctor?

A. Buproprion (Zyban)

B. Nicotine inhaler (Nicotrol)

C. Varenicline (Chantix)

D. Nicotine gum (Nicorette)

7-10. You obtain a fresh multidose vial of a bronchodilator from an automated drug dispensing cabinet for an asthmatic patient receiving continuous bronchodilator therapy (CBT). After you open the vial packaging and prepare it for mixing with sterile saline, the attending physician tells you that she is discontinuing the CBT. Which of the following should you do?

1. Use the cabinet's "Return" function to return the medication
2. Chart the reason why the medication was not used
3. Use the cabinet's "Waste" function to document wastage
A. 1 only
B. 1 and 2
C. 2 only
D. 2 and 3

WHAT YOU NEED TO KNOW: ESSENTIAL CONTENT

Accept and Verify Patient Care Orders

All respiratory care normally is provided by order of the patient's doctor. In some settings, orders also may originate from other licensed providers, such as nurse practitioners or physician assistants. Your state licensure regulations and institutional policies will dictate if you can accept orders from other health professionals. Orders must come from a provider with prescribing privileges. You cannot accept orders transmitted to you via unauthorized third parties, such as registered nurses. If an order is transmitted to you via a third party, you must verify the order in the patient's chart before proceeding. In most institutions, orders written by medical students must be countersigned by a physician before you carry them out. You also should not accept blanket orders, such as "continue previous medications" or "resume preoperative orders."

Regarding verbal or telephone orders, if "the doctor is in the house" and the situation is not an emergency, you should secure a regular written order. If a verbal order is required and you are authorized to take it, you must avoid transcription errors. The Joint Commission recommends the following procedure for taking verbal orders:

1. While speaking with the originator, write or type the order into the applicable section of the record, clearly identifying it as transmitted verbally.
2. Read the order back to the originator exactly as written, and clarify as needed.
3. Have the originator confirm the accuracy of the order as read back.
4. Write the time and date of the order with the name and credentials of originator, specify "read back and confirmed," and provide your signature and credentials.

Regardless of their source or route of transmission, it is your duty to ensure that all orders are accurate and complete. Although the components vary according to what is being prescribed, a complete written order generally includes the following information:

- Date and time of order (often with a expiration date)
- Name of therapy or diagnostic test being prescribed
- Requisite details for therapy (e.g., ventilator settings) or conditions for diagnostic testing
- Frequency of therapy or testing (if intermittent)
- Name, signature, and credentials of the originator

If the order is for a drug (including oxygen), it must also contain the drug name, administration route, and dose/concentration (for O_2, the liter flow or FIO_2).

If the order is for mechanical ventilation, it should include at least one and ideally both of the following:

- Desired range for $Paco_2$ and/or desired range for Pao_2 or oxygen saturation
- Ventilator setting to achieve the desired blood gas results (e.g., volume, rate, FIO_2, PEEP)

Should any of these elements be missing, the order is incomplete and you should contact the originator for clarification before implementation. The same procedure applies if the order falls outside institutional standards. For example, if the order specifies a drug dosage higher than that recommended for your patient or includes a ventilator mode or setting not normally applied in similar cases, you should contact the originator for clarification before proceeding.

Record Therapy and Results

Basic Rules for Medical Record Keeping

Good record keeping begins with careful attention to detail, requires proper use of terms and abbreviations, and involves knowledge of how to make needed corrections to a patient's record. Basic rules for record keeping include the following:

1. For paper records, write your entries legibly in the applicable chart section (see Chapter 1). Sign each entry with your first initial, last name, and credential/title (e.g., RRT, Resp Care Student), such as "S. Smith, RRT." Agency policy may require supervisors to countersign student entries.
2. Never use ditto marks.
3. Never erase written entries. Erasures call to question the information if used later for quality review or legal purposes. If you make a mistake, draw a line through it and print the word "error" above it. Then continue your charting as before.
4. Make entries after completing each patient task, and sign your name correctly after each entry.
5. Be exact in noting the time, effect, and results of all treatments and procedures.
6. Record patient complaints and general behavior. Describe the severity, type, location, onset, and duration of pain. Describe clearly and concisely the character and amount of secretions (see Chapter 2).
7. To prevent charting by someone else in an area you signed, avoid leaving blank lines; instead, draw a line through any empty lines.
8. Use only institutionally accepted abbreviations.
9. Never use future tense, as in "patient will receive treatment after lunch."
10. Spell correctly. If you are not sure about the spelling of a word, use a dictionary.

Each institution establishes its own accepted abbreviations, which you must follow. Due to variations among institutions, the NBRC avoids using all but the most common general abbreviations on its exams. However, *the NBRC does expect that you know all standard respiratory care abbreviations and symbols*. A complete list of the standard respiratory care abbreviations and symbols is published by the AARC in *Respiratory Care* and is available online at http://www.rcjournal.com/guidelines_for_authors/symbols.pdf.

Because of growing safety concerns about errors associated with written miscommunications, organizations such as The Joint Commission and Institute for Safe Medication Practices have established listings of abbreviations and symbols that clinicians should avoid in written documentation. **Table 7-1** provides examples of these "banned" terms, which generally apply to all handwritten orders and medication-related documentation. Note that these are examples only and that each institution maintains its own listing.

If an order contains a banned notation, you should confirm its intent before proceeding. The exception is when order confirmation would delay essential treatment or increase patient risk. In these cases, if you judge the order as being clear, complete, and otherwise correct, you should carry it out and obtain confirmation as soon as possible thereafter.

Specify the Therapy Administered

There is a common saying in health care that "If it wasn't charted, it wasn't done!" This saying has several important implications. First, if you fail to chart a therapy or medication you have provided, your patient may receive additional unnecessary or harmful treatments. Second, if a procedure is not charted, the hospital may not be able to get reimbursed for the services provided. Third, should any legal questions ever arise, the medical record becomes the primary source of evidence about the care provided.

Table 7-1 Examples of Abbreviations and Symbols to Avoid in Written Documentation

Do Not Use	Potential Problem	Preferred Term
U, u (for unit)	Mistaken as zero, four, or cc	Write "unit"
IU (for international unit)	Mistaken as IV (intravenous) or 10 (ten)	Write "international unit"
Q.D., QD, q.d., qd (once daily) Q.O.D., QOD, q.o.d., qod (every other day)	Mistaken for each other. The period after the Q can be mistaken for an "I" and the "O" can be mistaken for "I."	Write "daily" or "every other day"
Trailing zero (X.0 mg)	Decimal point is missed	Never write a zero by itself after a decimal point (X mg)
Lack of leading zero (.X mg)	Decimal point is missed	Always use a zero before a decimal point (0.X mg)
MS, MSO_4, $MgSO_4$	Confused for one another; can mean morphine sulfate or magnesium sulfate	Write "morphine sulfate" or "magnesium sulfate"
mg (for microgram)	Mistaken for mg (milligrams) resulting in 1000-fold dosing overdose	Write "mcg"
c.c. (for cubic centimeter)	Mistaken for U (units) when poorly written	Write "mL" or "milliliters"
> (greater than) < (less than)	Misinterpreted as the number "7" (seven) or the letter "L"	Write "greater than" Write "less than"
Abbreviations for drug names	Misinterpreted due to similar abbreviations for multiple drugs	Write drug names in full
Apothecary units	Unfamiliar to many clinicians; confused with metric units	Use metric units
@	Mistaken for the number "2" (two)	Write "at"

For all these reasons, *whenever you provide therapy or perform a diagnostic procedure, you must record all relevant details and, as necessary, communicate them to other members of the patient's healthcare team.* Only in this way will everyone involved in the patient's care know what was done when and how the patient responded. To that end, after each patient encounter you must record at least the following information:

1. Specific therapy or diagnostic test performed
2. Date and time of therapy or test
3. Medication name, dose, and concentration if applicable
4. Patient response to therapy or test results (covered in the next section)

A patient's refusal of therapy also must be charted, along with the reasons. You also should notify the patient's nurse orally whenever a treatment is refused.

Ventilator management represents a special case of record keeping, because it normally involves using a flow sheet. A typical ventilator flow sheet provides sequential row or column data entries that concisely combine information on the "therapy" (ventilator settings) and the patient's response (monitoring data).

Each institution usually develops its own ventilator flow sheet. Typically, each entry must specify the date and time at which the information was logged and by whom (signature or initials, depending on institutional policy). In terms of additional information, most institutions follow the recommendations established by the AARC in their clinical practice guideline on patient-ventilator system checks, as summarized in **Table 7-2**.

Table 7-2 Key Information Elements for Recording Patient-Ventilator System Checks (Flow Sheets)

Ventilator Settings	Patient Observation/Response
Should include but not be limited to the following:	Should include but not be limited to the following:
• F_{IO_2}	• Breath sounds
• Humidifier temperature setting (when applicable)	• Spontaneous respiratory rate, volume, and pattern
• Mode of ventilation	• Chest motion
• Set frequency	• Pallor, skin color
• Peak, mean, and baseline airway pressures and presence of auto-PEEP (if applicable)	• Patient's level of consciousness or remarks
• Set peak inspiratory pressure limit and pressure support level, if applicable	• ET tube stability, position, cuff pressure
• Set tidal volume (if applicable)	• Volume and consistency of secretions
• Delivered tidal volume (measured or calculated)	• Results of bedside PFT evaluations
• Set minute ventilation (if applicable)	• Any untoward effects of ventilator disconnection during bedside procedures
• Set inspiratory flow and waveform (if applicable)	• Documentation of oxygenation and ventilation status (e.g., ABGs, pulse oximetry, capnometry)
• Set I:E ratio, percent inspiration, or inspiratory and expiratory times	• Documentation of patient–ventilator synchrony
• Set sensitivity (if applicable)	• Documentation of time of last HME and/or circuit change
• Documentation of alarm settings and activation of appropriate alarms	• Condition of ancillary equipment (e.g., chest tube apparatus and manual resuscitator)

Noting and Interpreting the Patient's Response to Therapy

All documentation must include assessment of the results of your intervention and the patient's response to it. At a minimum, this means charting the outcomes of therapy or testing and recording any adverse patient reactions. In addition, for most encounters you should assess and record the patient's vital signs, breath sounds, and volume and quality of secretions (see Chapters 2 and 11 for details). If available, data derived from pulse oximetry, ECG monitoring, and capnography should be documented as well. Your charting responsibilities also require that you verify all computations and note any erroneous data.

In terms of documenting the effects of therapy, what you chart depends on (1) the procedure's expected outcomes, (2) the parameters you are monitoring, and (3) the measures available to evaluate the expected outcomes. In addition, the NBRC expects you to properly chart any adverse reactions exhibited by the patient during or after the procedure.

For most respiratory care procedures, the requisite information is provided in the practice guidelines published by the AARC and made available online at http://www.rcjournal.com/cpgs/ (a complete listing of the AARC guidelines is also provided in Appendix C in this text). Each guideline details the expected outcomes, variables to monitor, and adverse reactions that might occur. For example, were you to suction a patient receiving ventilatory support, the applicable AARC guideline would direct you to document whether one or more of the following outcomes was achieved:

- Removal of pulmonary secretions
- Improvement in appearance of ventilator graphics and breath sounds
- Decreased peak inspiratory pressure (PIP) with narrowing of PIP-Pplat (plateau pressure)
- Decreased airway resistance or increased dynamic compliance
- Increased tidal volume delivery during pressure control ventilation
- Improvement in arterial blood gas values or saturation

To monitor for adverse effects, you also would need to assess the following aspects of the patient's condition:

- Breath sounds
- O_2 saturation (skin color, SpO_2)
- Respiratory rate and pattern
- Hemodynamic parameters
- EKG, if available
- Sputum characteristics
- Cough effort
- Intracranial pressure (if indicated and available)
- Ventilator parameters (e.g., PIP, Pplat, V_T [tidal volume])

Based on the information provided by these additional monitoring parameters, you would include in your chart entry the occurrence of any of the following adverse effects:

- Hypoxemia
- Cardiac dysrhythmias
- Changes in blood pressure
- Cardiac or respiratory arrest
- Atelectasis
- Bronchospasm
- Bleeding/tissue trauma
- Elevated intracranial pressure

An alternative record keeping format that goes beyond simply charting outcomes and adverse reactions is the problem-oriented method, also called the SOAP format. This acronym stands for

S: Subjective data
O: Objective data
A: Assessment
P: Plan

Table 7-3 describes the components of the SOAP format, with examples of how such information typically would be recorded in the chart for a specific problem—in this example, an asthma patient's breathing effort.

Table 7-3 Components of the Problem-Oriented Method (SOAP) for Medical RecordKeeping

Element	Description	Charting Example
S: Subjective data	Qualitative information collected from the patient in response to questions or based on the judgment of the clinician	S = "Patient states his breathing is better today and he has not had to use his Proventil MDI."
O: Objective data	Objective data collected by the therapist via physical exam or instrumentation	O = "The patient's FEV_1 has increased from a low of 700 mL on admission to 2,500 mL (70% predicted) after the 10/5 3 PM treatment; minimal wheezing on auscultation."
A: Assessment	Conclusions based on the goal of therapy and the subjective and objective information gathered	A = "Patient's asthma appears under control and need for PRN MDI reliever medication has diminished."
P: Plan	Recommendations for how to proceed with the patient's respiratory care	P = "Recommend continuing therapy and discussing discharge planning and patient education with the patient's attending physician."

Whether or not your institution uses the problem-oriented approach, you should still use it when providing daily clinical care *and* when taking NBRC exams. **Figure 7-1** outlines this process. First, identify the patient's problem or the objective of the prescribed therapy. Then, collect the information needed to assess the patient (subjective and objective). Next, analyze this information by comparing your findings to the patient's problem or the therapy objective. Finally, develop your care plan, communicate it to others, and implement it after physician approval. As indicated in Figure 7-1, you should repeat the data collection and analysis as needed and modify or update your plan accordingly until the patient's problem is resolved or the objectives are achieved.

Many procedures require you to use or derive information based on computations. As with any chart data, these computations must be precise and accurate. First, never report data about which you are unsure. Second, if you mistakenly record inaccurate data, be sure to follow the rules for correcting charting errors, as previously described.

Several examples of NBRC-type questions designed to assess your skill in verifying computations and noting erroneous data are provided in Appendix A. There you will find good examples of questions that test your ability to (1) recognize and/or deal with conflicting data (*Data Just Don't Jive*), (2) recognize plainly incorrect data (*Errors, Errors Everywhere!*), and (3) identify and derive essential but missing information (*Don't Know What You're Missing!*).

To do well on these questions, you must first know how to apply the common formulas and equations likely to appear on the NBRC exams, as detailed in Appendix B. In addition, whenever a question involves any numeric data you should follow three key steps:

1. Inspect the data for obvious errors—that is, values that simply could not exist. An example would be a Pa_{O_2} of 200 torr on a patient breathing room air.
2. Inspect the data for discrepancies—that is, two or more values in conflict. An example would be a patient with a reported Pa_{O_2} of 50 torr and with an Sa_{O_2} of 95%.
3. Review the numbers to see what, if anything, is missing—missing data may be the key to solving the problem. An example would be assessing the mechanics of a patient receiving volume-controlled ventilation with a plateau pressure = 50 cm H_2O, PEEP = 10 cm H_2O, and V_T = 400 mL. Missing is the patient's compliance = 400 mL/(50 − 10) cm H_2O = 10 mL/cm H_2O (a very low value).

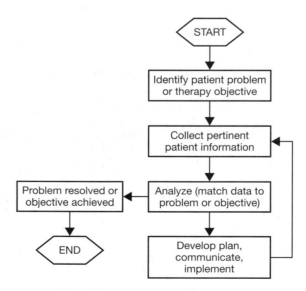

Figure 7-1 The Basic Problem-Oriented Approach to Patient Care.

Courtesy of: Strategic Learning Associates, LLC, Little Silver, New Jersey.

Communicating Information

Effective communication among health professionals can reduce errors, improve patient safety, and help ensure the quality of care. The NBRC assesses your communication skills in three areas:

1. Reporting the patient's clinical status
2. Coordinating the patient's care
3. Planning for patient discharge

If your written plan includes any recommendations to change therapy, you should immediately communicate this information to the prescribing physician. Likewise—in addition to being charted—any adverse effects to therapy should be communicated orally to the patient's physician and nurse. In general, the more serious the problem, the sooner these people should be informed. In particular, *if it is clear that the patient's vital signs are deteriorating, you should call for your institution's medical emergency/rapid response team.*

As a key member of the healthcare team, you should participate in coordinating your patient's care. Your responsibility is to work with the patient's nurse and/or physician to schedule therapy at times (1) least likely to conflict with other treatments, tests, or meals and (2) most likely to coincide with applicable drug administration. For example, you would avoid performing postural drainage on a postoperative patient immediately after a meal, but you would schedule the therapy after pain medication has been given. In contrast, you would wait until after sedatives have been withheld from a patient on a ventilator (a "sedation vacation") before implementing a spontaneous breathing trial.

Another key aspect related to coordinating care is the patient "handoff." Patient handoffs commonly include shift change reporting, temporarily taking over a colleague's patient assignments, receiving a patient in a specialized care unit, and having other clinicians take over during emergency procedures such as resuscitation. To provide accurate and concise information about the patient being handed off, most institutions use the **SBAR** method:

S	Situation	What is the patient's current condition?
B	Background	Which factors led to/underlie the patient's current condition?
A	Assessment	Which essential patient data (objective/subjective) apply?
R	Recommendation	Which action(s) do you propose?

To ensure that effective communication occurs, the recipient of the handoff should verify the received information via either repeat-back (for oral handoffs) or read-back (for written handoffs).

Applying Computer Technology to Medical Record Keeping

Computerized electronic medical record (EMR) systems are used to document patient care, monitor workload assignments, and ensure patient safety (e.g., for drug dispensing and order entry).

Security and Privacy

EMR security and privacy are regulated via provisions of the Health Insurance Portability and Accountability Act (HIPAA). HIPAA defines protected health information (PHI) and strictly limits its use to reasons of treatment, payment, and routine healthcare operations. The accompanying box summarizes some of the key privacy and security expectations for health professionals established under HIPAA.

Some Key HIPAA-Related Privacy and Security Considerations

- Access only that patient information needed to perform your job.
- Don't leave a patient's paper records open and available for prying eyes.
- Avoid discussing patient information with people who have no need to know or in public settings where you can be overheard.
- Provide only the minimal needed patient information on request, and only via methods approved by the patient.
- Never share computer passwords and log-on information or leave a computer unattended without logging off.
- Position workstations so that the screens are not visible to others.
- Keep patient information recorded on whiteboards to a minimum.
- Place fax machines used to receive patient information in secure locations.

Automated Alerts

Most EMR systems provide automated alerts. Some alerts warn of dangerous drug interactions; others track order dates. For example, if an order is about to expire, the EMR system will alert the physician to evaluate it for renewal. When such alerts occur, you should communicate with the patient's physician regarding continuation or modification of the current order and document this interaction in the record. Depending on institutional policy, EMR systems also may let you record a physician's verbal order and verify it electronically. Normally, this is followed by an alert to the prescribing physician to cosign the verbal order.

Automated Drug Dispensing

Automated drug dispensing cabinets (ADDCs) like the Pyxis MedStation are computerized systems designed to help reduce medication errors. ADDCs are stocked by the central pharmacy and interface with both the pharmacy and (if utilized) the EMR computer systems, which facilitates maintenance of drug inventories and usage tracking. Medication orders are received in the pharmacy as usual from physicians. After the pharmacist checks the order, it is sent to the ADDC, where authorized healthcare providers can withdraw the proper unit dose for administration to the identified patient. In hospitals with EMR systems, dispensed medications are electronically charted as administered (unless returned or wasted).

Proper use of an ADDC involves user authentication, removal of medications, returning and wasting medications, and logging off. The basic medication access procedure involves the following key steps:

- Log in using your user ID/password and/or biometric signature (e.g., fingerprint).
- Specify the patient, medication, quantity/dosage, and administration time.
- After the unit opens the applicable drawer, remove the medication, bar scan it (if required), and close the drawer.
- Log off/exit the system after all transactions are completed (*never leave an ADDC with an active screen*).
- Administer the mediation to the patient (bar scan it if required).
- Unless automatically recorded to the EMR, chart the medication in the patient's medication administration record *and* (if required) in the respiratory care or the general patient care notes (as per institutional policy).

If a withdrawn medication is not used (discontinued, dosage change, patient refusal), it must be returned to the ADDC using the "Return" function, which also credits the patient's account. A returned medication must be placed back in the ADDC in its original unopened package, with the reason it was not administered charted in the patient record.

If a medication is opened but not used or only partially used, it must be wasted (*not* saved for subsequent dosing). Typically, an ADDC "Waste" function documents medication wastage and creates an audit trail. As with returned medications, you must chart the reason why any prescribed drug was wasted.

Explaining Planned Therapy and Goals to Patients

The effectiveness of most respiratory care modalities depends on patient cooperation. Good patient cooperation requires that the patient understand both the procedure itself and its goals. Thus, to provide effective care, you must properly explain to your patients both what needs to be done and why.

Good communication with patients and their families is also an essential safety strategy. The more patients know about their care, the more likely it is that they will recognize any adverse events or potential treatment errors. You should always encourage patients and their family members to report any concerns they might have about the patient's condition, treatment, or any related safety issues. A particularly important safety issue for patients receiving respiratory care is infection control. You should always explain to your patients and their families all infection control measures they need to implement, including good hand hygiene, respiratory hygiene/cough etiquette, and any transmission-based precautions applicable to the patient's condition (Chapter 5).

An additional skill tested in this section of the NBRC exams is your ability to "translate" therapeutic goals and procedural descriptions into lay terms. To do so, you need to (1) know the methods and expected outcomes of the procedure and (2) use appropriate language with patients and their families. *The key is always to avoid using medical terminology.* **Table 7-4** provides examples of proper and improper patient explanations of planned therapy and its goals.

Communicating Results of Therapy and Altering Therapy According to Protocol(s)

Special considerations apply to record keeping when implementing respiratory care protocols. As recommended by the AARC, the main requirements for documenting protocols are as follows:

1. Date and time of protocol initiation
2. Pertinent medical history and physical examination
3. Pertinent diagnostic results
4. Management plan details
5. Physician notification criteria (i.e., guidelines for notification of patient status change)
6. Adverse reaction, if any, and remedial steps taken
7. Notification of physician, nurse, and other appropriate personnel
8. Required departmental documentation
9. Signature with credential

When implementing a protocol, make sure you are familiar with the limits or *boundaries* within which you are permitted to make independent adjustments, as well as any conditions

Table 7-4 Proper and Improper Patient Explanations for Incentive Spirometry

Improper Explanation	Proper Explanation
Ms. Smith, your doctor has ordered incentive spirometry treatments for you. These treatments will help you avoid getting atelectasis. The treatment requires that you perform a sustained maximum inspiratory maneuver, or SMI. This device will measure your inspiratory capacity as you perform the SMI.	Ms. Smith, your doctor has ordered deep breathing exercises for you. These exercises will help prevent your lungs from collapsing, which can lead to pneumonia. All you need to do is take a few slow, deep breaths in. I'll also encourage you to briefly hold your breath after you take in all the air you can, then slowly exhale. This little device will show us how well you are doing.

requiring physician notification. For example, in a mechanical ventilation protocol, you might find a boundary rule like this:

If more than 50% O_2 is needed to maintain the $Spo_2 \geq 88\%$, inform the ordering MD.

If you were implementing a protocol with this rule, as long as you could maintain a satisfactory Spo_2 with the $Fio_2 \leq 0.50$, you would be allowed to modify the O_2 setting on the ventilator. In contrast, if your assessment indicated that the patient needed more than 50% O_2, you would need to notify the physician and identify an alternative approach that might be outside this boundary, such as adding PEEP.

Educating the Patient and Family

You can expect questions on this part of the NBRC exams to cover providing education to patients and often family members on health management and smoking cessation.

Health (Disease) Management

Health (or disease) management programs provide care for patients with chronic disorders. These programs aim to develop patient self-management skills, improve compliance with treatment plans, reduce disease-related symptoms and hospitalizations, and enhance the quality of life. Most programs involve interdisciplinary teams with specialized expertise broadly covering all aspects of the patient's condition. RTs will most often be involved as team members in programs for patients with asthma or chronic obstructive pulmonary disease (COPD). **Table 7-5** outlines the key components and related activities common to health management programs designed for these patients.

Table 7-5 Common Components in Health Management Programs for Patients with Asthma or COPD

Component	Related Activities
Establishing a relationship with the patient/family	• Applying effective communications skills • Understanding the patient's disease experience • Assessing the patient's treatment preferences • Helping the patient and family know what to expect
Determining the severity of disease	• Obtaining a comprehensive patient history • Evaluating the patient's pulmonary function • Assessing the patient's quality of life
Reducing further risk/slowing progression	• Identifying/avoiding triggers that worsen symptoms • Having the patient quit smoking (*smoking cessation*) • Ensuring the patient receives needed immunizations • Involving the patient in a rehabilitation program (see Chapter 17)
Managing symptoms/reducing complications	• Setting healthy goals (personal action plans) • Providing self-management education/skill building • Involving family members in care delivery • Offering support for stress and negative emotions • Linking the patient to community resources
Providing ongoing follow-up (frequency based on disease severity)	• Retesting pulmonary function • Assessing symptom control/quality of life • Evaluating psychosocial issues such as depression • Determining the need for social/home health services

In terms of risk reduction—especially for COPD patients—the single most important strategy is to quit smoking (covered in more detail subsequently). Other triggers that both patients with asthma and COPD should avoid include outdoor air pollution, second-hand smoke, and household dusts, molds, and animal dander.

Ongoing management of disease symptoms aims to reduce exacerbations and the need for hospitalization, with *self-management education* being the key. General skills that self-management education should impart to patients with chronic respiratory disease include the following:

- Knowledge about the disease
- Ability to identify and avoid exposure to environmental triggers
- Ability to assess symptoms and know when to seek medical help
- Knowledge of prescribed medications and skill in their administration
- Maintenance of good nutrition and physical conditioning
- Ability to effectively communicate with providers
- Development of coping skills (to deal with frustration, fatigue, and other stressors)

Additional skills that patients with COPD may need to be taught include breath retraining and energy conservation methods, bronchial hygiene techniques, and the safe use of oxygen (see Chapter 17). Ultimately, if it is to be effective, self-management education must be tailored to the individual needs of each patient, including his or her health literacy, language, cultural beliefs, and ethnocultural practices.

Individualized educational activities should be based on *personal action plans*. An action plan is a collaborative goal-setting tool designed to help patients determine desired behavioral or lifestyle changes, plan on how to attain them, and establish follow-up mechanisms to assess progress and ensure goal achievement. The accompanying box provides an example of a simple action plan for a patient with COPD who wants to increase exercise tolerance.

Example of Personal Action Plan for a Patient with COPD

Goal	Begin exercising
Plan	
How	Walking
Where	Around the block (about ⅓ mile)
What	Initially once around; try to increase as tolerated
When	Before lunch
Frequency	4× per week
Potential barriers	O_2 cylinder cart is cumbersome
Plans to overcome barriers	Get more portable O_2 source
Follow-up	Maintain activity/distance logs (use pedometer)
	Discuss progress at next office visit (3 months)

Of course, depending on the goal and problem being addressed, you may need to refer the patient to another health professional who is better able to support the desired plan. For example, if the goal involved better eating habits, you likely would refer the patient to a clinical nutritionist.

Smoking Cessation Education

The first step in any well-planned education effort is assessing the patient's learning needs (see Chapter 2). In regard to smoking cessation, your assessment of learning needs ideally should reveal a desire to quit. For patients who appear hesitant to quit smoking, you will need to motivate them

Table 7-6 Using the Five R's to Motivate Patients to Quit Smoking

Component	Description
Relevance	Encourage the patient to express why quitting is personally **relevant**. Motivational information has the greatest impact if it is relevant to a patient's disease status or risk, family or social situation (e.g., children in the home), health concerns, age, sex, and other important patient characteristics (e.g., prior quitting experience, personal barriers to quitting).
Risks	Ask the patient to identify the **negative consequences** of smoking. Suggest and highlight those consequences most relevant to the patient. Acute risks include shortness of breath, worsening of asthma, pregnancy complications, impotence, and increased CO levels. Long-term risks include heart attacks and strokes, lung cancer, and COPD, among others. Environmental risks include lung cancer and heart disease in spouses; higher rates of smoking by children; increased risk for low-birth-weight infants; and increased risk of sudden infant death syndrome (SIDS) and asthma/respiratory infections in the children of smokers. Be sure to emphasize that smoking low-tar/low-nicotine cigarettes or use of smokeless tobacco, cigars, or pipes does not eliminate these risks.
Rewards	Ask the patient to identify potential **benefits** of quitting. Suggest and highlight those most relevant to the patient (e.g., quitting will improve health, sense of smell/taste and self-esteem; home, car, clothing, and breath will smell better; quitting will set a good example for kids; quitting will result in healthier babies and children; quitting will avoid exposing others to smoke; quitting will help improve tolerance for physical activities; quitting will reduce wrinkling/aging of skin).
Roadblocks	Ask the patient to identify **barriers** to quitting and note elements of treatment (problem solving, pharmacotherapy) that could address these barriers. Typical barriers might include withdrawal symptoms, fear of failure, weight gain, lack of support, depression, and enjoyment of tobacco.
Repetition	**Repeat** the motivational interventions as needed.

by explaining the health consequences of not quitting as well as the significant benefits that result from quitting. For these patients the U.S. Department of Health and Human Services recommends a strategy based on the five R's: *relevance, risks, rewards, roadblocks,* and *repetition* (**Table 7-6**).

Once the patient has expressed a desire to quit, you should recommend to the patient's physician implementation of a comprehensive treatment program that includes both pharmacologic support and counseling/behavioral therapies. Regarding pharmacologic therapy for smoking cessation, **Table 7-7** summarizes the common available medications, some of which require a physician prescription.

According to the U.S. Department of Health and Human Services, counseling and behavioral therapies that can significantly motivate patients to stop smoking include the following measures:

- Provision of practical counseling (problem-solving/skills training)
- Provision of "intra-treatment" social support
- Obtaining "extra-treatment" social support

Table 7-8 outlines and defines the major components involved in each of these strategies and provides practical examples of discussion points or suggestions to share with the patient.

Relapse from smoking cessation is a relatively common problem that may be detected via counseling sessions, interviews, or carbon monoxide breath analysis. In the case of relapse, patients should be encouraged to continue trying and informed that smokers who are highly motivated to quit and are persistent eventually achieve their goal.

Table 7-7 Pharmacologic Treatment for Tobacco Dependence

Drug	Precautions	Side Effects	Dosage	Duration
Varenicline (Chantix) *Prescription*	Nausea	Constipation Insomnia Headache Dry mouth	Days 1–3: 0.5 mg 1 time/day Days 4–7: 0.5 mg 2 times/day Days 8 to end: 1 mg 2 times/day	12 weeks
Bupropion (Zyban) *Prescription*	Seizure Eating disorders	Insomnia Dry mouth	150 mg each morning for 3 days, then 150 mg 2 times/day (begin treatment 1–2 weeks prior to quitting)	7–12 weeks post quitting; maintenance up to 6 months
Nicotine gum (Nicorette) OTC*	Dependency	Mouth soreness Dyspepsia	1–24 cigarettes/day: 2-mg gum, ≤ 24/day 25+ cigarettes/day: 4-mg gum, ≤ 24/day	Up to 12 weeks
Nicotine inhaler (Nicotrol) *Prescription*	Dependency	Local irritation of mouth and throat	6–16 cartridges/day (each cartridge delivers 4 mg of nicotine)	Up to 6 months
Nicotine nasal spray (Nicotrol NS) *Prescription*	Dependency	Nasal irritation	8–40 doses/day (one dose is 1 mg of nicotine requiring 2 sprays, one in each nostril)	3–6 months
Nicotine patch (Nicoderm CQ) OTC	Dependency	Local skin reaction	21 mg/day 14 mg/day 7 mg/day	4 weeks, then 2 weeks, then 2 weeks
* *OTC*, over the counter (does not require prescription)				

Table 7-8 Counseling and Behavioral Therapies for Smoking Cessation

Component	Discussion Points or Suggestions
Practical Counseling (Problem-Solving/Skills Training) Treatment	
Identify events, internal states, or activities that increase the risk of smoking or relapse.	• Negative mood • Being around other smokers • Drinking alcohol • Experiencing urges • Being under time pressure
Identify and practice coping or problem-solving skills. Typically, these skills are intended to cope with danger situations.	• Learning to anticipate and avoid temptation • Learning cognitive strategies that will reduce negative moods • Accomplishing lifestyle changes that reduce stress, improve quality of life, or produce pleasure • Learning cognitive and behavioral activities to cope with smoking urges (e.g., distracting attention)
Provide basic information about smoking and successful quitting.	• The fact that any smoking increases the likelihood of full relapse • Withdrawal symptoms typically peak within 1–3 weeks after quitting • Withdrawal symptoms include negative mood, urges to smoke, and difficulty concentrating • The addictive nature of smoking

(*continues*)

Table 7-8 Counseling and Behavioral Therapies for Smoking Cessation (*continued*)

Intra-treatment Supportive Interventions	
Encourage the patient in the quit attempt.	• Note that effective tobacco dependence treatments are now available • Note that half of all people who have ever smoked have now quit • Communicate belief in the patient's ability to quit
Communicate caring and concern.	• Ask how the patient feels about quitting • Directly express concern and willingness to help • Be open to the patient's expression of fears of quitting, difficulties experienced, and ambivalent feelings
Encourage the patient to talk about the quitting process.	Ask about: • Reasons the patient wants to quit • Concerns or worries about quitting • Success the patient has achieved • Difficulties encountered while quitting
Extra-treatment Supportive Interventions	
Train the patient in support solicitation skills.	• Show videotapes that model support skills • Practice requesting social support from family, friends, and coworkers • Aid the patient in establishing a smoke-free home
Prompt support seeking.	• Help the patient identify supportive others • Call the patient to remind him or her to seek support • Inform the patient of community resources such as hotlines and helplines
Help arrange outside support.	• Mail/email messages to supportive others • Call supportive others • Invite others to cessation sessions • Assign patients to be "buddies" for one another

COMMON ERRORS TO AVOID

You can improve your score by avoiding these mistakes:

- Never accept an incomplete order, a blanket order, or an order transmitted to you via an unauthorized third party.
- Never use medical or technical terms with patients or their families when explaining procedures or providing education.
- Never erase record entries; instead, always line it out and write "error" above the line-out (your institution may also require you to initial this entry).
- Avoid using any banned abbreviations and request clarification if an order contains them.
- Never allow unauthorized individuals access to any patient's healthcare information.

SURE BETS

In some situations, you can always be sure of the right approach to a clinical problem or scenario:

- Always read back and confirm a telephone order, and note the phone order in the chart.
- Always contact the physician and request an explanation before proceeding with any order that falls outside established standards.

- Always document each patient encounter with an assessment of the intervention and the patient's response.
- Always chart a patient's refusal of therapy and the reason, if provided.
- Always communicate any recommendations for a change in therapy directly to the prescribing physician as soon as possible.
- Always verify that the appropriate information has been received by those to whom you "hand off" a patient.
- Always notify the physician if any significant change occurs when managing a patient via a protocol.
- Always respect patients' privacy rights and their right of access to their own health information.
- Always recommend both counseling and pharmacologic support for patients who want to quit smoking.

PRE-TEST ANSWERS AND EXPLANATIONS

Following are this chapter's pre-test answers and explanations. Be sure to review each answer's explanation thoroughly to help you understand why it is correct. If the explanation is still unclear to you, review the chapter content.

7-1. **Correct answer: C.** Check to verify that a valid physician's order is present. All respiratory care is normally provided by order of the patient's personal doctor or attending physician. A progress note or plan is not the same as an order. Before initiating any therapeutic or diagnostic procedure, you need to check whether a valid physician order is present.

7-2. **Correct answer: D.** Line out the error, write the word "error," and correct and initial it. The ventilator flow sheet is part of the patient record and represents a legal document. Consequently, whenever errors are detected, the error should be lined out, the word "error" should be noted, the corrected information should be given, and the therapist correcting the error should write his or her initials.

7-3. **Correct answer: D.** Whenever a limit or boundary rule takes effect. When implementing a protocol, you must know the limits (also called boundaries) within which you are permitted to make independent adjustments, as well as know which conditions require physician notification. In general, if your assessment indicates that the patient's response strays outside any of the protocol's defined boundaries, you cannot proceed until you notify the ordering physician and determine a new course of action.

7-4. **Correct answer: C.** Contact the ordering physician for clarification. The minimum requirements for a proper prescription for respiratory care-related drugs include the following: (1) the drug name, (2) the drug dosage/concentration, (3) the frequency of administration, (4) the route of administration, and (5) the signature of the prescribing physician. Always seek clarification from the patient's physician if the order does not specify this necessary information.

7-5. **Correct answer: D.** In the patient's chart. The patient's chart is an official record of his or her ongoing progress and course of treatment. Consequently, the best way to routinely communicate a patient's clinical status is by accurately recording all essential information in the patient's medical record.

7-6. **Correct answer: D.** 1, 2, and 3. When noting an adverse change in a patient's condition, you should notify the nurse, contact the physician (if a therapy change is warranted), and record the reaction in the patient's chart. If the patient becomes unstable due to the adverse change, you should also stay with the patient until he or she is stable or help arrives. Recording this information in the medical record is a very important part of making sure that vital patient information is communicated among all healthcare professionals providing care to the patient.

7-7. **Correct answer: D.** 1, 2, and 3. If any adverse reaction is noted to a patient receiving therapy, the treatment should initially be stopped, the patient assessed, the problem corrected. Once the patient is stable, the therapy can be completed and documented. Documentation should include a description of the treatment (including any medications administered and their dosages), pre- and post-treatment assessment, and—in the event of an adverse response—nature of the problem and the way in which it was corrected.

7-8. **Correct answer: A.** Call for the institution's rapid response team. Any unexpected response to therapy or adverse effects noted when charting a patient encounter should be communicated orally to the patient's physician and nurse. In general, the more serious the problem, the sooner these key people should be informed. However, if it is clear that the patient's vital signs are deteriorating, do not wait to inform the doctor. Instead, call for your institution's rapid response or medical emergency team.

7-9. **Correct answer: D.** Nicotine gum (Nicorette). Of the medications listed, only nicotine gum is available without prescription (over-the-counter). It is always good to recommend to patients that they discuss taking *any* medications or dietary supplements with their physician.

7-10. **Correct answer: D.** 2 and 3. When using an ADDC, if a medication is opened but not used or only partially used, it must be wasted (not saved for subsequent dosing). Typically, an ADDC "Waste" function documents medication wastage and creates an audit trail. As with returned medication, you must chart the reason any medication was wasted.

POST-TEST

To confirm your mastery of this chapter's topical content, you should take the chapter post-test, available online at http://go.jblearning.com/respexamreview. A score of 80% or more indicates that you are adequately prepared for this section of the NBRC written exams. If you score less than 80%, you should continue to review the applicable chapter content. In addition, you may want to access and review the relevant Web links covering this chapter's content (courtesy of RTBoardReview. com), also online at the Jones & Bartlett Learning site.

CHAPTER 8

Maintain a Patent Airway/Care of Artificial Airways

Craig L. Scanlan
(previous version co-authored with Salomay R. Corbaley)

Maintaining the airway and caring for artificial airways are critical components of good respiratory care. It is for this reason that the NBRC devotes a specific section on its exams to this topic. You must be familiar with the many types of artificial airways available and know how to properly place, maintain, and remove these devices. In addition, because normal airway function depends on proper humidification, you must be proficient in this area.

OBJECTIVES

In preparing for the shared NBRC exam content, you should demonstrate the knowledge needed to:

1. Properly position a patient
2. Insert oropharyngeal and nasopharyngeal airways
3. Perform endotracheal intubation
4. Assess tube placement
5. Maintain position in the airway and appropriate cuff inflation of:
   a. Tracheal tubes
   b. Laryngeal mask airways and esophageal–tracheal Combitubes
6. Perform tracheostomy care
7. Change tracheostomy tubes
8. Maintain adequate humidification
9. Perform extubation

WHAT TO EXPECT ON THIS CATEGORY OF THE NBRC EXAMS

CRT exam: 7 questions: about 30% recall, 30% application, and 40% analysis
WRRT exam: 3 questions; 100% analysis
CSE exam: indeterminate number of questions; however, exam III-B knowledge can appear in both CSE Information Gathering and Decision-Making sections

PRE-TEST

Carefully respond to each of the following questions. After completing the pre-test, compare your answers to those provided at the end of this chapter. Then thoroughly review each answer's explanation to help understand why it is correct.

8-1. A patient suddenly loses consciousness. Which of the following is the first procedure you should perform to maintain an open airway in this patient?
A. Insert a laryngeal mask airway
B. Apply the jaw-thrust maneuver
C. Insert an oropharyngeal airway
D. Apply the head-tilt/chin-lift maneuver

8-2. A patient in the intensive care unit exhibits signs of acute upper airway obstruction and is concurrently having severe seizures that make it impossible to open his mouth. In this case, what is the adjunct airway of choice?
A. Oral endotracheal tube
B. Nasopharyngeal airway
C. Tracheostomy tube
D. Oropharyngeal airway

8-3. An oropharyngeal airway is *least* appropriate for a patient who:
  A. Is having seizures
  B. Requires manual ventilation
  C. Is conscious and alert
  D. Is heavily sedated

8-4. When ventilating a patient with a bag-valve resuscitator through a laryngeal mask airway (LMA), you note significant air leakage. Which of the following should be your first approach to eliminating this leakage?
  A. Bag slowly to reduce peak pressure
  B. Add more air to the cuff of the LMA
  C. Pull the tube out by 2–3 cm
  D. Lower the cuff pressure

8-5. Which of the following should be prescribed to provide adequate humidification to an intubated patient?
  A. Inspired gas with 100% relative humidity
  B. Inspired gas with an absolute humidity greater than 30 mg/L
  C. Inspired gas through a cold bubble humidifier
  D. Tracheobronchial suctioning

8-6. When checking for proper placement of an endotracheal tube in an adult patient on chest x-ray, it is noted that the distal tip of the tube is 3 cm above the carina. Which of the following actions is appropriate?
  A. None, because the tube is properly positioned in the trachea
  B. Withdraw the tube by 4–5 cm (using tube markings as a guide)

  C. Withdraw the tube by 1–2 cm (using tube markings as a guide)
  D. Advance the tube by 1–2 cm (using tube markings as a guide)

8-7. After insertion of an esophageal–tracheal Combitube, you begin ventilation through the #1 pharyngeal airway connection. Your partner reports an absence of breath sounds and the presence of gurgling over the epigastrium. To provide effective ventilation, what should you do?
  A. Deflate the large (#1) cuff
  B. Withdraw the Combitube by 3–4 cm
  C. Ventilate through the other (#2) tube
  D. Deflate the small (#2) cuff

8-8. Significant overinflation of an endotracheal tube cuff may cause which of the following?
  A. Laryngospasm
  B. Tissue damage
  C. Tachycardia
  D. Stridor

8-9. Which of the following devices are contraindicated for a patient whose upper airway has been bypassed?
  A. A heat and moisture exchanger (HME)
  B. A heated large-volume jet nebulizer
  C. A simple bubble humidifier
  D. A heated wick humidifier

8-10. The methylene blue test is used to confirm:
  A. "Leakage-type" aspiration
  B. Tracheal granuloma
  C. Infection
  D. Artificial airway obstruction

WHAT YOU NEED TO KNOW: ESSENTIAL CONTENT

Position Patients Properly

Proper patient positioning is a key in emergency airway management, is important in preventing ventilator-associated pneumonia (VAP), and can be helpful in managing conditions that cause hypoxemia or excessive respiratory tract secretions. **Table 8-1** summarizes the conditions requiring special positioning and the rationale for each.

Insert Oropharyngeal and Nasopharyngeal Airways

During resuscitation, if you cannot establish a patent airway by proper positioning alone, the pharynx may be obstructed by the tongue. If so, an oropharyngeal or nasopharyngeal airway can help overcome this problem. In addition to this use, both airways can serve other purposes.

Table 8-1 Conditions Necessitating Special Patient Positions

Condition or Situation	Position	Rationale
Resuscitation	Head-tilt/chin-lift maneuver (all rescuers)	Helps displace the tongue away from the posterior pharyngeal wall
	Jaw-thrust maneuver without head extension (healthcare provider)	Minimizes neck movement in patients with suspected C-spine injury
	Recovery position (lateral recumbent) with the patient placed on his or her side and with the lower arm in front of the body	Helps maintain a patent airway and reduces the risk of airway obstruction and aspiration in unresponsive adults with normal breathing and effective circulation
Endotracheal intubation	"Sniffing" position (i.e., neck hyperextended and pillow or towel under the head)	Aligns upper airway structures with larynx and trachea, facilitating tube insertion; *not to be used with suspected C-spine injury*
Prevent VAP	Elevating the head of the bed by 30° or more (unless contraindicated)	Helps prevent gastric reflux aspiration and improves the distribution of ventilation and the efficiency of diaphragmatic action
Acute respiratory distress syndrome (ARDS)	Prone position (consider only if ARDS ventilator protocol cannot provide satisfactory oxygenation)	Recruits collapsed lung units and shifts blood flow away from shunt regions, thereby improving V/Q balance and oxygenation
Unilateral lung disease	Left or right lateral decubitus position with the good lung down*	Improves oxygenation by diverting blood flow and ventilation to the dependent (good) lung
Postural drainage	Varies according to lobe or segment being drained (see Chapter 9 for details)	Vertical alignment of the lobar or segmental bronchus facilitates drainage into the mainstem bronchi for removal by coughing or suctioning
Directed coughing	Sitting or semi-Fowler's position, with knees slightly flexed, forearms relaxed, feet supported	Aids exhalation and facilitates thoracic compression during coughing

*Exceptions to the "keep the good lung down" rule include lung abscess or bleeding, in which the good lung is kept in the upward position to prevent blood or pus from entering the good lung. Likewise, in infants with unilateral pulmonary interstitial emphysema (PIE), the good lung normally is kept on top.

Oropharyngeal Airways

Oropharyngeal airways help prevent upper airway obstruction when providing bag-mask ventilation. They also may be used as a "bite block" in intubated patients who are heavily sedated or unconscious. In addition, oropharyngeal airways may be indicated in patients experiencing a seizure or when a comatose patient develops upper airway occlusion.

Size selection is based primarily on the patient's age (**Table 8-2**). Note that too large or small an airway can worsen obstruction. To avoid this problem, tailor the size to the patient by measuring from the corner of the mouth to the angle of the jaw.

To place and secure an oropharyngeal airway:

- Insert the airway either with the distal tip pointing up or from the side, and advance to the base of the tongue.
- Rotate the airway into the midline so that it holds the tongue away from the posterior pharynx.
- Avoid taping over the center opening of the airway (may be used to pass a suction catheter).

Table 8-2 Guidelines for Oropharyngeal and Nasopharyngeal Airway Sizes Based on Patient's Age

Patient Age or Size	Oropharyngeal Airway	Nasopharyngeal Airway
Premature infant	40 mm/00	NA
Newborn–1 year	50 mm/0	3 (12 Fr)
1–3 years	60 mm/1	3 (12 Fr)
3–6 years	60 mm/1	4 (16 Fr)
8 years	70 mm/2	5 (20 Fr)
12 years	70 mm/2	5 (20 Fr)
16 years	80 mm/3	6 (24 Fr)
Adult female	80 mm/3	6 (24 Fr)
Adult male	90 mm/4	7 (28 Fr)
Large adult	100 mm/5	8–9 (32–36 Fr)

After proper insertion, if airway obstruction is not relieved:

- Remove and reinsert the airway, and confirm that it extends past the base of the tongue.
- Recheck the size of the airway:
  - If the airway is too large/long, it will block the airway itself.
  - If it is too small/short, it can force the tongue against the posterior pharynx.

To avoid vomiting and aspiration, if the patient gags or otherwise does not tolerate the airway, remove it immediately. Instead, consider a nasopharyngeal airway or reposition the patient using the head-tilt/chin-lift or jaw-thrust maneuver.

Nasopharyngeal Airways

A nasopharyngeal airway also is used to prevent upper airway obstruction, most often when an oral airway is contraindicated—for example, when the patient is conscious, has a gag reflex, or has mouth or jaw trauma. These airways also are indicated for patients with upper airway obstruction who are having seizures that prevent opening the mouth, and those having undergone certain types of oronasal surgery such as pharyngoplasty or cleft palate repair. In addition, nasopharyngeal airways are used to prevent trauma in patients requiring frequent nasotracheal suctioning. You should avoid nasopharyngeal airways in patients with nasal trauma and when the nasal passages or nasopharynx is blocked or damaged (e.g., adenoid hypertrophy in children).

As with the oral device, sizing is based on the patient's age (Table 8-2). To individually tailor the size, measure from the nares to the earlobe (some devices have a movable ring to customize the length). Note that some designs have left and right versions, which typically are labeled "R" or "L," respectively, and can be readily identified by the different cut of their bevels (which always face medially). In general, you should select the largest diameter that will pass through the inferior meatus without force.

To place and secure a nasopharyngeal airway:

- Prior to insertion (if time permits), advance a suction catheter to see which meatus is more patent.
- Lubricate the airway with water-soluble jelly before inserting.
- Tilt the patient's head back slightly and advance the airway without force along the *floor* of the nasal passage (inferior meatus).
- After insertion, attach a safety pin to the flange to prevents slippage into the nose.
- If the patient experiences excessive bleeding or tissue trauma, notify the physician.

If a lubricated nasopharyngeal airway will not pass through the selected nasal passage, the patient may have a deviated septum. To overcome this problem, insert the airway through the opposite naris. If that is unsuccessful, select and insert a smaller airway.

When suctioning through a nasopharyngeal airway, always lubricate the catheter and secure the airway to prevent it from moving back and forth. Never lavage through a nasopharyngeal airway. If a lubricated catheter will not pass, first check whether mucosal swelling may be compressing the airway. If so, do not try to replace the airway, but instead notify the physician. Otherwise, either remove the airway and reinsert it in the other naris or replace it with a larger one.

Endotracheal Intubation

In the NBRC hospital, RTs must be skilled in intubation. For this reason, you can expect to see several questions on this procedure on the NBRC exams, either in this section or in the section covered in Chapter 16, which discusses assisting physicians with intubation. Here we focus on RTs performing the procedure.

Intubation Equipment

The first step in endotracheal (ET) intubation is gathering the needed equipment and confirming its function. Chapter 4 summarizes the general indications for, selection, use, and troubleshooting of ET tubes. The accompanying box lists the other needed equipment.

Equipment Needed for Routine ET Intubation

* indicates items typically included on an intubation tray.

- CDC personal protective equipment (e.g., gloves, gowns, masks, eyewear)
- Towels (for positioning)
- O_2 flowmeter and connecting tubing
- Bag-valve-mask (BVM) manual resuscitator
- Vacuum source/suction apparatus (e.g., regulator, portable pump)
- Suction catheters (e.g., flexible suction catheters, Yankauer tip)
- Local anesthetic spray*
- Water-soluble lubricating jelly*
- Laryngoscope handles (two) with assorted blades, batteries, and bulbs*
- ET tubes (at least three different sizes)*
- Stylet*
- Magill forceps*
- Syringe*
- Devices used to assess placement (e.g., EDD, CO_2 detector, capnograph, light wand)
- Tape and/or ET tube holder(s)*
- Oropharyngeal airways and/or bite blocks*

Table 8-3 provides guidelines for ET tube sizes and insertion lengths based on patient age and size. You should select an appropriate-size tube, but have available at least one size larger and one size smaller. Note that *uncuffed* tubes are recommended for premature infants or those weighing less than 3 kg. Otherwise, both cuffed and uncuffed ET tubes are acceptable for intubating infants and children. As with adults, if cuffed ET tubes are used on infants and children, cuff pressure must be monitored and limited according to manufacturer's specifications (usually 20–30 cm H_2O).

Table 8-3 ET Tube Size Guidelines and Insertion Lengths Based on Patient's Age

Patient Age/Size	ET Tube ID[a] (mm)	ET Tube Length[b] (cm)
Premature or < 3 kg	2.5–3.0 uncuffed	9–11
Newborn–1 year	3.0–4.0	11–12
1–3 years	4.0	11–13
3 years	4.5	12–14
5 years	5.0	13–15
6 years	5.5	14–16
8 years	6.0	15–17
12 years	6.5	17–19
16 years	7.0	18–20
Adult female	7.0–8.0	19–21
Adult male	8.0–9.0	21–23
Large adult	8.5+	23+

[a] ID = internal diameter. For infants and children, you estimate cuffed tube size ID = (age/4) + 3 and uncuffed size ID = (age/4) + 4 (*cuffed tubes must be slightly smaller*).
[b] From incisors to tube tip in the trachea; for the nasotracheal route (adults), add 2 cm to the insertion length.

Table 8-4 provides more detail on the accessory equipment needed for intubation, including its selection, use, and troubleshooting.

Intubation Procedure

The accompanying box outlines the key steps in oral intubation. The nasotracheal route is discouraged because (1) the incidence of VAP, sinusitis, and otitis media is higher; (2) smaller or longer ET tubes are required, which increases airway resistance; and (3) necrosis of the nasal septum and naris can occur.

Key Steps in Adult Orotracheal Intubation

1. Test laryngoscope and ET tube cuff.
2. Lubricate ET tube/stylet.
3. Position patient in sniffing position, and suction oropharynx.
4. Apply topical anesthetic.
5. Hyperoxygenate patient.
6. Insert laryngoscope, expose and lift epiglottis, and visualize vocal cords.
7. Insert ET tube between cords until cuff disappears (2–3 cm beyond cords).
8. Inflate the cuff to 20–30 cm H_2O.
9. Provide ventilation and 100% O_2.
10. Observe the patient's breathing, auscultate chest for symmetrical ventilation; auscultate epigastrium.
11. Verify tube placement (using breath sounds, chest wall movement, EDD, CO_2 detector, or capnography*).
12. Secure and stabilize tube, mark and record its length at incisors.
13. Confirm proper position tube by x-ray; reposition and resecure as needed.

*During resuscitation, the American Heart Association recommends continuous quantitative waveform capnography for confirmation and monitoring of ET tube placement and to assist in recognizing return of spontaneous circulation (ROSC). If capnography is not available, an EDD or CO_2 detector is acceptable.

Table 8-4 Accessory Equipment Needed for ET Intubation

Description	Selection and Use	Troubleshooting
Laryngoscope		
• Used to visualize the glottis • Consists of a handle with batteries and a blade with a light source	• Curved/MacIntosh blade inserted at base of tongue (vallecula); lifts epiglottis indirectly • Straight/Miller blade positioned under the epiglottis, which is directly lifted • Blade selection based on personal preference (most clinicians use a straight blade for infants) • Size based on age: premature infant: 0; infant: 1; 3–12 months: 1–1½; child: 2; adult: 3; large adult: 4	• To prevent aspiration, always make sure light bulb is tightly screwed in (not necessary with fiberoptic scopes) • If the bulb does not light: 　○ Recheck the handle/blade connection, then 　○ Replace the blade, then 　○ Replace the batteries, then 　○ Check/replace the bulb
Stylet		
• Adds rigidity and maintains the shape of an ET tube during insertion	• Used only for oral intubation	• To prevent trauma, make sure stylet tip does not extend beyond ET tube tip: 　○ Use a stylet flange or 　○ Bend stylet at a right angle at the ET tube adaptor
Magill Forceps		
• Used to manipulate the ET tube during nasal intubation by direct visualization	• Once the tip of the ET tube is in the oropharynx, insert the laryngoscope, and visualize the glottis • Use the forceps to grasp the tube just above the cuff and direct it between the cords	• To prevent trauma, never use forceps without direct visualization and avoid forceful movements
Squeeze-Bulb Esophageal Detection Device (EDD)		
• Self-inflating rubber bulb used to detect esophageal intubation • Not recommended for children younger than 1 year	• Connect squeezed bulb to ET tube • If bulb quickly reexpands, the tube is in an airway • If the bulb does not reexpand, tube is in esophagus	• Reexpansion does not confirm tracheal placement; always check breath sounds and confirm with x-ray
Colorimetric CO₂ Detector		
• Disposable CO_2 indicator used to confirm ET tube placement in airway	• Select correct type based on patient size/weight • Place between ET tube and bag-valve resuscitator • Correct tube position indicated when color changes from purple to tan/yellow as patient is ventilated	• Failure to change color can occur even with proper position during cardiac arrest (false negative) • Color change can occur with improper placement in mainstem bronchus (false positive)
Light Wand		
• A flexible stylet with a lighted bulb at the tip passed with the ET tube	• Characteristic glow ("jack-o'-lantern" effect) under the skin indicates tracheal placement • No glow if the tube is in esophagus	• Does not confirm proper tracheal position; always check breath sounds and confirm with x-ray
Bite Block/Tube Holder		
• Stabilizes oral ET tube, prevents biting on tube, minimizes movement/accidental extubation	• Options include: 　○ Oral airway taped to ET tube 　○ Flanged tube holder with straps	• Gagging response may require sedation • Can make oral care difficult

Key considerations related to ET tube placement include the following:

- To test the cuff, inflate it and observe for deflation; alternatively, immerse it in sterile saline and observe for leaks.
- The average oral tube length from teeth to tip in adults is 21–23 cm in males and 19–21 cm in females.
- After insertion and cuff inflation, listen for bilateral breath sounds and look for chest wall motion with ventilation.
- Stomach (epigastric) gurgling indicates esophageal intubation; correct it by removing tube and reintubating patient.
- Decreased breath sounds or chest movement on the left suggest intubation of the right mainstem bronchus; correct this problem by slowly withdrawing the tube until you confirm bilateral breath sounds.
- If a suction catheter will not pass after placement, the tube may be kinked or displaced out of the trachea; reposition it or reintubate the patient.
- Always provide 1–2 minutes of oxygenation and (if necessary) ventilation between intubation attempts.
- If available, use waveform capnography to confirm ET tube placement; acceptable alternatives include a squeeze-bulb EDD (good) or a colorimetric CO_2 detector (better).
- There are only two ways to *confirm* tube placement: chest x-ray or fiberoptic laryngoscopy. On x-ray, the ET tube tip should be about 4–6 cm above the carina, usually between T2 and T4.
- Because the ET tube moves up and down as the patient's head and neck moves, you should also check head and neck position when reviewing an x-ray for tube placement.
- If the ET tube is malpositioned, remove the tape and reposition the tube using the centimeter markings as a guide. Confirm the new position via either a chest x-ray or laryngoscopy.

Tracheotomy

Tracheotomy creates an opening or *stoma* through the neck tissues into the trachea, normally below the cricoid cartilage. The most common indications for tracheotomy are the need for long-term positive pressure ventilation or a permanent artificial airway.

Standard Tracheostomy Tubes

Tracheostomy (trach) tubes are placed through the stoma into the trachea and secured around the neck. Tubes are sized by *internal diameter* (ID) in millimeters using the International Standards Organization (ISO) system. **Table 8-5** provides general guidelines for trach tube selection based on the ISO system. Note that most trach tubes designed for infants and small children (ISO size 5 or smaller) have too narrow an ID to hold an inner cannula.

When a doctor selects a trach tube, primary consideration is given to the outside diameter (OD), especially for cuffed tubes. *A trach tube's outside diameter generally should be no more than two-thirds to three-fourths of the internal diameter of the trachea.* Bigger tubes will impede airflow around the cuff when deflated, while smaller tubes may require unacceptably high cuff pressures to achieve an adequate seal.

Key points in the placement and management of standard trach tubes include the following:

- To ease insertion and guard against tears, the cuff should be tapered back by gently "milking" it away from the distal tip as it is deflated.
- The blunt obturator prevents tissue trauma ("snowplowing") during insertion; remove it immediately after insertion but keep it at the bedside for tube reinsertion.
- If the tube has an inner cannula, slide it into the outer cannula and lock it into place.
  - To prevent blockage by secretions, regularly remove and clean the inner cannula.
  - Always kept a spare inner cannula at the bedside.

Table 8-5 Common Tracheostomy Tube Sizes

Patient Age or Size	ISO Size[a]	ID Without Inner Cannula (mm)	Approximate ID with Inner Cannula (mm)[b]	Approximate OD (mm)[b]
Premature infant	2.5	2.5	N/A	4.5
Newborn infant	3.0	3.0	N/A	5.0
	3.5	3.5	N/A	5.5
Toddler/small child	4.0	4.0	N/A	6.0
School-age child	4.5	4.5	N/A	7.0
	5	5	N/A	7.5
Adolescent/small adult	6	6	4–5	8.5
	7	7	5–6	9–10
Adult	8	8	6–7	10–11
	9	9	7–8	11–12
Large adult	10	10	8–9	13–14

[a] ISO standards require that both the inner diameter (ID) without inner cannula and its outside diameter (OD) in millimeters be displayed on the neck plate.
[b] Dimensions vary somewhat by manufacturer.

- The flange at the proximal end of some tubes can be adjusted to customize the fit and ensure proper position in the trachea (needed for severely obese patients or patients with abnormally thick necks).
- Secure the tube using cotton tape or hook-and-loop ties attached to the flange and around the patient's neck; ties should be changed as needed for comfort or cleanliness.
- To prevent disconnection, accidental extubation, or tracheal damage, always avoid pulling on or rocking the tube's 15-mm equipment connector.
- As with ET tubes, placement of trach tubes should be verified by x-ray or a fiberoptic scope.

Providing Tracheotomy Care

Optimal care of patients with trach tubes involves provision of adequate humidification, suctioning as needed, and regular cuff management. For patients with trach tubes, the NBRC also expects you to be skilled in basic tracheostomy care. In general, you should provide trach care whenever the stoma dressing becomes soiled. Key considerations involved when providing tracheotomy care include the following:

A. Equipment and supplies needed (most items are provided in trach care kits):
   - Replacement inner cannula
   - Clean trach ties or a replacement hook-and-loop tube holder
   - Precut sterile trach dressing (avoid plain gauze pads, as fibers may be aspirated into the airway)
   - Sterile trach brush, basin, cotton-tipped applicators, and gauze pads
   - Half-strength hydrogen peroxide
B. Basic procedure:
   1. Remove old dressing, being careful to keep tube in place.
   2. Clean around stoma site with the hydrogen peroxide and sterile applicators.
   3. Remove the inner cannula and insert the replacement.
      a. Clean the inner cannula in hydrogen peroxide with the trach brush.
      b. Rinse the inner cannula thoroughly with sterile water.
      c. Dry the inner cannula using a sterile gauze sponge.
   4. Replace the inner cannula.

5. Place a clean trach dressing under the flange.
6. Change the tube ties/holder as necessary.
    a. While changing tube ties or holders, *always have a second person hold tube in place*.
    b. *Never* fix ties with a bow knot; *always use a square knot*.
7. Ensure that the tube is secured in the proper position.

Changing Tracheostomy Tubes

In addition to providing trach care, in the NBRC "hospital" you are expected to be skilled in changing trach tubes. A tube change is indicated if the cuff is leaking or if the physician wants a different-size or different-type tube (e.g., a fenestrated or "talking" tube). The accompanying box outlines the key points involved in changing a trach tube.

Key Steps in Changing a Tracheostomy Tube

1. Perform a surgical hand scrub.

2. Follow appropriate barrier precautions, including use of sterile gloves.

3. Suction the patient before deflating the cuff (first above the cuff, then tracheal aspiration).

4. Remove the new tube from its package and place it on a sterile field.

5. Check the cuff for leaks; deflate cuff completely while "milking" it away from the distal tip.

6. Attach new, clean tracheostomy ties.

7. Remove the new tube's inner cannula, insert the obturator, and lubricate the tube/obturator tip.

8. Position the patient in semi-Fowler's position with the neck slightly extended.

9. Loosen or untie the old ties and fully deflate the cuff.

10. Remove any attached supporting equipment.

11. Remove the old tube and visually inspect the stoma for bleeding or infection.

12. Insert the new tube with a slightly downward and curving motion.

13. Remove the obturator and insert the inner cannula.

14. Inflate the cuff if ordered, ensure proper placement, and secure tube in place.

15. Restore the patient to the prior level of support.

Specialized Tracheostomy Airways

The NBRC exams also may assess your knowledge of two specialized tracheal airways: fenestrated trach tubes and trach buttons.

Fenestrated Tracheostomy Tubes

Fenestrated tubes are indicated (1) to facilitate weaning from a standard tube or (2) to support patients needing intermittent (e.g., nocturnal) ventilatory support. As illustrated in **Figure 8-1**, a fenestrated tube has an opening in the posterior wall of the outer cannula above the cuff. Removal of the inner cannula opens the fenestration. When the cuff is deflated and the tube's exterior opening is plugged, air can move freely between the trachea and upper airway through the fenestration and around the cuff. Removal of the plug allows access for suctioning, while reinsertion of the inner cannula closes the fenestration and allows for positive-pressure ventilation.

Troubleshooting of fenestrated tubes is similar to that for regular tubes. The most common problem with fenestrated tubes is malpositioning of the fenestration, such as between the skin and the stoma, or against the posterior tracheal wall. Tube malpositioning typically causes respiratory

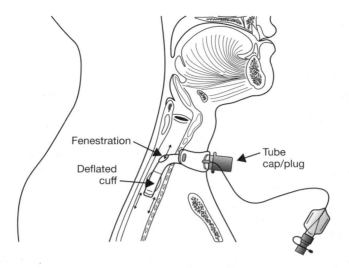

Figure 8-1 "Plugged" Fenestrated Tracheostomy Tube in Place with Cuff Deflated.

Courtesy of: Strategic Learning Associates, LLC, Little Silver, New Jersey.

distress when the tube is plugged and the cuff deflated. In most cases, repositioning the tube under bronchoscopic observation solves this problem. Alternatively, if the tube has an adjustable flange, modifying its position can help align the fenestration in the middle of the trachea.

Respiratory distress also can occur if the cuff is not completely deflated before plugging the tube. To avoid this problem:

- *Always make sure that the cuff is fully deflated before plugging the tube.*
- Attach a warning tag to the tube cap/plug.

If soft tissues obstruct the fenestration, you may feel resistance when inserting the inner cannula. To avoid tissue damage, never force the inner cannula during insertion. If you feel abnormal resistance when placing the inner cannula, withdraw it and notify the patient's physician immediately.

Tracheostomy Buttons

Trach buttons are small tubes used to maintain an open stoma after a trach tube is removed. The patient can eat, breathe, and cough normally, but the stoma is available to bypass laryngeal or upper airway obstruction, for suctioning, or for ventilatory support. Be aware of the following points regarding trach buttons' placement:

- The cannula is slightly flared at the outer end to prevent it from slipping into the trachea.
- The inner end is flanged to keep it in place against the tracheal wall.
- Spacers of various widths are used to adjust the cannula depth.
- A plug can seal the button, forcing the patient to breathe and cough via the upper airway.
- A standard connector can be used for positive-pressure ventilation; however, leakage will occur.
- A one-way valve that blocks expiration (e.g., Passy-Muir valve) can allow the patient to talk, eat, and cough normally.

To ensure continued patency, one should regularly pass a suction catheter through the button. If respiratory distress occurs with an unplugged button, it likely is protruding too far into the trachea and will need to be repositioned by changing the number of spacers. As with fenestrated trach tubes, proper placement is confirmed using fiberoptic bronchoscopy.

Tracheal Airway Cuff Management

Monitoring tracheal airway cuff pressures is a standard of care for respiratory therapy and a mandatory part of routine patient–ventilator system checks. Cuff pressures in excess of 25–30 cm H_2O can obstruct blood flow (ischemia), causing tissue ulceration and necrosis. Conversely, when cuff pressures are too low, leakage-type aspiration occurs, which can cause VAP. Thus the goal is to avoid tracheal mucosal damage without increasing the risk of VAP.

Cuff pressures should be monitored and adjusted regularly (e.g., once per shift) and more often if the tube is changed, if its position changes, if air is added to or removed from the cuff, or if a leak occurs. To measure and adjust cuff pressures, you need a calibrated manometer, a three-way stopcock, and a 10- or 20-mL syringe. Many institutions use a commercially available bulb device that combines the functions of these components. If using the three-way stopcock system:

1. Attach the syringe and manometer to the stopcock set so that all three ports are open.
2. Attach the third stopcock port to the cuff's pilot tube valve, being sure that the connection is leak free.
3. With the stopcock open to the syringe, manometer, and cuff, add or remove air while observing the pressure changes on the manometer.
4. If the patient is receiving positive-pressure ventilation, adjust the pressure to eliminate gurgling sounds at the cuff throughout inspiration (indicating a leak-free seal) but at a pressure no higher than 30 cm H_2O.
5. If the patient is breathing spontaneously, initially adjust the pressure to 15–20 cm H_2O, and then determine the lowest pressure needed to prevent aspiration.

To determine the lowest pressure needed to prevent aspiration in spontaneously breathing patients, you must perform the methylene blue test, normally by order of the physician. To perform this test:

1. Inflate the cuff to 15–20 cm H_2O.
2. Have the patient swallow a small amount of methylene blue dye that has been added to water.
3. Suction the patient's trachea through the artificial airway.

If you obtain blue-tinged secretions during suctioning, aspiration is occurring and you should increase the pressure by 5 cm H_2O and repeat the test. If aspiration still occurs and the cuff pressure is at the maximum 25–30 cm H_2O, you should recommend one or more of the following strategies to help minimize aspiration:

- Performing oropharyngeal suctioning (above the tube cuff) as needed.
- During or after oral feeding, elevating the head of the bed and temporarily increasing the cuff pressure.
- Switching the patient to a tracheal airway that continually aspirates subglottic secretions.
- Inserting a feeding tube into the duodenum (confirm its position by x-ray).

Additional fine points in the procedure that may appear on NBRC exams include the following:

- Most hospitals (including the NBRC "hospital") set 25 cm H_2O as the high-pressure limit.
- Attaching a manometer and syringe to a pilot tube line causes volume loss and lowers cuff pressure; for this reason, *you must always adjust the pressure—never just measure it.*
- Any change in ventilator settings that alters peak pressures may require pressure readjustment.
- Cuff pressures should be recorded as part of the airway management or ventilator documentation.

- Obtaining a leak-free seal at acceptable cuff pressures during mechanical ventilation may be difficult when (1) high peak pressures are required or (2) the tracheal tube is too small for the patient's airway. In these cases, it is best to keep pressures below 25–30 cm H_2O but recommend exchanging the airway for one that provides continuous aspiration of subglottic secretions (see Chapter 9).
- Even at pressures of 20–30 cm H_2O, low-pressure cuffs may still allow some leakage. Again, the solution is using a tube that provides continuous aspiration of secretions above the cuff.

Some clinicians recommend recording and tracking cuff inflation *volume* in addition to pressure. *Increases in inflation volume over time likely indicate tracheal dilation*, which can lead to permanent damage such as tracheomalacia. However, because this technique requires emptying the cuff, it can increase the likelihood of aspiration. Given that this hazard outweighs the potential benefits of this procedure, it is not recommended.

Two unique cuff designs can help avoid tracheal trauma: the Lanz tube and the Bivona Fome-Cuf (also called the Kamen-Wilkinson tube). The Lanz tube incorporates an external regulating valve and control reservoir that automatically maintains cuff pressure at about 30 cm H_2O. Bivona Fome-Cuf tubes have a foam cuff that seals the trachea at atmospheric pressure. With the Bivona Fome-Cuf tube:

- Prior to insertion, you *deflate* the cuff with a syringe and close off the pilot tube.
- Once the tube is positioned properly in the trachea, you open the pilot tube to the atmosphere and allow the foam to expand against the tracheal wall.

Troubleshooting Tracheal Airways

Basic troubleshooting of artificial airways is covered in Chapter 4. Here we cover three of the most critical problems in depth: (1) cuff leaks, (2) accidental extubation, and (3) an obstructed airway.

Cuff Leaks

Cuff leaks are among the most common problems with tracheal airways. In patients on a ventilator, a leak in the cuff or pilot tube can cause a loss of delivered volume or an inability to maintain the pre-set pressure. With both ventilator-managed and spontaneously breathing patients, cuff leaks also can lead to aspiration. Key points you need to address when dealing with leaks include the following:

- Small/slow leaks are evident when cuff pressures decrease between readings.
- Your first step is to try to reinflate the cuff, while checking the pilot tube and valve for leaks.
  - If the leak is at the one-way valve, attach a stopcock to its outlet.
  - If the leak is in the pilot tube, place a needle (with stopcock) in the pilot tube distal to the leak. Usually, one of these methods will allow you to reinflate the cuff and thus avoid reintubation.
- A large cuff leak ("blown cuff") makes it impossible to pressurize the cuff.
  - A patient on a ventilator with a blown cuff will exhibit a decrease in delivered V_T and/or inspiratory pressure; breath sounds typically decrease and gurgling may be heard around the tube.
  - A patient with a blown cuff normally requires reintubation; if the blown cuff is on an oral ET tube, using a tube exchanger will make reintubation easier.

Because the signs of partial extubation are similar to those occurring with a blown cuff, do not recommend reintubation until you confirm that a cuff leak is the problem.

- Before presuming a cuff leak, advance the tube slightly and reassess breath sounds.
- Next, rule out or correct any pilot tube or valve leakage.
- Finally, try to measure the cuff pressure.
- If you cannot maintain cuff pressure (confirming a large leak), the patient must be reintubated.

Accidental Extubation

Accidental extubation (including self-extubation) can be minimized by attention to tube fixation, avoidance of traction on the tube connector, maintenance of adequate sedation, and appropriate use of restraints.

Accidental extubation can occur even with proper attention to these measures. It can be partial or complete. Because partial extubation can mimic a blown cuff, the first step in dealing with this problem is to rule out a large cuff leak by quickly measuring the cuff pressure.

If partial extubation of an ET tube occurs, you should deflate the cuff, remove the securing tape, and try to reposition the tube back into the trachea. If this does not reestablish the airway, you will need to extubate the patient, provide bag-mask ventilation with O_2, and then consider reintubation.

If accidental extubation occurs in a patient with a trach whose tube is fresh:

- Call the attending physician or surgeon to replace the tube.
- Occlude the stoma with a sterile petroleum jelly gauze pad.
- Provide bag-mask ventilation with oxygen as needed.

In the NBRC "hospital," if the stoma is well established, you are expected to obtain a sterile tube of the same size or one size smaller and follow the previously described procedure for changing trach tubes.

Dealing with an Obstructed Airway

Tracheal tube obstruction can be caused by any of the following:

- Kinking of the tube
- The patient biting down on the tube (ET tubes only)
- Malpositioning of the tube tip against the tracheal wall (mainly trach tubes)
- Herniation of the cuff causing occlusion of the tube tip (rare)
- Compression of the tube due to cuff overinflation (mainly silicone ET tubes)
- Inspissated secretions, mucus, or blood clots plugging the tube lumen

Figure 8-2 provides a general algorithm for dealing with tracheal tube obstruction in patients receiving ventilatory support. Typically, such patients will exhibit signs of respiratory distress. However, because many problems can cause respiratory distress—including a malfunctioning ventilator—*the first step is always to remove the patient from the ventilator, provide manual ventilation with 100% O_2, and reassess the situation.* If no improvement is noted, you then progress through the algorithm, reassessing the adequacy of ventilation at each step.

Ultimately, you may reach the point at which the only viable solution is to remove the tube. Once you remove an obstructed tube, you should first try to reestablish ventilation and oxygenation, normally using a bag-valve resuscitator and face mask. For trach patients, you may need to close off the stoma with a petroleum jelly gauze pad. Once the patient is stabilized, a new tube can be reinserted.

Alternative Emergency Airways

Oral endotracheal intubation is the procedure of choice in emergency situations requiring airway protection and artificial ventilation. However, the NBRC expects you to be proficient with two alternative emergency airways: (1) the laryngeal mask airway and (2) the esophageal–tracheal Combitube.

Laryngeal Mask Airway

As depicted in **Figure 8-3**, a laryngeal mask airway (LMA) consists of a tube and a mask with an inflatable cuff that is blindly inserted into the pharynx. When properly positioned and with the cuff inflated, the mask seals off the laryngeal inlet. This effectively bypasses the esophagus and provides a direct route for bag-valve ventilation via a standard connector.

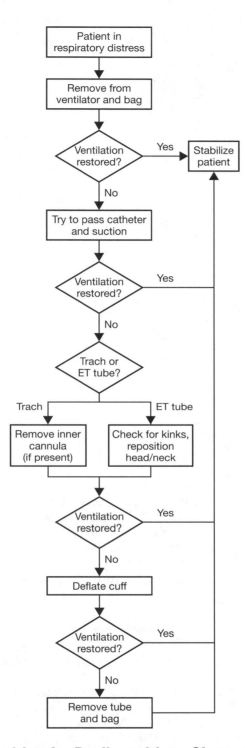

Figure 8-2 General Algorithm for Dealing with an Obstructed Artificial Tracheal Airway.

Courtesy of: Strategic Learning Associates, LLC, Little Silver, New Jersey.

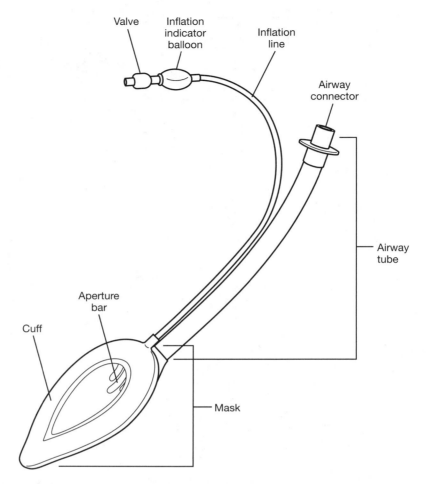

Figure 8-3 The Components of the Laryngeal Mask Airway. This device consists of a tube and a mask with an inflatable cuff. The tube provides a standard 15-mm airway connector for attaching equipment. The mask is inflated via an inflation line with a valve and a pilot indicator balloon, much like those used on ET tubes. The mask portion fits into the pyriform sinus, over the opening into the larynx. The aperture bars, used mainly in the reusable versions, help prevent the epiglottis from obstructing the inlet to the mask.

The LMA is used primarily by anesthesiologists as an alternative to ET intubation during surgery. Because it allows rapid airway access without laryngoscopy, it also is used for emergency airway management of unconscious patients in whom ET intubation cannot be performed or fails. Because the LMA does not prevent aspiration, users must take into account the risk of regurgitation. Unfortunately, gastric tubes do not eliminate and may even increase the risk of aspiration in patients with LMAs. For these reasons, when tracheal intubation cannot be performed and the risk of aspiration is high, the esophageal–tracheal Combitube may be a better choice.

You should avoid using an LMA to establish an airway in patients who are conscious, who have intact gag reflexes, or who resist insertion. You also should avoid using an LMA in patients needing tracheal suctioning. The LMA should not be inserted in patients with trauma or obstructive lesions in the mouth or pharynx. In addition, the LMA is a poor choice if ventilation requires high pressures because this will breach the mask seal around the larynx.

Proper sizing of the LMA is critical. **Table 8-6** provides guidance on LMA selection based on patient size and weight as well as the maximum cuff inflation volume for each size.

Table 8-6 Laryngeal Mask Airway Sizes and Maximum Cuff Inflation Volumes

Patient Size	Recommended LMA Size	Maximum Cuff Volume*
Neonate/infant: < 5 kg	1	4 mL
Infants: 5–10 kg	1½	7 mL
Infants/children 10–20 kg	2	10 mL
Children: 20–30 kg	2½	14 mL
Children: 30–50 kg	3	20 mL
Adults: 50–70 kg	4	30 mL
Adults: 70–100 kg	5	40 mL
Adults: > 100 kg	6	50 mL
*These are *maximum* volumes that should never be exceeded. The cuff should be inflated to 60 cm H_2O.		

Key points related to the use of the LMA are summarized as follows:

Preparation

- Choose an LMA appropriate for the patient's size and weight (Table 8-6).
- Always have a spare LMA ready for use; ideally, have one size larger and one size smaller available.
- Fully deflate the cuff by pulling back firmly on the deflating syringe until it forms a smooth wedge shape without wrinkles; insertion with a partially deflated cuff can obstruct the airway.
- Lubricate the posterior side of the mask using a water-soluble jelly.
- Preoxygenate the patient and implement standard monitoring procedures.

Insertion

- Use the "sniffing position" (head extension, neck flexion) for insertion.
- Use upward and posterior pressure with the fingers to keep the mask pressed against the rear of the pharynx (palatopharyngeal curve).
- Avoid excessive force during insertion.

Inflation

- Inflate the cuff to 60 cm H_2O; during inflation, avoid holding the tube, as this may prevent the mask from settling into the correct position.
- Cuff volumes vary according to the size of the patient and LMA; volumes less than the maximum (Table 8-6) are often sufficient to obtain a seal and achieve 60 cm H_2O cuff pressure.
- During cuff inflation, you should observe a slight outward movement of the tube.
- Avoid cuff pressures greater than 60 cm H_2O; higher pressures can cause malpositioning or tissue damage.

Assessing and Ensuring Correct Placement

- No portion of the cuff should be visible in the oral cavity.
- Chest expansion during inspiration, good breath sounds, and expired CO_2 indicate correct placement.
- Malpositioning can cause leakage (decreased tidal volumes/expired CO_2) or obstruction (prolonged expiration and/or increased peak inflation pressures).
- If the tube is malpositioned, deflate cuff and reposition or reinsert the LMA to achieve adequate ventilation.

Fixation

- Insert a bite block; *avoid oropharyngeal airways*, as they can cause malpositioning.
- Apply gentle pressure to tube while securing it with tape (presses the mask against the esophageal sphincter).
- Keep the bite block in place until the LMA airway is removed.

Providing Positive-Pressure Ventilation (PPV)

- To avoid leaks during manual ventilation, squeeze the bag slowly and try to keep inspiratory pressures below 20–30 cm H_2O.
- If a leak occurs during PPV:
  - Confirm that the airway is securely taped in place.
  - Readjust the airway position by pressing the tube downward.
  - Resecure the airway in its new position.
  - *Do not simply add more air to the cuff* (may worsen leakage by pushing cuff off larynx).

Troubleshooting

- If airway/ventilation problems persist, remove the LMA and establish an airway by other means.
- If regurgitation occurs, *do not remove the LMA*; instead:
  - Place patient in a head-down or side-lying (rescue) position and disconnect all ventilation equipment so that gastric contents are not forced into the lungs.
  - Reposition the LMA to ensure its distal end is pressing against the esophageal sphincter.
  - Suction through the airway tube.
  - Prepare for immediate tracheal intubation.

Removal

- Consider removing the LMA only after the patient's upper airway reflexes have returned.
- Prior to removing, gather suctioning and intubation equipment.
- Avoid suctioning the airway tube with the LMA in place (may provoke laryngospasm).
- Deflate the cuff and simultaneously remove the device.
- Verify airway patency and unobstructed ventilation.
- Perform oropharyngeal suctioning as needed.

Esophageal–Tracheal Combitube

Like the LMA, the esophageal–tracheal Combitube (ETC) is an alternative to endotracheal intubation for emergency ventilatory support and airway control, which is designed to be inserted blindly. The ETC is a common alternative to ET intubation in the prehospital/emergency setting. In the hospital, it is a good choice for patients who prove difficult to intubate due to trauma, bleeding, vomiting, or other factors that make visualization of the vocal cords impossible. Like the LMA, the ETC should not be inserted in conscious patients or those with intact gag reflexes. It is contraindicated for infants and small children and for patients with esophageal trauma or disease.

As depicted in **Figure 8-4**, the ETC is a double-tube, double-cuff airway. This design ensure effective ventilation regardless of whether the airway ends up in the esophagus or trachea. In either case, the pharyngeal balloon fills the space between the tongue and soft palate, thereby eliminating the need for a mask. If the airway is inserted into the esophagus, the distal cuff seals this passageway and ventilation occurs via the holes in the pharyngeal tube, below the pharyngeal cuff. If the ETC ends up in the trachea, it functions as an ET tube, with the distal cuff sealing the lower airway and preventing aspiration.

The ETC comes in two sizes. The 37-French version is recommended for patients 4 to 5 feet tall, with the 41-French version reserved for taller patients. However, the 37-French ETC generally suffices for patients 4 to 6 feet tall, so it is satisfactory for all but the largest patients.

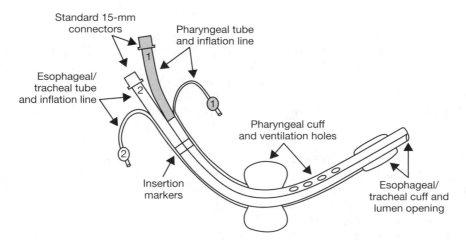

Figure 8-4 Esophageal–Tracheal Combitube. The #1 pharyngeal tube (longer blue connector) has a large volume cuff, ventilation holes distal to the cuff, and terminates in a dead end. The shorter, clear #2 tracheal/esophageal tube has a regular volume cuff and beveled opening at its tip. Both cuffs have inflation lines and pilot balloons, ringed insertion markers, and standard 15-mm connectors for attaching equipment at their proximal ends. Accessory equipment provided with the airway includes two inflation syringes (large and small), a suction catheter, and an aspiration deflection elbow (to deflect vomitus should regurgitation occur).

Courtesy of: Strategic Learning Associates, LLC, Little Silver, New Jersey.

The basic procedure for inserting the ETC is the same for both sizes, except for the cuff inflation volumes. Key steps are outlined in the accompanying box.

Procedure for Insertion of an Esophageal–Tracheal Combitube

1. Suction mouth and oropharynx, and preoxygenate patient.

2. Inflate cuffs with the applicable syringe to confirm integrity, and then fully deflate.

3. Lubricate the tube tip and pharyngeal balloon with water-soluble jelly.

4. Place patient's head in a *neutral position* and pull the mandible and tongue forward.

5. Place the ETC tip in the midline of the mouth and guide it along the palate and posterior pharynx using a curving motion (do not force tube; if resistance is felt, withdraw tube, reposition the patient's head, and try again).

6. Advance the ETC until the upper teeth or gums are aligned between the two black insertion markers.

7. If unable to insert within 30 seconds, ventilate the patient with O_2 for 1–2 minutes and try again.

8. Inflate the large/small cuffs (41 Fr: 100 mL/15 mL; 37 Fr: 85 mL/12 mL).

9. Begin ventilating through the longer blue #1 pharyngeal tube.

10. If there is good chest rise and breath sounds (or expired CO_2 is detected) without stomach gurgling (indicating esophageal placement), continue ventilating through the #1 tube.

11. Absent chest excursions, breath sounds or expired CO_2, with stomach gurgling indicates tracheal placement; in such a case, switch to the #2 tracheal/esophageal tube and reconfirm good ventilation.

12. If you cannot ventilate the patient through either tube, the ETC may be inserted too deep and obstructing the glottis; if so, withdraw tube 2–3 cm at a time while ventilating via connector #1 until breath sounds are heard.

13. If you still cannot provide good ventilation, remove the ETC and reestablish the airway by any alternative means available.

14. Once adequate ventilation is confirmed, secure tube with tape or a tube holder and continue providing essential life support.

Note that most Combitubes end up in the esophagus. *This is why initial attempts at ventilation should always be via the pharyngeal tube.* Once esophageal placement is confirmed, you can use the #2 tube to relieve any gastric distension due to positive-pressure ventilation. To do so, insert the provided suction catheter into the #2 tube to between the two insertion markers. Then connect the catheter to a vacuum source set to low for several minutes. Once the gastric distension is relieved, remove the catheter.

To switch a patient from an ETC to an oral ET tube, the airway must be in the esophagus. In this case, gather and prepare all equipment needed for intubation (Chapter 4), and aspirate any stomach contents through the #2 tube. Then deflate the large #1 pharyngeal cuff. This will allow for laryngoscopy while the #2 cuff keeps the esophagus occluded. Alternatively, if stomach contents have been aspirated, you can consider removing the ETC before proceeding with tracheal intubation.

Remove the ETC when the patient regains consciousness, begins biting or gagging on the tube, or requires tracheal intubation. Because regurgitation can occur with ETC removal, you must have suction equipment set up for immediate use. Normally, you roll the patient to the side (rescue position) before removing the ETC. You then fully deflate both cuffs until the pilot balloons are completely collapsed and gently remove the tube while suctioning the airway.

Maintaining Adequate Humidification

Humidity therapy is indicated either to humidify dry medical gases or to overcome the humidity deficit when bypassing the upper airway. In addition, providing adequate humidification can help mobilize secretions. Heated humidification also can be used to treat hypothermia and bronchospasm caused by inhaling cold air.

Humidification Needs

Table 8-7 specifies the humidification needs by type of therapy. Due to the effectiveness of the nose as a heat and moisture exchanger, temperature and humidity needs are less when delivering medical gases to the upper airway. Indeed, a humidifier normally is *not* needed when delivering O_2 to the upper airways in the following circumstances:

- With low-flow O_2 therapy ($\leq$ 4 L/min)
- Via air-entrainment devices providing less than 50% O_2
- Via O_2 masks in emergency situations or for short time periods

Table 8-7 Humidification Needs by Type of Therapy

Type of Therapy	Temperature Range	Relative Humidity	Minimum H₂O Content
O₂ Therapy			
O₂ therapy to nose/mouth (intact upper airway)	20–22°C	50%	10 mg/L
O₂ therapy via tracheal airway (bypassed upper airway)	34–41°C	100%	33–44 mg/L
Mechanical Ventilation			
Invasive ventilation (bypassed upper airway) with active (heated) humidification	34–41°C	100%	33–44 mg/L
Invasive ventilation (bypassed upper airway) with passive humidification (HME)	30–35°C	100%	≥ 30 mg/L
Noninvasive ventilation (via mask) with active humidification (heated *or* unheated humidifier)*	Based on patient comfort, tolerance, adherence, and underlying condition	50–100%	10–44 mg/L
*Passive humidification is not recommended for noninvasive ventilation.			

In contrast, if a patient's upper airway has been bypassed via intubation, you must overcome the humidity deficit by providing extra heat and humidity. *For this reason, the use of unheated active humidifiers is contraindicated in patients with bypassed upper airways.*

Selecting a Humidification Strategy

Figure 8-5 provides an algorithm for selecting the appropriate humidification strategy. Key information needed to make your decision includes (1) whether or not the patient has an artificial tracheal airway, (2) the thickness of secretions, (3) the gas flow, (4) the need for and duration of mechanical ventilation, and (5) the presence of contraindications against using an HME.

Spontaneously Breathing Patients

For patients with intact upper airways with normal secretions receiving O_2 at flows greater than 4 L/min, a simple unheated bubble humidifier is satisfactory. For patients with either thick secretions or a tracheal airway, bland aerosol therapy is the most common humidification option. **Table 8-8** itemizes the various airway appliances used to deliver bland aerosol and their best use. As with humidifiers, heat can be added to the nebulizer to increase water delivery.

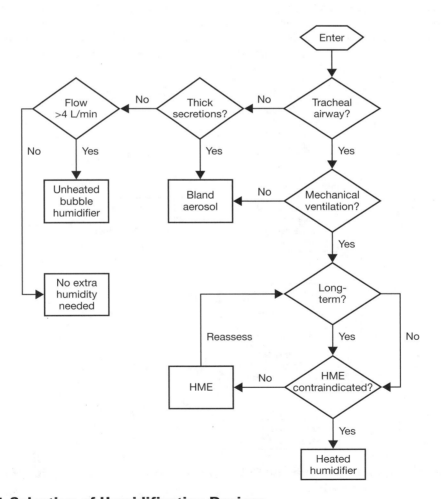

Figure 8-5 Selection of Humidification Devices.

Courtesy of: Strategic Learning Associates, LLC, Little Silver, New Jersey.

Table 8-8 Selection of Airway Appliances for Bland Aerosol Therapy

Airway Appliances	Best Use
Aerosol mask	Short-term application to most patients with intact upper airways
Face tent	Patients with intact upper airways who will not tolerate an aerosol mask; also for patients with facial trauma or burns
T-tube	Patients with an ET or trach tube needing a moderate to high F_{IO_2}
Trach mask	Patients with a trach for whom precise or high F_{IO_2} is not needed; also ideal when you need to avoid traction on the airway

Patients Requiring Invasive Mechanical Ventilation

All patients receiving ventilatory support via a tracheal airway require a humidifier in the ventilator circuit—either an active heated humidifier or a passive HME. **Figure 8-6** provides an algorithm for determining which device to use. In general, you can begin with an HME unless it is contraindicated (see the accompanying box). Because HME performance varies, *be sure that the device you select meets or exceeds the minimum water vapor content of 30 mg/L.* If an HME is contraindicated, start the patient on a heated humidifier.

HMEs increase deadspace by 30 to 70 mL. Thus, for infants and small children, you must be sure to select the correct size HME and adjust the V_T to compensate for the deadspace. HMEs also slightly increase flow resistance through the breathing circuit, which is not a problem for most adults. However, if mucus accumulates in the HME, resistance can increase over time, increasing airway pressures during volume-controlled ventilation and potentially decreasing delivered volumes during pressure-controlled ventilation. You can verify this problem by inspecting the HME and correct it by replacing the device with a new one.

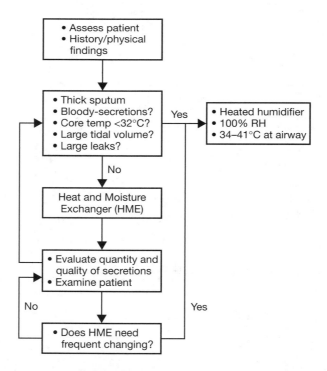

Figure 8-6 Decision Algorithm for Selecting Humidifier Systems for Patients with Artificial Tracheal Airways.

Adapted from: Branson RD, Davis K, Campbell RS, et al. Humidification in the intensive care unit: prospective study of a new protocol utilizing heated humidification and a hygroscopic condenser humidifier. *Chest.* 1993;104:1800–1805.

Contraindications Against Using HMEs

HMEs are contraindicated for patients with any of the following:

- Bloody or thick, copious secretions

- Body temperatures < 32°C

- High spontaneous minute volumes (> 10 L/min)

- Expired V_T < 70% of the delivered V_T

- ALI/ARDS receiving low V_T or hypercapnia respiratory failure

- Noninvasive ventilation via leakage-type breathing circuits

Should any contraindication arise during patient management, or if you need to change the HME more than four times per day, you should switch to a heated humidifier.

Heated passover humidifiers can be used alone or in combination with heated-wire circuits. When used alone, a heated humidifier always will cause condensation in the circuit. Heated-wire circuits provide better control over gas temperatures and prevent tubing condensation. However, reports have cited heated wires actually melting the delivery tubing and causing dangerous circuit leaks. To avoid this potentially serious problem, follow these guidelines:

1. Never use reusable wires with disposable breathing circuits.
2. Ensure that heating wires are threaded evenly along the tubing and not bunched up.
3. Never cover a heated-wire circuit with towels, drapes, or linens.

Patients Receiving Noninvasive Mechanical Ventilation

Some patients receiving noninvasive ventilation (NPPV) may also require extra humidification, especially those using oral interfaces or when ambient humidity levels are low. In addition, providing humidification during NPPV can improve patient adherence and comfort.

HMEs are contraindicated for patients receiving NPPV. The characteristic one-way flow and large leakage occurring during NPPV impairs the performance of these devices. Moreover, the added deadspace and flow resistance that HMEs impose can increase CO_2 levels and the work of breathing.

Because patients breathe through the upper airway during NPPV, a simple unheated passover humidifier usually will suffice. However, if supplemental O_2 is being provided or if the patient has problems with secretions retention, consider using a heated humidifier. Likewise, if the patient complains of dryness or discomfort even when using an unheated humidifier, consider heated humidification. To prevent condensation problems with these systems, be sure to place the humidifier *below* both the ventilator and the patient.

Perform Extubation

Removal of a tracheal tube should be considered only in those patients who meet the following criteria:

- Can maintain adequate oxygenation and ventilation without ventilatory support
- Are at minimal risk for upper airway obstruction
- Have adequate airway protection and are at minimal risk for aspiration
- Can adequately clear pulmonary secretions on their own

The patient's ability to maintain adequate oxygenation and ventilation should be demonstrated via a spontaneous breathing trial. To assess for upper airway obstruction, perform a *cuff-leak test*. To do so, after removing secretions above the tube cuff, fully deflate the cuff and completely occlude the tube at its outlet. If leakage occurs during spontaneous breathing (a "positive" test), then the airway likely is patent. A positive gag reflex and the ability of the patient to raise his or her head off the bed indicate adequate airway protection. In addition, the ability to clear secretions is evident if the patient is alert, coughs deeply on suctioning, and can generate a maximum expiratory pressure (MEP) greater than 60 cm H_2O.

Equipment needed to extubate a patient includes suction apparatus, a bag-valve-mask resuscitator, a bland aerosol mask setup, an SVN with racemic epinephrine available, and an intubation tray (in case reintubation is required).

Key considerations in performing extubation include the following:

- Place the patient upright if possible (semi-Fowler's position or higher).
- Suction the tube and pharynx to above the cuff.
- Provide 100% O_2 via a bag-valve system for 1–2 minutes after suctioning.
- Fully deflate the cuff and remove the securing tape or device.
- Insert a new catheter into the tracheal tube.
- Simultaneously have the patient cough while you apply suction and quickly pull the tube.
- Provide cool, humidified O_2 via aerosol mask at a higher FIO_2 than prior to extubation.
- Assess breath sounds, work of breathing, and vital signs.
- If stridor develops, recommend treatment with aerosolized racemic epinephrine.
- Initiate bronchial hygiene therapy or directed coughing.
- Recommend that the patient be NPO (except for sips of water) for 24 hours.
- Analyze arterial blood gases as needed.

The most serious complication that can occur with extubation is laryngospasm. Should laryngospasm occur, you should initially provide positive-pressure ventilation via a bag-valve-mask with 100% O_2. If laryngospasm persists, the doctor may need to paralyze the patient with a neuromuscular blocking agent and reintubate.

COMMON ERRORS TO AVOID

You can improve your score by avoiding these mistakes:

- Never place or keep an oropharyngeal airway in a conscious patient.
- Never use Magill forceps during intubation without direct visualization.
- Never tie tracheostomy ties with a bow; instead, always use a square knot.
- Never force insertion of a trach tube inner cannula, and do not pull on or rock it when attaching equipment.
- Never just measure cuff pressure; always adjust the pressure if it is not correct.
- Never use more than 60 cm H_2O to inflate an LMA cuff.
- Never cover a heated-wire breathing circuit with towels, drapes, or linens.
- Never extubate a patient without being prepared to reintubate.

SURE BETS

In some situations, you can always be sure of the right approach to a clinical problem or scenario:

- Always be sure a nasopharyngeal airway is well lubricated before insertion.
- Always keep an obturator and backup tubes (including one size smaller) at the bedside of trach patients.
- Unless otherwise indicated, maintain tracheal tube cuff pressures in the 20–30 cm H_2O range.
- If available, always use tracheal airways that provide for aspiration of subglottic secretions.
- Always suction the patient's oropharynx and area above the cuff before you extubate.
- Always provide 100% O_2 to adult patients prior to suctioning and both before and after extubation.
- Always regularly pass a suction catheter through artificial tracheal airways to ensure patency.
- Always make sure that the cuff of a fenestrated trach tube is fully deflated before plugging it.
- Always provide all patients receiving ventilatory support via an artificial tracheal airway with at least 30 mg/L water vapor.

PRE-TEST ANSWERS AND EXPLANATIONS

Following are this chapter's pre-test answers and explanations. Be sure to review each answer's explanation thoroughly to help you understand why it is correct. If the explanation is still unclear to you, review the chapter content.

8-1. **Correct answer: D.** Apply the head-tilt/chin-lift maneuver. The initial procedure used to maintain an open airway in an unconscious patient is the head-tilt/chin-lift maneuver. This maneuver helps displace the tongue away from the posterior pharyngeal wall.

8-2. **Correct answer: B.** Nasopharyngeal airway. When the mouth is unavailable for airway access, you should try the nose. In this case, a nasopharyngeal airway would help overcome the upper airway obstruction and is quickly and easily inserted.

8-3. **Correct answer: C.** Is conscious and alert. Oropharyngeal airways can provoke a gag reflex and possibly vomiting, so they should be avoided in conscious patients.

8-4. **Correct answer: A.** Bag slowly to reduce peak pressure. To avoid leaks during positive-pressure ventilation through an LMA, you should use slow inflation and keep peak pressures at less than 20–30 cm H_2O. If a leak persists in spite of these efforts, you should readjust the tube's position by pressing it downward and resecuring it. Avoid adding more air to the cuff, as this can worsen the leak by displacing the cuff away from the larynx.

8-5. **Correct answer: B.** Inspired gas with an absolute humidity greater than 30 mg/L. To provide adequate humidity to intubated patients, the absolute humidity should be at least 30 mg/L. Providing gas at lower levels of humidity to these patients can cause damage to the tracheal mucosa and impair mucociliary clearance.

8-6. **Correct answer: C.** Withdraw the tube by 1–2 cm (using tube markings as a guide). The tip of an ET or trach tube should be positioned 4–6 cm above the carina. If the tube is malpositioned, you should get permission to reposition the tube using the markings on the tube as a guide and as confirmed by x-ray or laryngoscopy. This often requires two people to prevent extubation.

8-7. **Correct answer: C.** Ventilate through the other (#2) tube. After insertion of an ETC, you normally begin ventilation through the #1 pharyngeal tube. If you detect no chest motion or breath sounds via this route, or if stomach gurgling is present, the tube is in the trachea and you should switch to using the shorter #2 esophageal/tracheal tube.

8-8. **Correct answer: B.** Tissue damage. Tracheal wall tissue damage can occur as a result of over-inflating the cuff of a tracheal tube, because pressures greater than 25–30 cm H_2O can cause tissue ischemia.

8-9. **Correct answer: C.** A simple bubble humidifier. When the upper airway has been bypassed, the only way to prevent large humidity deficits is to provide inspired gases at or near BTPS conditions. This is not possible with an unheated humidifier. Instead, either a heated humidifier, HME, or large-volume nebulizer must be used. These systems can control temperature and humidity levels and provide 100% relative humidity at or near body temperature.

8-10. **Correct answer: A.** "Leakage-type" aspiration. The methylene blue test can help determine if leakage aspiration is occurring. Methylene blue diluted in water is swallowed by the patient. Once the dye is introduced, the patient's trachea is suctioned. If blue-tinged secretions are retrieved, aspiration is occurring.

POST-TEST

To confirm your mastery of this chapter's topical content, you should take the chapter post-test, available online at http://go.jblearning.com/respexamreview. A score of 80% or more indicates that you are adequately prepared for this section of the NBRC written exams. If you score less than 80%, you should continue to review the applicable chapter content. In addition, you may want to access and review the relevant Web links covering this chapter's content (courtesy of RTBoardReview. com), also online at the Jones & Bartlett Learning site.

CHAPTER 9

Remove Bronchopulmonary Secretions

Albert J. Heuer
(previous version co-authored with Brian X. Weaver)

Many patients require assistance in removing bronchopulmonary secretions. In this section of the NBRC exams, you will be tested on this type of therapy, including postural drainage, percussion, and vibration, as well as directed coughing and the use of mechanical aids. Also included in this section are questions on the use of bland aerosols and drugs to facilitate secretion clearance. All of these techniques are ultimately intended to improve ventilation and gas exchange. As such, they represent a small but important component of the exams.

OBJECTIVES

In preparing for the shared NBRC exam content, you should demonstrate the knowledge needed to:

1. Perform postural drainage, percussion, and vibration
2. Instruct and encourage bronchopulmonary hygiene techniques
3. Perform airway clearance using mechanical devices
4. Clear secretions via suctioning
5. Administer aerosol therapy with prescribed medications

WHAT TO EXPECT ON THIS CATEGORY OF THE NBRC EXAMS

CRT exam: 4 questions, 25% recall and 75% application
WRRT exam: 3 questions; 100% analysis
CSE exam: Indeterminate number of questions; however, exam III-C knowledge is a prerequisite to success on CSE Decision-Making sections

PRE-TEST

Carefully respond to each of the following questions. After completing the pre-test, compare your answers to those provided at the end of this chapter. Then thoroughly review each answer's explanation to help understand why it is correct.

9-1. An adult male requires postural drainage of the posterior basal segments bilaterally. To properly position this patient, you should:
1. Elevate the foot of the bed 30 degrees
2. Keep the bed flat but put a pillow under the patient's hips
3. Have the patient lie supine with a pillow under the hips
4. Have the patient lie prone with a pillow under the hips

A. 1 and 2 only
B. 3 and 4 only
C. 1 and 4 only
D. 2 and 3 only

9-2. All of the following are needed for an effective cough *except*:
A. A closed glottis
B. A compression phase
C. Explosive exhalation
D. Low inspiratory volumes

9-3. Which of the following should you do to properly perform nasotracheal suctioning on an adult patient?
1. Lubricate the catheter
2. Apply suction for less than 15 seconds
3. Preoxygenate and postoxygenate the patient
4. Have the patient exhale and then hold breath
A. 1 and 4 only
B. 1, 2, and 3
C. 3 and 4 only
D. 1, 3, and 4

9-4. The administration of which aerosolized drug is most appropriate to thin secretions and help in the removal of a mucus plug?
A. Albuterol
B. Ipratropium bromide
C. Acetylcysteine
D. Racemic epinephrine

9-5. All of the following are proper patient instructions for positive expiratory pressure (PEP) *except*:
A. Take in a breath that is larger than normal, but don't fill lungs completely
B. Exhale forcefully and maintain expiratory pressure of at least 20 cm H_2O
C. After 10 to 20 breaths, perform 2 to 3 "huff" coughs, and rest as needed
D. Repeat the cycle four to eight times, not to exceed 20 minutes

9-6. A nurse is concerned that a patient with a neuromuscular disorder under her care cannot develop a good cough. Which of the following would you recommend as best able to aid this patient in clearing secretions?
A. Combining mechanical insufflation-exsufflation with suctioning
B. Applying forward waist flexion to aid expiratory flow
C. Implementing positive expiratory pressure (PEP) therapy
D. Employing the forced expiration technique (FET)

9-7. Which of the following bronchial hygiene techniques is most suitable for small infants?

A. Postural drainage, percussion, and vibration
B. Positive expiratory pressure
C. Aggressive suctioning with a 14-Fr catheter
D. High-frequency oscillation

9-8. You need to suction a 7-month-old orally intubated patient. For this patient, what are the appropriate pressure and time limits for this procedure?
A. Suction pressure range of −40 to −60 mm Hg, limiting the time to 30 seconds
B. Suction pressure range of −80 to −100 mm Hg, limiting the time to less than 10–15 seconds
C. Suction pressure range of −100 to −120 mm Hg and continuing until you observe secretions in the suction catheter
D. Suction pressure range of −60 to −80 mm Hg, limiting the time to less than 10–15 seconds

9-9. Which of the following are possible complications of postural drainage, percussion, and vibration?
1. Pulmonary barotrauma
2. Acute hypotension during procedure
3. Dysrhythmias
4. Fractured ribs
A. 1 and 3 only
B. 1, 2, and 3
C. 1, 2, 3, and 4
D. 2, 3, and 4

9-10. To remove accumulations of subglottic secretions from above the cuff of intubated patients, you should recommend which of the following?
A. Intrapulmonary percussive ventilation
B. Use of a tracheal tube with a suction port above the cuff
C. Aggressive tracheal suctioning with saline lavage
D. Frequent oropharyngeal suctioning with a Yankauer tip

WHAT YOU NEED TO KNOW: ESSENTIAL CONTENT

Selecting the Best Approach

Bronchial hygiene therapy involves a variety of methods. Important factors in determining which methods to use are the patient's age, preexisting conditions, and personal preference. **Table 9-1** indicates the recommended bronchial hygiene techniques for the most common disorders that require secretion clearance. In some cases, methods are combined to achieve optimal results.

Bronchial hygiene often is ordered by protocol, giving you discretion as to the selection and implementation of therapy and its evaluation. **Figure 9-1** provides a sample algorithm for a bronchial hygiene protocol that directs your decision-making based on the patient's diagnosis, volume of sputum produced, and ability to cough.

Postural Drainage, Percussion, Vibration, and Turning

Postural drainage, percussion, and vibration (PDPV) techniques help loosen and clear secretions from a patient's respiratory tract. This method can help reduce infection, enhance ventilation, and improve both pulmonary function and gas exchange. PDPV is indicated in conditions that increase the likelihood of secretion retention, mucus plugging, and atelectasis:

- Difficulty coughing or clearing the airways
- An inability to turn or change position
- Presence of an artificial airway
- Conditions that increase the volume or viscosity of secretions

Not all patients can undergo this rigorous procedure. **Table 9-2** summarizes the contraindications, hazards, and complications of PDPV.

The accompanying box outlines the key elements in the PDPV procedure. As indicated, you should monitor the patient's clinical status before, during, and after the therapy. Your monitoring of patients should include their overall appearance, vital signs, breathing pattern, and pulse oximetry. If the patient shows any signs of distress, you should stop the treatment, remain with and monitor the patient, and promptly notify the nurse and physician.

Key Elements in the Postural Drainage, Percussion, and Vibration Procedure

- Verify and evaluate order or protocol; determine lobes/segments to be drained by reviewing x-rays results, progress notes, and diagnosis; scan chart for any possible contraindications.
- Coordinate therapy (before meals/tube feedings or 1–1½ hours later and with pain medication, as needed).
- Assess vital signs, breath sounds, SpO_2, color, level of dyspnea, and ability to cooperate.
- Instruct patient in diaphragmatic breathing and coughing.
- Position patient for drainage, beginning with most dependent zones first.
- Maintain position for 10–15 minutes as tolerated.
- Perform percussion/vibration over identified areas.
- Encourage maintenance of proper breathing pattern.
- Encourage and assist patient with coughing; examine (collect) sputum.
- Reassess patient's response and tolerance; modify as needed.
- Reposition patient and repeat procedure as indicated and tolerated.
- Return patient to a comfortable position and reassess.
- Document outcomes.

Adapted from: Scanlan CL, West GA, von der Heydt PA, Dolan GK. *Respiratory therapy competency evaluation manual.* Boston: Blackwell Scientific; 1984.

Table 9-1 Bronchial Hygiene Techniques

Condition	Recommended Technique
Cystic fibrosis, bronchiectasis	
Infants	PDPV
3–12 years old	PEP, PDPV, HFO
> 12 years old	AD, PEP, PDPV, HFO
Adult, living alone	PEP, HFO (flutter valve)
Atelectasis	PEP, PDPV, T&R
Asthma (with mucus plugging)	PEP, PDPV, HFO
Neurologic abnormalities (spasticity, bulbar palsy, aspiration prone)	PDPV, suction, MI-E, T&R
Musculoskeletal weakness (muscular dystrophy, myasthenia, poliomyelitis)	PEP, MI-E, T&R
PDPV = postural drainage, percussion, and vibration; PEP = positive expiratory pressure; AD = autogenic drainage; MI-E = mechanical insufflation–exsufflation; HFO = high-frequency oscillation; T&R = turning and rotation.	

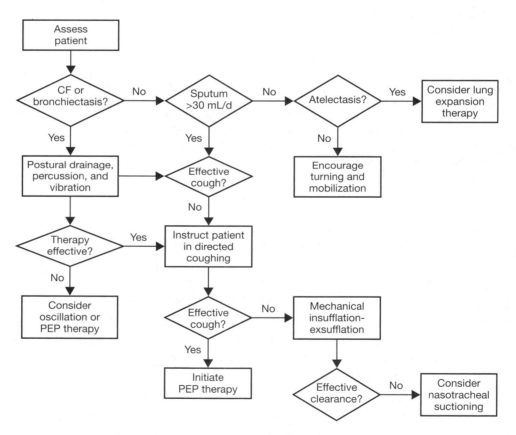

Figure 9-1 Example Algorithm for Bronchial Hygiene Therapy. CF = cystic fibrosis; PEP = positive expiratory pressure.

Adapted from: Burton GG, Hodgkin JE, Ward J. *Respiratory care: a guide to clinical practice* (4th ed.). Philadelphia: J. B. Lippincott; 1997.

Table 9-2 Contraindications, Hazards, and Complications of Postural Drainage, Percussion, and Vibration

Contraindications	Hazards and Complications
• Intracranial pressure (ICP) > 20 mm Hg	• Hypoxemia
• Head and neck injury until stabilized	• Increased ICP
• Active hemorrhage with hemodynamic instability	• Acute hypotension
• Recent spinal surgery	• Pulmonary hemorrhage
• Active hemoptysis	• Pain or injury to muscles, ribs, or spine
• Empyema or large pleural effusion	• Vomiting and aspiration
• Bronchopleural fistula	• Bronchospasm
• Pulmonary edema	• Dysrhythmias
• Pulmonary embolism	
• Rib fracture	
• Uncontrolled airway at risk for aspiration	

Figure 9-2 depicts the positions commonly used during PDPV, which align the affected area in the "up" position. With such positioning, gravity can help move secretions toward the large airways for removal. For example, to drain the posterior segment of the lower lobes, you would place the patient in the prone position with the foot of the bed raised by 18 inches.

To aid in secretion clearance, percussion and vibration are applied to the affected area. With percussion, cupped hands are used to deliver rapid, repetitive thumps to the chest wall over the targeted segment(s). As described subsequently, you also can use mechanical devices such as pneumatic or electrical percussors. However, there is little evidence that these devices are more effective than manual percussion. For this reason, your selection of percussion method should be guided by patient preference, convenience, and availability.

Vibration involves rapid shaking motion performed against the chest wall over the affected area *during expiration*. It may be performed manually or with a mechanical device. In combination with percussion and other secretion-clearance aids, vibration can help loosen the patient's secretions, particularly if they are copious and thick.

Instead of intermittent application of PDPV, some critical care units use turning and rotation protocols to help prevent retained secretions. This procedure involves rotating the patient's body around its longitudinal axis. Turning can be done manually (with pillows or a foam wedge) or using a specially equipped bed.

To assess the effectiveness of PDPV, you should monitor several indicators. Changes in the chest x-rays and vital signs, including SpO_2, can all be monitored noninvasively. Sputum production and auscultation also provide a good gauge to determine effectiveness. In general, when the sputum production drops below 30 mL/day and the patient can generate an effective spontaneous cough, PDPV is no longer indicated and should be discontinued.

Provide Instruction in and Encourage Bronchopulmonary Hygiene Techniques

PDPV simply moves secretions into the patient's large airways. From there, secretions normally are cleared by spontaneous coughing. Because not all patients can cough effectively, they may need coaching. If patients cannot cough effectively, artificial removal techniques (i.e., suctioning or mechanical exsufflation) may be required.

Directed Cough and Related Methods

Cough-related training techniques that the NBRC expects you to be familiar with include directed coughing, the forced expiratory technique, the abdominal thrust maneuver, and autogenic drainage.

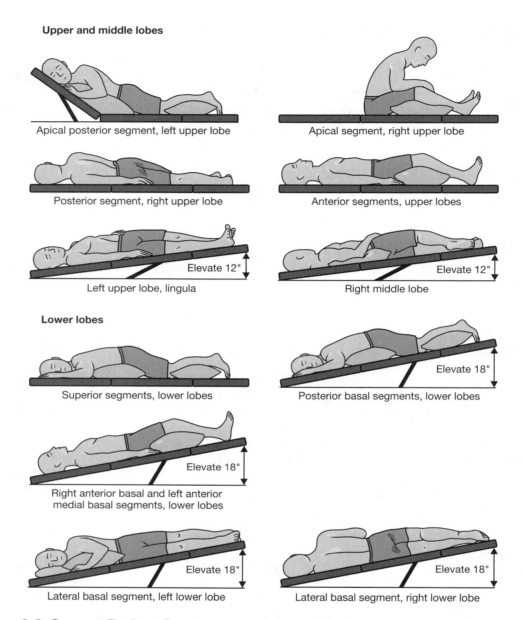

Upper and middle lobes

Apical posterior segment, left upper lobe

Apical segment, right upper lobe

Posterior segment, right upper lobe

Anterior segments, upper lobes

Left upper lobe, lingula — Elevate 12"

Right middle lobe — Elevate 12"

Lower lobes

Superior segments, lower lobes

Posterior basal segments, lower lobes — Elevate 18"

Right anterior basal and left anterior medial basal segments, lower lobes — Elevate 18"

Lateral basal segment, left lower lobe — Elevate 18"

Lateral basal segment, right lower lobe — Elevate 18"

Figure 9-2 Correct Patient Positions for Postural Drainage.

Source: Potter PA, Perry AG. Patient positions for postural drainage. In Kozier BJ, Erb G, Berman AJ, Snyder S. *Fundamentals of nursing: concepts, process and practice* (4th ed.). St. Louis: Mosby; 1997. Courtesy of Elsevier Ltd.

A normal cough has three phases: (1) deep inspiration, (2) compression against a closed glottis, and (3) explosive exhalation. Often patients have trouble with one or more of these phases. Due to pain, many postoperative patients have trouble with both the inspiratory and expiratory phases. Obviously coordinating coughing sessions with pain medication can help these patients cough more effectively, as can splinting the incision site with a pillow or using modified cough techniques. Patients with neuromuscular disorders also may have trouble generating both a deep inspiration and a forceful exhalation. In these cases, the deep inspiration can be provided by manual bag-mask/mouthpiece inflation, with the expiratory component facilitated using either an abdominal thrust or manual chest compression (a "quad cough"). Alternatively, mechanical insufflation–exsufflation can be used with these patients (discussed later in this chapter).

The *forced expiratory technique* (FET) or "huff cough" is an alternative to the explosive exhalation normally created by compression of air against a closed glottis. The FET method consists of two or three forced exhalations, or huffs, *with the glottis open*, followed by a rest period. This process is repeated until the secretions have been mobilized and cleared. The FET is best suited for postoperative patients for whom explosive exhalation is very painful, and patients with COPD who are prone to airway closure during regular coughing.

The *abdominal thrust* maneuver augments expiratory flow by quick application of pressure to the upper abdomen in synchrony with the patient's own cough effort. The motion should be upward toward the epigastrium, not the belly. This technique is contraindicated in pregnant women, patients with abdominal trauma or surgical incisions, and those with acute abdominal pathology. In these cases, the pressure can be applied to the lateral costal margins instead of the abdomen. However, this alternative approach is contraindicated for patients with osteoporosis or flail chest.

Autogenic drainage is usually combined with directed coughing. This procedure consists of three phases. In phase 1, the goal is to loosen mucus by having the patient taking a breath to TLC. During phase 2, the patient breathes at a low volume to allow mucus to build in the airways. During the third and final phase, the patient "stacks" three breaths on top of each other, followed by a cough. To maximize its benefits, autogenic drainage should be performed in a sitting position. In addition, patients should be taught to control their expiratory flows to prevent airway collapse. Although this procedure may be as effective as PDPV, it can be difficult for some patients to learn and apply.

The accompanying box outlines the key elements involved in directed coughing, including incorporation of the FET and abdominal thrust maneuver, as needed.

Key Elements in the Directed Coughing and Related Procedures

- Assess patient.
- Explain and/or demonstrate procedure and confirm patient understanding.
- Position patient in semi-Fowler's position (or side-lying position) with knees bent.
- Instruct patient in effective use of diaphragm and demonstrate cough phases.
- Demonstrate how to splint incision (postoperative patients).
- Encourage deep inspiration, inspiratory hold, and forceful exhalation.
- Observe, correct common errors, and reinstruct as needed.
- Modify technique as appropriate:
  - Forced expiratory technique
  - Abdominal thrust
  - Autogenic drainage
  - Manually assisted bag-valve inspiration
- Reassess patient and repeat procedure as indicated and tolerated.
- Collect and examine sputum.
- Return patient to a comfortable position.
- Document outcomes.

Mechanical Devices to Facilitate Secretion Clearance

Several mechanical devices may be used to aid clearance of secretions, all of which can appear on NBRC exams. Note that irrespective of the device used, effective secretion clearance still requires rigorous implementation of bronchial hygiene therapy, including directed coughing.

Handheld Percussors and Vibrators

Handheld mechanical percussors and vibrators are used to aid secretion clearance in children and adults (for infants, use small percussion cups or a percussion "wand"). You adjust the force to achieve the desired impact, using the higher frequencies (20–30 Hz) for vibration. As compared to manual "clapping," these devices deliver consistent rates and impact force and do not cause user fatigue. They also are useful when home caregivers cannot perform manual percussion. However, these devices are no more effective than manual methods for facilitating secretion clearance.

High-Frequency Chest Wall Oscillation/Compression (RRT-Specific Content)

High-frequency chest wall oscillation or compression systems consist of an inflatable vest and an air-pulse generator that produces rapid positive-pressure bursts. You can adjust both the pulse strength and frequency, typically from 5–20 Hz. These systems are used primarily on patients with chronic conditions causing retained secretions, such as cystic fibrosis. They are particularly useful for home care patients who do not have caregiver support.

To assemble and use a chest wall oscillation system:

1. Select the appropriate-size vest and fit it snuggly to the patient during a deep inhalation.
2. Connect the air hoses to the air-pulse generator and vest.
3. Select the mode, frequency, pressure, and treatment time and activate the unit (a remote control is available for independent patient use).

If a vest system fails to oscillate, make sure that the remote control is on; if oscillation is inadequate after adjustment, check all tubing connections and the vest's fit.

Mechanical compressions also can be applied *internally* via a technique called intrapulmonary percussive ventilation (IPV). IPV treatment is similar to intermittent positive-pressure breathing (IPPB) therapy, except that high-frequency (100–300/min) percussive bursts of gas are provided during breathing. Percussion is manually activated via a button and adjusted to ensure visible/palpable chest wall vibrations. Typically, saline solution (normal or hypertonic) is aerosolized during the IPV procedure, with the device requiring a fill volume of 20 mL. As with vest systems, patients can use IPV independently, and the treatment has the added benefit of providing aerosolized drug delivery. If an IPV device fails to properly function, make sure that there is an adequate source of gas pressure and that all connections are leak free.

Positive Expiratory Pressure Devices

Positive expiratory pressure (PEP) therapy is another method used to aid secretion clearance. PEP therapy also can be used to help prevent or treat atelectasis and to reduce air trapping in asthma and COPD. When used in conjunction with a nebulizer, some PEP devices can facilitate bronchodilator administration as well.

PEP therapy should not be used on patients who cannot tolerate any increased work of breathing, are hemodynamically unstable, or suffer from bullous emphysema, high intracranial pressure, untreated pneumothorax, sinusitis, epistaxis, or middle ear problems.

There are three types of PEP devices, summarized in **Table 9-3**. All of these devices typically generate between 6 to 25 cm H_2O pressure during exhalation and allow unrestricted inspiration. **Figure 9-3** depicts the two most common vibratory PEP devices, the Flutter valve and Acapella.

Because PEP therapy is no more effective than other methods of bronchial hygiene, you should select the approach that best meets the patient's needs and preferences. Because some PEP devices are flow sensitive, selection may also need to take into account the patient's flow capabilities. *If the goal is to help mobilize retained secretions, then a vibratory PEP device probably is the best choice.* If concurrent aerosol therapy is indicated, all devices except the Flutter valve and Threshold PEP device provide adaptors for attaching a nebulizer.

Key considerations in applying PEP therapy include the following:

1. The patient should sit upright or in a semi-Fowler's position, with the abdomen unrestricted.
2. Initially set PEP to its lowest level, as per manufacturer's recommendations (e.g., the largest orifice, the lowest spring tension or flow).

Table 9-3 Positive Expiratory Pressure Devices

Type of PEP Device	Mechanism to Generate PEP	Example
Flow resistor	Patient exhales against a fixed orifice (size is based on patient age and expiratory flow)	TheraPEP system
Threshold resistor	Patient exhales against an adjustable counterweight, spring-loaded valve, or reverse Venturi	EZPap[a] Threshold PEP device
Vibratory PEP	Patient exhales against a threshold resistor with an expiratory valve oscillating at 10–30 Hz	Flutter valve Quake[b] Acapella

[a] The EZPap device also provides positive pressure on inspiration.
[b] Pressure oscillations with the Quake device are generated by rotating a crank that opens and closes the expiratory orifice.

3. Slowly increase the PEP to between 10 to 20 cm H_2O as per manufacturer's recommendations (e.g., a smaller orifice, increased spring tension or flow, higher device angle [for the Flutter valve]).
4. With vibratory PEP, vibrations should be felt over the central airways during exhalation.

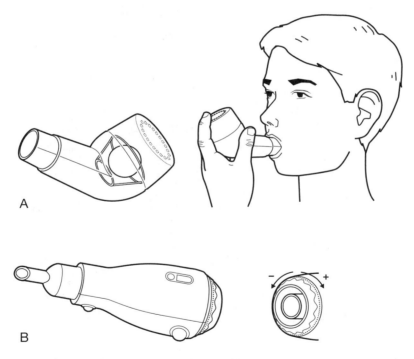

Figure 9-3 The Pipe-Shaped Flutter Valve and Acapella Device. (A) The pipe-shaped Flutter valve contains a steel ball that sits atop a cone-shaped orifice covered by a perforated cap. When a patient exhales through the mouthpiece, the weight of the ball creates expiratory pressures between 10 and 25 cm H_2O. Due to the angle of orifice, the ball rapidly rises and falls, which creates the pressure oscillations. Flutter valve PEP levels increase when the device is raised above horizontal and with higher expiratory flows. (B) The Acapella device uses a counterweighted lever and magnet to produce PEP and airflow oscillations. As exhaled gases pass through the device, flow is intermittently blocked by a plug attached to the lever, producing the vibratory oscillations. PEP levels are adjusted using a knob located at the distal end of the device. To increase PEP, you turn this knob clockwise.

5. Have the patient perform sets of 10–20 slow, moderately deep inspirations with short breath holds followed by active (but *not* forced) exhalations (I:E ratio = 1:3 to 1:4).

6. After each cycle of 10–20 breaths, assist the patient with the appropriate directed coughing technique/bronchial hygiene therapy.

7. Repeat the cycle four to eight times, not to exceed a total session time of 20 minutes.

If a PEP device fails to generate pressure, the most likely problem is a leak, which is easily corrected by tightening all connections. Unexpectedly high pressures also can occur in these devices if the outlet port is obstructed—for example, by the patient's hand or bedding. To overcome this problem, make sure the outlet port remains open.

Home care patients should be taught to properly maintain their PEP device according to the manufacturer's recommendations. Most PEP devices can be cleaned in warm, soapy water, followed by a good rinse and complete air drying.

Mechanical Insufflation–Exsufflation

Mechanical insufflation–exsufflation (MI-E), also known as cough assist, involves application of alternating positive and negative pressure to the airway to help increase expiratory flows and remove secretions. **Figure 9-4** depicts the device used for MI-E. MI-E is indicated for patients with weak cough effort (expiratory pressures less than 60 cm H_2O), such as those with neuromuscular conditions causing respiratory muscle weakness. Contraindications include a history of bullous emphysema, susceptibility to pneumothorax, and recent barotrauma.

MI-E can be applied to spontaneously breathing patients via a mask or mouthpiece and via a standard 15-mm adaptor for those patients with tracheal airways. The inspiratory and expiratory time and pressure can be manually adjusted or preset for models with auto mode. Key elements in the procedure are summarized in the following box.

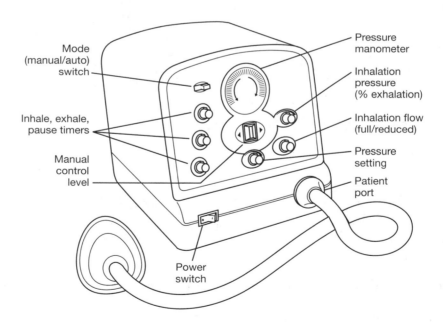

Figure 9-4 Cough-Assist or Mechanical Insufflation–Exsufflation Device. The mask and large-bore tubing attach to the patient port. The power switch turns the unit on and off. The mode switch toggles between automatic and manual modes. The pressure setting varies the inhalation and exhalation pressures together, while the inhalation pressure knob adjusts this value to a percentage of the exhalation pressure. Inhalation flow can be switched between full and reduced. Three timers allow adjustment of the inhalation, exhalation, and pause time. A pressure manometer calibrated in cm H_2O displays the pressure changes.

Key Elements in the Mechanical Insufflation–Exsufflation Procedure

- Test equipment by turning it on, occluding the circuit, and toggling between inhalation and exhalation.

- Adjust initial inhalation/exhalation pressures to between 10 and 15 cm H_2O.

- Connect circuit interface to patient's airway.

- Set inhalation pressure between 15 and 40 cm H_2O and exhalation pressure between 35 and 45 cm H_2O (the lowest effective pressures should be used).

- Administer 4–6 cycles of insufflation and exsufflation.

- Remove visible secretions from airway or tubing.

- Reassess patient.

- Return patient to prescribed support therapy.

- Document outcomes.

Clearance of Secretions via Suctioning

If directed coughing techniques and the use of adjunct devices prove ineffective, you may need to consider suctioning. Suctioning is used as needed on all patients with artificial tracheal airways. In addition, patients with certain neuromuscular disorders or those with conditions that increase the volume or viscosity of secretions may require suctioning.

Chapter 4 provides details on the selection, use, and troubleshooting of suctioning equipment, including both vacuum systems and suction apparatus. Here we focus on the procedures used to remove retained secretions.

Several clinical clues indicate the need for suctioning:

- Presence of a weak, loose cough
- Auscultation revealing rhonchi
- Direct observation of secretions in the mouth or oropharynx
- Tactile fremitus (vibrations felt on the chest wall)
- Patient feedback suggesting retained secretions

For patients receiving mechanical ventilation, an increase in peak pressure (volume control ventilation) or a decrease in delivered volume (pressure control ventilation) may indicate the presence of secretions. Less specific indications for excessive secretions include deterioration in Spo_2 or arterial blood gases and a chest x-ray indicating atelectasis.

Suctioning can be dangerous. Potential hazards and complications associated with the various suctioning methods include oxygen desaturation/hypoxemia, tissue trauma/bleeding, bronchospasm, cardiac dysrhythmias, hypertension or hypotension, cardiac or respiratory arrest, increased ICP, and infection. Careful implementation of safety measures before, during, and after the procedure, as well as careful monitoring throughout, can minimize these potential risks. In most cases, the danger associated with *not* clearing retained secretions far outweighs these potential hazards.

Oropharyngeal Suctioning

Oropharyngeal suctioning involves the removal of secretions, vomit, or food particles from the oral cavity and pharynx. For this reason, you normally use a rigid catheter with a larger-diameter lumen, such as a Yankauer suction tip (**Figure 9-5**). With a Yankauer tip, you can reach the back of the oropharyngeal cavity and remove both secretions and particulate matter.

Suctioning via a Tracheal Airway

Two general methods are used for suctioning of patients with tracheal airways: open suctioning and closed ("in-line") suctioning. Open suctioning is performed using a suction kit and sterile technique; it requires disconnecting the patient from supporting equipment. Closed suctioning employs

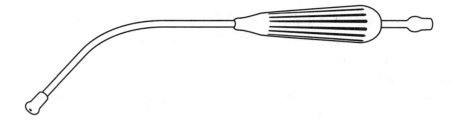

Figure 9-5 Yankauer Suction Tip.

a closed in-line catheter system; it requires neither sterile technique nor disconnecting the patient from support. The accompanying box outlines the essential elements common to these methods.

Key Elements in the Tracheal Suctioning Procedure

- Perform suctioning only when indicated, *not* routinely.
- Decontaminate hands and apply standard/transmission-based precautions.
- Assess patient oxygenation continuously via Sp_{O_2}.
- Preoxygenate and postoxygenate patients with 100% O_2 (10% above baseline for neonates) for at least 30–60 seconds.
- Use an inline/closed-suction system on patients receiving ventilatory support.
- Select a catheter that occludes less than 50% of the ET tube internal diameter (less than 70% in infants).
- Maintain sterile technique with open suctioning; maintain asepsis with the inline/closed technique.
- Use the lowest vacuum pressure needed to evacuate secretions.
- Limit the duration of suctioning to less than 15 seconds.
- Use shallow suctioning (insert the catheter just beyond the tube tip—about 2 cm in adults).
- Do *not* routinely lavage the patient with saline (its use is controversial)
- Immediately terminate the procedure if a serious adverse event is observed.
- Restore patient to prior status.
- Assess and document outcomes.

Adapted from: Scanlan CL, West GA, von der Heydt PA, Dolan GK. *Respiratory therapy competency evaluation manual.* Boston: Blackwell Scientific; 1984.

When setting vacuum pressure, you should select the lowest level needed to effectively remove the secretions. For centrally piped vacuum systems, the recommended starting range for adults is between –100 and –120 mm Hg; the initial range for children is –80 to –100 mm Hg. Negative pressure applied to the infant airway generally should be limited to –60 to –80 mm Hg.

To ensure that there is adequate space for gas to flow around the catheter and prevent atelectasis, always select a suction catheter that occludes less than 50% of the ET tube internal diameter (ID) (less than 70% in infants). **Table 9-4** provides general guidelines for selecting suction catheters with tracheal tubes in the 2.5- to 9.5-mm ID range.

Table 9-4 Guidelines for Selection of Suction Catheter Size

Tracheal Tube (ID mm)	Suction Catheter (OD French)
2.5–3.0	5
3.0–4.0	6
4.0	6
4.5	8
5.0	8
5.5	10
6.0	10
6.5	12
7.0	12
8.0	14
8.5	16
9.0	16
> 9.0	16
8.5–9.5	16

Alternatively, you can quickly estimate correct catheter size in French units (Fr) by doubling the internal diameter of the tracheal tube and selecting the next smallest catheter size. For example, to suction a patient with a 6.0-mm tracheal tube:

2 × 6 = 12
Next smallest catheter size = 10 Fr

Figure 9-6 depicts the key components of an inline closed-suction system for use on ventilator patients (a separate model is available for spontaneously breathing patients with trach tubes). Key points to help ensure effectiveness and safety when using this device include the following:

- Select the correct type of catheter (systems for trach patients have shorter catheters).
- Always set the pressure on the suction regulator with the thumb valve fully depressed.

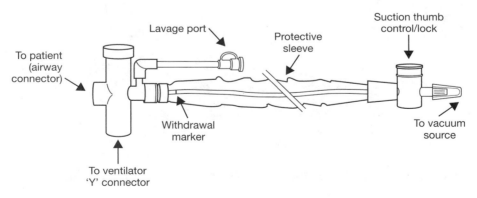

Figure 9-6 Closed-Suction System.

Courtesy of: Strategic Learning Associates, LLC, Little Silver, New Jersey.

- Apply closed suctioning to patients receiving ventilatory support only with a mode that either (1) provides continuous circuit flow or (2) will trigger and provide flow during suctioning.
- Stabilize the airway when suctioning by keeping a firm hold on the T-piece.
- To avoid bunching of the sleeve from limited insertion depth, advance the catheter from, at, or near the airway connection in increments of approximately 2 inches.
- Always fully withdraw the catheter when finished (indicated by visualizing the black marking ring); if the catheter is not fully withdrawn, airway pressure and work of breathing may increase.
- Be careful not to withdraw the catheter too far (can allow gas from the ventilator to enter the sleeve).
- Always lock the thumb valve in the off position when finished; otherwise, accidental suction may be applied.
- To clear the catheter after withdrawal, instill at least 5 mL of saline through the lavage port while applying continuous suctioning; always cap the lavage port after use.
- Change the system as per the manufacturer's recommendations or institutional protocol; daily changes do not decrease the risk of ventilator-associated pneumonia (VAP).

A common problem in intubated patients is leakage of subglottic secretions past the tracheal tube cuff. These secretions can contaminate the lower respiratory tract and are thought to contribute to development of VAP. For this reason, many VAP protocols call for continuous aspiration of subglottic secretions (CASS). As depicted in **Figure 9-7**, this is accomplished using specially designed tracheal tubes that incorporate a suction port just above the cuff. You connect this port via a suction line to a standard wall vacuum unit and set it to apply continuous low suction, normally 20 mm Hg. To avoid any confusion over the various connecting lines (e.g., cuff inflation line, feeding lines), you should clearly label the CASS suction port.

Nasotracheal Suctioning

Nasotracheal suctioning is the method most commonly used to clear secretions in patients who do not have artificial airways and cannot cough effectively. In general, this method should be considered only when other efforts to remove secretions have failed. Contraindications to nasotracheal

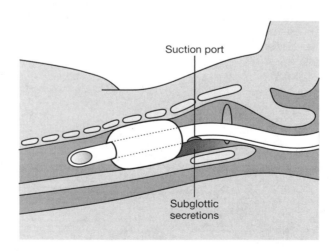

Figure 9-7 Endotracheal Tube Designed for Continuous Aspiration of Subglottic Secretions.

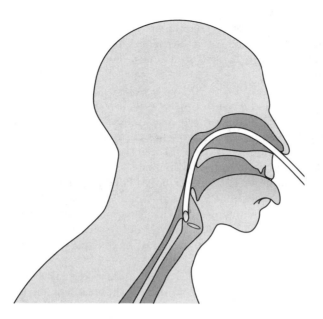

Figure 9-8 Patient Positioning for Insertion of a Nasotracheal Suction Catheter.

suctioning include occluded nasal passages; nasal bleeding; epiglottitis or croup (both absolute contraindications!); upper respiratory tract infections; nasal, oral, or tracheal injury or surgery; a coagulopathy or bleeding disorder; and laryngospasm or bronchospasm.

With a few exceptions, nasotracheal suctioning is similar to open tracheal suctioning. To minimize the risk of spreading nasopharyngeal bacteria into the lungs, many protocols specify that patients should blow their noses and rinse their mouths and throats with an antiseptic mouthwash prior to the procedure. To avoid airway trauma, lubricate the catheter with a sterile, water-soluble jelly before insertion. If frequent suctioning is required, you can minimize trauma by using a nasopharyngeal airway. In this case, lubricate the catheter with sterile water, not water-soluble jelly.

To increase the likelihood of the catheter entering the trachea, have the patient assume a modified sniffing position (**Figure 9-8)**, with the neck slightly hyperextended and the tongue displaced forward. If the patient cannot displace the tongue, you can manually pull it forward using a gauze pad. You should then advance the catheter slowly during inspiration (to ensure abduction of the vocal cords). In most patients, vigorous coughing confirms that you have passed through vocal cords and are in the trachea.

Assessment

The effectiveness of suctioning can be assessed by the amount of secretions removed, as well as by changes in breath sounds, vital signs, and oxygenation. For a patient being mechanically ventilated in the volume-control mode, removal of retained secretions usually reduces peak airway pressures, whereas patients receiving pressure-control ventilation may experience an increase in delivered volume. Ultimately, the benefits of bronchial hygiene, including suctioning, may be seen in improved aeration on the chest x-ray and an overall improvement in clinical status.

Administer Aerosol Therapy with Prescribed Medications

Bland Aerosols

Bland aerosol administration (water or normal saline) is indicated for spontaneously breathing patients with bypassed upper airways and those patients needing assistance in mobilizing secretions. For these situations, the aerosol frequently is heated. However, when used to treat upper airway edema such as that caused by laryngotracheobronchitis or to manage post-extubation swelling, bland aerosols are delivered unheated (actually below room temperature due to evaporative cooling). Hypertonic saline or high-density ultrasonic water aerosols may be used to promote secretion clearance for sputum induction.

Due to its potential to cause bronchoconstriction in some patients, bland aerosol therapy is contraindicated in those individuals with a history of airway hyperresponsiveness. Other potential hazards of bland aerosol therapy include infection, caregiver exposure to contagious microorganisms, overhydration, and airway edema or bronchoconstriction.

Details on the specific equipment used for bland aerosol therapy are given in Chapter 4. To provide continuous bland aerosol therapy for patients whose upper airways have been bypassed, you generally use a heated large-volume jet nebulizer filled with sterile water (note that this method is neither as effective nor—due to infection risk—as safe as using a heated humidifier). For upper airway edema, an *unheated* large-volume nebulizer is applied until clinical evidence of edema has subsided. If the goal is to induce coughing and obtain a sputum sample, consider either jet nebulization of a hypertonic saline solution (typically 5%) or delivery of a high-density ultrasonic water aerosol.

Assessment of patients receiving bland aerosol therapy depends on both the rationale for its administration and the stability and severity of the condition being treated. Parameters to monitor typically include the following:

- Patient comfort and presence/absence of dyspnea
- Breath sounds and tactile fremitus
- Respiratory rate and pattern
- Skin color and pulse O_2 saturation
- Sputum quantity, color, and consistency

Administration of Prescribed Agents

Administration of aerosolized medications is covered in detail in Chapter 10. In this section of the NBRC exams, the focus is primarily on the use of inhaled drugs to facilitate removal of bronchopulmonary secretions. The drugs commonly used to mobilize and remove secretions are classified into the following categories: bronchodilators, steroids, mucolytics, and diluting agents. These agents and their roles in bronchial hygiene are summarized in **Table 9-5**.

Bronchodilators such as albuterol dilate the airways, which when coupled with the thinning action of mucolytics may aid secretion clearance. The most commonly used mucokinetic agents are acetylcysteine (Mucomyst) and dornase alpha (Pulmozyme). These agents are often used in patients with conditions such as cystic fibrosis or those with abnormally thick secretions not easily managed

Table 9-5 Selected Aerosol Agents Used to Facilitate Secretion Clearance

Agent	Classification	Example Agent	Role in Bronchial Hygiene
Bronchodilators	Beta agonists	Albuterol	Dilates airways
	Parasympatholytics	Ipratropium bromide	Dilates airways
Steroids	Corticosteroids	Fluticisone	Anti-inflammatory action helps maintain airway patency and reduce mucus production
Mucokinetics	Mucolytics	Acetylcysteine Dornase alpha	Thins mucus (Note: acetylcysteine can cause bronchospasm and typically should administered in combination with a bronchodilator)
Diluting agents	Expectorants	Hypertonic saline	Dilutes mucus by drawing fluid into the airway

with bland aerosol therapy. Two other types of aerosolized agents that may be helpful in secretion removal are corticosteroids and diluting agents such as hypertonic saline. By reducing airway inflammation, inhaled steroids help maintain airway patency and may reduce secretions production. Diluting agents such as aerosolized saline work by thinning secretions.

When combinations of these agents are used to aid secretions clearance, they are typically administered in the following sequence: (1) open the airways with a bronchodilator, (2) clear the secretions with a mucolytic or diluting agent (combined with directed coughing), and then (3) decrease further inflammation with an inhaled steroid.

COMMON ERRORS TO AVOID

You can improve your score by avoiding these mistakes:

- Avoid performing head-down postural drainage positions in patients with high intracranial pressures (more than 15–20 mm Hg), unstable head/neck injury, active hemorrhage, or hemodynamic instability.
- Avoid performing percussion and vibration therapy immediately before or after meals.
- Do not apply abdominal thrusts to patients with abdominal trauma or surgical incisions or to pregnant women.
- Avoid using PEP therapy devices on patients with acute exacerbations of asthma or COPD, or on any patient who cannot tolerate added work of breathing.
- Never perform endotracheal suctioning "routinely" (e.g., every hour); instead, suction only when secretions are present.
- Avoid routine instillation of saline into the airway prior to endotracheal suctioning.
- Do not use excessive suction pressures on patients. In general, suction pressures should never exceed –120 mm Hg for adults, –100 mm Hg for children, and –80 mm Hg for infants.
- Avoid applying suction to the airway for more than 15 seconds for each attempt.

SURE BETS

In some situations, you can be sure of the right approach to a clinical problem or scenario:

- Always monitor a patient before, during, and immediately following bronchial hygiene therapy, including the patient's overall appearance, vital signs, breath sounds, and SpO_2.
- If an adverse reaction occurs during therapy, always stop the treatment, stay with and monitor the patient, and notify the nurse and physician.
- Always splint surgical incision sites with a pillow to help patients generate a more effective cough.
- Always remember that patients with a weak cough, rhonchi, or fremitus (vibrations) on the chest wall may need bronchial hygiene therapy.
- Always preoxygenate a patient with an F_{IO_2} of 100% (10% above the baseline F_{IO_2} in neonates) for at least 30–60 seconds before each suction attempt and monitor oxygenation via pulse oximetry.
- Always give preference to the inline closed-suctioning technique in patients receiving continuous mechanical ventilation, especially those requiring high F_{IO_2}s and PEEP.
- Always consider recommending the addition of bland aerosol and the administration of bronchodilators and mucolytics if percussion, vibration, PEP therapy, and cough assistance alone are not effective.
- Always remember that the effectiveness of bronchial hygiene therapy can be assessed through an improvement in breath sounds, vital signs, oxygenation, and overall appearance.

PRE-TEST ANSWERS AND EXPLANATIONS

Following are this chapter's pre-test answers and explanations. Be sure to review each answer's explanation thoroughly to help you understand why it is correct. If the explanation is still unclear to you, review the chapter content.

9-1. Correct answer: C. 1 and 4 only. To drain the posterior basal segments, place the patient in the prone Trendelenburg position (30° downward tilt), with a pillow under the hips.

9-2. Correct answer: D. Low inspiratory volumes. The effectiveness of a cough requires proper integration of three phases: the inspiratory component, the compression phase, and the explosive exhalation. Strong abdominal muscles to generate large volumes with glottis closure will generate a good cough.

9-3. Correct answer: B. 1, 2, and 3. When applying nasotracheal suctioning, the patient should be both preoxygenated and postoxygenated, and the suction catheter should be prelubricated. As with tracheal suctioning in general, the time for applying suction should not exceed 15 seconds.

9-4. Correct answer: C. Acetylcysteine (Mucomyst). Acetylcysteine breaks the disulfide bonds in mucus, thereby helping thin and mobilize secretions in patients with mucus plugs.

9-5. Correct answer: B. Exhale forcefully and maintain expiratory pressure of at least 20 cm H_2O. Patients performing PEP therapy should sit comfortably. After taking in a moderately deep breath, they should exhale actively, *but not forcefully*, to create a positive pressure of 10-20 cm H_2O. Ideally, expiration should be 3 to 4 times longer than inspiration. The maneuver should be performed for 10–20 breaths, then followed by the appropriate coughing technique and rest as needed. The cycle should be repeated four to eight times, not to exceed 20 minutes.

9-6. Correct answer: A. Combining mechanical insufflation-exsufflation with suctioning. In patients who cannot generate an effective cough due to muscle weakness, mechanical insufflation/exsufflation is a good airway clearance option. In this technique, the device provides a positive pressure breath, followed immediately by application of negative airway pressure. This can help increase the volume and velocity of expired air, and may help move secretions toward the trachea, where they can be suctioned out.

9-7. Correct answer: A. Postural drainage, percussion, and vibration. Of the choices available, the bronchial hygiene technique most suitable for small infants is postural drainage, percussion, and vibration. Positive expiratory pressure, high-frequency oscillation, and aggressive suctioning would be potentially harmful.

9-8. Correct answer: D. Suction at a pressure range of –60 to –80 mm Hg, limiting the time to less than 15 seconds. The normal pressure range for adults is –100 to –120 mm Hg, for children –80 to –100 mm Hg, and for infants –60 to –80 mm Hg. The patient should be preoxygenated with 100% oxygen for at least 30–60 seconds, and the total suction time should be limited to no more than 15 seconds on each attempt.

9-9. Correct answer: D. 2, 3, and 4. Major hazards and complications of postural drainage, percussion, and vibration include hypoxemia; acute hypotension during the procedure; pulmonary hemorrhage; pain or injury to muscles, ribs, or spine; vomiting and aspiration; bronchospasm; and dysrhythmias.

9-10. **Correct answer: B.** Use of a tracheal tube with a suction port above the cuff. A common problem in intubated patients is leakage of subglottic secretions past the tracheal tube cuff, which can contaminate the lower respiratory tract and contribute to the development of VAP.

POST-TEST

To confirm your mastery of this chapter's topical content, you should take the chapter post-test, available online at http://go.jblearning.com/respexamreview. A score of 80% or more indicates that you are adequately prepared for this section of the NBRC written exams. If you score less than 80%, you should continue to review the applicable chapter content. In addition, you may want to access and review the relevant Web links covering this chapter's content (courtesy of RTBoardReview. com), also online at the Jones & Bartlett Learning site.

Achieve Adequate Respiratory Support

CHAPTER 10

Craig Scanlan and Al Heuer

Achieving adequate respiratory support is one of many critical roles performed by respiratory therapists (RTs). This chapter includes important NBRC exam content related to specialized ventilator strategies, including high-frequency ventilation, disease-specific protocols, and newer modes of mechanical ventilation such as airway pressure-release ventilation (APRV), as well as new inhaled drugs.

OBJECTIVES

In preparing for the shared NBRC exam content, you should demonstrate the knowledge needed to:

1. Instruct a patient in deep breathing, incentive spirometry, and inspiratory muscle training
2. Initiate and adjust:
   a. IPPB therapy
   b. Conventional and high-frequency mechanical ventilation
   c. Noninvasive ventilation
   d. Elevated baseline pressure (e.g., CPAP, PEEP)
3. Select ventilator graphics (e.g., waveforms, scales)
4. Apply disease-specific ventilator protocols
5. Initiate and modify weaning procedures
6. Administer drugs via inhalation *(liquid aerosol and dry powder)* and endotracheal instillation
7. Administer oxygen
8. Position patients to minimize hypoxemia
9. Prevent procedure-associated hypoxemia

WHAT TO EXPECT ON THIS CATEGORY OF THE NBRC EXAMS

CRT exam: 8 questions, about 25% recall, 60% application, and 15% analysis
WRRT exam: 5 questions; 100% analysis
CSE exam: Indeterminate number of questions; however, exam III-D knowledge is a prerequisite to success on both CSE Information Gathering and Decision-Making sections

PRE-TEST

Carefully respond to each of the following questions. After completing the pre-test, compare your answers to those provided at the end of this chapter. Then thoroughly review each answer's explanation to help understand why it is correct.

10-1. While suctioning a patient receiving ventilatory support, you note the heart rate increases abruptly from 92–145 beats per minute. Which of the following actions is appropriate?

A. Recommend an IV dose of atropine before suctioning

B. Instill lidocaine (Xylocaine) into the trachea before suctioning

C. Increase the oxygen concentration immediately before suctioning

D. Give the patient two MDI puffs of beclomethasone before suctioning

10-2. A patient with ARDS is receiving ventilatory support with 100% oxygen and 25 cm H_2O PEEP at the recommended high limit of the protocol (Pplat > 30 cm H_2O, V_T = 4 mL/kg) but remains dangerously hypoxemic. Which of the following should you recommend?
A. Increase the mandatory rate
B. Put the patient in the prone position
C. Administer a paralytic agent
D. Increase the pressure limit

10-3. Which of the following is the appropriate load to establish for patients receiving inspiratory muscle training?
A. At least 33% of the predicted inspiratory capacity (IC)
B. At least 10–15 mL/kg of predicted body weight (PBW)
C. At least 30% of the maximum inspiratory pressure (MIP/PI_{max})
D. At least –25 cm H_2O, as measured by a calibrated manometer

10-4. To obtain the most effective ventilation, a patient with severe emphysema should be instructed to:
A. Inhale slowly
B. Exhale slowly
C. Hold every third breath
D. Breathe as deeply as possible

10-5. For which of the following patients would you carefully monitor cardiovascular function during application of intermittent positive-pressure breathing (IPPB)?
1. A patient with low blood pressure
2. A patient with poor vasomotor tone
3. A patient with cardiac insufficiency
A. 1 and 2 only
B. 2 and 3 only
C. 1 and 3 only
D. 1, 2, and 3

10-6. An adult patient in respiratory failure has the following ABGs on a simple O_2 mask at 8 L/min: pH = 7.19; $Paco_2$ = 68 torr; HCO_3 = 28 mEq/L; Pao_2 = 85 torr. The attending physician orders intubation and ventilatory support. Which of the following modes of support are appropriate?

1. Volume control A/C at rate of 12/min
2. Volume control SIMV at rate of 12/min
3. CPAP with 10 cm H_2O pressure
A. 1 or 2 only
B. 2 or 3 only
C. 1 or 3 only
D. 1, 2, or 3

10-7. A physician asks you to decrease the $Paco_2$ of a patient receiving high-frequency oscillation ventilation (HFOV). You should consider all of the following adjustments *except*:
A. Increasing the power/amplitude
B. Decreasing the frequency
C. Deflating the ET tube cuff
D. Decreasing the bias flow

10-8. A patient with congestive heart failure is coughing up large quantities of pink, frothy sputum. ABG values on simple mask O_2 at 7 L/min are as follows:

pH	7.44
$Paco_2$	29 torr
Hco_3	20 mEq/L
BE	–3 mEq/L
Pao_2	46 torr
Sao_2	76%

Which of the following treatments would you recommend?
A. Nonrebreathing mask at 12 L/min and postural drainage therapy
B. Intermittent positive-pressure breathing (IPPB) with compressed air
C. Starting intrapulmonary percussive ventilation to clear secretions
D. Mask continuous positive airway pressure (CPAP) with 80% O_2

10-9. During CPR, an intravenous line cannot be started on the patient. The physician wants to administer nalaxone to counteract a morphine overdose. Which alternative route of administration would you recommend?
A. Nasogastric tube
B. Feeding tube
C. Intraosseous route
D. Endotracheal tube

10-10. Data for a patient being mechanically ventilated are as follows:

Ventilator Settings		Blood Gases	
Mode	Vol Ctrl A/C	pH	7.55
VT	900 mL	$Paco_2$	20 torr
Set rate	10	Hco_3	17 mEq/L
Actual rate	20	Pao_2	125 torr
Fio_2	0.35	Sao_2	99%

Based on this information, you would suggest which of the following?
- **A.** Add 5 cm H_2O PEEP
- **B.** Add deadspace to the ventilator breathing circuit
- **C.** Change to volume control SIMV at a rate of 10/min
- **D.** Lower the Fio_2 to 0.25

10-11. During a patient–ventilator check in the ICU, you observe the following settings and monitored parameters on a 70-kg (154-lb) patient receiving ventilatory support:

Mode	Vol Ctrl SIMV
VT	600 mL
Mandatory rate	10
Total rate	38
PEEP	8 cm H_2O
Minute volume	10 L/min

Which of the following actions would you recommend at this time?
- **A.** Switch to assist/control mode
- **B.** Decrease the mandatory rate
- **C.** Add pressure support
- **D.** Increase the PEEP level

10-12. Data for a 63-kg (140-lb) patient receiving ventilatory support with 10 cm PEEP are as follows:

Ventilator Settings		Blood Gases	
Mode	Vol Ctrl SIMV	pH	7.45
VT	600 mL	$Paco_2$	36 torr
Rate	10	Hco_3	25 mEq/L
Fio_2	0.70	Pao_2	55 torr
PEEP	5 cm H_2O	Sao_2	100%

Which of the following changes should you recommend at this time?
- **A.** Lower the VT
- **B.** Increase the rate
- **C.** Increase PEEP
- **D.** Decrease the Fio_2

10-13. Which of the following best describes the way a patient should perform incentive spirometry?
- **A.** The patient should exhale maximally and hold it for at least 5 seconds
- **B.** The patient should inhale normally and hold it for several seconds
- **C.** The patient should hold a maximum inspiratory capacity (IC) breath for at least 5 seconds
- **D.** The patient should repeat maximum inspiratory and expiratory efforts for 10–15 seconds

10-14. Which of the following ventilator graphics displays would be the best choice to identify the presence of auto-PEEP?
- **A.** Volume versus time display
- **B.** Pressure versus time display
- **C.** Flow versus time display
- **D.** Pressure versus volume display

10-15. You are called to the ER to help in the assessment and care of a patient admitted with severe pulmonary edema. While starting an intravenous line, the physician tells you to give the patient O_2. How should you provide oxygen to this patient?
- **A.** Nonrebreathing mask at 15 L/min
- **B.** Nasal cannula at 6 L/min
- **C.** Simple face mask at 7 L/min
- **D.** 50% air-entrainment mask

10-16. A patient receiving bilevel positive airway pressure for acute respiratory failure has a Pao_2 of 48 torr on 65% O_2 with IPAP = 20 cm H_2O and EPAP = 5 cm H_2O. To raise this patient's Pao_2, which change should you recommend?
- **A.** Increasing the Fio_2 to 0.80
- **B.** Increasing IPAP to 25 cm H_2O
- **C.** Increasing EPAP to 10 cm H_2O
- **D.** Decreasing IPAP to 15 cm H_2O

10-17. You are asked to assess whether a 65-kg (143-lb) patient with a neuromuscular disorder receiving pressure control SIMV is ready for weaning. After obtaining the following data during a bedside spontaneous breathing assessment, what would you recommend next?

Spontaneous VT	250 mL
Minute ventilation	10 L/min
Vital capacity	650 mL
MIP/NIF	–20 cm H_2O

A. Beginning a spontaneous breathing T-piece trial

B. Postponing weaning and reevaluating the patient

C. Beginning weaning using a pressure support protocol

D. Beginning weaning by decreasing the SIMV rate

10-18. A doctor institutes volume control A/C ventilation for an 80-kg (176-lb) patient with ARDS. Which of the following is the maximum pressure you should aim to achieve in this patient?

A. 50 cm H_2O peak pressure

B. 30 cm H_2O plateau pressure

C. 40 cm H_2O peak pressure

D. 50 cm H_2O plateau pressure

10-19. A 95-kg (209-lb) patient receiving mechanical ventilation has the following ventilator settings and arterial blood gas results:

Ventilator Settings		Blood Gases	
Mode	Vol Ctrl SIMV	pH	7.26
VT	750 mL	$Paco_2$	56 torr
Set rate	4	Hco_3	22 mEq/L
Spon rate	0	Pao_2	92 torr
Fio_2	0.55	Sao_2	96%

Which of the following should you recommend?

A. Increasing the inspiratory time

B. Increasing the tidal volume to 800 mL

C. Decreasing the Fio_2 to 0.50

D. Increasing the SIMV rate

10-20. After initiating a spontaneous breathing trial for a patient receiving ventilatory support, you note a 15-torr rise in the $Paco_2$, an increase in the rate of breathing from 20–35, and accessory muscle use. What should you recommend?

A. Continuing the trial and carefully monitoring the patient for an additional 30 minutes

B. Ending the trial and returning the patient to a full ventilatory support mode

C. Adding 10 cm H_2O pressure support and obtaining another ABG to assess the effect

D. Ending the trial and restoring the patient to partial support to exercise the diaphragm

WHAT YOU NEED TO KNOW: ESSENTIAL CONTENT

Instruct Patients in Deep Breathing/Muscle Training

Deep breathing, incentive spirometry, and respiratory muscle training are used to aid in secretion clearance, prevent or treat postoperative atelectasis, and improve aerosol drug delivery as well as improve the efficiency of ventilation and exercise tolerance.

Breathing Exercises

There are two types of inspiratory breathing exercises: diaphragmatic (abdominal) breathing and lateral costal breathing. Both are intended to promote effective use of the diaphragm, with less emphasis on the accessory muscles. As an added benefit, inspiratory breathing exercises can improve the efficiency of ventilation by increasing VT and decreasing the rate of breathing.

Key steps in teaching diaphragmatic breathing include the following:

1. Place the patient in a semi-Fowler's position, with forearms relaxed and knees bent.
2. Position your hand on the patient's upper abdomen, below the xiphoid.

3. Encourage the patient to inhale slowly through the nose and "push out" against your hand.
4. Provide progressive resistance to the abdominal movement until end-inspiration.
5. Repeat this exercise (with rest as needed) until satisfactory movement is achieved.

In teaching patients, you should first demonstrate this technique on yourself, while explaining both the "why" and "how" to the patient. Your goal is to get patients to perform these exercises on their own. In the rehabilitation setting, patients can create the resistance using a small weight (about 5 lb) placed over the upper abdomen and progressively increase the load as their diaphragm becomes stronger.

Lateral costal breathing exercises are a good alternative to the diaphragmatic method, especially for patients who have undergone abdominal surgery. The technique is similar to that used in teaching diaphragmatic breathing, but with the resistance applied by both hands "cupping" the lower rib edges. As you apply increasing resistance during inspiration, you instruct the patient to slowly "breathe around the waist" and push out against your hands.

The expiratory breathing technique is also important, especially for patients with COPD. Exhalation through pursed lips increases "back-pressure" in the airways during exhalation and can help lessen air trapping and prolong expiratory times, thereby decreasing the rate of breathing. In combination, these effects can improve ventilation and may help diminish dyspnea. Patients should aim for an expiratory time that is at least 2–3 times longer than inspiration.

Incentive Spirometry

Incentive spirometry (IS) uses simple disposable indicator devices to help patients perform slow, deep breaths accompanied by a breath hold (a sustained maximal inspiration). This technology is used primarily in the acute care setting for patients at risk for or diagnosed with atelectasis, typically those who have undergone thoracic or abdominal surgery. IS cannot be effectively performed on patients who cannot cooperate or generate an inspiratory capacity that is at least one-third of their predicted values. The primary hazard of IS is discomfort due to pain.

Chapter 4 provides details on the selection, use, and troubleshooting of incentive spirometry equipment. The accompanying box summarizes the key points to keep in mind when administering incentive spirometry.

Key Elements in the Incentive Spirometry Procedure

- Verify and evaluate order or protocol; review chart for pertinent information.
- Coordinate therapy with other therapies and with pain medication, as needed.
- Assess vital signs, breath sounds, SpO_2, color, level of dyspnea, and ability to cooperate.
- Instruct the patient in proper method:
  - Full inspiratory capacity (IC) with 5- to 10-second breath hold
  - Adequate recovery time between breaths to avoid hyperventilation
  - Perform 6–10 times per hour
- Have the patient confirm understanding via a return demonstration.
- Assist patient in splinting any thoracic/abdominal surgical incisions to minimize pain.
- Measure the achieved volume.
- Instruct the patient to cough; observe for any sputum production.
- Notify appropriate personnel, and make recommendations or modifications to the patient care plan.
- Document outcomes.

Adapted from: Scanlan CL, West GA, von der Heydt PA, Dolan GK. *Respiratory therapy competency evaluation manual.* Boston: Blackwell Scientific; 1984.

After preliminary patient instruction and confirmation of proper breathing technique, you should encourage the patient to increase the volume goal. Other key points that can help ensure effective outcomes with IS include the following:

- If ordered for a surgical patient, initial instruction ideally should occur preoperatively.
- To accurately measure volumes, attach a one-way breathing valve and respirometer to the IS device.
- If the patient cannot cooperate or cannot generate an IC greater than 33% of predicted, recommend intermittent positive-pressure breathing (IPPB) as an alternative.
- If the patient also has retained secretions, recommend addition of bronchial hygiene to the regimen.
- Recommend discontinuation when clinical signs indicate resolution of atelectasis (e.g., resolution of fever, improvement in breath sounds, normal chest x-ray, improved oxygenation).

Inspiratory Muscle Training

Inspiratory muscle training (IMT) can help COPD patients manage their dyspnea, increase their exercise tolerance, and enhance their health-related quality of life. IMT also may improve diaphragm function in patients with certain neuromuscular disorders and may aid in weaning ventilator-dependent patients.

There are two types of IMT devices: flow and threshold resistors. Both are similar in concept to the resistors used to deliver positive expiratory pressure (PEP) therapy, as discussed in Chapter 4. However, with IMT the patient *inhales* against the resistor. Spring-loaded threshold resistors are preferred for IMT because they can be adjusted to a specific negative pressure, which ensures a constant muscle load independent of flow.

Key points needed to ensure effective outcomes with IMT include the following:

- Before implementing IMT, train the patient in proper diaphragmatic breathing.
- Measure the patient's maximum inspiratory pressure (MIP/PI_{max}) with a calibrated manometer.
- Encourage slow breathing (fewer than 10–12 breaths/minutes) through the device with minimal initial resistance.
- Once the patient becomes accustomed to the device, slowly increase resistance until the inspiratory pressure is 30% or more of the MIP/PI_{max}.
- After confirming the load setting and the patient's ability to independently perform the procedure, instruct the patient to perform 10- or 15-minute exercise sessions once or twice per day.
- Encourage the patient to maintain a detailed treatment log, including session dates and durations.
- If the MIP does not improve, interview the patient and inspect the log to determine why (usually noncompliance).

Table 10-1 summarizes IMT parameter recommendations from various sources. Note in particular that patients will progressively lose any health-related benefit if they cease training.

Initiate and Adjust Mechanical Ventilation

IPPB Therapy

Intermittent positive-pressure breathing is the application of positive-pressure breaths to a patient as a short-duration treatment modality. IPPB is indicated to:

- Improve lung expansion in patients with atelectasis who cannot use other methods, such as incentive spirometry
- Aid in delivery of aerosolized drugs (usually when other methods have failed)
- In rare situations, provide short-term ventilatory support (now provided mainly via noninvasive ventilators)

Table 10-1 Recommended Inspiratory Muscle Training Parameters

Parameter	Consideration	Recommendation
Mode	Type of device	Threshold or flow resistor (calibrated threshold preferred; if using a flow resistor, attach a manometer to the device's monitoring port)
Intensity	Load against which the person is exercising	Minimum of 30% of PI_{max} (lower initial intensity may be needed with COPD patients); increase PI_{max} by 5% per week as tolerated
Frequency/duration	Number of sessions/day	1–2 sessions per day, depending on patient exercise tolerance
	Length of sessions	Total of 30 minutes per day (divided over 1–2 sessions); initial sessions may need to be limited to 3–5 minutes
	Number of days/week	4–6 days of sessions per week according to patient tolerance
	Weeks of training	Continue indefinitely to maintain training benefits; functional improvement usually requires at least 5 weeks of training

Table 10-2 specifies the major contraindications and hazards associated with IPPB. Among the contraindications listed, only an untreated tension pneumothorax is an absolute contraindication.

IPPB machines are either pneumatic or electrically powered pressure-cycled devices. Pneumatic IPPB devices typically are driven by oxygen and use air entrainment to enhance flow and lower the FIO_2. Electrically powered devices use a small compressor to deliver room air to the patient. All IPPB devices provide user control over the peak inspiratory (cycling) pressure and incorporate a small-volume nebulizer to deliver aerosolized drugs. Some devices provide additional control over the sensitivity or trigger level, inspiratory flow and flow waveform, and expiratory flow (i.e., expiratory retard). Airway interfaces common to all IPPB devices include mouthpieces, flanged mouthpieces, masks, and 15-mm ET tube adaptors. Flanged mouthpiece or masks are used for patients unable to maintain a seal with a simple mouthpiece.

With the exception of FIO_2 control, which device you use to deliver IPPB is less important than your skill in its application. Key points in ensuring effective IPPB therapy include the following:

- After assembly, confirm proper operation of the equipment.
- Assess the patient before therapy (vital signs and breath sounds).
- Record the relevant outcome measure at baseline:
  - Tidal volume and inspiratory capacity for treating atelectasis
  - Peak flow or $FEV_1\%$ for bronchodilator therapy

Table 10-2 Contraindications and Hazards/Complications Associated with IPPB

Contraindications	Hazards/Complications
• Tension pneumothorax (untreated)	• Increased airway resistance/work of breathing
• Intracranial pressure (ICP) > 15 mm Hg	• Barotrauma, pneumothorax
• Hemodynamic instability	• Nosocomial infection
• Recent facial, oral, or skull surgery	• Hyperventilation or hypocarbia
• Tracheoesophageal fistula	• Hyperoxia when oxygen is the gas source
• Recent esophageal surgery	• Gastric distension
• Active hemoptysis	• Impedance of venous return
• Radiographic evidence of bleb	• Air trapping, auto-PEEP, overdistended alveoli

- Adjust settings initially to approximately 10–15 cm H_2O with moderate flow.
- Have patient maintain tight seal with mouthpiece (apply nose clips, mouth flange, or mask as needed).
- Instruct patient to inhale slightly until the breath triggers and allow the machine to augment inspiration; measure and note inspired volumes.
- Adjust the sensitivity as needed to facilitate triggering.
- Adjust the pressure and flow until the VT is 2–3 times the baseline value without patient discomfort.
- Instruct the patient to avoid forceful exhalation and breathe slowly (to prevent hyperventilation).
- Reassess the patient's vital signs, breath sounds, and IC and/or expiratory flows.
- Observe for adverse reactions.

To check the IPPB device's function, manually trigger the machine on and confirm that it cycles off when the circuit is obstructed. If the machine does not cycle off with the circuit obstructed, check for leaks in the tubing connections. If the device includes a rate control, make sure it is off. If delivering inhaled medications, make sure that the nebulizer is on and that aerosol is being produced. Start therapy with an initial sensitivity of approximately –2 cm H_2O, with the cycle pressure set between 10 and 15 cm H_2O and with a moderate flow (if adjustable).

In terms of FIO_2, you should try to match it to the patient's O_2 therapy prescription, if any. With pneumatic units, you can deliver either 100% O_2 or an air mixture with an FIO_2 varying between 0.40 and 0.60. The air-mix control also affects the amount and pattern of inspiratory flow. In the air-mix modes, flow is higher and the pattern of flow more normal (decelerating ramp). When air mix is off, available flow is less. In addition, some devices set to deliver pure source gas provide a less desirable square wave (constant) flow pattern.

To provide a precise FIO_2 a with pneumatically powered IPPB unit, you must attach it to an O_2 blender and set the device to deliver pure source gas (turn off air mix). Moderate but inexact O_2 concentrations can be achieved with electrically powered IPPB units by bleeding 100% O_2 into the delivery circuit.

During therapy, you should carefully observe the IPPB unit's pressure manometer during breathing. As indicated in **Figure 10-1**, the goal is to achieve quick and near-effortless on-triggering, followed by a relatively rapid pressure rise and ending in a short plateau (pattern A). In pattern B, airway pressure drops below zero after the breath starts. This "scalloping" of the pressure waveform indicates that the patient's flow exceeds that provided by the machine (i.e., there is inadequate flow to meet the patient's demand). If you observe this condition, you should either coach the patient to relax and let the machine do the work or increase the inspiratory flow. Pattern C demonstrates a different problem. Here the large drop in airway pressure below zero *before the breath starts* indicates improper triggering, which usually is corrected by increasing the sensitivity. The same situation

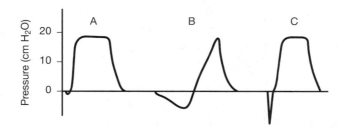

Figure 10-1 Graphic Depiction of IPPB Pressure Patterns. (A) A normal pattern with quick on-triggering, followed by a relatively rapid pressure rise and ending in a short plateau. **(B)** "Scalloping" of the pressure waveform after machine triggering indicating inadequate flow. **(C)** A large drop in airway pressure below zero before the breath starts, indicating inadequate sensitivity or a malfunctioning breathing valve.

Courtesy of: Strategic Learning Associates, LLC, Little Silver, New Jersey.

can occur if the IPPB valve malfunctions or is sticking. A malfunctioning valve usually indicates improper assembly, whereas a sticking value most often signifies accumulation of dirt or aerosolized drug residue on its surface. In either case, the device should be replaced with one that properly triggers on and cycles off. For more details on the various modifications you can make to tailor IPPB therapy to meet individual patient needs, refer to Chapter 12.

Continuous Mechanical Ventilation Settings

To do well on the NBRC credentialing exams, candidates must be able to properly select appropriate modes and set and adjust ventilator parameters. The accompanying box summarizes the key points to keep in mind when initiating ventilatory support.

Key Elements in Initiating Mechanical Ventilation

- Verify and evaluate order or protocol; scan chart for indications and precautions.
- Evaluate the patient's vital signs, breath sounds, and applicable monitored parameters (e.g., ECG, SpO_2).
- Connect the ventilator to an emergency electrical outlet and applicable gas supply (usually 50 psi air and O_2).
- Turn on the ventilator, test circuit, and verify proper ventilator function.
- Select appropriate ventilator mode and settings, including initial alarm parameters.
- Analyze and confirm FiO_2.
- Connect patient to ventilator and confirm ventilation (chest rise, return tidal volume).
- Reassess the patient, including comfort, oxygenation, ventilation, mechanics, and hemodynamics.
- Adjust ventilator settings to ensure adequate ventilation and oxygenation and patient–ventilator synchrony.
- Record pertinent data in the patient's chart and departmental records.
- Notify appropriate personnel and make any necessary recommendations or modifications to the care plan.

Adapted from: Scanlan CL, West GA, von der Heydt PA, Dolan GK. *Respiratory therapy competency evaluation manual.* Boston: Blackwell Scientific; 1984.

Chapter 6 covers procedures for verifying proper ventilator function. Chapters 11–13 discuss how to evaluate and monitor a patient's responses to mechanical ventilation and modify this support accordingly. Here we focus on selecting the appropriate ventilator mode, setting initial ventilator parameters, and making basic adjustments to ensure adequate ventilation and oxygenation.

Selecting the Ventilatory Support Modes

The NBRC "hospital" expects candidates to be familiar with all common ventilator modes, including control mode, assist/control (A/C) mode, synchronous intermittent mandatory ventilation (SIMV), pressure support (PS), continuous positive airway pressure (CPAP), and bilevel positive airway pressure (BiPAP). You also may be expected to understand dual breath modes such as pressure-regulated volume control (PRVC) as well as a bilevel mode called airway pressure-release ventilation (APRV).

Table 10-3 describes each of these modes of ventilation, specifies their appropriate use, and defines their advantages and disadvantages. In the NBRC hospital, you generally should start an intubated patient in respiratory failure on *full ventilatory support*, with the ventilator initially responsible for the full minute volume and workload. Full ventilatory support modes include volume- or pressure-controlled A/C or normal-rate SIMV (with or without pressure support). However, as the patient improves, you typically will implement modes that require spontaneous breaths (*partial ventilatory support*), with the goal always being restoration of full spontaneous breathing as soon as possible. If however the physician wants to avoid intubation but still provide a patient with ventilatory support, you should select or recommend noninvasive ventilation using bilevel positive airway pressure (as discussed later in this chapter).

Table 10-3 Modes of Ventilatory Support

Description	Recommend or Use	Advantages	Disadvantages
Pure Control Mode (Patient Triggering Not Allowed)			
• Patient breathes at rate and time interval set on ventilator • No patient triggering • All machine (mandatory) breaths • Provides full support • May control either volume (VC) or pressure (PC)	• When full support is needed but the rate and/or pattern must be controlled or patient effort eliminated; examples include inverse I:E ratio ventilation, permissive hypercapnia, and hyperventilation in brain injury	• Rate, ventilatory pattern, and $Paco_2$ are controlled • Eliminates work of breathing (as long as patient makes no efforts) • Allows for "abnormal" patterns such as inverse I:E ratio	• Poorly tolerated • Patient efforts cause asynchrony ("fighting the ventilator") and increased work of breathing • May require heavy sedation or neuromuscular paralysis
Assist/Control Mode (A/C)			
• Ventilator provides a guaranteed rate, which the patient can exceed by triggering additional breaths • All machine (mandatory) breaths • Provides full ventilatory support • Can be VC or PC	• When full ventilatory support is needed but patient's breathing rate results in acceptable $Paco_2$	• Patient controls own breathing rate and CO_2 level • May avoid need for sedation or paralysis • Guaranteed rate if patient's rate falls	• Hyperventilation can occur at high triggering rates (due to anxiety, fear, pain, or hypoxemia) • Asynchronous breathing due to improper sensitivity or flow settings may increase work of breathing and O_2 consumption • May worsen auto-PEEP in COPD patients
Synchronous Intermittent Mandatory Ventilation (SIMV)			
• Patient breathes spontaneously between machine breaths • Provides full support at normal rates and partial support at lower rates • Machine breaths may be VC or PC • Spontaneous breaths may be pressure supported	• When full ventilatory support is needed but patient's spontaneous breathing rate would result in hyperventilation on A/C • To incrementally lower support levels (weaning)	• Allows graded levels of support • Spontaneous breathing allowed; patient controls rate and pattern • Decreased need for sedation • Less "fighting" of ventilator • Lower mean pressures than with A/C	• Hypoventilation is a hazard at low rates (adequate minute volume not ensure) • Asynchronous breathing can still occur during machine breaths (improper sensitivity or flow)

(continues)

Table 10-3 Modes of Ventilatory Support (*continued*)

Description	Recommend or Use	Advantages	Disadvantages
Pressure Support Ventilation (PS)			
• Patient-triggered, pressure-limited, flow-cycled spontaneous breaths • V_T depends on pressure level and patient effort • Normally provides partial support; provides full support only if pressure level yields normal V_T (PSV_{max})	• To overcome imposed work of breathing caused by small artificial airways (low PSV) • To boost the spontaneous V_T of patients receiving SIMV • To incrementally lower support levels (for weaning)	• Patient controls rate of breathing, inspiratory time, and flow • Results in lower rate, higher V_T, less muscle activity, and lower O_2 consumption than pure spontaneous breathing • Improves respiratory muscle conditioning; facilitates weaning	• Without backup rate, hypoventilation can occur • Variable V_T and $\dot{V}_E$ • Unless rise time can be adjusted, asynchrony may occur • In COPD patients, flow cycling to end-inspiration may either require active effort or be prolonged
Pressure-Regulated Volume Control (PRVC)			
• Pressure control A/C ventilation in which the pressure limit automatically adjusts breath-to-breath to maintain a target tidal volume	• For patients requiring the lowest possible pressure and a guaranteed consistent V_T • For patients requiring variable inspiratory flow • For patients with changing C_{LT} or Raw	• Lower PIP than VC or PC A/C; lower incidence of barotrauma • Pressure automatically adjusts to changing C_{LT} and Raw • Near-constant V_T • Patient controls rate and $\dot{V}_E$ • Automatic decrease in ventilatory support as the patient improves • Decelerating flow pattern	• Variable patient effort will result in variable V_T and possible asynchrony • Severe increase in Raw or decrease in C_{LT} may result in high/unsafe PIP or reduced V_T • When patient demand is increased, pressure level may diminish when support is most needed • As pressure drops, Pmean drops, possibly causing hypoxemia • May cause or worsen auto-PEEP
Continuous Positive Airway Pressure (CPAP)			
• Positive airway pressure throughout spontaneous breathing • May be provided by either demand-flow or continuous-flow systems	• For patients with CHF/pulmonary edema (short-term use) • For patients with sleep apnea (nocturnal use) • To treat refractory hypoxemia in patients with adequate spontaneous ventilation	• Provides increased PaO_2 for a given FIO_2 • Can increase lung compliance and decrease work of breathing	• Increases mean pleural pressure, ICP, and pulmonary vascular resistance • Decreases venous return • Increases incidence of barotrauma • Hypoventilation (adequate $\dot{V}_E$ not guaranteed) • Continuous flow systems make volume monitoring difficult

Table 10-3 Modes of Ventilatory Support (continued)

Bilevel Positive Airway Pressure (BiPAP)		
• Patient-triggered, pressure-limited breaths with positive pressure maintained throughout the expiratory phase (equivalent to PS with CPAP) • V_T depends on pressure difference (IPAP – EPAP) and patient effort	• To avoid intubation of patients in respiratory failure (e.g., COPD) • To avoid reintubation of patients failing spontaneous breathing trials • For patients with CHF or pulmonary edema • For patients with sleep apnea (especially central sleep apnea)	• Fewer hazards than invasive ventilatory support • Patient controls rate of breathing, and inspiratory time and flow • Requires cooperative patient with adequate secretion clearance • Some systems have limited F_{IO_2} ($\leq$ 60%) or pressure ($\leq$ 40 cm H_2O) capabilities • Airway interface problems can cause discomfort, tissue trauma, and leaks
Airway Pressure-Release Ventilation (APRV)		
• Equivalent to CPAP with intermittent releases in pressure to baseline • Technically time-triggered, pressure-limited, time-cycled ventilation with spontaneous breathing • Often referred to as "inverted IMV" (based on graphic appearance)	• For patients with acute lung injury (ALI)/ARDS, especially when Pplat > 30 cm H_2O • For patients with refractory hypoxemia due to collapsed alveoli • For patients with massive atelectasis	• Lower PIP/Pplat than VC, PC A/C • Less hemodynamic impact than A/C • Reduced risk of lung injury • Allows for spontaneous breathing throughout the ventilatory cycle • Improves V/Q matching and oxygenation • May decrease physiologic deadspace and lower V_E needs • Reduces the need for sedation/paralysis • V_T delivery depends on C_{LT}, Raw, and patient effort • Provides partial support only (relies on spontaneous breathing to help remove CO_2) • Caution should be used with hemodynamically unstable patients • Auto-PEEP is usually present • Asynchrony can occur if spontaneous breaths are out of phase with release time

C_{LT} = total lung + thorax compliance; Raw = airway resistance.

In terms of using volume or pressure control for mandatory breaths, in the NBRC hospital either option is satisfactory as long as the volume or pressure setting minimizes the possibility of overdistending the lungs (i.e., creating barotrauma or volutrauma). **Table 10-4** compares the basic advantages and disadvantages of volume and pressure control of mandatory breaths. *To help avoid lung injury due to overdistension, patients requiring plateau pressures greater than 30 cm H_2O during volume control ventilation should probably be switched to pressure control at a safe pressure limit (i.e., 30 cm H_2O or less).*

Selecting the Initial Ventilator Settings

Table 10-5 outlines the typical settings used to initiate full ventilatory support in the A/C or SIMV modes for adult patients. In terms of selecting tidal volumes, settings in the 6–10 mL per kilogram of predicted body weight (PBW) range are used in the NBRC hospital, *except for patients with acute hypoxemic respiratory failure* (see the NHLBI ARDS protocol later in this chapter). To compute the PBW, use the applicable gender-specific formula:

$$\text{Male PBW (kg)} = 50 + 2.3 \text{ [height (in.)} - 60]$$
$$\text{Female PBW (kg)} = 45.5 + 2.3 \text{ [height (in.)} - 60] \quad \cdot$$

For example, the PBW for a 6-foot (72-inch)-tall male patient would be calculated as follows:

$$\text{PBW (kg)} = 50 + 2.3 \text{ [72} - 60]$$
$$\text{PBW (kg)} = 50 + 27.6 \cong 78 \text{ kg}$$

Using 8 mL/kg for this patient (a good rule of thumb value!) would yield a starting volume of approximately 625 mL. Note that using PBW as opposed to actual body weight is necessary to avoid excessive volumes. Based on this understanding, were this 6-foot-tall patient to actually weigh 120 kg (265 lb), *we would still apply a VT in the 600–800 mL range*, and definitely *not* 1200 mL!

Airway pressure-release ventilation is a unique mode with unique settings. As depicted in **Figure 10-2**, patients receiving APRV breathe spontaneously at a high baseline pressure termed P_{high} (the inflation pressure, equivalent to CPAP). However, after a set time interval termed T_{high}, this pressure is released, or allowed to drop down to a lower deflation pressure termed P_{low}. This drop in pressure causes the patient to exhale, which facilitates CO_2 removal, with the length of this release termed T_{low}. P_{low} generally is set in the 0–8 cm H_2O range with P_{high} set to provide an inflation volume of 4–8 mL/kg PBW but kept below 30–35 cm H_2O. Initially T_{high} is set in the 3–5 seconds range, with T_{low} typically adjusted to between 0.2 and 0.8 seconds, resulting in approximately 10–20 inflations/deflation cycles per minute. The initial F_{IO_2} settings for APRV are the same as for traditional full support modes.

Table 10-4 Comparison of Volume Control and Pressure Control of Mandatory Breaths

Breath Control	Advantages	Disadvantages
Volume control (VC)	• Maintains constant VT with changes in CLT and Raw • Changes in CLT and Raw easy to detect	• Applied pressure can rise as CLT falls, risking barotrauma • Fixed flow pattern can cause asynchrony
Pressure control (PC)	• Variable flow aids patient synchrony • Less risk of barotrauma with decreasing CLT	• VT varies with changes in CLT and Raw • Changes in CLT and Raw difficult to detect
VT = tidal volume; CLT = total lung + thorax compliance; Raw = airway resistance.		

Table 10-5 Typical Initial Settings for Full Ventilatory Support of Adults

Parameter	Typical Settings
Tidal volume (if VC or PRVC)	• 6–10 mL/kg PBW; keep Pplat ≤ 30–35 cm H_2O • 4–6 mL/kg in ALI/ARDS (ARDS protocol)
Pressure limit (if PC)	• 20–30 cm H_2O with aim to achieve expired V_{TS} as above
Rate	• 8–24/min
Trigger/sensitivity	• Pressure triggering: 1–2 cm H_2O < baseline • Flow triggering: 1–3 L/min < baseline
Flow, I-time, I:E	Set to achieve I:E ≤ 1:1 (e.g., 1:2, 1:3) and prevent auto-PEEP
Flow waveform	• VC: square or decelerating with flow sufficient to prevent scalloping of inspiratory pressure curve (use flow compensation if available) • PC: adjust rise time to achieve end-of-breath pressure plateau without spiking
Pressure support (SIMV only)	5–10 cm H_2O as needed to overcome artificial airway resistance and maintain an acceptable spontaneous rate (< 25/min) and work of breathing
F_{IO_2}	• Initially 60–100% if Sao_2 or Pao_2 data not available • Then as needed to maintain Pao_2 ≥ 60 torr or Sao_2 ≥ 92% • ARDS: F_{IO_2}/PEEP combinations (ARDS protocol)
PEEP	• Initially 5–10 cm H_2O, then as needed to maintain Sao_2 ≥ 92 with F_{IO_2} ≤ 50% • ARDS: F_{IO_2}/PEEP combinations (ARDS protocol) • As needed to balance auto-PEEP
VC = volume control ventilation; PC = pressure control ventilation; PBW = predicted body weight; ARDS = acute respiratory distress syndrome; ARI = acute lung injury; Pplat = plateau pressure.	

Making Preliminary Adjustments to Ventilator Settings

In adjusting ventilator settings, your primary goals are to (1) achieve acceptable arterial blood gases and (2) maximize patient comfort and patient–ventilator synchrony. To achieve acceptable arterial blood gases, you should focus on normalizing the pH and oxygenation. Chapters 11 and 12 address ways to detect abnormal patient–ventilator synchrony (i.e., asynchrony) and correct it.

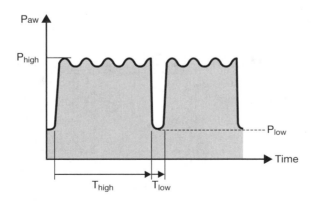

Figure 10-2 Representative Pressure Versus Time Plot for Airway Pressure-Release Ventilation.

Normalizing the pH

To normalize the pH, you adjust the minute ventilation, which alters the $Paco_2$. **Table 10-6** outlines the methods commonly used to alter pH and $Paco_2$ for the various ventilator modes. In most cases, the goal is a pH between 7.35 and 7.45. However, depending on the patient's underlying problem, you may allow the pH to go as low as 7.30 or as high as 7.50. Note also that in normalizing the pH of some patients, the resulting $Paco_2$ may be abnormal. For example, in a patient with COPD who has chronic CO_2 retention (compensated respiratory acidosis), a normal pH may be achieved with $Paco_2$ levels of 55 torr or higher. In contrast, in a patient with severe (uncorrected) diabetic ketoacidosis and respiratory failure, a normal pH may be achieved only via forced hyperventilation—that is, with a lower than normal $Paco_2$.

Because you alter the minute ventilation to adjust the pH, you can do so by changing the rate or the delivered V_T. In all modes, the base machine rate is set. In volume-control modes, the delivered V_T is set. In pressure-control modes, you alter the delivered V_T by increasing or decreasing the driving pressure, termed ΔP (= PIP – PEEP). The following guidelines apply to making such changes:

- In most modes, to adjust the pH you first adjust the machine rate, keeping it in the range of 8–24/min.
- If rate adjustments alone do not normalize the pH, then you alter the delivered V_T.
- In altering the delivered V_T, try to keep it between 4 and 10 mL/kg PBW with a Pplat less than 30–35 cm H_2O.
- If the pH remains below 7.30 and the rate, delivered V_T, and Pplat are at their recommended high limits, consider permissive hypercapnia.

Normalizing Oxygenation

To ensure normal oxygenation, you need to do the following:

1. Adjust/maintain an acceptable Pao_2 and SaO_2.
2. Check and confirm an acceptable Hb content (≥10 g/dL).
3. Check for and confirm adequate circulation.

Table 10-6 Altering the pH and Paco$_2$ of Adult Patients Receiving Ventilatory Support

Mode	To Decrease Paco$_2$/Increase pH	To Increase Paco$_2$/Decrease pH
Volume Control		
A/C	• Increase machine rate (≤ 24/min)	• Decrease machine rate (≥ 8/min)
	• Increase set V$_T$ (keep Pplat < 30–35 cm H$_2$O)	• Add deadspace
SIMV	• Increase machine rate (≤ 24/min)	• Decrease machine rate (≥ 8/min)
	• Increase set V$_T$ (keep Pplat < 30–35 cm H$_2$O)	• Decrease machine V$_T$
	• Add/increase pressure support	• Decrease pressure support
Pressure Control		
A/C	• Increase machine rate (≤ 24/min)	• Decrease machine rate (≥ 8/min)
	• Increase ΔP (PIP – PEEP)	• Decrease ΔP (PIP – PEEP)
SIMV	• Increase machine rate (≤ 24/min)	• Decrease machine rate (≥ 8/min)
	• Increase ΔP (PIP – PEEP)	• Decrease ΔP (PIP – PEEP)
	• Add/increase pressure support	• Decrease pressure support
PS	• Increase ΔP	• Decrease ΔP
BiPAP	• Increase machine rate (≤ 24/min)	• Decrease machine rate (≥ 8/min)
	• Increase ΔP (IPAP – EPAP)	• Decrease ΔP (IPAP – EPAP)
APRV	• Increase release frequency (↓T$_{high}$)	• Decrease release frequency (↑T$_{high}$)
	• Increase ΔP (P$_{high}$ – P$_{low}$)	• Decrease ΔP (P$_{high}$ – P$_{low}$)

For most patients, acceptable ABG values for oxygenation are $PaO_2 \geq 65$ torr and $SaO_2 \geq 92\%$. Note, however, that in patients with either COPD or ALI/ARDS, we can accept PaO_2 values as low as 55 torr as long as we can keep the arterial saturation at or above 88%.

General guidelines for initial adjustment of PaO_2/SaO_2 are as follows:

- If an acceptable PaO_2/SaO_2 can be maintained on less than 50% O_2, normalize oxygenation by altering the FIO_2.
- If an acceptable PaO_2/SaO_2 cannot be maintained on less than 50% O_2, normalize oxygenation by altering the baseline pressure (CPAP, PEEP, EPAP, P_{low}).
- If PaO_2/FIO_2 ratio is 200 or less (see Chapter 11) or if 50% or more O_2 with PEEP of 12 cm H_2O or more is insufficient to maintain acceptable PaO_2/SaO_2 values, you should recommend the NHLBI ARDS protocol (covered later in this chapter).
- When oxygenation improves, first decrease F_IO_2 until it is 0.50 or less, and then lower PEEP.

Noninvasive Ventilation

Noninvasive ventilation is the delivery of assisted mechanical ventilation without the need for an artificial tracheal airway. **Table 10-7** lists the major advantages and limitations of noninvasive ventilation.

There are two primary types of noninvasive ventilation: negative pressure and positive pressure. Noninvasive negative-pressure devices include the iron lung or tank ventilator, chest curiass, and pneumosuit. Most noninvasive positive-pressure ventilation (NPPV) is delivered using ventilators capable of providing and independently regulating the pressure support and CPAP levels. *Application of NPPV requires that the patient have control over his or her upper airway function, be able to manage secretions, and be cooperative and motivated.* **Table 10-8** lists the indications and contraindications for NPPV.

Because the airway interface defines NPPV, technically any ventilator or mode can be applied noninvasively. However, pressure-support ventilation has become the norm for providing NPPV. When NPPV combines pressure support with an elevated baseline pressure, this approach is commonly called bilevel positive airway pressure. The two pressure levels are the peak or IPAP pressure (inspiratory positive airway pressure) and the baseline or EPAP pressure (expiratory positive airway pressure—equivalent to CPAP). BiPAP can be delivered by most ICU ventilators, but more commonly is provided by devices designed specifically for this purpose.

Table 10-9 outlines the typical initial settings and basic ways to adjust NPPV. Additional key pointers related to application of NPPV include the following:

- Confirm that the patient is alert and has intact upper airway function/secretions control.
- Position the patient in a high semi-Fowler's (sitting) position if possible.
- Choose the best interface (generally an oronasal or "full" face mask for acute respiratory failure).

Table 10-7 Advantages and Limitations of Noninvasive Ventilation

Advantages	Limitations
• Avoidance of intubation-related trauma	• Can be used only in cooperative patients
• Preservation of airway defenses	• Does not provide direct airway access
• Lower incidence of nosocomial pneumonia	• Increases the risk of secretion retention
• Permits normal speech and eating	• Requires more caregiver time (initially)
• Reduces the need for sedation	
• Facilitates the weaning process	
• Shorter duration of ventilation/length of hospital stay	
• Reduces costs	

Table 10-8 Indications and Contraindications for NPPV

Indications	Contraindications
• Reverse hypercapnic respiratory failure (pH > 7.20) • Reverse hypoxemic respiratory failure (P/F ratio < 200) • Treat acute cardiogenic pulmonary edema • Facilitate earlier weaning/extubation of COPD patients from invasive support • Support patients with chronic hypoventilation syndromes • Alleviate breathlessness and fatigue in terminally ill patients	• Respiratory arrest • pH < 7.20 • Uncooperative patient • Inability to protect airway or clear secretions • Upper airway obstruction • Hemodynamic instability/hypotension • Uncontrolled arrhythmias • Active upper gastrointestinal bleeding • Facial burns or trauma • Need for airway protection, high risk for aspiration

- Establish initial settings (Table 10-9).
- Hold the NPPV interface in place (without strapping) until the patient becomes accustomed to it.
- Keep IPAP levels less than 20–25 cm H_2O (esophageal opening pressure).
- Assess for improvement in blood gases, resolution of dyspnea, tachypnea, or accessory muscle use.
- Adjust ventilation ($Paco_2$, pH) via IPAP and ΔP.
- Adjust oxygenation (Pao_2/Sao_2) via Fio_2 and EPAP.
- If any factor that is a contraindication to NPPV develops, or if oxygenation or ventilation worsens, consider intubation and conventional invasive mechanical ventilation.

Table 10-9 Initial Settings and Basic Adjustments for NPPV

Parameter	Initial Settings and Basic Adjustments
Tidal volume	Function of patient effort and ΔP (IPAP – EPAP); aim for 6–8 mL/kg
Pressure limit	Initial IPAP = 10–15 cm H_2O; adjust to normalize pH/$Paco_2$
Rate	Guarantee minimum of 8/min
Trigger/sensitivity	If adjustable: 1–2 cm H_2O < baseline pressure or 1–3 L/min < baseline flow
Flow, I-time, or I:E	N/A for spontaneous breaths; in timed modes, start with %I-time in the 20–30% range
Flow waveform	If adjustable, set rise time to achieve the end-of-breath pressure plateau without spiking
Fio_2	As needed to maintain $Pao_2 \geq 65$ torr or $Sao_2 \geq 92\%$
PEEP	Initial EPAP = 5 cm H_2O; adjust to maintain $Pao_2 \geq 65$ torr or $Sao_2 \geq 92\%$ Keep ΔP (IPAP – EPAP) ≥ 5 cm H_2O
To adjust pH/$Paco_2$	To ↓ $Paco_2$ or ↑ pH: ↑ IPAP To ↑ $Paco_2$ or ↓ pH: ↓ IPAP
To adjust Pao_2/Sao_2	If simple V/Q imbalance and $Fio_2 < 0.50$, raise Fio_2 If shunting is present ($Pao_2 \leq 50$ torr and $Fio_2 \geq 0.50$), increase EPAP (keep $\Delta P \geq 5$ cm H_2O) When oxygenation improves, first decrease Fio_2 until ≤ 0.50, then lower EPAP

Elevated Baseline Pressure (CPAP, PEEP, EPAP, P$_{low}$)

Whereas CPAP is a mode of ventilatory support, PEEP is an "add-on" that can be applied to any mode. Both methods maintain the baseline airway pressure above atmospheric pressure. Strictly speaking, CPAP involves *spontaneous breathing at an elevated baseline pressure*. CPAP is indicated to treat sleep apnea and acute cardiogenic pulmonary edema, as well as to manage refractory hypoxemia in infants with respiratory distress syndrome. Low levels of PEEP (5–10 cm H_2O) also are applied to most patients receiving full or partial ventilatory support to maintain the FRC and prevent atelectasis. Higher levels of PEEP are applied as needed to patients with acute hypoxemic respiratory failure (P/F ratio < 200) to reduce shunting and allow for lower FIO_2s (to avoid oxygen toxicity). High levels of CPAP or PEEP (as high as 30–40 cm H_2O) also are used briefly or intermittently to reopen collapsed alveoli (see the discussion of recruitment maneuvers later in this chapter). Finally, in patients with dynamic hyperinflation, externally applied PEEP can help decrease auto-PEEP and improve patient–ventilator synchrony.

CPAP and PEEP can have detrimental effects. Both increase mean pleural pressures. Higher mean pleural pressures can increase intracranial pressure (ICP) and pulmonary vascular resistance, and decrease venous return and cardiac output. In addition, CPAP and PEEP can increase the risk of barotrauma.

The use of CPAP to manage sleep apnea is discussed in detail in Chapter 17. When using CPAP to treat cardiogenic pulmonary edema, you apply 5–20 cm H_2O and adjust this pressure as needed to maintain an adequate PaO_2/SpO_2 and eliminate the signs of pulmonary edema. When CPAP is used to manage infants with respiratory distress syndrome, you typically start CPAP at 5 cm H_2O and gradually increase it as needed to meet the following goals:

- Stabilize FIO_2 requirements ($FIO_2 \leq 0.50$ with $PaO_2 > 50$ torr)
- Reduce the work of breathing as indicated by:
  ○ A decrease in respiratory rate
  ○ A decrease in the severity of retractions, grunting, and nasal flaring
- Improve lung aeration (as indicated by chest x-ray)

Deciding when to apply PEEP is easy; determining how much PEEP to use is difficult. The problem is that too little PEEP may not overcome shunting, while too much can cause overdistension, worsen preexisting lung injury, and decrease O_2 delivery to the tissues. "Optimal" PEEP represents the end-expiratory pressure level that maximizes patient benefits while minimizing risks.

Currently, there are four ways to determine optimal PEEP, any of which might appear on the NBRC exams. These four different methods define optimal PEEP as the pressure level that:

1. Maximizes O_2 delivery to the tissues
2. Yields the highest static total compliance (C$_{LT}$)
3. Provides the maximum volume change for a given ∆P
4. Exceeds the lower inflection point (LIP) on the pressure–volume curve

Method 1 is based on the fact that oxygen delivery to the tissues is a function of the patient's cardiac output (CO) and arterial O_2 content (CaO$_2$):

$$O_2 \text{ delivery} = CO \times CaO_2$$

In general, as PEEP levels rise, so does the patient's arterial O_2 content (good!). However, the higher the PEEP level, the greater the potential negative impact on cardiac output (bad!). Based on these relationships, PEEP is optimized when the desired increase in CaO$_2$ is not offset by decreases in CO. To make this determination, the patient must have a pulmonary artery catheter in place so that you can measure both cardiac output and the mixed venous O_2 content. You then apply incremental levels of PEEP while simultaneously measuring these parameters and the arterial O_2 content via an A-line. O_2 delivery is computed at each PEEP increment, with optimal PEEP defined as that level with the highest O_2 delivery.

Methods 2 through 4 all use measures of respiratory mechanics to determine optimal PEEP. The conventional technique involves raising PEEP while simultaneously measuring the patient's static compliance during volume control ventilation. An example of this type of PEEP study as it might appear on the NBRC exams is depicted here:

PEEP (cm H$_2$O)	V$_T$ (mL)	PIP (cm H$_2$O)	Pplat (cm H$_2$O)
0	600	30	20
5	600	36	24
10	600	41	27
15	600	45	33
20	600	49	41

First, you can disregard the peak pressure (PIP)—it is there to confuse you. What you are interested in is the difference between the plateau pressure and the positive end-expiratory pressure: Pplat – PEEP. *Because the tidal volume is constant, the smaller this difference, the greater the compliance.* This relationship is demonstrated here:

Pplat (cm H$_2$O)	PEEP (cm H$_2$O)	Pplat – PEEP (cm H$_2$O)	C$_{LT}$ (mL/cm H$_2$O)
20	0	20	30
24	5	19	32
27	10	17	35
33	15	18	33
41	20	21	29

Based on this method, the optimal PEEP for this patient would be 10 cm H$_2$O, the level yielding the highest static compliance (35 mL/cm H$_2$O).

What if the patient is receiving pressure-control ventilation? In this case you can use method 3, which applies the same basic concept as just discussed. With this method, however, *rather than maintain a constant volume, you maintain a constant* ΔP (PIP – PEEP), typically 15–25 cm H$_2$O. You then assess the exhaled V$_T$, with the largest increase representing the optimal PEEP. For obvious reasons, this approach is called the *equal pressure method.* An example of the equal pressure method for determining optimal PEEP as it might appear on the NBRC exams is depicted here:

PEEP (cm H$_2$O)	PIP (cm H$_2$O)	V$_T$ (mL)
5	20	390
10	25	410
15	30	430
20	35	380

Using method 3, the optimal PEEP for this patient is 15 cm H$_2$O, corresponding to the maximum volume change for a given ΔP (430 mL).

The last method for determining optimal PEEP (method 4) requires plotting of a static pressure–volume curve for the patient's respiratory system, as depicted in **Figure 10-3**. Note first that the slope of any line on this graph equals compliance ($\Delta V/\Delta P$). Second, note that the curve exhibits the typical "S" shape, with a low slope (low compliance) at low pressures and volumes, changing over to a steep slope (high compliance) at moderate volumes and pressures, and then changing back to a low slope (low compliance) at high pressures and volumes. In theory, the low compliance at low lung volumes is due to the high opening pressures required to expand collapsed alveoli. As

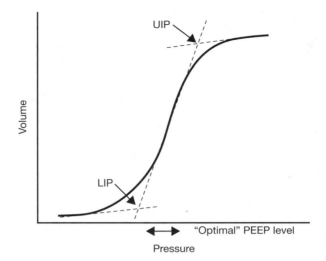

Figure 10-3 Idealized Static Pressure–Volume Curve of the Respiratory System. The points at which the slope of the curve changes are called inflection points. (Note that these points are not on the curve itself, but extrapolated from tangents of the curve.) Optimal PEEP is the lowest pressure needed to exceed LIP. LIP = lower inflection point representing the changeover from low to high compliance at low lung volume (also called Pflex); UIP = upper inflection point representing the changeover from high compliance to low compliance at high lung volume.

more and more alveoli open (alveolar recruitment), the curve steepens and enters the "sweet spot" for efficient mechanics of breathing, where compliance is at a maximum. However, like any elastic structure, the lungs eventually reach their limit of expansion, signaled by a rapid leveling off of the pressure–volume curve at high volumes—that is, overdistension. Here any small increase in volume results in a large increase in pressure.

The lower inflection point (LIP or sometimes Pflex) of the curve corresponds to the changeover from low to high compliance at low lung volume, representing maximum alveolar recruitment. Based on these concepts, optimal PEEP is the *lowest pressure* needed to exceed LIP or Pflex. Clinically, we maintain PEEP at 2–3 cm H_2O above the LIP or Pflex to keep alveoli open, while avoiding overdistension.

Selecting Ventilator Graphics

The ventilator graphics display incorporated into most critical care ventilators provides the following essential monitoring capabilities:

- Checking/confirming and fine-tuning ventilator function
- Assessing patients' respiratory mechanics
- Evaluating patients' responses to therapy
- Troubleshooting patient–ventilator interaction

The interpretation and use of ventilator graphics are covered in detail in Chapters 11 and 12. Here we address only which graphic displays to select according to the information you need.

There are two major types of ventilator graphics: scalar (time-based) and X-Y (loops). As depicted in **Figure 10-4**, scalar graphics plot pressure, volume, or flow on the Y-axis against time on the X-axis. On most ventilators, you can set the graphics screen to display one or more of these three parameters. Most ventilators also allow you to change the time scale (sweep speed) when displaying scalar graphics. Changing the time scale by selecting a faster speed gives you a closer look at individual breath waveforms, whereas selecting a slow sweep speed can help you identify trends.

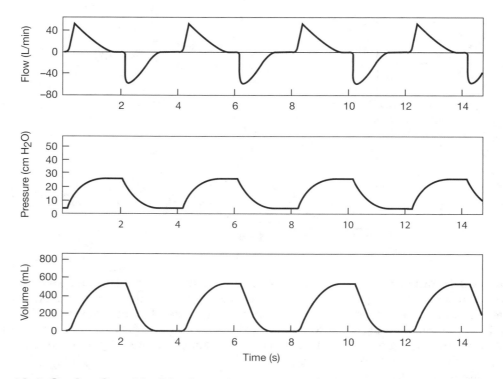

Figure 10-4 Scalar Graphic Display of Flow, Pressure, and Volume Versus Time.
The flow and pressure waveform indicate pressure control ventilation with 4 cm H$_2$O PEEP.

X-Y or loop graphics simultaneously display two variables plotted on the X- and Y-axes. The two most common loop graphics are pressure (X-axis) versus volume (Y-axis) and volume (X-axis) versus flow (Y-axis). **Figure 10-5** depicts a representative X-Y plot of volume versus pressure. **Table 10-10** provides guidance on which graphic display to select, based on your monitoring needs.

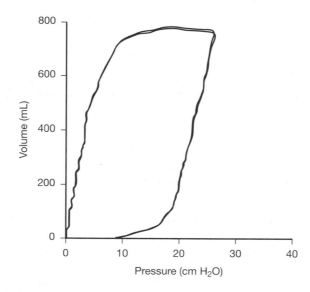

Figure 10-5 X-Y Graphic Display of Pressure–Volume Loop During Mechanical Ventilation. The right-side upswing is the inspiratory portion, with the downswing to the left being the expiratory return to baseline pressure (in this example 0 cm H$_2$O).

Table 10-10 Common Usage for Scalar and X-Y Loop Graphic Displays

Display	Uses
Scalar Graphics	
Flow versus time	• Identify presence of auto-PEEP (expiratory) • Identify flow starvation (VC) • Assess/adjust rise time (PC, PSV) • Identify asynchrony
Pressure versus time	• Confirm PIP and PEEP level • Visually assess mechanics using PIP-Pplat ($\approx$ Raw) and Pplat – PEEP ($\approx$ CLT) • Assess sensitivity/trigger response • Identify asynchrony
Volume versus time	• Identify leaks • Identify asynchrony
X-Y Loop Graphics	
Pressure (X-axis) versus volume (Y-axis)	• Assess overall work of breathing • Identify overdistension • Assess trigger work • Adjust PSV levels
Volume (X-axis) versus flow (Y-axis)	• Assess bronchodilator response • Identify presence of auto-PEEP • Identify leaks

Applying Disease-Specific Ventilator Protocols

The NBRC expects you to be familiar with selected disease-specific protocols, the most important of which is the National Heart, Lung, and Blood Institute (NHLBI) ARDS protocol. This protocol helps increase survival of patients with acute respiratory distress syndrome by maintaining adequate oxygenation while preventing ventilator-associated lung injury. You should consider implementing this protocol for any patient who exhibits an acute onset of respiratory distress not associated with heart failure and meets the following criteria:

- P/F ratio < 300 (see Chapter 11)
- Bilateral diffuse infiltrates on x-ray consistent with pulmonary edema
- No clinical evidence of left atrial hypertension/left ventricular failure

Basic ventilator setup and adjustment are as follows:

1. Calculate the patient's predicted body weight (see the male/female formulas given earlier in this chapter).
2. Select any ventilator mode but try to ensure an I:E $\leq$ 1:1.
3. Set the initial VT to 8 mL/kg PBW.
4. Reduce VT by 1 mL/kg at intervals $\leq$ 2 hours until VT = 6 mL/kg PBW.
5. Set the initial rate to approximately the baseline $\dot{V}$E (no greater than 35/min).
6. Adjust the VT and rate to achieve the pH and plateau pressure goals.

To ensure adequate oxygenation, the goal is to maintain a Pao_2 between 55 and 80 torr or an Spo_2 between 88% and 95%. To achieve these targets, you use at least 5 cm H_2O PEEP. You then consider incremental Fio_2/PEEP combinations such as those suggested in **Table 10-11** to achieve adequate oxygenation.

Table 10-11 Suggested Incremental Fio₂/PEEP Combinations to Achieve Adequate Oxygenation

	Conservative Approach (Higher Fio₂/Lower PEEP)													
Fio₂	0.30	0.40	0.40	0.50	0.50	0.60	0.70	0.70	0.70	0.80	0.90	0.90	0.90	1.0
PEEP	5	5	8	8	10	10	10	12	14	14	14	16	18	18–24
	Aggressive Approach (Lower Fio₂/Higher PEEP)													
Fio₂	0.30	0.30	0.40	0.40	0.50	0.50	0.60	0.60	0.70	0.80	0.80	0.90	1.0	1.0
PEEP	12	14	14	16	16	18	18	20	20	20	22	22	22	24
Source: NIH NHLBI ARDS Clinical Network Mechanical Ventilation Protocol Summary.														

To help prevent lung injury, you should keep the plateau pressure at 30 cm H_2O or less, and measure it every 4 hours and after each change in PEEP or VT. The following guidelines apply to adjusting Pplat:

- If Pplat > 30 cm H_2O, decrease VT in 1 mL/kg steps to a minimum of 4 mL/kg.
- If Pplat < 25 cm H_2O and VT < 6 mL/kg, increase VT by 1 mL/kg until Pplat > 25 cm H_2O or VT = 6 mL/kg.
- If Pplat < 30 cm H_2O and breath stacking/dysynchrony occurs, consider increasing VT in 1 mL/kg steps to 7–8 mL/kg if Pplat remains < 30 cm H_2O.

In terms of acid–base balance, the goal is to keep the pH between 7.30 and 7.45. If the pH rises above 7.45 (rare), you should decrease the ventilator rate. Otherwise:

- If pH > 7.15 but < 7.30: increase the rate until pH > 7.30 or Paco₂ < 25 (maximum rate = 35/min).
- If pH < 7.15: increase the rate to 35/min.
- If rate = 35/min and pH < 7.15: increase VT in 1 mL/kg steps until pH is greater than 7.15 (Pplat target may be exceeded); consider $NaHCO_3$ administration.

Weaning patients off the NHLBI ARDS protocol is described in a subsequent section of this chapter.

Initiating and Adjusting High-Frequency Ventilation

High-frequency ventilation is mechanical ventilation at frequencies between 150 to 900 breaths per minute, with tidal volumes as small as 1-2 mL/kg (significantly less than the anatomic deadspace). Gas transport at such low volumes likely involves various mechanisms, including bulk convection, "pendulluft," shear-type dispersion, and molecular diffusion. Because less pressure is transmitted to the distal airways and alveoli, high frequency ventilation decreases the risk of ventilator-associated lung injuries, such as barotrauma and bronchopulmonary dysplasia or BPD. High-frequency ventilation also may improve gas exchange in the presence of air leaks.

High-frequency ventilation is indicated primarily for patients with hypoxemic respiratory failure who have not responded to more conventional methods of improving oxygenation. Common scenarios include patients with severe IRDS/ARDS with or with air-leak syndrome. Additional indications specific to neonates include BPD, meconium aspiration, pulmonary interstitial edema, congenital diaphragmatic hernia, and pulmonary hypoplasia. Relative contraindications include hypotension/unstable cardiovascular status, the presence of air trapping/dynamic hyperinflation, and (among neonates) intracranial hemorrhage. Moreover, based on current evidence, high-frequency ventilation should not be applied if conventional ventilation can provide effective patient support.

The two primary mode of high-frequency ventilation in current use are high-frequency oscillation ventilation (HFOV) and high-frequency jet ventilation (HFJV). Gas delivery during HFOV is driven by an electromagnetic piston that oscillates a rubber diaphragm, much like a stereo speaker. Because the diaphragm pushes gas forward *and* draws gas back though the circuit, both inspiration and exhalation are active. Gas delivery during HFJV is controlled by an interrupter valve that rapidly opens and closes, causing intermittent "jets" or bursts of gas to be applied to the airway. With HFJV, inspiration is active but exhalation is passive.

In the U.S., the CareFusion (Sensormedics) 3100A is the mostly commonly HFOV device used with infants and small children (a separate model, the 3100B, is available for larger children and adults). The Bunnell LifePulse is the most commonly used device to deliver HFJV, with its application limited to infants and small children. Unlike the free-standing CareFusion HFOV device, the Bunnell LifePulse *always* is used in tandem with a conventional ventilator, which provides the background PEEP and IMV breaths as needed for alveolar recruitment and stabilization.

Table 10-12 compares HFOV and HFJV as delivered by these two different ventilators, including commonly recommended initial settings used on neonates, the parameters typically monitored, and how to adjust ventilation and oxygenation. In terms of adjusting ventilation or PaCO$_2$, the *primary* control variable for both HFOV and HFJV is ΔP, or the difference between the high and low oscillation/jet pressures. As with conventional ventilation, changes in frequency also can affect ventilation, but with lesser effect. Interestingly, frequency changes during HFOV affect CO$_2$ elimination in a manner opposite to that observed during conventional ventilation—that is, decreasing the HFOV frequency tends to lower the PaCO$_2$, while increasing the HFOV frequency tends to raise the PaCO$_2$. In terms of adjusting oxygenation, the *primary* control variables during both HFOV and HFJV are the mean airway pressure (Pmean) and FIO_2.

Table 10-12 Comparison of High-Frequency Oscillation and High-Frequency Jet Ventilation (Neonatal Application)

HFOV (CareFusion 3100A)	HFJV (Bunnell LifePulse)
Description	
Rapid "push-pull" of small volumes applied to airway via oscillating diaphragm (active inspiration *and* exhalation)	Rapid application of small bursts of gas to the airway via an interrupter valve (active inspiration with passive exhalation)
Ventilator Control Variables (Ranges)	
Frequency (3–15 Hz; 180–900/min)	Jet Ventilator
% I-time (30–50%)	Frequency (240-660/min; 6–11 Hz)
Bias flow (0–40 L/min)	PIP (8–50 cm H$_2$O)
Power/amplitude (1–10)	I-time (0.02–0.034 sec)
Pmean 3–45 cm H$_2$O	FIO_2 (.21–1.0; via external blender)
FIO_2 (.21–1.0 via external blender)	Companion (Standard) Ventilator
	PEEP (varies by device)
	FIO_2 (.21–1.0 to match jet ventilator)
	IMV breaths (varies by device)
Circuit	
External blender and heated humidifier system controls FIO_2 and conditions source gas	External blender and heated cartridge-type humidifier controls FIO_2 and conditions source gas
Specialized three-valve circuit delivers source gas, controls Pmean, and limits applied pressure (see Chapter 4 for details)	External box with electronically controlled "pinch valve" to provide gas bursts
	Special adapter placed between standard ventilator circuit "Y" and ET tube; provides jet port and pressure monitoring adapter

(continues)

Table 10-12 Comparison of High-Frequency Oscillation and High-Frequency Jet Ventilation (Neonatal Application) (*continued*)

HFOV (CareFusion 3100A)	HFJV (Bunnell LifePulse)
Typical Initial Settings for Neonates	
Frequency 10–15 Hz	Jet Ventilator
% I-time 33% (I:E 1:2)	Frequency 420/min (7 Hz)
Bias flow 10–20 L/min	PIP 0–2 cm H_2O < PIP on CMV
Power/amplitude 2-4[a]	I-time 0.02 sec
Pmean 10–20 cm H_2O[b]	Standard Ventilator
FIO_2 as needed for adequate PaO_2/SaO_2	PEEP
(*Note*: the larger the patient, the *lower* the frequency and the *higher* the applied bias flow, amplitude, and Pmean)	7–12 cm H_2O or
	2–4 cm H_2O < Pmean on CMV
	FIO_2 as needed for adequate PaO_2/SaO_2 IMV breaths
	Frequency 0-3/min
	I-time = 0.4–0.6 sec
	PIP 20–50% < HFJV PIP
Monitored Parameters	
Frequency	PIP
% I-time	ΔP
Pmean	P_{mean}
ΔP	PEEP
	Servo pressure[c]
	I:E ratio
Adjusting $PaCO_2$ (Ventilation)	
To Raise $PaCO_2$	To Raise $PaCO_2$
↓ power/amplitude (ΔP)	↓ PIP (ΔP)
↑ frequency	↑ frequency
To Lower $PaCO_2$	To Lower $PaCO_2$
↑ power/amplitude (ΔP)	↑ PIP (ΔP)
↓ frequency	↓ frequency
↑ % I-time	
Adjusting PaO_2 (Oxygenation)	
To Increase PaO_2/SaO_2	To Increase PaO_2/SaO_2
↑ Pmean	↑ Pmean (↑ PIP + PEEP equally so $\Delta P = K$)
↑ FIO_2	↑ FIO_2
↑ % I-time	↑ I-time
To Decrease PaO_2/SaO_2	↑ frequency (↑ I:E)
↓ FIO_2	To Decrease PaO_2/SaO_2
↓ Pmean	↓ Pmean (↓ PIP + PEEP equally so $\Delta P = K$)
	↓ FIO_2

[a] Adjust to get chest "wiggle"
[b] Set 1–5 cm H_2O higher than Pmean on VC or PC ventilation
[c] Pressure needed to maintain the desired PIP; rough indicator of changes in pulmonary mechanics
Hz = Hertz or cycles per second; PIP = peak inspiratory pressure; Pmean = mean airway pressure; CMV = conventional mechanical ventilation; ΔP = difference between high and low oscillation or jet applied pressures; % I-time = percent of total cycle time devoted to inspiration; K = constant.

Initiate and Modify Weaning Procedures

Patients receiving mechanical ventilation for respiratory failure should undergo a weaning assessment whenever the following criteria are met:

1. Evidence for some reversal of the underlying cause of respiratory failure
2. Adequate oxygenation (e.g., P/F ≥ 150–200, PEEP ≤ 5–8 cm H_2O, FiO_2 ≤ 0.4–0.5)
3. pH ≥7.25
4. Hemodynamic stability (no myocardial ischemia or significant hypotension)
5. The capability to initiate an inspiratory effort

In terms of the method for weaning acutely ill patients who meet these criteria, daily *spontaneous breathing trials* (SBTs) provide the quickest route for discontinuing mechanical ventilation. Tracking measures such as vital capacity and MIP/NIF while the patient is receiving ventilatory support can provide useful insights into weaning potential. However, a carefully monitored SBT provides the most valid information for deciding whether a patient can stay off the ventilator.

Spontaneous breathing modes used in SBT weaning protocols include (1) straight T-tube breathing, (2) CPAP, (3) pressure support, and (4) pressure support plus CPAP (i.e., BiPAP). Based on current evidence, no one approach appears to be better than the others. However, provision of CPAP during weaning can help improve breath triggering in patients who experience auto-PEEP.

SBT protocols vary somewhat by institution and unit—for example, surgical versus medical ICU. **Figure 10-6** provides a decision-making algorithm for a typical spontaneous breathing trial protocol. All such protocols involve initial assessment of the patient to ensure that he or she is ready to wean, using criteria such as those delineated above. The next step normally is application of a brief (2–5 minutes) supervised period of carefully monitored spontaneous breathing. During this "screening" phase, you assess the patient's breathing pattern, vital signs, and comfort level. If the patient tolerates the screening phase, you continue the SBT for at least 30 minutes, but no more than 120 minutes.

Objective physiologic measures indicating a successful SBT include the following:

- Acceptable gas exchange
  - SpO_2 ≥ 85–90% or PaO_2 ≥ 50–60 torr
  - pH ≥ 7.30
  - Increase in $PaCO_2$ ≤ 10 torr
- Stable hemodynamics
  - Heart rate < 120–140/min; change < 20%
  - Systolic blood pressure < 180–200 mm Hg and > 90 mm Hg; change < 20%
  - No vasopressors required
- Stable ventilatory pattern
  - Respiratory rate ≤ 30–35/min
  - Change in respiratory rate < 50%

If these objective indicators are not met, you should return the patient to a sufficient level of ventilatory support to maintain adequate oxygenation and ventilation and prevent muscle fatigue. Even when the patient meets these physiologic measures, you may need to discontinue the SBT if you note one or more of the following subjective indicators of intolerance or failure:

- Change in mental status (e.g., somnolence, coma, agitation, anxiety)
- Onset or worsening of discomfort
- Diaphoresis
- Signs of increased work of breathing:
  - Use of accessory respiratory muscles
  - Thoracoabdominal paradox

If a patient fails an SBT, you should work with the physician to determine the cause(s). Once these factors are identified and corrected, you should resume performing an SBT every 24 hours.

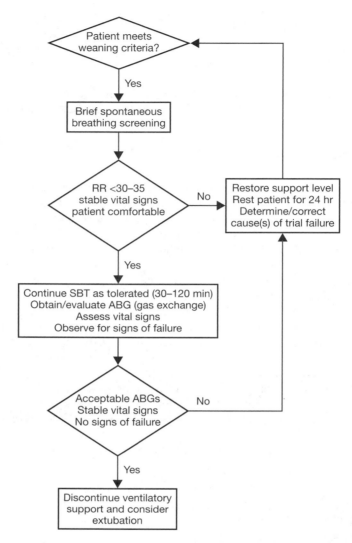

Figure 10-6 Example Algorithm for a Spontaneous Breathing Trial Protocol.

If the patient can maintain acceptable physiologic parameters and is able to tolerate the SBT for its full duration, you can consider extubation. The decision whether to proceed with extubation should be a separate consideration, based on assessment of the patient's airway patency and protective reflexes. Chapter 8 provides details on when and how to extubate a patient.

The NHLBI ARDS protocol follows these basic principles but uses a progressive transitioning from CPAP to pressure support to true unassisted spontaneous breathing. Details on this portion of the ARDS protocol are provided in the accompanying box.

NHLBI ARDS Protocol: Weaning Component

Criteria Indicating Readiness for a Spontaneous Breathing Trial

- $F_{IO_2} \leq 0.40$ and PEEP ≤ 8 cm H_2O, or $F_{IO_2} \leq 0.50$ and PEEP ≤ 5 cm H_2O

- PEEP and $F_{IO_2} \leq$ previous day's settings

- Patient has acceptable spontaneous breathing efforts (↓ vent rate by 50% for 5 minutes to detect effort)

- Systolic BP ≥ 90 mm Hg without vasopressors

- No neuromuscular blocking agents or blockade

Procedure

Initiate a spontaneous breathing trial of up to 120 minutes with $F_{IO_2} < 0.5$ and PEEP < 5 cm H_2O:

1. Place patient on T-piece, trach collar, or CPAP ≤ 5 cm H_2O with PS < 5 cm H_2O.

2. Assess for tolerance as follows for up to 2 hours:

   a. $Sp_{O_2} ≥ 90\%$ and/or $Pa_{O_2} ≥ 60$ mm Hg

   b. Spontaneous $V_T ≥ 4$ mL/kg PBW

   c. Respiratory rate ≤ 35/min

   d. pH ≥ 7.3

   e. No respiratory distress (distress = 2 or more of the following)

      ○ HR > 120% of baseline

      ○ Marked accessory muscle use

      ○ Abdominal paradox

      ○ Diaphoresis

      ○ Marked dyspnea

3. If tolerated for at least 30 minutes, consider extubation.

4. If not tolerated, resume preweaning settings.

Adapted from: National Heart, Lung, and Blood Institute, ARDS Clinical Network. *Mechanical ventilation protocol summary.* 2008. Available at: http://www.ardsnet.org.

Weaning from HFOV focuses mainly on oxygenation needs. As oxygenation improves in the adult HFOV patient, you should first lower the F_{IO_2} to 0.40, then slowly reduce Pmean by 2–3 cm H_2O every 4–6 hours until it is 20 cm H_2O or less. At this point, you should consider switching the patient to pressure control at a pressure limit less than or equal to 30 cm H_2O and PEEP of 10–12 cm H_2O. Thereafter, weaning should follow a standard SBT protocol, as previously described.

Administer Medications

One of your most frequent tasks as an RT is administration of bronchodilators, anti-inflammatory agents, mucolytics, or anti-infective agents to patients via the inhalation route. Depending on the preparation of these drugs, they may be delivered as either liquid or dry-powder aerosols. In certain circumstances, you may also administer specific drugs directly into the lungs via endotracheal instillation.

Aerosolized Drugs

Chapter 4 covers the selection, use, and troubleshooting of aerosol drug delivery systems, including small-volume nebulizers, metered-dose inhalers, dry-powder inhalers, and accessory equipment. Here we focus on the specific drugs available to you and offer general pointers regarding their administration.

Table 10-13 provides details on the most common drugs you may administer by aerosol, including their generic and brand names; available preparations; recommended adult doses; onset, peak, and duration of action; and recommended frequency of administration.

Regarding use of the beta-adrenergic (beta-agonist) bronchodilators, keep the following key points in mind:

- All beta-adrenergics have some cardiovascular and CNS effects; in general, you should select those with the least beta$_1$ and most beta$_2$ effects (e.g., albuterol or its isomer levalbuterol).
- Beta-adrenergics are best used as relievers of bronchospasm; corticosteroids should be used to control reactive airway disease.
- If also administering steroids, mucokinetics, or anti-infective agents by inhalation, always give the bronchodilator first.

Table 10-13 Medications Commonly Administered by the Inhalation Route

Generic Name	Brand Name(s)	Delivery and Preparation	Adult Dose and Frequency	Action	Comments
Beta-Adrenergic (Beta-Agonist) Bronchodilators					
Albuterol	Proventil Ventolin	SVN 0.5% MDI (90 mcg/puff) DPI (200 mcg/cap)	0.5 mL every 4–6 hr 2 puffs every 4–6 hr 1 puff every 4–6 hr	Onset: 5 min Peak: 30–60 min Duration: 3–8 hr (medium)	Mild CV/CNS side effects; can be mixed with cromolyn or ipratropium
Bitolterol	Tornalate	SVN 0.2% MDI (37 mcg/puff)	1.25 mL 3–4 times/day 2 puffs every 6 hr	Onset: 3–4 min Peak: 30–60 min Duration: 5–8 hr (medium)	Mild CV/CNS side effects; *do not* mix with other drugs
Epinephrine	Adrenalin	SVN 1% (1:100)	0.25–0.5 mL PRN	Onset: 3–5 min Peak: 5–20 min Duration: 1–3 hr (short)	Strong CV/CNS side effects
Formoterol	Foradil	DPI 25 mcg/puff	1 puff 2 times/day	Onset: 1–3 min P Peak: 30–60 min Duration: 12 hr (long)	Use only if inhaled steroids do not control the asthma; patients should seek treatment if symptoms worsen
Levalbuterol	Xopenex	SVN 0.31, 0.63, 1.25 mg in 3 mL diluent MDI 45 mcg/puff	3.0 mL 3 times/day 2 puffs every 4–6 hr	Onset: 15 min Peak: 1–1/2 hr Duration: 5–8 hr (medium)	Mild CV/CNS side effects
Metaproterenol	Alupent Metaprel	SVN 5% MDI (650 mcg/puff)	0.2–0.3 mL 2–3 puffs every 4–6 hr	Onset: 5–30 min Peak: 1/2–1 hr Duration: 1–6 hr (medium)	Mild CV/CNS side effects
Pirbuterol	Maxair	MDI (200 mcg/ puff)	2 puffs every 4–6 hr	Onset: 5 min Peak: 0.5–1 hr Duration: 3–5 hr (medium)	Mild CV/CNS side effects
Racemic epineph- rine	Vaponefrin Micronephrin	SVN 2.25%	0.25–0.5 mL PRN	Onset: 3–5 min Peak: 5–20 min Duration: 0.5–2 hr (short)	Used for upper airway inflammation (croup, post extubation); can cause "rebound" edema

Table 10-13 Medications Commonly Administered by the Inhalation Route

Salmeterol	Serevent	MDI 25 mcg/puff DPI 50 mcg/puff	2 puffs 2 times/day 1 puff 2 times/day	Onset: 10–20 min Peak: 3 hr Duration: 12 hr (long)	Use only if inhaled steroids do not control the asthma; patients should seek treatment if symptoms worsen
Terbutaline sulfate	Bricanyl	DPI 500 mcg/puff	2 puffs every 4–6 hr	Onset: 5–30 min Peak: 0.5–1 hr Duration: 3–6 hr (medium)	Mild CV/CNS side effects
Anticholinergic Bronchodilators					
Ipratropium bromide	Atrovent Atrovent HFA	SVN 500 mcg/vial MDI 17 mcg/puff	1 vial 3–4 times/day 2 puffs every 6 hr	Onset: 15–30 min Peak: 1–2 hr Duration: 4–5 hr	Avoid eye contact with aerosol (can cause or worsen narrow-angle glaucoma); contraindicated in patients hypersensitive to atropine
Tiotropium bromide	Spiriva	DPI 18 mcg/capsule	2 puffs 1 time/day	Onset: 30 min Peak: 3–4 hr Duration: ≥ 24 hr	Avoid eye contact with aerosol (can cause or worsen narrow-angle glaucoma); contraindicated in patients hypersensitive to atropine
Adrenergic + Anticholinergic Combinations					
Ipratropium + albuterol	Combivent DuoNeb	SVN 2.5 mg albuterol + 0.5 mg ipratropium MDI 90 mcg albuterol + 18 mcg ipratropium	3 mL (unit dose) 3–4 times/day 2 puffs 3–4 times/day	As per component (see above)	As per component (see above)
Corticosteroids					
Beclomethasone	Vanceril Beclovent	MDI 40 mcg/puff MDI 80 mcg/puff	2 puffs 2 times/day	Varies	Have patient rinse mouth with water after therapy to prevent pharyngitis and oral candidiasis

(*continues*)

Table 10-13 Medications Commonly Administered by the Inhalation Route (*continued*)

Generic Name	Brand Name(s)	Delivery and Preparation	Adult Dose and Frequency	Action	Comments
Budesonide	Pulmicort	DPI 200 mcg/puff SVN 0.25/0.5 mg/2 mL	1–3 puffs 2 times/day 2 mL (unit dose) 2 times/day	Onset: within 24 hr Duration: varies	Have patient rinse mouth with water after therapy to prevent pharyngitis and oral candidiasis
Flunisolide	AeroBid	MDI 250 mcg/puff	2 puffs 2 times/day	Varies	Have patient rinse mouth with water after therapy to prevent pharyngitis and oral candidiasis
Fluticasone propro-nate	Flovent Flovent Rotadisk	MDI 44/110/220 mcg/puff DPI 50/100/250 mcg	2 puffs 4 times/day 100 mcg inhalation 2 times/day	Onset: within 24 hr Duration: 2–3 days	Have patient rinse mouth with water after therapy to prevent pharyngitis and oral candidiasis
Triamcinolone acetonide	Azmacot	MDI 100 mcg/ puff	2 puffs 3–4 times/day	Varies	Have patient rinse mouth with water after therapy to prevent pharyngitis and oral candidiasis
Corticosteroids + Adrenergic Combinations					
Fluticasone + salmeterol	Advair Diskus	100, 250, or 500 mcg fluticasone + 50 mcg salmeterol	1 puff 2 times/day	As per component (see above)	As per component (see above)
Mast Cell Stabilizers					
Cromolyn sodium	Intal	MDI 800 mcg/puff SVN 20 mg/2 mL amp	2–4 puffs 3–4 times/day 1 ampule 3–4 times/day	Onset: 20–30 min Duration: 2–6 hr	Not for acute bronchospasm; can be mixed with albuterol
Mucokinetics					
Acetylcysteine	Mucomyst	10/20% (4-, 10-, 30-mL vials)	6–10 mL 10% 3–4 times/day (dilute 20% for equivalency)	Decreases sputum viscosity on contact	Can cause bronchospasm; give bronchodi-lator first

Table 10-13 Medications Commonly Administered by the Inhalation Route (*continued*)

Dornase alpha	Pulmozyme	2.5 mL single-use ampule (1.0 mg/mL)	1 ampule/day or 2 times/day	Decreases sputum viscosity on contact	Can cause bronchospasm; give bronchodilator first; do not mix with other drugs
Hypertonic saline	N/A	3–7%	4-6 mL 2 times/day	In patients with cystic fibrosis, rehydrates airway surface's liquid layer and induces cough; may have anti-inflammatory and anti-infective properties	Give bronchodilator first; good choice for CF patients intolerant of dornase alpha
Anti-infectives					
Colistimethate polymyxin E	Colistin Coly-Mycin	150-mg vials (powder); add 2 mL sterile H₂O	37.5–150 mg every 8–12 hr	Antipseudomonal agent	Requires valved nebulizer (Pari LC Plus)
Tobramycin	Tobi	300 mg in 5-mL saline ampule	300 mg every 12 hr for 28 days, then 28 days off	Antipseudomonal agent	Many side effects; do not mix with other drugs; give bronchodilator first; requires valved nebulizer (Pari LC Plus)
Cayston	Aztreonam	75-mg unit dose vial reconstituted with 1 mL 0.17% saline	3 times/day for 28 days, then 28 days off	Antipseudomonal agent	Give bronchodilator first; requires Altera mesh nebulizer
Zanamivir	Relenza	DPI 5 mg/blister	10 mg (2 blisters) 2 times/day for 5 days	Stops viral replication (influenza A and B)	Not for use in asthma or COPD patients; if bronchospasm develops, stop therapy and treat immediately

CF = cystic fibrosis; CV = cardiovascular; DPI = dry powder inhaler; mcg = microgram; MDI = metered dose inhaler; SVN = small volume nebulizer

- In acute exacerbations of asthma, repeat the standard dose every 20 minutes (up to 3 times) or provide continuous nebulization until symptoms are relieved.
- Long-acting beta-adrenergics such as salmeterol (Serevent) should be used for asthma only if inhaled steroids do not provide control of symptoms.
- For maintenance therapy of bronchospasm in patients with COPD, consider an anticholinergic such as ipratropium or tiotropium.

In terms of administration of inhaled corticosteroids, you need to remember the following essentials:

- Inhaled corticosteroids control inflammation and are the first-line drugs for mild persistent asthma.
- With the exception of budesonide (Pulmicort), common inhaled steroid preparations are all intended for used in a metered-dose inhaler (MDI) or dry-powder inhaler (DPI); therefore, proper technique is critical.
- Rinsing the mouth after therapy is essential to prevent pharyngitis and oral candidiasis.
- Use of spacers or valved holding chambers with MDI-delivered steroids minimizes pharyngeal deposition and the incidence of pharyngitis and candidiasis.

In administering mucokinetics, you need to be aware of the following issues:

- All mucokinetics are irritating to the airway; to prevent bronchospasm, always precede treatment with a bronchodilator.
- Acetylcysteine can be instilled directly into the airway via ET tube.
- Mucokinetics should be administered in combination with bronchial hygiene to facilitate secretions removal.

Regarding use of inhaled anti-infective agents, keep in mind the following key points:

- Aerosolized antibiotics (Colistin, Cayston, Tobramycin) are generally indicated only in patients with cystic fibrosis (CF) and suspected or confirmed *Pseudomonas aeruginosa* pulmonary infections.
- If the patient is receiving several inhaled medications, the recommended order is bronchodilator first, followed by mucolytic, then bronchial hygiene therapy, then steroids, and finally the aerosolized antibiotics.

Endotracheal Instillation

Selected drugs can be administered as liquids or "instilled" directly into the lungs via a tracheal airway. You may be asked to instill lidocaine, epinephrine, atropine, or naloxone ("L-E-A-N") in emergency situations when IV access is not available. Guidelines for endotracheal instillation of these agents include the following:

- Make sure the dose administered is 2–2.5 times greater than the IV dose.
- Dilute the drug dose with 10 mL of sterile water or saline for injection.
- Put the patient in a supine position (not Trendelenberg).
- Halt chest compressions.
- Instill the drug through a catheter that passes beyond the ET tube tip.
- Immediately after instillation, provide 5–10 rapid inflations via a bag-valve resuscitator.

Other than mucokinetics, the only other respiratory agent you may be asked to administer by endotracheal instillation is surfactant. Surfactant preparations are administered prophylactically to infants at high risk of developing respiratory distress syndrome (RDS), or as rescue therapy for those infants with clinical evidence of RDS. When administering surfactant to these patients, be sure to do the following:

- Recommend a chest x-ray before instillation to confirm ET tube position.
- Suction the infant prior to administration if necessary.
- Monitor the patient's SpO_2 and ECG continuously.

- Use a 5-Fr feeding tube or suction catheter to instill the solution.
- Insert the installation catheter up to, but not past, the tip of the ET tube.
- Split the dose in half, and instill half a dose into each dependent bronchus (turning the infant from side to side).
- Administer the dose as rapidly as tolerated.
- After administration, bag the infant for 1–2 minutes.
- Carefully monitor blood gases and chest wall movement during the first 3 hours after dosing.
- Adjust the ventilator settings and F_{IO_2} as appropriate (the patient may transiently require higher levels of ventilatory support).
- If possible, avoid suctioning for 6 hours following instillation.

Treating and Preventing Hypoxemia

You should suspect hypoxemia whenever a patient exhibits one or more of the following signs or symptoms:

- Tachypnea or tachycardia
- Dyspnea
- Cyanosis
- Hypertension or peripheral vasoconstriction
- Disorientation/confusion, headache, or somnolence

You should also suspect hypoxemia in cases in which poor oxygenation is common, such as in postoperative patients and those suffering from carbon monoxide or cyanide poisoning, shock, trauma, or acute myocardial infarction. Documented hypoxemia exists regardless of the patient's condition when the patient's Pa_{O_2} is less than 60 torr or the arterial saturation is less than 90% on room air.

Treating Hypoxemia

You normally treat suspected or documented hypoxemia by administering oxygen. However, when hypoxemia is caused by shunting, O_2 therapy alone is insufficient to remedy it. You know that hypoxemia is due to significant shunting when the P/F ratio (Chapter 12) drops below 200 or you cannot maintain satisfactory arterial oxygenation on 50% or more oxygen (i.e., $Pa_{O_2} \leq 50$ torr on $F_{IO_2} \geq 0.50$). In these cases, the recommended treatment normally is CPAP or PEEP, as previously discussed. An additional method that can help raise the Pa_{O_2} level in patients suffering from refractory hypoxemia is to use patient positioning to decrease shunting.

Chapter 4 provides some detail regarding the selection and use of O_2 therapy devices. However, once the proper device is selected, the following guidelines apply to titrating O_2 therapy:

- In otherwise normal patients, adjust the flow and F_{IO_2} to the lowest level needed to maintain normal oxygenation (i.e., Pa_{O_2} of 80–100 torr with saturation $\geq 92\%$).
- If you cannot maintain normal oxygenation on less than 50% oxygen, accept a $Pa_{O_2} \geq 55$–60 torr with a $Sa_{O_2}/Sp_{O_2} \geq 88\%$.
- When treating patients with carbon monoxide poisoning, cyanide poisoning, acute pulmonary edema, shock, trauma, or acute myocardial infarction in emergency settings, provide the highest possible F_{IO_2}.
- For patients with chronic hypercapnia, aim to keep the Pa_{O_2} in the 55–60 torr range to prevent depression of ventilation.
- In low-birth-weight or preterm infants at risk for retinopathy of prematurity, your goal should be a Pa_{O_2} in the 50–80 torr range.

Patient positioning can be used to alter the distribution of ventilation and perfusion, and thereby improve oxygenation without raising the F_{IO_2}. Patient positioning may also decrease the incidence of pneumonia in certain patients. **Table 10-14** describes positioning techniques you need to be familiar with and their appropriate use.

Table 10-14 Patient Positioning Techniques to Minimize Hypoxemia

Position	Use/Recommend	Comments
Semi-Fowler's position (head of the bed elevated 30° or more)	To minimize ventilator-associated pneumonia in patients receiving mechanical ventilation	• Use on all ventilator-supported patients unless contraindicated • Helps prevent aspiration • Improves the distribution of ventilation • Enhances diaphragmatic action
Lateral rotation therapy	To prevent or minimize respiratory complications associated with immobility in bedridden patients	• Employs a bed or air mattress system that automatically turns the patient from side to side • Improves drainage of secretions within the lung and lower airways • Increases the FRC (by increasing the critical opening pressure to the independent lung)
"Keeping the good lung down"	To improve oxygenation in patients with unilateral lung disease	• Patient is positioned in the left or right lateral decubitus position with the good lung down • Improves oxygenation by diverting most blood flow and ventilation to the dependent (good) lung • Exceptions in which the good lung is kept up include (1) lung abscess or bleeding and (2) unilateral pulmonary interstitial emphysema in infants
Prone positioning	To improve oxygenation in patients with ARDS and refractory hypoxemia	• Improves oxygenation by shifting blood flow to better-aerated lung regions; may also improve diaphragmatic action • Facilitated by devices that support the chest and pelvis, leaving the abdomen freely suspended • Trial of "proning" is recommended in patients with ARDS if oxygenation is inadequate on $FIO_2 \geq 0.6$ and PEEP ≥ 10 cm H_2O • Not all patients will benefit from this positioning; a significant increase in PaO_2 (more than 10 torr) in first 30 minutes is a good indicator of success (if tolerated) • Not recommended for patients whose heads cannot be in a face-down position, for those who have circulatory problems, for those with a fractured pelvis, and for those who are morbidly obese • Major risks include extubation and dislodgement of intravascular catheters

Prevent Procedure-Associated Hypoxemia

Hypoxemia is a complication associated with many procedures you perform as an RT, including postural drainage, suctioning, and exercise testing. In addition, in patients being treated for acute lung injury or ARDS, hypoxemia can occur whenever the patient is removed from CPAP/PEEP.

The first rule in preventing this type of hypoxemia is to ensure that the patient is adequately oxygenated before implementing the procedure. For this reason, you should always monitor the patient's SpO_2 with a pulse oximeter prior to, during, and after any procedure that can cause hypoxemia. If a patient develops mild hypoxemia during a procedure, you should increase the FIO_2. If, however, a patient develops moderate to severe hypoxemia during a procedure, you should immediately stop what you are doing and provide the patient with as high an FIO_2 as possible.

Suctioning is a special case, because it involves both removal of oxygen and reduction of lung volume. For this reason, you should hyperoxygenate the patient for 30–60 seconds before suctioning and limit suction time to no more than 10–15 seconds. Patients receiving ventilatory support, especially with CPAP/PEEP, require additional consideration when being suctioned. First, use the hyperoxygenation button provided on most ICU ventilators, which typically provides 100% O_2 for 1–2 minutes without loss of CPAP/PEEP. Second, consider using an inline/closed catheter suction system, especially in patients with pre-existing hypoxemia. This allows you to suction patients while they are still receiving ventilatory support, including CPAP/PEEP. An alternative is to use a special swivel adapter that provides a self-sealing port through which you can pass a standard suction catheter (or bronchoscope) while the patient is still on the ventilator.

Of special concern are those patients receiving low tidal volumes to protect against ventilator-associated lung injury—that is, patients being managed via the ARDS protocol. These patients are particularly prone to loss of lung volume. In these cases, you need to restore or maintain the patient's lung volume. The method by which you restore lung volume is called a *recruitment maneuver*. A commonly used recruitment maneuver involves applying a high level of PEEP for a set period of time. One common implementation of this maneuver involves the following steps:

1. Ensure hemodynamic stability.
2. Set the F_{IO_2} to 1.0.
3. Wait 10 minutes.
4. Apply 30–40 cm H_2O PEEP (or 10 cm H_2O above the plateau pressure).
5. Maintain the pressure for 30–45 seconds.
6. Return the ventilator to the previous settings.

You will know that the recruitment is successful if the patient's oxygenation is restored or improved and either the static compliance increases or the slope of the patient's pressure–volume loop increases.

COMMON ERRORS TO AVOID

You can improve your score by avoiding these mistakes:

- Never use or recommend incentive spirometry for patients who cannot cooperate.
- Never administer IPPB to a patient with an untreated tension pneumothorax.
- Never use NPPV for patients who do not have control over their upper airway or cannot manage their secretions.
- Whenever possible, avoid plateau pressures greater than 30 cm H_2O during mechanical ventilation.
- Do not use or recommend high-frequency oscillation ventilation for patients with obstructive lung disease.
- Do not use or recommend mast cell stabilizers (cromolyn sodium) for patients with acute bronchospasm.
- Never mix tobramycin (Tobi) with other drugs for inhalation.
- Avoid suctioning (if possible) for 6 hours following surfactant instillation.
- Never withhold supplemental oxygen from a patient who needs it.

SURE BETS

In some situations, you can be sure of the right approach to a clinical problem or scenario:

- To confirm patient understanding of muscle training, incentive spirometry, or IPPB, always require a "return demonstration" by the patient.
- To prevent hyperventilation during IPPB, always instruct the patient to breathe slowly.
- When initiating mechanical ventilation, always use a high F_{IO_2} (0.60–0.90) until an ABG can be obtained.

- Except with ARDS patients, when initiating mechanical ventilation, set the initial V_T to 8–10 mL/kg PBW when targeting volume or set the pressure limit to 20–30 cm H_2O when targeting pressure.
- To adjust a patient's $Paco_2$/pH during mechanical ventilation, always change the rate first; change the V_T/pressure limit only if rate changes exceed the recommended adult limits (8–24 breaths/min and up to 35/min for adults with ARDS).
- Unless contraindicated, always use an oronasal/"full" face mask when initiating NPPV for patients with acute respiratory failure.
- To avoid esophageal opening/gastric distension, always keep IPAP levels during NPPV below 20–25 cm H_2O.
- Whenever a patient's cardiac output or blood pressure falls when the PEEP level is raised, decrease PEEP back to its prior setting.
- Always give the bronchodilator first when it is ordered in combination with a mucokinetic or anti-infective agent.
- To prevent pharyngitis and oral candidiasis with inhaled steroids, always have patients rinse their mouth out after administration of these medications.
- When treating patients with carbon monoxide poisoning, cyanide poisoning, acute pulmonary edema, shock, trauma, or acute myocardial infarction in emergency settings, always provide the highest possible Fio_2.

PRE-TEST ANSWERS AND EXPLANATIONS

Following are this chapter's pre-test answers and explanations. Be sure to review each answer's explanation thoroughly to help you understand why it is correct. If the explanation is still unclear to you, review the chapter content.

10-1. **Correct answer: C.** Increase the oxygen concentration immediately before suctioning. Most cardiac arrhythmias during suctioning are due to arterial hypoxemia. The best way to prevent or minimize arterial hypoxemia during suctioning is to preoxygenate the patient for 1–2 minutes and to keep suction time to less than 10–15 seconds.

10-2. **Correct answer: B.** Put the patient in the prone position. In patients with a generalized decrease in lung volume (as in ARDS), use of the prone position can improve oxygenation by shifting blood flow to lung regions that are better aerated and by facilitating better movement of the diaphragm.

10-3. **Correct answer: C.** At least 30% of the maximum inspiratory pressure (MIP/PI_{max}). For inspiratory training to be effective, the load against which the patient breathes must be sufficient to increase muscle strength—generally at least 30% of the MIP/PI_{max}.

10-4. **Correct answer: B.** Exhale slowly. Patients with severe emphysema tend to have highly compliant (floppy) airways. To help prevent airway collapse and air trapping, these patients should be instructed to exhale slowly. Teaching these patients to purse their lips while exhaling also can help prevent airway collapse by creating low levels of positive pressure.

10-5. **Correct answer: D.** 1, 2, and 3. IPPB can impede venous return to the heart by increasing intrathoracic pressures. Patients with poor venomotor tone or those who are already hypotensive due to conditions such as shock or cardiac insufficiency are particularly prone to this effect. A patient's cardiovascular status should be assessed before administering IPPB.

10-6. **Correct answer: A.** 1 or 2 only. The mode of ventilatory support initially chosen depends mainly on the patient's underlying pathophysiologic problem. When a patient's respiratory failure is associated with hypercapnia due to inadequate alveolar ventilation—as in this case—either the A/C or SIMV mode (with equivalent rate settings) should be employed.

10-7. **Correct answer: D.** Decreasing the bias flow. Increasing the HFOV power/amplitude is usually the first step to increase CO_2 elimination and lower the Pa_{CO_2}. *Decreasing* the frequency can also lower the Pa_{CO_2} (note that frequency changes during HFOV affect CO_2 elimination in a manner opposite to that observed during conventional mechanical ventilation). If hypercapnia is severe despite use of the maximum power/amplitude and lowest frequency settings, you can also consider creating a cuff leak to enhance CO_2 removal. Decreasing the bias flow tends to lower the Pmean and negatively affect oxygenation.

10-8. **Correct answer: D.** Mask continuous positive airway pressure (CPAP) with 80% O_2. A patient with congestive heart failure who is coughing up pink, frothy sputum is likely suffering from acute cardiogenic pulmonary edema. The blood gas indicates a fully compensated respiratory alkalosis secondary to severe hypoxemia (due to the pulmonary edema). The goal is to restore adequate oxygenation and maintain alveolar inflation. High concentrations of oxygen combined with noninvasive positive pressure (mask CPAP or BiPAP) are generally indicated in such instances. The positive pressure (1) helps keep alveoli open, (2) reduces venous return to the right heart, and (3) lowers pulmonary vascular pressures. These effects, in turn, decrease fluid movement into the interstitial space and alveoli and improve oxygenation.

10-9. **Correct answer: D.** Endotracheal tube. Some medications can be delivered via endotracheal tube. Specifically, cardiovascular medications and lidocaine, epinephrine, atropine, and nalaxone ("L-E-A-N") can be delivered via endotracheal tube safely.

10-10. **Correct answer: C.** Change to the SIMV mode with a set rate of 10 breaths/min. The blood gas indicates a partially compensated respiratory alkalosis, most likely the result of the patient initiating 10 machine breaths above the set rate. By changing to SIMV the patient's additional spontaneous breaths (above 10/min) not trigger extra machine breaths, thereby reducing the minute ventilation, raising the Pa_{CO_2} and lowering the pH.

10-11. **Correct answer: C.** Add pressure support. The key problem is the patient's rapid spontaneous breathing rate and low spontaneous tidal volume. The spontaneous tidal volume = [total minute volume – set minute volume]/[total rate – set rate] = [10,000 – 6000]/[38 – 10] = 4000/28 = 143 mL. To increase the spontaneous VT, you should add pressure support.

10-12. **Correct answer: C.** Increase PEEP. The goal of PEEP is to achieve adequate oxygenation with a safe F_{IO_2}. In this case, the F_{IO_2} is dangerously high, but shunting persists. Given the Pa_{O_2} of 55 torr, the PEEP level should be increased.

10-13. **Correct answer: C.** The patients should hold a maximum inspiratory capacity (IC) breath for at least 5 seconds. The "sustained maximum inspiration" underlying incentive spirometry is essentially an inspiratory capacity maneuver, followed by a 5-10 second breath hold.

10-14. **Correct answer: B.** Of the available options, the best choice to identify the presence of auto-PEEP would be a flow versus time display. When displaying flow versus time, auto-PEEP would be indicated when the expiratory flow waveform fails to return to baseline before the next machine breath. A volume versus flow X-Y loop also can be used to detect auto-PEEP.

10-15. **Correct answer: A.** Nonrebreathing mask at 15 L/min. When treating patients with carbon monoxide poisoning, cyanide poisoning, acute pulmonary edema, shock, trauma, or acute myocardial infarction in emergency settings, always provide the highest possible F_{IO_2}. Of the devices listed, only the nonrebreathing mask can deliver high F_{IO_2} levels.

10-16. **Correct answer: C.** Increasing EPAP to 10 cm H_2O. This patient's hypoxemia is due to shunting ($Pa_{O_2} \leq 50$ torr, $F_{IO_2} \geq 0.50$). If shunting is present when you are administering NPPV for acute respiratory failure, you should increase the EPAP level, while being sure to keep ΔP (IPAP – EPAP) ≥ 5 cm H_2O.

10-17. **Correct answer: B.** Postponing weaning and reevaluating the patient. Although the patient's vital capacity and MIP/NIF are borderline adequate, the tidal volume is very low (less than 4 mL/kg). The (missing) spontaneous breathing rate is too high (calculated as 10 L/min ÷ 0.250 L/breath = 40 breaths/min). This yields a rapid shallow breathing index of 40/0.25 = 160, which is far above the threshold of 105. You should recommend postponing weaning and reevaluating the patient at a later time.

10-18. **Correct answer: B.** 30 cm H_2O plateau pressure. According to the NHLBI protocol, the target volume for ARDS patients is 4–6 mL/kg, with a maximum plateau (alveolar) pressure of 30 cm H_2O. The ventilator rate should initially be set to match the prior $\dot{V}E$, but can be increased as needed up to a maximum of 35 breaths/min.

10-19. **Correct answer: D.** Increasing the SIMV rate. The blood gas indicates uncompensated respiratory acidosis. To lower the $Paco_2$ and raise the pH, the patient's minute ventilation needs to be increased. Because the tidal volume is in the acceptable range (about 8 mL/kg), the best way to increase this patient's minute ventilation would be to increase the SIMV rate.

10-20. **Correct answer: B.** Ending the trial and returning the patient to a full ventilatory support mode. In this case, the rise in $Paco_2$ exceeds the limit (10 torr) for acceptable gas exchange; the increased rate of breathing and the greater accessory muscle use suggest intolerance of the procedure. For these reasons, you should return the patient to full ventilatory support.

POST-TEST

To confirm your mastery of this chapter's topical content, you should take the chapter post-test, available online at http://go.jblearning.com/respexamreview. A score of 80% or more indicates that you are adequately prepared for this section of the NBRC written exams. If you score less than 80%, you should continue to review the applicable chapter content. In addition, you may want to access and review the relevant Web links covering this chapter's content (courtesy of RTBoardReview.com), also online at the Jones & Bartlett Learning site.

Evaluate and Monitor the Patient's Objective and Subjective Responses to Respiratory Care

Narciso E. Rodriguez

This chapter covers basic noninvasive and invasive assessment procedures, as well as techniques that the NBRC expects you to apply when evaluating a patient's response to therapy. Heavy emphasis in this section should be given to high-level mastery of this content, as the majority of NBRC exam questions will involve either application or analysis.

OBJECTIVES

In preparing for the shared NBRC exam content, you should demonstrate the knowledge needed to:

1. Recommend and review chest radiographs
2. Obtain blood samples
3. Interpret the results of the following tests:
   a. Blood gas, pulse, and hemoximetry analyses
   b. Capnography
   c. Transcutaneous monitoring
   d. Hemodynamic assessment (covered in Chapters 2–4)
4. Measure and record vital signs
5. Monitor cardiac rhythms
6. Evaluate fluid balance (covered in Chapter 13)
7. Interpret bronchoprovocation studies
8. Recommend blood tests (covered in Chapter 4)
9. Observe for changes in sputum characteristics
10. Auscultate the chest and interpret breath sounds
11. Observe for patient–ventilator asynchrony
12. Adjust and check alarm systems
13. Measure F_{IO_2} and/or oxygen flow
14. Monitor and assess airway pressures
15. Interpret ventilator graphics

WHAT TO EXPECT ON THIS CATEGORY OF THE NBRC EXAMS

CRT exam: 15 questions; about 20% recall, 50% application, and 30% analysis
WRRT exam: 9 questions; 100% analysis
CSE exam: indeterminate number of questions; however, exam III-E knowledge underlies most CSE Information Gathering sections

PRE-TEST

Carefully respond to each of the following questions. After completing the pre-test, compare your answers to those provided at the end of this chapter. Then thoroughly review each answer's explanation to help understand why it is correct.

11-1. The emergency department physician asks you to review a chest x-ray from a patient with history of severe emphysema. Which of the following findings would you expect to observe on this film?
1. A wide mediastinum
2. An increase in peripheral vascular markings
3. A lowered, flattened diaphragm
4. An increased radiolucency in the lung fields
5. Presence of bullae and blebs

A. 2 and 3 only
B. 3, 4, and 5 only
C. 2, 3, and 5 only
D. 1, 2, 3, 4, and 5

11-2. When using a pulse oximetry device, what is the most common source of error and false alarms?
A. Patient motion artifact
B. Presence of HbCO
C. Presence of vascular dyes
D. Ambient light detection

11-3. A patient receiving volume control A/C ventilation is making asynchronous breathing efforts against the ventilator's controlled breaths. What will be the result?
A. Decreased ventilatory drive
B. Increased physiologic deadspace
C. Increased work of breathing
D. Acute metabolic acidosis

11-4. A patient on a 30% aerosol oxygen mask has the following ABG results:

pH	7.54
$Paco_2$	27 torr
Pao_2	80 torr
HCO_3	23 mEq/L
BE	−2 mEq/L

Which of the following is the correct interpretation of this ABG?

A. Acute alveolar hyperventilation without hypoxemia
B. Partially compensated respiratory alkalosis
C. Respiratory acidemia with hypoxemia
D. Hypochloremic metabolic alkalosis

11-5. You find a patient receiving volume control SIMV with a preset rate of 12 breaths/min, a V_T of 500 mL, and a PEEP of 10 cm H_2O. You note a peak inspiratory pressure of 50 cm H_2O for each mechanical breath. Which of the following alarm settings are appropriate for this patient?
1. Low exhaled minute volume at 8 L/min
2. Inspiratory:expiratory (I:E) ratio alarm at 1:1
3. High inspiratory pressure limit at 65 cm H_2O
4. Low PEEP/CPAP pressure alarm at 5 cm H_2O

A. 1, 2, and 3 only
B. 2 and 3 only
C. 2, 3, and 4 only
D. 1 and 4 only

11-6. Arterial hemoglobin saturation should be kept above what level to guarantee adequate oxygen delivery to the tissues?
A. 60%
B. 70%
C. 80%
D. 90%

11-7. A new medical resident asks for your help in calculating the static lung compliance for an ICU patient receiving volume control A/C ventilation. The patient has the following settings and monitoring data:

V_T	700 mL
Rate	12/min
Peak pressure	50 cm H_2O
Plateau pressure	30 cm H_2O
PEEP	10 cm H_2O
Mechanical deadspace	100 mL

What is the patient's static lung compliance?

A. 18 mL/cm H_2O
B. 35 mL/cm H_2O
C. 22 mL/cm H_2O
D. 26 mL/cm H_2O

11-8. A doctor wants your recommendation on how to monitor the cardiopulmonary status of a patient undergoing a bronchoscopy procedure during moderate sedation. Which of the following should you recommend?
A. Pulmonary function testing
B. Noninvasive pulse oximetry
C. Frequent ABGs via radial puncture
D. Transcutaneous Pao_2 monitoring

11-9. A patient receiving 30% O_2 has a Pao_2 of 66 torr and $Paco_2$ of 32 torr. Which of the following best describes this patient's oxygenation status?
- **A.** A mild disturbance of oxygenation consistent with hypoventilation
- **B.** A mild disturbance of oxygenation consistent with a V/Q imbalance
- **C.** A moderate disturbance of oxygenation consistent with acute lung injury
- **D.** A severe disturbance of oxygenation consistent with ARDS

11-10. A mechanically ventilated patient is being monitored by a capnograph in the ICU. The nurse calls you STAT to the room and you note that the $Petco_2$ dropped suddenly from 36 torr to 0 torr. All of the following are possible causes of this finding *except*:
- **A.** Ventilator disconnection
- **B.** Increased cardiac output
- **C.** Obstructed artificial airway
- **D.** Cardiac arrest

11-11. During a patient–ventilator system check, you notice the following airway pressures on an adult mechanically ventilated patient receiving 5 cm H_2O of PEEP:

	Time		
Measure	**0400**	**0500**	**0600**
Peak pressure (cm H_2O)	42	47	53
Plateau pressure (cm H_2O)	32	36	42

Knowing that no ventilator setting changes have been made, what is the most likely cause of these changes?

- **A.** The patient is developing bronchospasm.
- **B.** The patient's lungs are becoming more compliant.
- **C.** The patient is performing a Valsalva maneuver.
- **D.** The patient is developing atelectasis.

11-12. Common arterial sites used for percutaneous arterial blood sampling include all of the following *except*:
- **A.** Carotid
- **B.** Radial
- **C.** Brachial
- **D.** Femoral

11-13. On reviewing the ABG report on a patient, you note a $Paco_2$ of 25 torr, a base excess (BE) of −10 mEq/L, and a pH of 7.35. How would you characterize this acid–base abnormality?
- **A.** Compensated metabolic acidosis
- **B.** Acute (uncompensated) metabolic acidosis
- **C.** Compensated respiratory alkalosis
- **D.** Acute (uncompensated) respiratory alkalosis

11-14. You have just inserted an arterial catheter into the radial artery of an ICU patient. What is a good indication that the catheter has been successfully inserted in an artery?
- **A.** Presence of collateral circulation
- **B.** A good blood return
- **C.** Ability to flush the line
- **D.** Proper blood pressure waveform

11-15. A blood sample obtained from the distal port of a PA catheter has a Po_2 of 95 torr and a %HbO_2 of 97%. Which of the following statements could explain these results?
1. The catheter balloon remained inflated during sampling.
2. The catheter is misplaced in the right ventricle.
3. The blood sample was withdrawn too quickly.
4. The patient has an abnormally low cardiac output.
- **A.** 1, 2, and 3 only
- **B.** 2, 3, and 4 only
- **C.** 1 and 3 only
- **D.** 1 and 4 only

11-16. You need to provide continuous monitoring of the Fio_2 for a ventilator that uses a heated humidifier delivery system. The only analyzer available is a galvanic fuel cell analyzer. Where should you place the analyzer's sensor?
- **A.** Downstream/after the heated humidifier
- **B.** On the expiratory side of the circuit
- **C.** Upstream/before the heated humidifier
- **D.** As close to the patient as possible

11-17. Capillary blood sampling commonly is used with infants to assess
1. Ventilation
2. Oxygenation
3. Acid–base status
   A. 1, 2, and 3
   B. 2 and 3 only
   C. 1 and 2 only
   D. 1 and 3 only

11-18. After performing a modified Allen's test on the left hand of a patient, you note that his palm and fingers do not become pink for more than 15 seconds after releasing pressure on the ulnar artery. At this point, what should you do?
A. Use the left brachial site for sampling
B. Repeat the test on the right hand
C. Use the femoral site for sampling
D. Go ahead and draw the sample from that site

11-19. A 20-year-old, 65-kg (143-lb) patient is receiving volume control SIMV with a set rate of 14 breaths/min, a total rate of 14 breaths/min, a V_T of 500 mL, and an F_{IO_2} of 0.50. ABG results are as follows:

pH	7.52
Pa_{CO_2}	26 torr
HCO_3	23 mEq/L
Pa_{O_2}	94 torr

What are the appropriate recommendations for you to make?

A. Decrease the SIMV rate
B. Add mechanical deadspace
C. Decrease the F_{IO_2}
D. Add pressure support

11-20. You observe a sudden drop in the peak inspiratory pressure when monitoring a patient receiving volume control A/C ventilation. Which of the following may explain this change?
1. A defective exhalation valve
2. A torn ET tube cuff
3. A high V_T setting
4. Patient disconnection
   A. 2 and 4 only
   B. 3 only

C. 1, 2, and 4 only
D. 2, 3, and 4 only

11-21. The ER physician asks you to evaluate a trauma patient who was the victim of a house fire. To properly evaluate the cardiopulmonary status of this patient, you would evaluate all of the following *except*:
A. Breath sounds
B. Pulse O_2 saturation
C. Sensorium
D. Breathing pattern

11-22. While a surgical resident is inserting a chest tube on a patient in ICU, you notice the following changes in vital signs:

Heart rate	129/min (up from 103/min)
BP	155/90 mm Hg (up from 132/88 mm Hg)
Respiratory rate	38/min (up from 22/min)
Temperature	99.3°F

At this point, what should you recommend?

A. Paralyzing the patient
B. Repositioning the chest tube
C. Calling for the rapid response team
D. Assess the patient for pain

11-23. A patient with a size 8.0 tracheostomy tube is being suctioned by the nurse. While suctioning the patient, you observe several PVCs on the patient's monitor. What should you recommend that the nurse do?
A. Use a larger suction catheter
B. Preoxygenate the patient with 100% O_2
C. Sedate the patient prior to suction
D. Suction less often

11-24. A pulmonologist asks you to assess airway responsiveness during a PFT exam. He wants to rule out asthma from chronic bronchitis in a patient who is experiencing nocturnal wheezing. You should consider all of the following tests *except*:
A. Thoracic gas volume
B. Exercise challenge test
C. Histamine challenge test
D. Methacholine challenge test

11-25. A comatose patient breathing room air has an a/A ratio of 0.85 but is hypoxemic. What is the likely cause of the hypoxemia?

A. Laboratory error
B. V/Q imbalance
C. Hypoventilation
D. Pulmonary shunting

WHAT YOU NEED TO KNOW: ESSENTIAL CONTENT

Recommend and Review Chest Radiographs

Chest x-rays are used to evaluate lung and thoracic structures. You should *recommend* a chest x-ray to identify pathologic lung or chest abnormalities; assess disease progression; and locate lines, catheters, and tube positions. Descriptions of the most common normal and abnormal x-ray findings are delineated in **Table 11-1**.

The chest x-ray also is the best way to confirm proper placement of tracheal airways. However, you always should do your best to verify tube placement before a chest x-ray is taken. To do so,

Table 11-1 Common Chest X-Ray Findings in Adults

Condition	Radiograph Findings
Abnormalities of the chest wall	• Broken ribs: consider flail chest • Kyphoscoliosis/lordosis: causes lung restriction and decreases lung volumes
Acute respiratory distress syndrome (ARDS)	• Nonhomogeneous bilateral lung opacities (white-out) and infiltrates with normal heart size consistent with pulmonary edema
Airway complications	• Right (common) or left mainstem intubation; opposite lung tends to collapse • Tracheal narrowing (tracheal stenosis) or tracheal dilation (tracheomalacia) • Tracheal edema and inflammation: croup ("steeple sign" on AP film) and epiglottis ("thumb sign" on lateral neck x-ray) • Mucus plugging; causes affected lobe or segment to collapse
Atelectasis	• Increased radiopacity (whiteness) in the film • Air bronchograms due to tissue collapse around opened airways • Elevated hemidiaphragm on the affected side • Shift of trachea and mediastinum toward the affected side
Consolidation or infiltration	• Air bronchograms: airways silhouette surrounded by collapsed tissue • Increased radiopacity (whiteness) of the affected area
Congestive heart failure (CHF)	• Increased vascular markings • Cardiomegaly: increased heart size (cardiothoracic ratio > 50%) • Presence of pleura effusions/Kerley B lines
Emphysema (COPD)	• Lowered, flattened diaphragms • Decreased lung and vascular markings (hyperaeration, radiolucency) • Increased retrosternal air space (lateral film) • Presence of bullae/blebs (pockets of air in the lung parenchyma) • Narrow mediastinum
Pleura effusion	• Homogeneous areas of increased density that are position dependent, confirmed by a lateral decubitus x-ray • Loss of sharp costophrenic angles • Presence of a meniscus at the fluid–air interface

(continues)

Table 11-1 Common Chest X-Ray Findings in Adults (*continued*)

Condition	Radiograph Findings
Pneumothorax	• Loss of peripheral lung markings • Air between the lung margin and chest wall (radiolucent space) • Mediastinal shift to the opposite side • Diaphragm may be depressed on the affected side • Sulcus sign (deepening of the costophrenic angles observed on supine films)
Pulmonary edema	• Fluffy or patchy densities in the perihilar areas and in gravity-dependent lower lung fields • May be accompanied by cardiomegaly, pleural effusions, and air bronchograms

confirm bilateral breath sounds and absent epigastric sounds, and obtain a positive result using a CO_2 colorimetry device or capnograph. Subsequently, a chest x-ray should show the tube tip about 4–6 cm above the carina or between T2 and T4 (adults), which minimizes the chances for tube movement down into the bronchi (endobronchial intubation) or up into the larynx (extubation).

You also should be able to recommend proper x-ray positions according to the patient scenario. Posteroanterior (PA) films are recommended for ambulatory patients, who stand upright during maximum inspiration. The anteroposterior (AP) projection is most commonly used for ICU portable films. On an AP film, the heart shadow is magnified and typically the film quality is inferior to the PA technique. Lateral views (in combination with AP or PA films) are helpful in assessing for free fluid in the pleural space (pleural effusion).

Obtaining Blood Samples

Indications for blood gas and hemoximetry sampling and analysis are detailed in Chapter 3. Chapter 6 reviews sample analysis and related quality control procedures. Here we focus on the key elements involved in obtaining the samples and interpreting the results.

Arterial Sampling by Puncture

The radial artery is the preferred site for obtaining arterial blood for two reasons: (1) it is located near the skin surface and is not close to any large veins, and (2) the ulnar artery provides for collateral circulation. Other potential sites for sampling include the brachial, femoral, and dorsalis pedis arteries. These sites carry greater risk and should be used only by those with the proper training.

Key points in performing a radial arterial puncture for ABG analysis include the following:

- Choose the nondominant wrist first.
- Assess collateral circulation by performing the modified Allen's test (**Figure 11-1**).
  - If collateral circulation is not present on the initial side, assess the other wrist.
  - If both sides lack collateral circulation, use the brachial artery.
- After needle withdrawal, compress the site until the bleeding stops. Patients with a prolonged PT, PTT, or International Normalized Ratio (INR) may require longer compression times.
- After hemostasis is ensured, apply a sterile bandage over the puncture site; recheck the site after 20 minutes and document the procedure.
- Apply the methods outlined in Chapter 6 to avoid preanalytic errors.

Obtaining Blood Samples from Vascular Lines

If you need to obtain repeated arterial samples over several days or need to continually monitor blood pressure, you should recommend placement of an indwelling arterial catheter, or "A-line." In the NBRC hospital, RTs may be responsible for the insertion and care of arterial lines. The accompanying box outlines the key elements involved in inserting an arterial line. Chapter 5 provides details on infection control procedures for indwelling catheters.

Either direct cannulation or the guidewire (Seldinger) technique are used to insert the catheter. With direct cannulation, you puncture the artery with a needle sheathed in a catheter. Once blood is observed "flashing" at the needle hub, the catheter sheath is advanced over the needle into

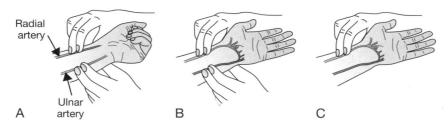

Radial artery

Ulnar artery

A   B   C

Figure 11-1 Modified Allen's Test. (A) Patient's hand is clenched while you obstruct flow to both the radial and ulnar arteries for about 5 seconds. **(B)** The patient opens his or her hand while you maintain pressure; the hand should appear blanched. **(C)** Upon release of pressure on the ulnar artery, the palmar surface should flush within 5–10 seconds and color should be restored. Prolonged delay before flushing indicates decreased ulnar artery flow.

Adapted from: Shapiro BA, Harrison RA, Walton JR. *Clinical application of blood gases* (2nd ed.). Chicago, IL: Year Book Medical; 1977.

the artery, and the needle is removed. With the Seldinger technique, you puncture the artery with a needle, then thread a small guidewire through the needle into the vessel. Next, you remove the needle, leaving the guidewire in place. Finally, you advance the catheter over the guidewire into the artery and remove the guidewire.

Figure 11-2 shows the basic equipment used to maintain an indwelling arterial catheter. Once inserted, this catheter is connected to a continuous flush device. The flush device keeps the line open via a continuous low flow of fluid through the system. To maintain continuous flow, the IV bag must be pressurized to 300 mm Hg, usually by a hand bulb pump. A pressure transducer, connected to the flush device, provides an electrical signal to a monitor, which displays the arterial pressure waveform. A sampling port (not shown in Figure 11-2) typically is included to allow intermittent blood withdrawal.

Two different procedures are used to obtain blood samples from vascular lines: the three-way stopcock method and the in-line closed reservoir method (**Table 11-2**). Given that closed reservoir sampling minimizes blood waste, reduces the potential for contamination, and better protects against exposure to bloodborne pathogens than the stopcock method, it is becoming the standard approach in many intensive care units.

When obtaining a blood sample from a PA or Swan-Ganz catheter (mixed venous blood), the following points must be considered:

- To avoid contamination with arterialized blood and falsely high O_2 levels, the sample must be drawn *slowly* from the catheter's distal port *with the balloon deflated*.
- Attention must be paid to the IV infusion rate through the catheter to prevent sample dilution.
- When obtaining arterial and mixed venous samples to calculate cardiac output (using the Fick equation), *both* samples must be drawn *at the same time*.

Key Elements Involved in Arterial Line Insertion

- Ensure that a "time-out" is performed before the procedure.
- Ensure that monitoring system is set up and calibrated, with lines properly flushed.
- Scrub the insertion site with chlorhexidine and cover area with sterile drape.
- Puncture skin at point of pulsation at 30-degree angle, with needle bevel and hub arrow up.
- Advance catheter into position, connect to transducer tubing, and flush the line.
- *Confirm proper arterial waveform on monitor*; reposition catheter if needed.
- Secure line to prevent traction on catheter.
- Cover line insertion point with a clear sterile dressing.
- Recheck for adequacy of distal blood flow and patient comfort.
- Instruct patient on line use and safety considerations.

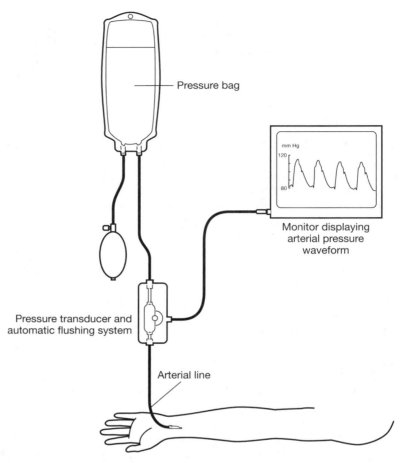

Pressure bag

mm Hg
120
80

Monitor displaying
arterial pressure
waveform

Pressure transducer and
automatic flushing system

Arterial line

Figure 11-2 Indwelling Arterial Catheter System.

Adapted from: Wilkins RL, Stoller JK, Scanlan CL, eds. *Egan's fundamentals of respiratory care* (8th ed.). St. Louis, MO: Mosby; 2003. Courtesy of Elsevier Ltd.

Table 11-2 Procedures for Obtaining Blood Samples from an Arterial Line (Adult Patient)

Three-Way Stopcock Sampling	In-line Closed Reservoir Sampling
• Swab sample port with chlorhexidine, povidone-iodine, or alcohol.	• Slowly draw blood into the reservoir to the needed fill volume.
• Attach waste syringe and turn stopcock off to flush solution/bag.	• Close the reservoir shut-off valve.
• Aspirate 5–6 mL blood (at least 6 times the "dead" volume).	• Swab sample port with chlorhexidine, povidone-iodine, or alcohol.
• Turn stopcock off to the port.	• Attach the blunt/needleless sampling syringe to the valved sampling port.
• Remove waste syringe and properly discard it.	• Aspirate the needed volume of blood.
• Secure heparinized syringe to port, reopen stopcock, collect sample.	• Open the reservoir shut-off valve.
• Turn stopcock off to the port, remove syringe.	• Slowly depress reservoir plunger to reinfuse blood into patient.
• Flush line until clear.	• Reswab sample port and flush line until clear.
• Turn stopcock off to patient, briefly flush sampling port, reswab sample port.	• Confirm restoration of arterial pulse pressure waveform.
• Turn stopcock off to the port and confirm restoration of arterial pulse pressure waveform.	

Obtaining a Capillary Blood Sample

Capillary blood gas sampling is used in infants and toddlers when a blood sample is needed to assess ventilation and acid–base status but arterial access is not available. Capillary sampling is less invasive, quicker, and easier to perform than arterial puncture. This sampling technique is contra-indicated when accurate analysis of oxygenation is needed and in neonates less than 24 hours old.

When obtaining a capillary blood sample:

- Gather the needed equipment: lancet, alcohol pad, sterile gauze, adhesive bandage, and preheparinized capillary tube with tube caps, and (if more than 30 minutes' delay will occur before analysis of the sample) a bag with ice slush.
- Select the site (e.g., heel, great toe, earlobe). Avoid inflamed, swollen, or edematous tissue or cyanotic or poorly perfused areas. For heel sticks, avoid the posterior curvature and puncture the lateral sides only (see **Figure 11-3**).
- Use a warm cloth or warming pack to warm the site for 3–5 minutes to no higher than 42–45°C.
- Puncture the skin with the lancet and wipe away the first drop of blood.
- Allowing the free flow of blood, collect the sample from the middle of the blood drop (do not squeeze the site).
- Fill the tube, cap its ends, and send it for analysis.

Arterial Blood Gas Interpretation

When assessing blood gas results, we recommend that you *first* assess acid–base status and then separately evaluate oxygenation.

Acid–Base Status

Follow these steps to properly assess the acid–base components of an arterial blood gas:

1. Categorize the pH (increased, decreased, or normal).
2. Determine the respiratory involvement ($Paco_2$ increased, decreased, or normal).
3. Determine the metabolic involvement (HCO_3 increased, decreased, or normal).
4. Assess for compensation.

Chapter 1 reviews normal ABG parameters and describes how to identify the four *primary* acid–base disturbances using just the pH and $Paco_2$. Here we focus on assessing *compensation* for these primary disturbances and identifying combined acid–base problems.

Blood pH is controlled by a balance between the buffering and excretion of fixed acids by the kidneys and the elimination of CO_2 by the lungs. Specifically, pH is determined by the ratio of the blood buffer/base bicarbonate (HCO_3) to the dissolved CO_2 in the blood:

$$pH \propto \frac{HCO_3^-}{Paco_2}$$

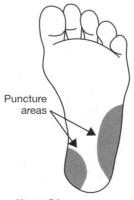

Puncture areas

Figure 11-3 Capillary Blood Sampling Sites.

Table 11-3 Primary Acid–Base Disorders and Compensatory Responses

Acid–Base Disorder	Primary Event	Compensatory Response	Base Excess
Respiratory acidosis	$\downarrow pH = \dfrac{HCO_3}{\uparrow Paco_2}$	$\leftrightarrow pH = \dfrac{\Uparrow HCO_3}{\uparrow Paco_2}$	> +2 mEq/L
Respiratory alkalosis	$\uparrow pH = \dfrac{HCO_3}{\downarrow Paco_2}$	$\leftrightarrow pH = \dfrac{\Downarrow HCO_3}{\downarrow Paco_2}$	< –2 mEq/L
Metabolic acidosis	$\downarrow pH = \dfrac{\downarrow HCO_3}{Paco_2}$	$\leftrightarrow pH = \dfrac{\downarrow HCO_3}{\Downarrow Paco_2}$	< –2 mEq/L
Metabolic alkalosis	$\uparrow pH = \dfrac{\uparrow HCO_3}{Paco_2}$	$\leftrightarrow pH = \dfrac{\uparrow HCO_3}{\Uparrow Paco_2}$	> +2 mEq/L

$\uparrow$ = primary increase; $\downarrow$ = primary decrease; $\Uparrow$ = compensatory increase; $\Downarrow$ = compensatory decrease; $\leftrightarrow$ restoration.

Compensation occurs when the system *not* affected by the primary disturbance attempts to restore the pH back to normal. Using respiratory acidosis as an example, if the lungs retain CO_2, the $Paco_2$ rises (the primary event). Based on the balance between base (HCO_3) and acid (dissolved CO_2), an increase in the $Paco_2$ will lower the blood pH (respiratory acidosis). To compensate, the system *not affected* (the kidneys) tries to restore the pH by increasing blood levels of HCO_3 (the compensatory response). As HCO_3 levels rise, the pH is restored back toward normal. **Table 11-3** summarizes these changes (primary events and compensatory responses).

By combining assessment of the $Paco_2$ and BE ($\pm$ 2 mEq/L), you can quickly identify whether compensation is occurring. *Compensation is occurring if both the $Paco_2$ and BE are abnormally high or low.* To determine which disturbance is primary, you look at the pH (see **Table 11-4**). If the pH is less than 7.40, the primary problem is the one causing acidosis. If the pH exceeds 7.40, the primary problem is the one causing alkalosis.

You can also use the pH to determine whether compensation is full or partial. Compensation is "full" if the pH is in the normal range (7.35–7.45); otherwise, compensation is termed "partial." In general, renal/metabolic compensation for primary respiratory disorders is slow (hours to days), whereas respiratory compensation for primary renal/metabolic disorders is fast (minutes). Indeed, *a failure of the lungs to quickly compensate for a primary renal/metabolic acid–base disturbance indicates impaired pulmonary function.*

When the $Paco_2$ and BE diverge in opposite directions (one abnormally high and the other abnormally low), a combined acid–base disturbance exists. A high $Paco_2$ and low BE define a combined respiratory *and* metabolic acidosis, while a low $Paco_2$ and high BE define a combined respiratory *and* metabolic alkalosis.

Evaluating Oxygenation

For monitoring and assessment of the patient's response to O_2, the Pao_2 and Sao_2 results always need to be compared against the patient's Fio_2. Four common indices are used to perform this assessment: (1) the alveolar to arterial O_2 tension gradient [$P(A\text{-}a)o_2$]; (2) the ratio of Pao_2 to Fio_2 (Pao_2/Fio_2, or P/F ratio); (3) the ratio of arterial to alveolar Po_2 (Pao_2/Pao_2 or a/A ratio); and (4) the

Table 11-4 Using Base Excess to Assess for Compensation

Paco₂	BE	pH	Acid–Base Disturbance
> 45 torr	> +2 mEq/L	> 7.40	Compensated *metabolic* alkalosis
		< 7.40	Compensated *respiratory* acidosis
< 35 torr	< –2 mEq/L	> 7.40	Compensated *respiratory* alkalosis
		< 7.40	Compensated *metabolic* acidosis

oxygenation index (OI). We also recommend applying a simple rule of thumb when assessing oxygenation in the NBRC "hospital."

Alveolar to Arterial O_2 Tension Gradient or $P(A\text{-}a)O_2$

To calculate a patient's alveolar–arterial O_2 tension gradient, you must first compute the alveolar oxygen tension (P_{AO_2}). To do so, apply the alveolar air equation:

$$P_{AO_2} = F_{IO_2} (P_B - P_{H_2O}) - 1.25 \times P_{aCO_2}$$

At sea level (the likely condition on the NBRC exam), this equation simplifies to

$$P_{AO_2} = F_{IO_2} (713) - 1.25 \times P_{aCO_2}$$

As an example, if a patient breathing 100% O_2 ($F_{IO_2} = 1$) has a P_{aO_2} of 250 torr and a P_{aCO_2} of 60 torr, the $P_{A O_2}$ would be computed as

$$P_{AO_2} = 1.0 (713) - 1.25 \times 60$$
$$P_{AO_2} = 713 - 75$$
$$P_{AO_2} = 638 \text{ torr}$$

To compute the $P(A\text{-}a)O_2$, simply subtract the P_{aO_2} from the calculated P_{AO_2}. Continuing our example:

$$P(A\text{-}a)O_2 = 638 - 250$$
$$P(A\text{-}a)O_2 = 388 \text{ torr}$$

The following key points pertain to interpreting the $P(A\text{-}a)O_2$:

- A normal $P(A\text{-}a)O_2$ on room air is about 5–10 torr.
- A normal $P(A\text{-}a)O_2$ on 100% O_2 is about 25–65 torr.
- Every 100 torr $P(A\text{-}a)O_2$ on 100% equals about a 5% shunt.

In our example, the $P(A\text{-}a)O_2$ of 388 torr is clearly abnormal, indicating the presence of almost a 20% intrapulmonary shunt ($388/100 = 3.8 \times 5 = 19\%$).

Ratio of P_{aO_2} to F_{IO_2} or P/F Ratio

Because the $P(A\text{-}a)O_2$ is time consuming to compute and varies with the F_{IO_2}, most clinicians prefer using the P/F ratio to assess oxygenation. Continuing the example, our patient's P/F ratio would be computed as follows:

$$P_{aO_2}/F_{IO_2} = 250/1.0 = 250$$

A P/F ratio between 200 and 300 indicates a mild disturbance of oxygenation (such as V/Q imbalance). A ratio between 100 and 200 indicates a moderate disturbance of oxygenation (due to shunting) consistent with acute lung injury (ALI). Finally, a P/F ratio less than 100 indicates a severe disturbance of oxygenation/severe shunting consistent with ARDS.

Ratio of P_{aO_2} to P_{AO_2} or a/A Ratio

The arterial-to-alveolar tension ratio (P_{aO_2}/P_{AO_2}) or a/A ratio is another oxygenation index. Like the $P(A\text{-}a)O_2$, the a/A ratio requires calculation of the P_{AO_2}. The a/A ratio for healthy individuals exceeds 0.75. An a/A ratio between 0.35 and 0.75 is caused by V/Q mismatch, with ratios less than 0.35 indicating intrapulmonary shunting.

Oxygenation Index

For patients receiving mechanical ventilation, some clinicians use a more comprehensive indicator of oxygenation status called the oxygenation index (OI), which was originally used in neonatal medicine to predict mortality and the need for extracorporeal membrane oxygenation (ECMO). The OI combines the P/F ratio (actually its inverse) with the mean airway pressure or MAP, which strongly correlates with the patient's oxygenation needs. You calculate the OI using the following equation:

$$OI = \frac{MAP \times F_{IO_2} \times 100}{Pa_{O_2}}$$

In adults with ARDS, OI values greater than 8 coincide with P/F ratios less than 200 (signifying ALI). In general, OI values greater than 20 indicate a severe oxygenation disturbance for which nonconventional modes of ventilation such as high-frequency oscillation should be considered. OI values greater than 40 are associated with very high mortality and are used to justify the need for ECMO in infants.

Oxygenation Rule of Thumb

A simple approach to assessing oxygenation (and one that will serve you well on the NBRC exam) is the 60/60 rule of thumb. This rule states that if the Pa_{O_2} is less than 60 torr on an F_{IO_2} greater than 0.60, then there is a severe disturbance in oxygenation, due mainly to shunting (refractory hypoxemia). A variation of this rule uses a Pa_{O_2} less than 50 torr on an F_{IO_2} greater than 0.5 to indicate refractory hypoxemia (the 50/50 rule). Note that both conditions correspond to a P/F ratio less than or equal to 100.

Causes of Hypoxemia and Appropriate Treatments

Table 11-5 describes the three major causes of hypoxemia, the basis for their classification, and their treatment. V/Q imbalances are the primary mechanism causing hypoxemia in most common lung diseases, such as asthma, bronchitis, and emphysema. V/Q imbalances generally respond well to O_2 therapy. In contrast, when hypoxemia is due to shunting, PEEP or CPAP is needed to improve oxygenation.

Evaluating CO-Oximetry Results

Table 11-6 provides the reference ranges for laboratory CO-oximetry analysis.
Essential points regarding the interpretation of CO-oximetry results include the following:

- Elevated blood HbCO levels can be caused by exposure to tobacco smoke, faulty gas furnaces, automobile exhaust, or smoky fires. *In these situations, standard pulse oximetry will provide falsely high values* and should not be used to assess for hypoxemia.

Table 11-5 Causes, Recognition, and Treatment of Hypoxemia

Cause of Hypoxemia	Basis for Conclusion	Recommended Treatment
Hypoventilation	• Hypercapnia • $P(A-a)O_2$ difference: normal • a/A, P/F ratios: normal	Increase ventilation
V/Q imbalance	• Normal Pa_{CO_2} • Pa_{O_2} > 60 torr with F_{IO_2} < 0.6 • P/F ratio: 200–300 • a/A ratio: 0.35–0.75	Increase F_{IO_2}
Shunt	• Pa_{CO_2} may be normal or abnormal • Pa_{O_2} < 60 torr with F_{IO_2} > 0.6 • $P(A-a)$ difference: > 300 torr (100% O_2) • P/F ratio: < 200 • a/A ratio: < 0.35	Add PEEP or CPAP

Table 11-6 Reference Ranges for Laboratory CO-Oximetry Analysis

Component	Whole Blood	Normal Values
Total Hb	Newborn	14.0–24.0 g/dL
	Adult male	13.5–16.5 g/dL
	Adult female	12.0–15.0 g/dL
Sao$_2$ (%HbO$_2$)	Arterial	92–99% (room air)
O$_2$ content (Cao$_2$)	Arterial	15–23 mL/dL
%HbCO	Nonsmokers	< 1.5% of total Hb
	Smokers	1.5–5.0% of total Hb
	Heavy smokers	5.0–9.0% of total Hb
%MetHb		< 3% of total Hb
%SHb		0%

- Elevated metHb may be hereditary or acquired through exposure to certain chemicals (e.g., nitrites, nitrates, chlorates, quinones, benzenes, nitrotoluenes) or drugs (benzocaine, nitroglycerin, nitroprusside).
- If the sum of the abnormal hemoglobins (HbCO + metHb + SHb) exceeds 15%, the O$_2$ carrying capacity of the blood is severely reduced.
- The presence of vascular dyes and high lipid intake (e.g., parenteral nutrition) can falsely decrease total Hb and Sao$_2$.
- Elevated bilirubin levels (common in infants) can falsely increase total Hb, HbO$_2$, and metHb levels.

Obtaining and Interpreting Pulse Oximetry Data

Pulse oximetry measures arterial hemoglobin saturation using noninvasive plethysmographic and spectrophotometric methods. Chapter 3 outlines the indications for pulse oximetry. Chapter 4 provides details on the setup, assembly, and troubleshooting of these devices. Here we focus on how to obtain good pulse oximetry data and the interpretation of this vital information.

When assessing and monitoring a patient with a pulse oximeter, the following steps are important to remember:

- Select a site for probe application, checking for adequate perfusion. Remove the patient's nail polish if necessary and clean the site with an alcohol prep pad.
- Attach the probe to the selected site and allow for proper stabilization. Observe the oximeter pulse rate and correlate it with palpated heart or ECG rate. Evaluate also for proper waveform or strength signal (if available).
- Document and interpret the pulse rate, Spo$_2$, and Fio$_2$ being delivered (and turn trend monitoring on for overnight oximetry, if ordered).
- Always interpret the Spo$_2$ in combination with Hb/Hct levels. For example, a patient with an Spo$_2$ of 97% and severe anemia (Hb < 7 g/dL) is predisposed to tissue hypoxia due to reduced blood O$_2$ content.
- Whenever possible, pulse oximetry values should be calibrated against CO-oximetry analysis of a baseline arterial blood sample.

Standard pulse oximeters provide relatively accurate (±2–4%) estimates of oxyhemoglobin saturation, as long as there are no abnormal hemoglobins present and the perfusion is good. The Spo$_2$ normally is greater than 93–95% on breathing room air. Levels less than 90% indicate the need for supplemental O$_2$ therapy (consider the margin of error). To relate the Spo$_2$ to the approximate Pao$_2$, use the "40-50-60/70-80-90" rule of thumb. According to this rule, Hb saturations of 70%, 80%, and 90% are about equal to Pao$_2$ values of 40, 50, and 60 torr, respectively. Drops in Spo$_2$ are usually the result of cardiac, pulmonary, or combined cardiopulmonary disease. Significant declines (more than 4–5%) during exercise or sleep are abnormal.

Table 11-7 Factors Causing Erroneous SpO_2 Readings

Factor	Potential Error
Presence of HbCO (e.g., smoke inhalation injury)	Falsely high $\%HbO_2$
Presence of high levels of metHb	Falsely low $\%HbO_2$ if $SaO_2 > 85\%$
	Falsely high $\%HbO_2$ if $SaO_2 < 85\%$
Anemia (low hematocrit)	Falsely low $\%HbO_2$
Vascular dyes (e.g., methylene blue)	Falsely low $\%HbO_2$
Dark skin pigmentation and nail polish	Falsely high $\%HbO_2$ (3–5%)
Ambient light	Varies (e.g., falsely high $\%HbO_2$ in sunlight); may also cause falsely high pulse reading
Poor perfusion and vasoconstriction	Inadequate signal; unpredictable results

Source: Scanlan CL. Analysis and monitoring of gas exchange. In Wilkins RL, Stoller JK, Scanlan CL, eds. *Egan's fundamentals of respiratory care* (8th ed.). St. Louis, MO: Mosby; 2003.

The most common source of errors and false alarms with pulse oximetry is motion artifact. To minimize this problem, consider relocating the sensor to an alternative site. **Table 11-7** outlines other factors that can cause erroneous SpO_2 readings and the expected direction of error. Note also that pulse oximeters provide little useful data when the PaO_2 rises above 100 torr (hyperoxia).

Obtaining and Interpreting Capnography Data

Capnography involves the measurement and display of CO_2 concentrations during breathing. Chapter 3 outlines the indications for capnography. Chapter 6 provides details on the setup and calibration of capnographs. Here we focus on interpretation of basic capnography data.

In healthy individuals, P_{ETCO_2} averages 1–5 torr less than arterial CO_2. **Table 11-8** differentiates between the causes of sudden and gradual changes in P_{ETCO_2} readings.

Most capnographs provide continuous breath-by-breath display of inspired and exhaled CO_2 concentrations. **Figure 11-4** depicts the components of the normal CO_2 waveform for one full breathing cycle. Note that in patients with COPD, CHF, auto-PEEP, V/Q mismatch, and pulmonary emboli, a clear alveolar plateau phase may never occur. **Table 11-9** describes the most common scenarios found during capnography.

Table 11-8 Conditions Associated with Changes in P_{ETCO_2}

	Rise in P_{ETCO_2}	Fall in P_{ETCO_2}
Sudden change	• Sudden increase in cardiac output (e.g., return of spontaneous circulation [ROSC] during CPR) • Sudden release of a tourniquet • Injection of sodium bicarbonate	• Sudden hyperventilation • Sudden drop in cardiac output/cardiac arrest* • Massive pulmonary/air embolism • Circuit leak/disconnection* • Esophageal intubation* • ET/trach tube obstruction or dislodgement*
Gradual change	• Hypoventilation • Increased metabolism/CO_2 production • Rapid rise in temperature (malignant hyperthermia)	• Hyperventilation • Decreased metabolism/CO_2 production • Decreased pulmonary perfusion • Decrease in body temperature

*Can result in a P_{ETCO_2} of 0 torr.

Source: Scanlan CL. Analysis and monitoring of gas exchange. In Wilkins RL, Stoller JK, Scanlan CL, eds. *Egan's fundamentals of respiratory care* (8th ed.). St. Louis, MO: Mosby; 2003.

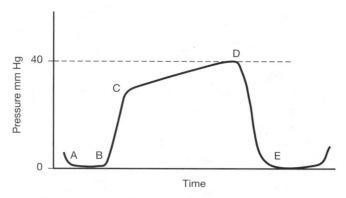

Figure 11-4 Normal End-Tidal CO$_2$ Waveform. A to B: Exhalation of pure deadspace gas. No exhaled CO$_2$ present. B to C: Combination of deadspace and alveolar gas. Exhaled CO$_2$ begins to rise. C to D: Alveolar plateau, exhalation of alveolar CO$_2$. PETCO$_2$ normally is measured at the end of the alveolar plateau. D to E: Inhalation of fresh gas (%CO$_2$ drops to zero).

Table 11-9 Common PETCO$_2$ Waveform Descriptions

Event	Example Capnogram	Possible Causes
Sudden decrease of exhaled CO$_2$ to zero baseline		• Esophageal intubation • Disconnection from ventilator • Ventilator malfunction/failure • Obstructed/kinked ET tube
Gradual decrease of exhaled CO$_2$ waveform		• Hyperventilation • Hypothermia • Sedation • Hypovolemia • Decreased CO$_2$ production
Gradual increase of exhaled CO$_2$ waveform		• Hypoventilation • Rising body temperature • Partial airway obstruction • Rewarming after surgery • Seizure, shivering, pain • Bicarbonate administration • COPD exacerbation • Increased cardiac output
Rise in waveform baseline		• Addition of mechanical deadspace to ventilator circuit

Table 11-10 Resolving Problems When Using Capnographs

Problem	Cause	Action
CO_2 values are erratic	Mechanically ventilated patient breathing spontaneously	No action needed
	Airway/circuit leak	Check for/correct cuff or ventilator circuit leaks
	Sampling line leak (sidestream units only)	Check for/correct sampling line connections
	Water or sputum blocking the sensor window (mainstream units only)	Clean or replace sensor; recalibrate device
CO_2 values higher or lower than expected	Physiological cause	Check patient
	Ventilator malfunction	Check ventilator and patient
	Improper calibration	Recalibrate unit
	Sampling line kinked/clogged (sidestream units only— gives "0" reading)	Unkink/unclog or replace sampling line
	Condensation trap full (sidestream units only)	Empty or replace moisture trap
	BTPS setting OFF (CO_2 values will be falsely high)	Turn BTPS correction ON

Several problems commonly occur when using capnographs. **Table 11-10** describes these common problems, their likely causes, and the appropriate actions to resolve them.

Interpreting Transcutaneous Monitoring Data

Chapter 3 lists the indications for transcutaneous monitoring of arterial P_{O_2} and P_{CO_2}, while Chapter 4 describes the setup and assembly, use, and troubleshooting of these devices. Here the focus is on interpretation of transcutaneous monitoring data.

Regarding P_{tcCO_2}, research indicates that it closely approximates Pa_{CO_2} under most clinical conditions. The close correlation between P_{tcCO_2} and Pa_{CO_2} makes this measure useful in assessing real-time changes in ventilation during mechanical ventilation. On the other hand, P_{tcO_2} is equivalent to Pa_{O_2} only in well-perfused patients and when Pa_{O_2} is less than 100 torr. The P_{tcO_2} value underestimates the Pa_{O_2} value in perfusion states causing vasoconstriction (e.g., low cardiac output, shock, and dehydration) and when Pa_{O_2} is greater than 100 torr. P_{tcO_2} also underestimates Pa_{O_2} in children and adults (due to their thicker skin) and when the sensor is underheated, when the sensor is placed on a bony surface, or too much pressure or contact gel is applied.

Due to the many factors affecting the correlation between P_{tcO_2} and Pa_{O_2}, most clinicians recommend that continuous measurement of this parameter be used primarily for trend monitoring, with the P_{tcO_2} maintained in the 50–80 torr range in neonates. If more precision is needed, it is recommended that the P_{tcO_2} be "calibrated" against a simultaneous Pa_{O_2} measurement. If the Pa_{O_2} value is substantially higher than the P_{tcO_2} and Pa_{O_2} values, poor peripheral circulation is the likely cause.

One well-accepted application is to assess if right-to-left shunting is occurring through the ductus arteriosus (patent ductus arteriosus [PDA]). In the presence of a PDA, the preductal P_{tcO_2} (measured on the right upper chest) typically runs at least 15 torr higher than the postductal P_{O_2} (measured either transcutaneously on the lower abdomen or thigh or via an umbilical artery ABG). A similar assessment can be made via dual pulse oximetry with probes placed on the right hand (preductal) and either foot (postductal).

Transcutaneous monitors also can provide a relative indication of local perfusion at the sensor site. This evaluation is done by tracking the power required to maintain the sensor's preset temperature. When perfusion increases, the underlying blood removes more heat from the tissues, which requires more power to the heating element. When perfusion decreases, less power is needed to maintain the sensor temperature.

Hemodynamic Assessment

Indications for invasive hemodynamic monitoring are listed in Chapter 3. Chapter 2 describes how to interpret vascular pressure and flow data, while Chapter 4 outlines the most frequently encountered problems with indwelling catheters and explains how to solve them.

Measuring and Recording Vital Signs

Regular measurement of vital signs is essential in evaluating and monitoring a patient's response to therapy. Changes in patient status usually are accompanied by changes in the patient's vital signs. For example, a 20% increase in heart rate above baseline when giving a bronchodilator treatment usually indicates an adverse reaction to the medication. Decreasing the dosage or changing to another bronchodilator may avoid this problem.

Normal values for vital signs are provided in Chapter 1. **Table 11-11** outlines the common causes of abnormal vital signs and their recommended solutions.

Table 11-11 Troubleshooting Changes in Vital Signs

Abnormal Vital Sign	Possible Cause	Recommendations
Increased heart rate (tachycardia)	• Anxiety/pain • ↓ Pao_2, ↓ or ↑ $Paco_2$ • Medications • Trauma • Fever • Failure to wean from mechanical ventilation • Ventilator asynchrony	• Relieve anxiety; treat pain • Stabilize blood gases • Treat the fever and the cause of the fever • If failure to wean, return to previous settings • Check patient–ventilator system synchrony; obtain and evaluate ABG • Recommend negative chronotropic agents (e.g., adenosine, calcium-channel blockers, beta blockers)
Decreased heart rate (bradycardia)	• Hypothermia • Medications • Cardiac disease • Cardiopulmonary arrest	• Provide warm blanket and fluids • Evaluate cardiac status (ECG, cardiac enzymes) • Recommend positive chronotropic agents (e.g., atropine, epinephrine, dopamine) • Perform CPR if needed
Increased blood pressure (hypertension)	• Anxiety/pain • Response to ↓ Pao_2, ↓ $Paco_2$ • Medications • Cardiovascular disease • Trauma (sympathetic response)	• Reassure; alleviate fear; relieve and treat pain • Obtain and evaluate ABG • Assess for cardiovascular events • Evaluate patient for cardiovascular risk factors • Recommend antihypertensive medications
Decreased blood pressure (hypotension)	• Hypovolemia • Trauma (bleeding) • Medications • Cardiovascular collapse	• Fluid resuscitation • Surgical intervention to stop hemorrhage • Recommend vasoactive drugs to increase BP (dopamine) • Provide CPR if necessary
Fever	• Infection • ↑ metabolic rate caused by ↑ work of breathing • Overheated humidifier	• Treat infection; review precautions • Check for mucus plugs; assess ETT position • Check sensitivity and patient–ventilator settings • Check temperature of humidifier heater

(continues)

Table 11-11 Troubleshooting Changes in Vital Signs (*continued*)

Abnormal Vital Sign	Possible Cause	Recommendations
Increased respiratory rate (tachypnea)	• Anxiety/pain	• Reassure; alleviate fear; relieve and treat pain
	• Altered ventilator settings	• Check patient–ventilator settings
	• ↓ Pao_2 or ↑ $Paco_2$	• Obtain and evaluate ABG
	• Failure to wean during mechanical ventilation	• If failure to wean, return to previous settings
	• Ventilator asynchrony	• Check patient–ventilator settings; adjust settings or recommend sedation
	• Change in metabolic needs	• Evaluate patient's metabolic rate
Decreased respiratory rate (bradypnea)	• Sleep	• Normal observation
	• Oversedation	• Reverse sedation or provide support
	• ↓ $Paco_2$	• Restore normal ventilatory status
	• Respiratory failure/arrest	• Provide airway support and CPR if necessary

Monitoring Cardiac Rhythms

Cardiac dysrhythmias can be classified as being lethal (causing death) and nonlethal. Chapter 15 covers the identification and protocol-based (ACLS) management of lethal rhythms. In this chapter, we provide a brief discussion of nonlethal dysrhythmias, along with example ECG rhythm strips.

Tachycardia (*Figure 11-5*)

- Identified in the ECG rhythm strip as:
  - Rate 100–180 beats/min (adults)
  - PR interval usually < 0.2 sec
  - A P wave for every QRS complex
  - Shortened R-R interval (< 0.60 sec) with normal QRS complexes
- For common causes and treatment recommendations, review the previous section on vital signs.

Bradycardia (*Figure 11-6*)

- Identified in the ECG rhythm strip as:
  - Rate < 50 beats/min (adults)
  - Regular rhythm with a normal PR interval
  - Normal P waves followed by regular QRS complexes
  - A prolonged (> 1 sec) R-R interval
- For common causes and treatment recommendations, review the previous section on vital signs.

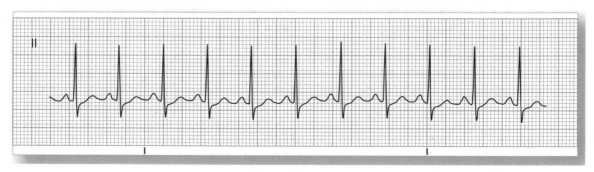

Figure 11-5 Example of Sinus Tachycardia (Rate ≈ 130/min).

Source: Garcia T, Miller GT. *Arrhythmia recognition: the art of interpretation.* Sudbury, MA: Jones and Bartlett; 2004.

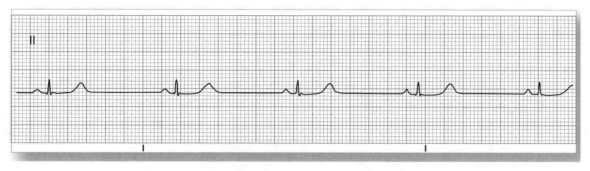

Figure 11-6 Example of Sinus Bradycardia (Rate ≈ 45/min).

Source: Garcia T, Miller GT. *Arrhythmia recognition: the art of interpretation.* Sudbury, MA: Jones and Bartlett; 2004.

Atrial Fibrillation (*Figure 11-7*)

- Identified in the ECG rhythm strip as:
  - Irregular rhythm
  - Variation in interval and amplitude in the R-R interval (more than 10% variation)
  - Absent P wave with "fibrillatory" base line
- Atrial fibrillation can be a side effect of β-adrenergic drugs. If it occurs during treatment, stop the treatment, stabilize the patient, and notify the physician.
- If this rhythm was already present before the therapy, assess the patient's heart rate and history, and consult with the patient's nurse and physician before administering treatment.

Atrial Flutter (*Figure 11-8*)

- Identified in the ECG rhythm strip as:
  - The classic "sawtooth" pattern seen in between the QRS complexes
  - The absence of a PR interval
- Causes and treatment recommendations are the same as with atrial fibrillation.

Premature Ventricular Contractions (PVCs) (*Figure 11-9*)

- Identified in the ECG rhythm strip as:
  - Abnormal QRS complexes (> 0.12 sec in width)
  - Underlying rhythm usually regular but becomes irregular with a PVC
  - No P wave present before the PVC
  - T waves deflected in the opposite direction following the PVC
- PVCs can be caused by anxiety, caffeine, tobacco, alcohol, and certain drugs such as β-agonists and theophylline.

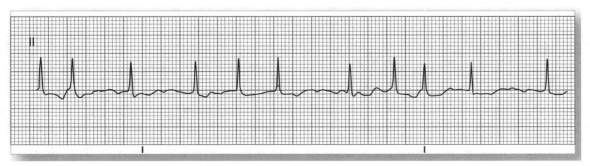

Figure 11-7 Example of Atrial Fibrillation.

Source: Garcia T, Miller GT. *Arrhythmia recognition: the art of interpretation.* Sudbury, MA: Jones and Bartlett; 2004.

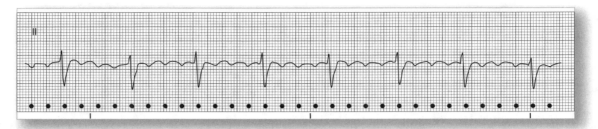

Figure 11-8 Example of Atrial Flutter with 4:1 Conduction Ratio.

Source: Garcia T, Miller GT. *Arrhythmia recognition: the art of interpretation.* Sudbury, MA: Jones and Bartlett; 2004.

- PVCs also can be caused by myocardial ischemia, acidosis, electrolyte imbalance, hypoxia, and direct myocardium stimulation.
- Many respiratory procedures can cause hypoxemia or myocardial stimulation. If PVCs occur while you are performing any respiratory procedure, stop what you are doing, provide supplemental oxygen to stabilize the patient, and notify the physician immediately.

Evaluating Fluid Balance

Chapter 13 covers the common signs of fluid balance alteration and management strategies that you can recommend to address abnormal intake and output.

Interpreting Bronchoprovocation Studies

Bronchoprovocation studies are used to identify and assess airway responsiveness (see Chapter 3 for a complete listing of indications). **Table 11-12** describes some of the techniques most commonly used to assess airway hyperreactivity.

Recommending Blood Tests

Normal values for laboratory blood tests are discussed in Chapter 1, while Chapter 3 gives examples of the most common lab tests you may want to recommend based on selected patient scenarios.

Observing and Interpreting Changes in Sputum Characteristics

Sputum assessment is discussed in detail in Chapter 2. The NBRC expects candidates to be able to relate a patient's sputum characteristics to the need for specific diagnostic tests or treatments. For example, if you determine that a patient has mucopurulent or purulent sputum (indicating a

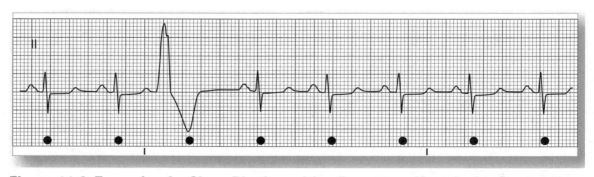

Figure 11-9 Example of a Sinus Rhythm with a Premature Ventricular Contraction.

Source: Garcia T, Miller GT. *Arrhythmia recognition: the art of interpretation.* Sudbury, MA: Jones and Bartlett; 2004.

Table 11-12 Common Bronchial Challenge Tests

Test	Description
Methacholine challenge	• Assesses changes in airway caliber with increasing concentrations of methacholine. • Patients with hyperreactive airways will show early changes at low dosages. • A 20% decrease in FEV_1 is considered a positive result. • The methacholine concentration at which a 20% decrease in FEV_1 occurs is called the "provocative concentration," or PC_{20}. The lower the PC_{20}, the worse the airway hyperreactivity.
Histamine challenge	• Uses histamine sulfate instead of methacholine. • Flushing and headaches are two common side effects from histamine inhalation. • Performed in a similar fashion as the methacholine test. • A 20% decrease in FEV_1 is considered a positive result.
Exercise challenge	• Indicated to assess exercise-induced bronchospasm (EIB). • A treadmill or a cycle ergometer can be used. • Bronchospasm usually occurs 5–10 minutes after cessation of the exercise. • A drop in FEV_1 of 10–15% is consistent with increased airway sensitivity.

potential pulmonary infection), you should recommend a chest x-ray, Gram stain, and culture and sensitivity testing. Depending on the lab results, you might also recommend antibiotic therapy. If, in contrast, you observe a patient with pink, watery, frothy sputum and signs or symptoms of congestive heart failure (indicating acute pulmonary edema), you should recommend high concentrations of O_2, ideally with CPAP or BiPAP, along with diuresis and possibly an inotropic agent.

Auscultating the Chest and Interpreting Breath Sounds

The NBRC exams typically incorporate breath sounds within patient monitoring and assessment scenarios. To score high on related questions, you need to pay close attention to any "clues" and always evaluate the breath sounds in the clinical context in which they are given.

Normal breath sounds are described in Chapter 2. Here we focus on abnormal or *adventitious* breath sounds. Most adventitious breath sounds are classified as being either *continuous* or *discontinuous*. High-pitched continuous sounds are called *wheezes*, whereas low-pitched continuous sounds are called *rhonchi*. Another abnormal continuous, loud, high-pitched sound heard primarily over the larynx and trachea during inhalation is *stridor*. Discontinuous sounds are intermittent, crackling, or bubbling sounds of short duration. The term *crackles* (rales) is used for discontinuous breath sounds. **Table 11-13** summarizes the likely mechanisms, characteristics, and causes of these adventitious breath sounds.

Observing for Patient–Ventilator Asynchrony

Patient–ventilator asynchrony occurs when a patient's breathing efforts are no longer in synchrony with that of the ventilator. The most common manifestations of patient–ventilator asynchrony include agitation and respiratory distress. In its most severe form, patients experiencing asynchrony may appear to be fighting or "bucking" the ventilator. Agitation can be recognized by irregular patient movements or facial signs of pain, discomfort, or distress. Additional physical signs of respiratory distress include tachypnea, diaphoresis, nasal flaring, accessory muscles use, intercostal retractions, ribcage–abdominal paradox, tachycardia, and blood pressure changes. Asynchrony also is often evident when viewing the ventilator's graphic display monitor (see Chapter 12 for more detail).

Table 11-13 Adventitious Breath Sounds

Lung Sounds	Likely Mechanism	Characteristics	Causes
Rhonchi	Airflow through mucus	Course, discontinuous	Pneumonia, bronchitis, inadequate cough
Wheezes	Rapid airflow through partially obstructed airways	High pitched; usually expiratory	Asthma, congestive heart failure, bronchitis
Stridor	Rapid airflow through obstructed upper airway	High pitched, monophonic; commonly inspiratory	Croup, epiglottitis, post-extubation edema
Pleural friction rub	Inflamed pleural surfaces rubbing together during breathing	Creaking or grating sound heard mainly during inhalation (can occur during both phases of breathing)	Pleurisy
Crackles: inspiratory and expiratory	Excess airway secretions moving with airflow	Coarse; often clear with coughing	Bronchitis, respiratory infections
Crackles: early inspiratory	Sudden opening of proximal bronchi	Scanty, transmitted to mouth; not affected by cough	Bronchitis, emphysema, asthma
Crackles: late inspiratory	Sudden opening of peripheral airways	Diffuse, fine; occur initially in the dependent regions	Atelectasis, pneumonia, pulmonary edema, fibrosis

Once you confirm patient–ventilator asynchrony, you should identify its underlying cause(s), while simultaneously making efforts to alleviate the patient's respiratory distress:

- Ensure adequate ventilation and oxygenation by disconnecting the patient from the ventilator and providing manual ventilation with 100% O_2. Removing the patient from the ventilator and manually supporting ventilation and oxygenation can help identify the cause of respiratory distress.
- Once the patient is stabilized, perform more detailed assessment and management.
- If the patient's distress resolves upon disconnection, the likely cause is ventilator related. If the patient's distress continues, it indicates a patient-related problem.

Patient-Related Problems

Airway obstruction (partial or complete) can lead to serious patient–ventilator asynchrony. If airway obstruction is not the problem, you should perform a rapid assessment of the patient to determine other potential causes of distress (e.g., bronchospasm, pulmonary edema, pneumothorax, anxiety, pain, air trapping). If death appears imminent, you should follow the applicable disease-specific or ACLS protocol before undertaking further patient assessment. Once the patient has been stabilized, you can undertake more detailed assessment and management.

Ventilator-Related Problems

Table 11-14 summarizes the most common ventilator-related problems causing respiratory distress and outlines how to identify them.

Adjusting and Checking Alarm Systems

Ventilator alarms indicate potential ventilator malfunction or untoward changes in patient status. Some alarms are preprogrammed (e.g., loss of power, gas supply loss, or ventilator malfunction), whereas others are set by the clinician (e.g., high/low pressure limit, high/low PEEP, high/low minute ventilation). **Table 11-15** summarizes some of the most common alarms found in a patient–ventilator system, their recommended settings, and their possible causes.

Table 11-14 Identifying Common Ventilator-Related Problems

Problem/Need	Problem Manifestation
Inadequate F_{IO_2}	• Oxygen analyzer alarm • Low oxygen pressure alarm • Low patient Sp_{O_2} • Clinical signs and symptoms of hypoxemia
Trigger/sensitivity problems	• Auto-PEEP • Patient–ventilator asynchrony • Large drops in pressure at the beginning of inspiration (see the section on ventilator waveforms) • Increased work of breathing

Flow problems	During volume control ventilation:
	  • Post-trigger patient effort (flow starvation)
	  • Patient–ventilator asynchrony
	  • Increased work of breathing
	  • "Scooping" or "scalloping" of the inspiratory pressure waveform
	During pressure control ventilation:
	  • Too much flow: spiking of the inspiratory pressure waveform (left "dog ear")
	  • Insufficient flow: "scooping" or "scalloping" of the inspiratory pressure waveform (lack of plateau)

Rate problems	During A/C ventilation:
	  • Inverse I:E ratio alarm
	  • Signs of auto-PEEP due to very low I:E ratios
	During SIMV:
	  • Spontaneous rate > 20–25/min
	  • Signs of muscle fatigue/weakness

Excessive tidal volume/pressure limit	• "Beaking" of pressure–volume loop (indicating overdistension)
Inadequate minute volume	• Hypercapnia • Minute ventilation < 4–6 L/min for adults
Mode	• Increased work of breathing, respiratory distress, and ventilator asynchrony • Inability to normalize blood gases, lung mechanics, and other physiology parameters
Auto-PEEP	• Flow not returning to zero at the end of exhalation • Trigger/sensitivity problems • Increased work of breathing and/or respiratory distress or ventilator asynchrony

In general, all noninvasive positive pressure ventilators used in the acute care setting must have a low-pressure/disconnect and power failure alarm. Most have a separate apnea alarm and some include high/low-volume and high-pressure alarms. Clinicians should respond to these alarms in the same manner as with invasive ventilatory support, with emphasis always on ensuring adequate patient ventilation and oxygenation.

Table 11-15 Clinical Alarms Commonly Used During Adult Mechanical Ventilation

Alarm	Recommended Alarm Parameters	Possible Causes
Ventilator Malfunction Alarms		
Loss of power	Preprogrammed	• Accidental power cord disconnection • Backup battery failure • Tripped circuit breaker • Institutional power failure
Gas supply loss	Preprogrammed	• Failure to connect gas lines • Gas lines connected to low pressure outlet (e.g., flowmeters) • High-pressure line failure
O_2 analyzer alarm	Usually preprogrammed ($\pm$5–6% of setting)	• Gas source failure (air or O_2) • Analyzer needs to be calibrated or replaced • Sudden changes in delivered F_{IO_2} (100% suction)
Patient Status Alarms		
Apnea delay alarm	20 seconds	• Sedation/anesthesia • Low metabolic rate • Low set respiratory rate
Low-pressure alarm	8 cm H_2O or 5–10 cm H_2O below PIP (use PIP of pressure supported breaths during SIMV)	• Disconnection • Airway/circuit leaks • Alarm set above pressure supported breath PIP • Improved compliance and/or resistance
High-pressure limit	50 cm H_2O or 10–15 cm H_2O above PIP (use mechanical breaths' PIPs during SIMV)	• Increased resistance/decreased compliance • Airway obstruction (partial/complete) • Cough/secretions, mucus plugs • Patient–ventilator asynchrony • Anxiety, restlessness, pain
Low PEEP/CPAP	3–5 cm H_2O below set PEEP	• Disconnection • Airway/circuit leaks
Low exhaled V_T	100 mL or 10–15% below set V_T or spontaneous V_T during SIMV	• Disconnection • Airway/circuit leaks • Pulmonary leaks (bronchopleural fistula) • Shallow breathing during spontaneous breaths • Coughing • Patient–ventilator asynchrony
Low $\dot{V}_E$	4–5 L/min or 10–15% below minimum SIMV or A/C set $\dot{V}_E$	• Same causes as "low exhaled V_T" • Sedation/anesthesia • Low metabolic rate
High $\dot{V}_E$	10–15% above baseline $\dot{V}_E$	• Increased metabolic rate (e.g., fever) • Tachypnea • Anxiety, restlessness, pain • Patient waking up from anesthesia/sedation

(*continues*)

Table 11-15 Clinical Alarms Commonly Used During Adult Mechanical Ventilation (*continued*)

Alarm	Recommended Alarm Parameters	Possible Causes
Temperature	2°C above and below set temperature; not to exceed 41°C	• Dry water chamber • Tubing condensation • Defective wiring, probes, and chamber • Heater malfunctioning • Environmental temperature changes • High minute ventilation and/or high ventilator flow

Adapted from: Shelledy DC. Initiating and adjusting ventilatory support. In Wilkins RL, Stoller JK, Kacmarek RM, eds. *Egan's fundamentals of respiratory care* (9th ed.). St. Louis, MO: Mosby; 2009.

Measuring FIO_2 and Liter Flow

According to AARC guidelines, all O_2 delivery systems should be checked at least daily. O_2 analysis is particularly important in the care of neonates, due to the risks of O_2 toxicity and retinopathy of prematurity (ROP). To protect against equipment failure causing either hypoxemia or hyperoxia, you should also monitor FIO_2 values continuously during mechanical ventilation.

Consider these key points when measuring a patient's FIO_2:

- Properly calibrate the O_2 analyzer (see Chapter 6).
- If continuously monitoring FIO_2 in a ventilator circuit, place the probe before/upstream to any active humidification systems. This will avoid erroneous readings due to condensation on the sensor.
- When analyzing the FIO_2 in a pediatric or neonatal O_2 enclosure, place the probe close to the infant's face at the bottom of the enclosure (because O_2 is heavier than N_2, it tends to settle).
- If the device is being used for continuous monitoring, set the analyzer's alarms to ±5% of the prescribed FIO_2.

Monitoring and Assessing Airway Pressures

During mechanical ventilation, you typically monitor the peak inspiratory pressure (PIP), the baseline or PEEP level, and the difference between the two (PIP − PEEP, called the *driving pressure* or ΔP). Depending on the patient, you also may monitor (1) the inspiratory pause or plateau pressure (Pplat), (2) the difference between PIP and Pplat, (3) the expiratory pause pressure, and (4) the mean airway pressure (Pmean or MAP). **Figure 11-10** depicts the key pressures that you should monitor and assess during mechanical ventilation.

Peak Inspiratory Pressure

During volume control ventilation, the delivered volume is held constant; therefore, PIP will rise if either the patient's lung/thoracic compliance (CLT) decreases or the airway resistance (Raw) increases. Conversely, PIP will decrease if Raw falls or CLT increases.

During pressure control ventilation, you set the PIP, holding ΔP constant during each breath. With ΔP held constant, the VT will decrease when CLT falls and increase when CLT rises. The effects of changes in Raw during pressure control depend on the inspiratory time and flow. If the airway and alveolar pressures *do not* equilibrate by the end of the breath (flow continues), the VT will decrease when Raw rises and increase when Raw falls. However, if airway and alveolar pressures do equilibrate by the end of the breath (flow ceases), changes in Raw will not affect the delivered VT.

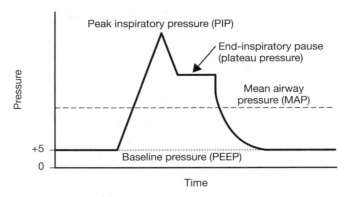

Figure 11-10 Key Pressures that Are Monitored and Assessed During Positive-Pressure Ventilation.

Courtesy of: Strategic Learning Associates, LLC, Little Silver, New Jersey.

Changes you make during volume control ventilation also can affect PIP and ΔP, independent of changes in the patient's Cʟᴛ and Raw. Specifically, whenever you change the ventilator's flow, volume, or PEEP settings, you will alter both PIP and ΔP. PIP rises when you increase either the set flow or volume. Conversely, PIP decreases when you decrease the set flow or volume. Last, adding or removing PEEP raises or lowers the whole airway pressure baseline (and thus PIP) by an equivalent amount. **Table 11-16** summarizes these factors and their effect on PIP during volume control ventilation.

Inspiratory Pause or Plateau Pressure

During an inspiratory pause or plateau, flow stops but the exhalation valve remains closed, holding the delivered volume in the lungs. Thus, during volume control ventilation, PIP will drop and hold at a lower level, called the plateau pressure, or Pplat (see Figure 11-10). Under these static conditions, any pressure due to flow resistance is eliminated, with the resulting pressure equivalent to the

Table 11-16 Factors Affecting Peak Pressure During Volume Control Ventilation

	Increases PIP	**Decreases PIP**
Patient factors	Increased airway resistance: • Bronchospasm • Airway edema • Mucus plugging • Kinked tubing	Decreased airway resistance: • Bronchodilator therapy • Resolution of other obstruction (e.g., swelling, secretions, airway edema)
	Decreased compliance: • Pulmonary edema • Surfactant deficiency • Atelectasis • Pneumothorax • Endobronchial intubation • Pneumonia	Increased compliance: • Resolution of pulmonary edema • Reexpansion of lung/lobes • Surfactant instillation • Resolution of pneumonia
Ventilator factors	• Increased flow • Increased Vᴛ • Increased PEEP	• Decreased flow • Decreased Vᴛ • Decreased PEEP

alveolar pressure at that volume. Because the plateau pressure (*minus* PEEP) represents the force stretching the alveoli, it is an important safety measure. To prevent ventilator-associated lung injury, you should always try to prevent Pplat from rising much higher than 30 cm H_2O.

Application of an inspiratory pause maneuver during volume control ventilation also separates or "partitions out" the pressures due to flow resistance form those due to elastic resistance/compliance. Specifically:

PIP – Pplat = pressure due to flow resistance (Raw)

Pplat – PEEP = pressure due to elastic resistance (C_{LT})

Simple trend analysis of these pressure differences helps in monitoring a patient's pulmonary mechanics. For example, with a constant V_T, flow, and baseline PEEP, if the PIP and Pplat pressures rise by an equal amount (i.e., no change occurs in PIP – Pplat), the patient's compliance is decreasing. In contrast, if Pplat remains constant but PIP rises over time, the patient's airway resistance is increasing. If more quantitative data are required, these two pressure differences can be used to actually estimate the patient's airway resistance and lung/thoracic compliance.

Estimating Airway Resistance and Lung/Thoracic Compliance

With a constant inspiratory flow (square wave flow pattern), you can estimate airway resistance according to the following formula:

$$Raw = \frac{PIP - Pplat}{\dot{V}\left(\frac{L}{sec}\right)}$$

Normal adult Raw ranges from approximately 0.5–2.5 cm H_2O/L/sec. Depending on their size and length, artificial tracheal airways can add 3–10 cm H_2O/L/sec or more to this value. An increase in Raw to more than 10–15 cm H_2O/L/sec in an intubated patient with otherwise normal lungs signals abnormal airway narrowing due to factors such as increased secretions, bronchospasm, pulmonary vascular congestion, or partial occlusion of the artificial airway (see Table 11-16).

As previously described, during an inspiratory hold of a volume-controlled breath, the difference between Pplat and the baseline or PEEP pressure is the force needed to maintain the lungs and thorax at the delivered volume under static conditions. By dividing the *corrected* tidal volume V_{T_c} by this pressure difference, we derive a close estimate of total lung and chest wall compliance (C_{LT}), called *static or effective compliance*:

$$C_{LT} = \frac{V_{T_c}}{Pplat - PEEP}$$

When interpreting and assessing static compliance, the following points must be considered:

- Normal C_{LT} ranges between 60 and 100 mL/cm H_2O (seldom observed in patients receiving ventilatory support).
- Diseases of the lung parenchyma such as pneumonia, pulmonary edema, and any chronic diseases causing fibrosis are all associated with decreased static compliance.
- Acute changes, such as atelectasis, pulmonary edema, ARDS, or lung compression due to a tension pneumothorax, may cause a rapid drop in C_{LT} (see Table 11-16).
- When C_{LT} is less than 25–30 mL/cm H_2O, as may occur in severe ARDS, the work of breathing is very high and can lead to muscle fatigue and respiratory failure, thus making weaning difficult.

The accompanying box provides an example of these computations, including interpretation of changes over time for an adult patient receiving volume control ventilation. Note that you usually need to convert the ventilator flow from L/min to L/sec to compute airway resistance (L/min ÷ 60 = L/sec).

Due to the variable flow occurring during pressure control ventilation, only the patient's C_{LT} can be accurately estimated by these methods, and then only if the flow ceases before the end of inspiration (confirmed by graphic analysis of the flow scalar). Under these circumstances, $C_{LT} = V_T/(PIP - PEEP)$. Note that computer analysis of the pressure–volume curves during breathing can provide automated estimates of Raw and C_{LT}. However, the NBRC expects candidates to be able to perform these computations manually and interpret their results.

End-Expiratory Pause Pressure (Measuring Auto-PEEP)

Like an inspiratory pause, an end-expiratory pause creates a condition of no flow. Under these static conditions, airway and alveolar pressures equilibrate. Thus an end-expiratory pause pressure also equals alveolar pressure, but at the end of exhalation.

Normally, alveolar pressure should be the same as the baseline airway pressure/PEEP at the end of exhalation. However, if any gas remains trapped in the alveoli (dynamic hyperinflation or air

---

Example of Compliance and Resistance Computations with Interpretation

Scenario

An adult patient receiving volume control ventilation exhibits the following parameters over time:

Parameter	7:00 AM	8:00 AM	9:00 AM	10:00 AM
V_T (mL, corrected)	500	500	500	500
Inspiratory flow (L/min)	40	40	40	40
PIP (cm H_2O)	50	55	60	65
Pplat (cm H_2O)	30	30	30	30
PEEP (cm H_2O)	5	5	5	5

Problems

1. What is the patient's static compliance and airway resistance at 7:00 AM?
2. What major change in this patient's lung mechanics is occurring over these 4 hours?

Solutions

1. Compute static compliance and airway resistance at 7:00 AM.

Compliance:

$$C_{LT} = \frac{V_{TC}}{Pplat - PEEP} = \frac{500\,mL}{30\,cm\,H_2O - 5\,cm\,H_2O} = \frac{500\,mL}{25\,cm\,H_2O} = 20\,mL/cm\,H_2O$$

Airway Resistance:

First convert L/min to L/sec:

$$L/min \div 60 = L/sec$$
$$40\,L/min \div 60 = 0.67\,L/sec$$

Then compute the airway resistance:

$$Raw = \frac{PIP - Pplat}{\dot{V}} = \frac{50\,cm\,H_2O - 30\,cm\,H_2O}{0.67\,L/sec} = \frac{20\,cm\,H_2O}{0.67\,L/sec} = 29.9\,cm\,H_2O/L/sec$$

2. Identify the major change in this patient's lung mechanics over these 4 hours:

- Pplat – PEEP remains constant, so compliance remains unchanged (at 20 mL/cm H_2O).
- PIP – Pplat increases from 20 cm H_2O to 35 cm H_2O, so airway resistance is increasing.

trapping), the alveolar pressure will exceed the airway baseline pressure. As indicated in **Figure 11-11**, if at this point you stop the flow and institute a pause, the airway pressure will equilibrate with the *higher* alveolar pressure, causing a momentary rise in the pressure baseline. This rise in baseline pressure corresponds to the level of residual pressure (and volume) "trapped" in the alveoli that does not fully escape during exhalation. We call this residual pressure *auto-PEEP*. Auto-PEEP can negatively affect ventilator triggering, increase patient–ventilator asynchrony, and impose additional work of breathing on the patient. For causes and management of auto-PEEP, refer to Chapters 12 and 13.

Mean Airway Pressure

The Pmean or MAP is the average pressure applied to the airway over time (refer to Figure 11-10). Factors affecting Pmean during mechanical ventilation that you can control include the mode, rate, VT or PIP set, inspiratory pressure waveform, I:E ratio, and PEEP level.

All else being equal, you will observe higher Pmean values when there are more machine breaths per minute (higher rates), larger VT or PIP values, "square" inspiratory pressure patterns, higher I:E ratios, and higher PEEP levels. Conversely, you will observe lower Pmean values when there are fewer machine breaths and more spontaneous breaths (e.g., SIMV), lower VT or PIP values, nonsquare pressure patterns, lower I:E ratios, and lower PEEP settings.

As Pmean increases, so does the functional residual capacity (FRC). In disease states associated with alveolar collapse and shunting, increases in FRC tend to improve oxygenation and raise the Pao_2. Thus, adjusting Pmean is one more method (in addition to adjusting Fio_2 and PEEP) you can use to alter patient oxygenation. Unfortunately, high Pmean levels also can decrease venous return and cardiac output and increase the risk of pulmonary barotrauma.

Interpreting Ventilator Graphics

You can use ventilator graphics/waveforms to assess or detect ventilator modes, patient–ventilator asynchrony, adverse events, and responses to therapy. Here we focus on the basic characteristics of ventilator waveforms. Chapter 12 extends this discussion by focusing on the significance of abnormal waveforms and the actions required to correct the problems they reveal.

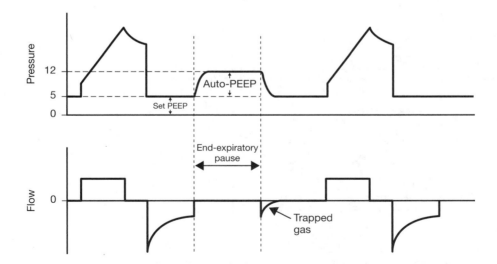

Figure 11-11 Implementation of an End-Expiratory Pause to Measure Auto-PEEP.
Occlusion of the expiratory valve toward the end of expiration causes equilibration between the alveoli and airway. A rise in airway pressure above the baseline/PEEP level indicates the presence of auto-PEEP. The amount of auto-PEEP is calculated as the difference between the end-expiratory pause pressure and the PEEP pressure—in this case, 12 – 5 = 7 cm H_2O. At the end of the pause, the expiratory valve opens and the remaining trapped gas is exhaled.

Courtesy of: Strategic Learning Associates, LLC, Little Silver, New Jersey.

The most common ventilator waveforms you will observe are the volume, pressure, and flow patterns over time (*scalar graphics*), and the pressure–volume and flow–volume *loops*. **Tables 11-17** through **11-20** provide *idealized* representations of the most common normal configurations and characteristics of these waveforms.

Table 11-17 Idealized Representation of Normal Volume Versus Time Waveforms

Idealized Waveform	Characteristics
Normal volume–time graphic 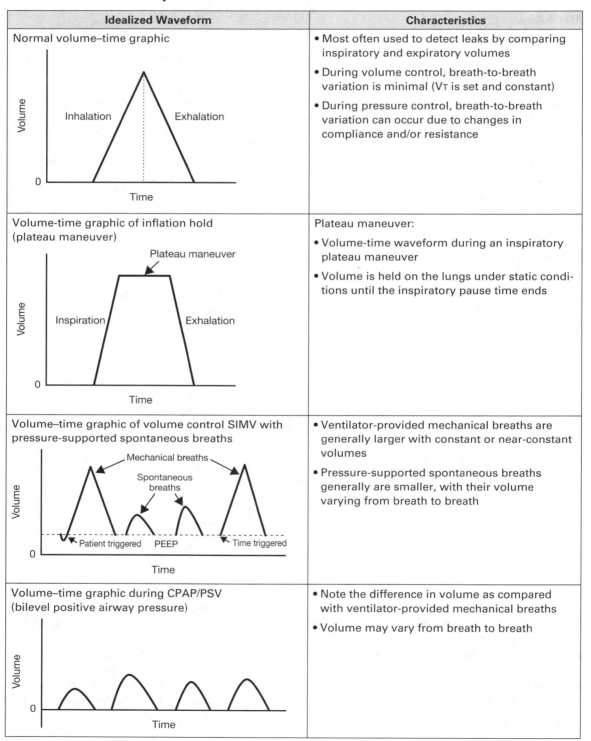	• Most often used to detect leaks by comparing inspiratory and expiratory volumes • During volume control, breath-to-breath variation is minimal (V_T is set and constant) • During pressure control, breath-to-breath variation can occur due to changes in compliance and/or resistance
Volume-time graphic of inflation hold (plateau maneuver)	Plateau maneuver: • Volume-time waveform during an inspiratory plateau maneuver • Volume is held on the lungs under static conditions until the inspiratory pause time ends
Volume–time graphic of volume control SIMV with pressure-supported spontaneous breaths	• Ventilator-provided mechanical breaths are generally larger with constant or near-constant volumes • Pressure-supported spontaneous breaths generally are smaller, with their volume varying from breath to breath
Volume–time graphic during CPAP/PSV (bilevel positive airway pressure)	• Note the difference in volume as compared with ventilator-provided mechanical breaths • Volume may vary from breath to breath

Table 11-18 Idealized Representation of Normal Pressure Versus Time Waveforms

Idealized Waveform	Characteristics
Pressure–time graphic during volume control ventilation 	• Pressure waveform may vary from breath to breath due to changes in the patient's lung/thoracic compliance and resistance • Can be used to assess for proper sensitivity settings of the assisted breaths if pressure trigger is being used • During pressure triggering, the absence of a trigger effort indicates a mechanical, time-triggered breath
Pressure–time graphic with inflation hold (plateau) during volume control ventilation 	• During an inspiratory hold maneuver, the plateau pressures will reflect true alveolar pressures during static conditions • Use to calculate patient's resistance and compliance
Pressure–time graphic of volume control SIMV with pressure support 	• Ventilator-provided mechanical breaths have higher PIP than pressure-supported spontaneous breaths • Can be used to assess proper sensitivity for pressure triggering of assisted breaths
Pressure–time graphic of pressure control ventilation (PCV) 	• The pressure remains constant throughout inspiration until the breath ends—hence the square shape of the waveform • Because the pressure limit remains constant for each mechanical breath, all breaths have the same PIP

(continues)

Table 11-18 Idealized Representation of Normal Pressure Versus Time Waveforms (*continued*)

Idealized Waveform	Characteristics
Pressure–time graphic of PCV with different rise times 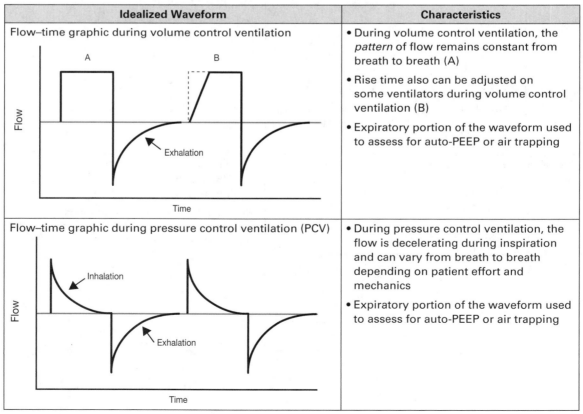	• Rise time to PIP (usually expressed as a percentage of I-time) can be adjusted during PCV • Changes in rise time will alter the length of the PIP plateau • Rise time adjustments are used to improve patient–ventilator synchrony or fine-tune ventilator settings
Pressure–time graphic of CPAP	• All breaths are spontaneous • Patient breathes during inspiration and exhalation at a baseline airway pressure above zero • Pressure support can be added to augment spontaneous tidal volumes

Table 11-19 Idealized Representation of Normal Flow Versus Time Waveforms

Idealized Waveform	Characteristics
Flow–time graphic during volume control ventilation	• During volume control ventilation, the *pattern* of flow remains constant from breath to breath (A) • Rise time also can be adjusted on some ventilators during volume control ventilation (B) • Expiratory portion of the waveform used to assess for auto-PEEP or air trapping
Flow–time graphic during pressure control ventilation (PCV)	• During pressure control ventilation, the flow is decelerating during inspiration and can vary from breath to breath depending on patient effort and mechanics • Expiratory portion of the waveform used to assess for auto-PEEP or air trapping

Table 11-20 Most Common Mechanical Ventilator Loops and Their Characteristics

Idealized Waveform	Characteristics
Pressure–volume loops 	• Graphic representation of the pressure needed to deliver a certain volume; helps you assess "at a glance" compliance and resistance. • Compliance is given by the slope of the curve. The greater the slope (loop A), the higher the compliance (compare to loop C, where higher pressure is required to deliver a smaller V_T—that is, a lesser slope indicates lower compliance). • Airway resistance is assessed by the width of the loop. The thinner the loop (C), the less airway resistance. A thicker loop (B) indicates increased airway resistance.
Flow–volume loops 	• Helps you classify the nature of the airway impairment as either restrictive (reduced volumes), obstructive (reduced flows), or both. • Loop A shows an obstructive patient with reduced expiratory flows and normal volume. • Loop B shows a restrictive process with normal expiratory flows but reduced tidal volume. • Also used to assess pre/post response to bronchodilator therapy during mechanical ventilation.

COMMON ERRORS TO AVOID

You can improve your score by avoiding these mistakes:

- Avoid placing O_2 analyzers downstream/after a heated humidifier in ventilator circuits; humidity and water vapor pressure may affect the analyzer's readings.
- Avoid performing capillary sampling in neonates less than 24 hours old.
- Avoid radial punctures for ABGs if the Allen's test indicates lack of collateral ulnar flow. Repeat the test on the opposite hand. If ulnar flow inadequate on that side also use the brachial artery instead.
- Avoid drawing blood from a distal port of a pulmonary catheter too fast or with the balloon inflated because sample contamination with arterial blood may occur.
- Do not use standard pulse oximetry to assess oxygenation in a patient suspected of carbon monoxide (CO) poisoning due to smoke inhalation. In such cases, the SpO_2 will be falsely high. Recommend CO-oximetry instead, or use a multi-wavelength pulse oximeter.
- Do not use a capillary blood gas test to assess oxygenation.

SURE BETS

In some situations, you can be sure of the right approach to a clinical problem or scenario:

- Always target a Hb saturation of more than 90–92% to maintain proper tissue oxygenation.
- Always use pressure monitor alarms for acutely ill patients receiving noninvasive positive-pressure ventilation (NPPV) or those requiring long-term 24-hour NPPV support.
- Always warm up the site for a capillary blood test before performing the puncture to allow for vasodilation and arterialization of the blood.
- P/F ratios less than 200 indicate shunting and the need for PEEP/CPAP.
- A healthy adult patient receiving 100% O_2 at sea level should have a PaO_2 of approximately 650 torr.
- When assessing changes in peak inspiratory pressures during volume control ventilation, always evaluate the plateau pressure to determine if a change in resistance or a change in compliance is the primary cause.
- Always set the high/low CPAP/PEEP pressure alarms at ±3–5 cm H_2O above and below the set pressure, respectively.
- Always confirm SpO_2 accuracy by correlating the heart rate, assessing pulse strength, and evaluating the SpO_2 waveform (if available).
- When interpreting blood gases, always assess ventilation (pH, $PaCO_2$) and oxygenation (PaO_2, SaO_2) separately.
- Always perform an Allen's test when drawing an ABG from the radial artery site.
- Normal breath sounds heard at abnormal locations are always an abnormal finding.
- Always use a chest radiograph (or bronchoscopic visualization) to confirm proper tracheal placement of an endotracheal tube; use bilateral breath sounds and a positive CO_2 test (colorimetry or capnography) only as a preliminary indicator of proper placement.

PRE-TEST ANSWERS AND EXPLANATIONS

Following are this chapter's pre-test answers and explanations. Be sure to review each answer's explanation thoroughly to help you understand why it is correct. If the explanation is still unclear to you, review the chapter content.

11-1. **Correct answer: B.** 3, 4, and 5 only. Flat diaphragms and increased radiolucency throughout the lung fields are common chest x-ray findings in COPD, as are a *decrease* in peripheral vascular markings, an *increased* retrosternal airspace, and a *narrow* mediastinum.

11-2. **Correct answer: A.** Patient motion artifact. The most common source of pulse oximetry errors and false alarms is motion artifact. Securing the sensor properly or relocating the sensor to an earlobe or toe can help minimize this problem.

11-3. **Correct answer: C.** Increased work of breathing. Controlled ventilation is poorly tolerated by many patients, often resulting in asynchrony. Asynchrony can increase the work of breathing, and with it, the O_2 consumption of the respiratory muscles. Sedation or paralysis may be required when controlled ventilation is necessary.

11-4. **Correct answer: A.** Acute alveolar hyperventilation without hypoxemia. The high pH value indicates alkalemia. The low $PaCO_2$ value indicates hyperventilation, consistent with the high pH (respiratory alkalosis). The normal HCO_3 and BE levels indicate *no* metabolic involvement; hence compensation has *not* begun yet (acute process). The PaO_2 is in the acceptable range at a low FIO_2 (no hypoxemia present).

11-5. **Correct answer: C.** 2, 3, and 4 only. The high-pressure-limit alarm should be set about 10–15 cm H_2O above the peak airway pressure of the mechanical-controlled breaths. The low-PEEP/CPAP alarm should always be set at 3–5 cm H_2O or 20% below the set baseline pressure. A low-exhaled-volume alarm should be triggered when either the V_T or $\dot{V}_E$ falls 20% below preset values (6 L/min in this question). I:E ratio alarms are used to detect inverse ratios caused by an increased respiratory rate, commonly seen during patient–ventilator asynchrony.

11-6. **Correct answer: D.** 90%. Normal Sao_2 should be more than 93–95% breathing room air. Levels below 90% indicate the need for O_2 therapy. Drops in O_2 saturation are usually the result of cardiac, pulmonary, or combined cardiopulmonary disease. *Hb saturation data must always be interpreted with knowledge of Hb/Hct levels.* For example, a patient with an Spo_2 of 97% and severe anemia (Hb < 7 g/dL) is still suffering from hypoxemia, due to reduced blood O_2 content.

11-7. **Correct answer: B.** 35 mL/cm H_2O. Static compliance equals corrected tidal volume divided by the plateau pressure – PEEP. In this instance, static compliance = 700/(30 – 10) = 700/20 = 35 mL/cm H_2O.

11-8. **Correct answer: B.** Noninvasive pulse oximetry. Besides vital signs, pulse oximetry is the standard of care when monitoring patients during moderate sedation procedures. More expensive, invasive techniques such A-line insertion are required only when more critical, invasive procedures are being done.

11-9. **Correct answer: B.** A mild disturbance of oxygenation consistent with a V/Q imbalance. The patient is hyperventilating so hypoventilation can be ruled out. The P/F ratio is 220 (66/0.3). P/F ratios between 200 and 300 indicate mild disturbances of oxygenation, usually due to V/Q imbalances. Ratios between 100 and 200 indicate a moderate disturbance due to shunting, consistent with acute lung injury. A P/F ratio less than 100 indicates a severe disturbance of oxygenation and severe shunting consistent with ARDS.

11-10. **Correct answer: B.** Increased cardiac output. Causes of a $Petco_2$ of zero may include (1) a large system leak or disconnection, (2) esophageal intubation, (3) cardiac arrest, and (4) a totally obstructed/kinked artificial airway. Increased cardiac output would lead to an *increase* in end-tidal CO_2.

11-11. **Correct answer: D.** The patient is developing atelectasis. The cause of the increased PIP cannot be increased airway resistance because the (peak – plateau) pressure difference remains constant at approximately 10 cm H_2O. What is changing is Pplat – PEEP, which is increasing due to a gradual rise in Pplat. This indicates a decrease in either lung or thoracic compliance. Atelectasis, which causes consolidation, decreases lung compliance. Bronchospasm causes an increase in airway resistance, which increases PIP – Pplat.

11-12. **Correct answer: A.** Carotid. Carotid arteries are never to be used for arterial puncture. The radial artery is the preferred site for arterial sampling. Other sites include the brachial, femoral, and dorsalis pedis arteries. These sites carry greater risk and should be used only by healthcare providers with proper training.

11-13. **Correct answer: A.** Compensated metabolic acidosis. First, you should recognize that compensation is occurring because *both* the $Paco_2$ and BE are abnormally low. Second, because the pH is less than 7.40, you can conclude that the primary problem is the one causing acidosis—in this case, the low BE (–10 mEq/L). Therefore, the low $Paco_2$ must represent compensation for the low BE.

11-14. **Correct answer: D.** Proper blood pressure waveform. The best indication that an arterial line has been properly inserted (and the line connected to the transducer/monitor) is the return of arterial blood pressure values accompanied by a good arterial waveform.

11-15. **Correct answer: C.** 1 and 3 only. When obtaining a mixed venous sample, if the balloon is inflated or the sample is withdrawn too quickly, you may contaminate the venous blood with blood from the pulmonary capillaries (oxygenated blood). The result is always a falsely high oxygen level. Rapid flow of IV fluid can also dilute the blood sample and affect oxygen content measures.

11-16. **Correct answer: C.** Upstream/before the heated humidifier. Inaccurate readings can occur with O_2 analyzers due to either condensed water vapor or pressure fluctuations. Galvanic cells are particularly sensitive to condensation. To avoid this problem, place the analyzer sensor upstream/ before the humidifier.

11-17. **Correct answer: D.** 1 and 3 only. Capillary blood gas sampling is used in infants and toddlers when a blood sample is needed to assess ventilation and acid–base status but arterial access is not available. Capillary sampling does not provide an accurate analysis of oxygenation.

11-18. **Correct answer: B.** Repeat the test on the right hand. The results of the initial Allen's test indicate lack of collateral circulation on the left hand. You should repeat the Allen's test on the opposite hand and proceed accordingly. Brachial puncture should be considered if the Allen test fails to show proper collateral circulation in both radial arteries.

11-19. **Correct answer: A.** Decrease the SIMV rate. The ABG results suggest normal oxygenation with an uncompensated respiratory alkalosis due to hyperventilation. The fact that there is no spontaneous ventilation (total rate = set rate) indicates suppression of the respiratory drive, probably due to hypocapnea. To stimulate the patient to breathe spontaneously, you need to eliminate the hypocapnea. During SIMV, this is best done by decreasing the ventilator's set rate. Adding mechanical deadspace generally is contraindicated in the SIMV mode.

11-20. **Correct answer: C.** 1, 2, and 4 only. During volume control ventilation, a sudden fall in peak inspiratory pressure can be caused by any of the following events: (1) improved compliance or resistance; (2) a decrease in either the volume or flow setting; and (3) patient–ventilator system leaks, such as an ET tube cuff leak, a malfunctioning exhalation valve, or tubing disconnection/leak.

11-21. **Correct answer: B.** Pulse O_2 saturation. Due to the patient's involvement in a house fire, you should immediately suspect the presence of carbon monoxide (CO) poisoning. Carbon monoxide's high affinity for hemoglobin will cause profound hypoxemia. Standard pulse oximetry cannot measure HbCO levels. To assess HbCO levels, you must use CO-oximetry.

11-22. **Correct answer: D.** Assess the patient for pain. After undergoing an invasive procedure, patients often develop surgical pain. Abnormal vital signs (usually on the high side of normal) are a common indication of the presence of pain. Assessing the patient for pain and providing for proper pain management is the right course of action.

11-23. **Correct answer: B.** Preoxygenate the patient with 100% O_2. Hypoxemia is a common cause of PVCs. Several respiratory procedures can cause hypoxemia and PVCs. Preoxygenating the patient with 100% O_2 for 30–60 seconds before suctioning can help reduce/prevent hypoxemia. Using a larger catheter, sedating the patient, and suctioning less often will not prevent hypoxemia.

11-24. **Correct answer: A.** Thoracic gas volume. Tests used to assess for airway hyperresponsiveness include methacholine bronchoprovocation, histamine challenge, and an exercise test. These tests also are indicated to screen individuals who may be at risk from environmental or occupational exposure to allergens. Thoracic gas volume (via body box) does not assess for airway responsiveness and reactivity.

11-25. **Correct answer: C.** Hypoventilation. A normal a/A ratio rules out V/Q imbalances or shunting as the cause of the hypoxemia. When breathing room air, a patient can develop hypoxemia with severe hypoventilation and still have a normal a/A ratio. Typically this would occur when the P_{CO_2} rises above 60–70 torr, which also could explain the patient's comatose state.

POST-TEST

To confirm your mastery of this chapter's topical content, you should take the chapter post-test, available online at http://go.jblearning.com/respexamreview. A score of 80% or more indicates that you are adequately prepared for this section of the NBRC written exams. If you score less than 80%, you should continue to review the applicable chapter content. In addition, you may want to access and review the relevant Web links covering this chapter's content (courtesy of RTBoardReview. com), also online at the Jones & Bartlett Learning site.

CHAPTER 12

Independently Modify Therapeutic Procedures Based on the Patient's Response

Albert J. Heuer

This chapter discusses how you can help determine the need to modify therapy, as well as the most common types of changes that you may independently implement in a given situation. Other changes that you may only recommend (because they require a physician's order) are described in Chapter 13. The following objectives have been established for this chapter to ensure that you are ready for NBRC exams.

OBJECTIVES

In preparing for the shared NBRC exam content, you should demonstrate the knowledge needed to:

1. Terminate treatment based on therapeutic goal attainment, adverse effects, or end-of-life considerations
2. Modify treatment techniques, including IPPB; incentive spirometry; aerosol, oxygen, and specialty gas (heliox, nitric oxide) therapies; and bronchial hygiene and suctioning
3. Adjust or alter artificial airway management techniques according to patient needs
4. Monitor, modify, and adjust both invasive and noninvasive mechanical ventilation settings to optimize oxygenation, ventilation, and patient synchrony
5. Initiate procedures for weaning (covered in Chapter 10)

WHAT TO EXPECT ON THIS CATEGORY OF THE NBRC EXAMS

CRT exam: 18 questions; mostly application and analysis, with two recall questions
WRRT exam: 9 questions; all analysis
CSE exam: indeterminate number of questions; however, exam III-F knowledge is a prerequisite to success on CSE Information Gathering sections

PRE-TEST

Carefully respond to each of the following questions. After completing the pre-test, compare your answers with those provided at the end of this chapter. Then thoroughly review each answer's explanation to help understand why it is correct.

12-1. While suctioning a patient, you observe an abrupt change in the ECG waveform being displayed on the cardiac monitor and a drop in SpO_2. Which of the following actions should you take?
   A. Change to a smaller catheter and repeat the procedure
   B. Stop suctioning and immediately administer oxygen

   C. Decrease the amount of negative pressure being used
   D. Instill 10 mL normal saline directly into the trachea

12-2. After you initiate bronchodilator aerosol therapy via IPPB to a patient with asthma, she becomes fatigued and short of breath. You note increased use of accessory muscles, an increase in heart rate from 90–122, and other signs of mild to moderate distress. Which of the following is the appropriate action at this time?

A. Stop the treatment and immediately chart this untoward reaction

B. Decrease the flow and have the patient exhale more forcibly

C. Increase the pressure limit and get the patient to breathe slower

D. Stop the treatment and stay with the patient until she improves

12-3. A patient is receiving appropriate oxygen therapy via a simple mask at 5 L/min but complains that the mask is confining and interferes with eating. Which of the following oxygen-delivery devices is a suitable alternative?

A. Nasal cannula at 4–5 L/min

B. Nasal cannula at 2 L/min

C. Nonrebreather mask at 10 L/min

D. A 28% Venturi mask at 6 L/min

12-4. During an IPPB treatment being given to a 66-year-old patient with COPD, you note signs of further air trapping during exhalation. Which of the following changes in technique should you consider?

1. Instructing the patient to prolong exhalation

2. Increasing the inspiratory flow rate

3. Increasing the preset pressure limit

4. Mechanically retarding exhalation

A. 1, 2, and 3

B. 2 and 4 only

C. 2, 3, and 4

D. 1, 2, and 4

12-5. You notice that the air-entrainment ports of a Venturi mask are occluded by a patient's bedding. What effect would this have on total flow and F_{IO_2}?

A. Increase total output flow and decrease F_{IO_2}

B. Increase both total output flow and F_{IO_2}

C. Decrease both total output flow and F_{IO_2}

D. Decrease total output flow and increase F_{IO_2}

12-6. To prevent hypoxemia during suctioning of an orally intubated adult patient, you should do which of the following?

A. Press the alarm silence button prior to suctioning

B. Set vacuum pressure to 100–120 mm Hg prior to suctioning

C. Administer 100% O_2 through the ventilator for 30–60 seconds prior to suctioning

D. Maintain the set F_{IO_2} and increase PEEP prior to suctioning

12-7. A 48-year-old male is orally intubated and is receiving mechanical ventilation with an 8.0-mm endotracheal (ET) tube secured in place. Cuff pressure is measured at 35 cm H_2O. Which step should you take?

A. Recommend reintubation with a smaller ET tube

B. Withdraw the ET tube 1–2 cm and reassess breath sounds

C. Recommend the physician perform a percutaneous tracheotomy

D. Lower the cuff pressure to less than 25 cm H_2O and assess for leaks

12-8. An adult patient is receiving volume control A/C ventilation with a heat and moisture exchanger (HME) in place. Over the course of 4 hours, the peak pressure has increased by 12 cm H_2O, but the plateau pressure is unchanged. It also has become more difficult to suction the patient's tracheal secretions. What should you recommend at this time?

A. Switching to the SIMV mode

B. Changing to a heated humidifier

C. Instilling normal saline before suctioning

D. Switching to a closed catheter suction system

12-9. After initiating volume control A/C ventilation, the inverse I:E ratio alarm is triggered. Which of the following should be increased to correct this problem?

A. Inspiratory flow

B. Pressure limit

C. Tidal volume

D. Respiratory rate

12-10. A college student is brought to the emergency department following a motor vehicle accident. He is tachypneic and tachycardic. He is receiving oxygen via a nonrebreathing mask at 10 L/min. You observe that the mask bag fully deflates on each inspiration. Which action should you take?

A. Change to a simple mask at 4 L/min

B. Increase the flow to 12–15 L/min

C. Change to a nasal cannula at 8 L/min

D. Continue therapy and monitor SpO_2

12-11. A physician orders O_2 therapy per protocol for an otherwise healthy postoperative patient who has a PaO_2 of 52 torr on room air. After initiating a nasal cannula at 2 L/min and repeating an arterial blood gas, the patient's PaO_2 is now 59 torr. Which action should you take?

A. Increase the oxygen flow and reassess the patient

B. Intubate the patient and institute mechanical ventilation

C. Decrease the oxygen liter flow and reassess the patient

D. Institute continuous positive airway pressure by mask

12-12. A 70-year-old male patient in the Emergency Department (ED) complains of shortness of breath, chest pain, and diaphoresis. Being busy with a anxious child in the adjoining cubicle, the ED physician asks you to implement care for the elderly man. Your initial action should include all of the following except:

A. Assess the patient's clinical status, including SpO_2

B. Quickly provide a moderate to high FIO_2

C. Promptly inform the nurse and physician of the patient's status

D. Measure the patient's maximum inspiratory pressure

12-13. You are asked to assess a 16-year-old girl with a severe head cold who is receiving 4 L/min O_2 via nasal cannula. The patient is alert and awake and is complaining that she cannot breathe through her nose. Her SpO_2 is 84%. Which action should you take?

A. Decrease the O_2 flow until the patient is more comfortable

B. Increase the O_2 flow until the SpO_2 equals or exceeds 90%

C. Change to a simple mask at 5–7 L/min

D. Recommend an arterial blood gas before considering any changes

12-14. A physician prescribes incentive spirometry for a postoperative patient who complains of dizziness when performing five inspiratory maneuvers in a row. Which action should you take?

A. Recommend that the therapy be discontinued

B. Coach the patient to pause before each maneuver

C. Switch to volume-oriented IPPB therapy

D. Begin oxygen therapy via protocol

12-15. A toddler is receiving volume control A/C ventilation. To minimize volume loss due to compression and tubing expansion, which of the following should you select?

A. Longer breathing circuit

B. Low-compliance tubing

C. Large-diameter tubing

D. Smaller-diameter ET tube connector

12-16. A recently intubated 25-year-old female patient receiving volume control SIMV has no breath sounds over the left side of her chest. Her SpO_2 on 40% O_2 has dropped from 96% to 90%. At the same time, the peak inspiratory pressure on the ventilator has increased from 35–45 cm H_2O. You note a tube length marking of 26 cm at the teeth. Which action should you take?

A. Increase the FIO_2 and the flow rate

B. Recommend a stat chest x-ray

C. Administer a bronchodilator

D. Retract the ET tube by 3–4 cm

12-17. An 88-year-old patient is having a problem holding the small-volume nebulizer mouthpiece for her bronchodilator treatment. Which action should you take?

A. Change to a dry-powder inhaler (DPI)

B. Change to a metered-dose inhaler (MDI)

C. Hold the nebulizer for the patient

D. Change to an aerosol mask

12-18. A patient coughs vigorously while receiving postural drainage and percussion on the superior segment of the left lower lobe. You then note that the sputum is mixed with a large amount of bright red blood. Which action should you take?

A. Stop the treatment, stabilize the patient, and inform the physician

B. Continue the treatment and make a note of the sputum in the chart

C. Give the patient O_2 by simple mask and continue the treatment

D. Quickly discard the sputum so the patient does not see it and become upset

12-19. During inhaled nitric oxide therapy at 6 ppm, the NO, NO_2, and O_2 analyzer readings all suddenly drop to 0. Which action should you take?
  A. Check and replace the nitric oxide cylinder
  B. Check and reconnect/replace the gas sampling line and filter
  C. Increase the concentration of NO to 10 ppm
  D. Flush the system with 100% O_2

12-20. A patient is receiving IPPB therapy for atelectasis with a set pressure of 25 cm H_2O. During therapy, the patient's pulse becomes thready and his blood pressure drops from 120/80 mm Hg to 90/50 mm Hg. Which action should you take?
  A. Decrease the IPPB pressure to 10 cm H_2O and monitor the patient
  B. Increase the IPPB pressure to 45 cm H_2O and continue the treatment
  C. Discontinue the treatment and notify the physician
  D. Change the treatment to intermittent CPAP with 10 cm H_2O PEEP

12-21. Prior to beginning an adrenergic bronchodilator treatment on an adult patient, you record a resting heart rate of 132/min. Which of the following is the correct action in this case?
  A. Double the drug diluent and prolong the administration time
  B. Have the patient self-administer the aerosol treatment
  C. Postpone therapy until you are able to contact the ordering physician
  D. Use half the standard dosage listed in the package insert

12-22. Following administration of a bland aerosol treatment, auscultation reveals rhonchi throughout the patient's middle and upper lung fields. Which action should you take?
  A. Encourage the patient to cough
  B. Recommend administration of a bronchodilator

  C. Recommend discontinuation of therapy
  D. Discontinue the treatment and administer oxygen

12-23. An adult patient being weaned from volume control A/C is placed on 10 cm H_2O pressure support ventilation with 5 cm H_2O CPAP. With the patient breathing at a rate between 25 and 28 breaths/min, the high respiratory rate alarm keeps sounding. Which action should you take?
  A. Recommend sedating the patient
  B. Increase the high-pressure alarm to 50 cm H_2O
  C. Increase the high-rate alarm to 30–35/min
  D. Stop weaning the patient immediately

12-24. While monitoring a patient during a spontaneous breathing trial, you note increased patient agitation, increased heart rate (from 85–110/min) and respiratory rate (from 15–34/min), and PVCs increasing to an average of 4 per minute. Which action should you take?
  A. Encourage the patient to relax and continue careful monitoring
  B. Request that the patient be given a stat bolus of lidocaine
  C. Reconnect the patient to the ventilator with the prior settings
  D. Request that the patient be given a strong sedative/hypnotic

12-25. After a patient has been on an aerosol from an ultrasonic nebulizer for 5 minutes, she begins to wheeze. What should you do at this time?
  A. Recommend that the patient be given IV epinephrine
  B. Stop the treatment, monitor the patient, and notify the physician
  C. Add 0.5 mL (2.5 mg) of albuterol to the nebulizer solution
  D. Switch the ultrasonic nebulizer source gas to 100% O_2

WHAT YOU NEED TO KNOW: ESSENTIAL CONTENT

Terminating Treatment Based on the Patient's Response to Therapy

In general, therapy should be terminated when the patient's safety is in question, when the therapeutic objectives have been fully met, when the therapy is clearly not achieving the intended goals, or in certain end-of-life situations. During therapy, patient safety is paramount! All patients must be monitored for adverse effects before, during, and after therapy. A good rule of thumb when a serious adverse effect is suspected is to follow these steps, starting with the "Triple S Rule": **S**top the therapy, **S**tay with the patient, **S**tabilize the patient. If in a hospital, notify the nurse and physician immediately and call a "code blue" or rapid response team (RRT), as appropriate. If in an alternative-care site such as during home care, call for help and dial 911.

Modifying Treatment Techniques

There are a host of other instances in which it may be appropriate for you to independently modify therapy based largely on the patient's response. The following sections summarize the most common situations warranting modification of treatment techniques and identify the recommended actions.

Modifying Incentive Spirometry

Incentive spirometry (IS) involves the use of a simple device to promote lung expansion. The success of this therapy depends heavily on patient cooperation and participation. Incentive spirometry measures and monitors inspired volumes and helps target goals for the patient to achieve. The equipment used for IS is discussed in more detail in Chapter 4. While IS therapy is relatively simple, sometimes modifications are needed to achieve clinical objectives. **Table 12-1** summarizes common problems and situations that may occur with IS, their likely causes, and modifications that may be helpful in resolving the problems.

Modifying Intermittent Positive-Pressure Breathing

Intermittent positive-pressure breathing (IPPB) therapy involves the application of positive pressure to the airway during inhalation to hyperinflate the lungs, help treat or prevent atelectasis, or aid in

Table 12-1 Common Modifications for Incentive Spirometry

Problem/Situation	Possible Cause(s)	Recommended Modification(s)
No volume or flow recorded on device, despite inspiratory effort from patient	Equipment assembled incorrectly, tubing or mouthpiece disconnected, patient exhaling instead of inhaling	Recheck equipment assembly and tube/mouthpiece connection, replace unit, and reinstruct patient
Patient cannot generate sufficient inspiratory effort to record volume or flow	Insufficient patient instruction, patient unable to follow directions or generate sufficient inspiratory effort	Reinstruct patient, coach patient to breathe in more deeply, consider another modality (e.g., IPPB)
Mild lightheadedness, dizziness, tingling fingers	Hyperventilation	Coach patient to breathe more and pause between maneuvers
Patient not showing clinical improvement, despite proper implementation of therapy	Incorrect diagnosis; consider diagnosis other than atelectasis or hypoventilation (e.g., pneumonia)	Call physician and recommend additional or alternative treatment (e.g., antibiotics or IPPB)
Patient cannot achieve enough flow to activate the incentive indicator	An obstructive disorder that prevents the patient from generating the flow needed to use a flow-oriented device	Recommend a volume-oriented device or one designed for patients with obstructive disorders

secretion clearance. IPPB therapy can also be used to administer and enhance the deposition of aerosolized drugs such as bronchodilators or mucolytics. With IPPB therapy, you as the RT decide on the patient interface (e.g., mask, mouthpiece) and can control and modify the gas source, FIO_2, sensitivity, inspiratory/expiratory flow, and peak pressure. The initiation of IPPB therapy, contraindications, and hazards are discussed in Chapter 10, and the equipment used is described in Chapter 4. **Table 12-2** outlines the common problems that you may experience when administering IPPB, along with the recommended modifications to correct these problems.

Modifying Bland Aerosol Therapy

Bland aerosol therapy is indicated to treat upper airway edema, laryngotracheobronchitis, and subglottic and postextubation edema. It also may help overcome a humidity deficit in patients with a bypassed upper airway or who are otherwise at risk for retained secretions. Bland aerosol therapy also is used for sputum induction procedures.

Table 12-2 Common Modifications for IPPB Therapy

Problem/Situation	Possible Cause(s)	Recommended Modification(s)
Pressure does not rise after triggering	Major leak/poor airway seal	Fix any circuit leaks, coach patient to achieve a tight mouth seal, use nose clips, consider a flanged lip seal or mask; if using an artificial airway, check cuff pressure and tube connection, and adjust terminal flow, if available
The machine does not cycle off at end-inspiration	Major leak or poor airway seal	See modifications above
	IPPB valve malfunction	Troubleshoot/clean IPPB valve
Insufficient measured exhaled V_T (one-third or more than the patient's predicted IC)	Insufficient pressure setting on the machine	Gradually increase the pressure to achieve targeted V_T
Evidence of air trapping (patients with COPD or asthma)	Increased expiratory airway resistance	Have patient slow exhalation or retard it using a flow resistor on the exhalation port
	Insufficient expiratory time	Coach patient to breathe more slowly
Mild dizziness, lightheadedness, and parasthesia (tingling in the extremities)	Hyperventilation	Coach patient to breathe more slowly (fewer than 8–10 breaths/min) and/or pause between breaths; reassess exhaled V_T and lower set pressure
Clinical evidence of worsening hypoxemia (e.g., decreasing SpO_2)	Inadequate FIO_2	Switch to device capable of high FIO_2
		Provide 100% O_2 (turn off air mix)
	Patient–machine asynchrony	Coach patient to "breathe with the machine"
		Adjust flow for desired I:E ratio
	Excessive mucus	Pause therapy and clear secretions
Patient not responding to drugs aerosolized during IPPB	Insufficient inspiratory time	Decrease the flow
	Dose wasted during expiration	Nebulize drug during inspiration only
Patient not showing clinical improvement, despite proper implementation of therapy	Incorrect diagnosis; consider diagnosis other than atelectasis or hypoventilation (e.g., pneumonia)	Call physician and recommend additional or alternative treatment (e.g., antibiotics)

Bland aerosol is usually generated by large-volume jet nebulizers; however, you may occasionally use other devices such as ultrasonic equipment. In regard to large-volume jet nebulizers, it is important that you remember the inverse relationship that exists between FIO_2 and total flow with air-entrainment devices. Specifically, as you increase the FIO_2, less air is entrained and total output flow decreases. Some of the questions on the NBRC exams will likely involve insufficient output flow of these devices at FIO_2s more than 40–45%. In other instances, you may need to modify this therapy. **Table 12-3** summarizes key problem situations that may warrant adjustments as well as the specific actions needed to resolve them.

Modifying Aerosol Drug Therapy

In addition to modifying bland aerosol therapy, you may also need to make modifications to optimize delivery of aerosolized medications. Changes in the drug, dosage, and frequency require a physician's order and are discussed in Chapter 13. However, as an RT, you can usually modify either the delivery device or the patient's breathing pattern to optimize drug delivery. The most common modifications of this type are described in **Table 12-4**.

Table 12-3 Common Modifications for Bland Aerosol Therapy

Problem/Situation	Possible Cause(s)	Recommended Modification(s)
Insufficient aerosol output flow despite $FIO_2 < 40$–45%	Insufficient input flow from flowmeter	Increase input flow from flowmeter
	Condensation in circuit	Drain condensate from circuit and add a water trap
Insufficient aerosol output at $FIO_2 > 40$–45%	High FIO_2 setting means little air entrainment and low output	Use high-output nebulizer or dual-nebulizer setup
Patient hypoxemia, despite nebulizer being properly set up	Insufficient flow output at $FIO_2 > 40$–45%	Use high-output nebulizer or dual-nebulizer setup
		If a T-piece is used, add a reservoir to its distal end
Risk of infection	Contaminated reservoir	Change nebulizer and do not drain condensate into reservoir
FIO_2 notably higher than setting and output flow decreased	Condensate in tubing	Drain condensate and add a water trap
	Obstructed entrainment port	Remove obstruction from entrainment port
Increase in airway swelling once aerosol therapy initiated	Increased edema due to absorption of moisture	Consider using a humidifier instead of an aerosol device
Aerosol output irritating to patient	Cold aerosol output may be irritating to patient's airway	Consider changing to a heated nebulizer
Despite cool aerosol therapy, patient exhibits signs of retained secretions	Insufficient aerosol delivery	Consider using a heated aerosol
	Too low a flow	Increase input flow
	Insufficient patient hydration	Recommend increased fluids, if tolerated
Insufficient output of ultrasonic nebulizer for sputum induction	Amplitude setting too low on ultrasonic device	Increase amplitude setting
Excessive aerosol output from ultrasonic nebulizer	Amplitude setting too high	Decrease amplitude setting

Table 12-4 Common Modifications for Aerosol Drug Therapy

Problem/Situation	Possible Cause(s)	Recommended Modification(s)
Inability to properly actuate or use a metered-dose inhaler (MDI), resulting in insufficient drug delivery	Inability to physically activate the device due to functional limitations	Switch to an actuator-assisted device
	Inability to coordinate breathing pattern with device actuation	Coach patient on proper breathing pattern, use a spacer or holding chamber, and consider a small-volume nebulizer (SVN)
Aerosolized medication ordered via MDI but patient is tachypneic (respiratory rate > 20)	Respiratory distress, pain, or anxiety	Use SVN; coach patient to breathe more slowly, with an intermittent breath hold; monitor patient and advise physician and nurse regarding tachypnea
Patient cannot hold mouthpiece in place for the SVN, use an MDI with spacer, or trigger a breath-actuated nebulizer	Patient is debilitated, cognitively impaired, or restrained; has facial weakness; or is otherwise unable to keep mouthpiece in place	If drug is available in other forms, use a mask with the SVN or MDI with spacer and mask
Patient unable to generate sufficient flows to use a dry-powder inhaler (DPI)	Patient is debilitated, weak, cognitively impaired, or otherwise unable to generate sufficient inspiratory flows	Use an aerosol mask with SVN
Patient receiving supplemental O_2 develops hypoxemia while receiving aerosolized medications via SVN	Inadvertent decrease in F_{IO_2} while receiving aerosolized medication	Maintain F_{IO_2} during therapy, and ensure that SVN tubing is connected to oxygen (not air)
	Paradoxical or other adverse response to therapy	Give supplemental O_2 as appropriate, monitor patient, and advise nurse and physician
Physician orders 3 mL of 20% acetylcysteine mucolytic, but only 10% formulation is available	Limited pharmacy stock	Use double the volume (6 mL) of the half-as-potent 10% acetylcysteine to achieve the equivalent dose of the drug
Patient develops severe irritation to the mouth and throat while taking inhaled steroids	Pharyngitis or oral thrush as a side effect of inhaled steroids	Instruct patient to rinse mouth after receiving inhaled steroids and add a spacer if MDI is being used
Patient has low respiratory rate, causing wasting of medication	Wasted medication is nebulized during prolonged pauses between breaths	Use a breath-actuated nebulizer
Use of a SVN in-line with ventilator circuit alters machine function	Added flow from nebulizer affects triggering and some monitoring functions (e.g., volume)	Use a small-volume ultrasonic or mesh nebulizer to deliver the drug (these devices do not add to or alter flow)

Modifying Oxygen Therapy

Once O_2 therapy has been ordered by the physician and initiated, there are instances when you should independently modify the mode of delivery or the flow. In certain circumstances, you may even change the F_{IO_2} in accordance with a preapproved O_2 therapy protocol. Although this technique is less common, an oxygen blender may also be used to deliver a desired F_{IO_2}. **Table 12-5** outlines the most common circumstances warranting modification of oxygen therapy.

Table 12-5 Common Modifications for Oxygen Therapy

Problem/Situation	Possible Cause(s)	Recommended Modification(s)
Patient remains hypoxemic after initiation of nasal O_2 therapy	Patient is a "mouth breather"	Switch to a Venturi or simple mask
	Cannula nasal prongs are blocked with secretions	Replace cannula
	Patient needs higher F_{IO_2}	Contact physician for an order to increase or use higher F_{IO_2} as permitted per protocol
	O_2 device connected to air	Ensure that the device is connected to an O_2 flowmeter
Patient complains of nasal or mouth dryness	Insufficient humidity causing drying of mucosa	Add a humidifier, particularly if input flow of nasal cannula is 4 L/min or more
Patient on simple mask at 5 L/min taking food orally	Cannot eat with mask on	Switch to nasal cannula at equivalent flow
Patient requires a low to moderate F_{IO_2} but has a high/variable minute volume	Standard nasal cannula not suitable for patients with high/variable minute volume	Switch to a high-flow device such as a Venturi mask or high-flow nasal cannula
Patient has high minute ventilation and needs a high F_{IO_2}	Inability to meet high inspiratory flow demands at high F_{IO_2}	Consider a high-flow nebulizer or high-flow nasal cannula
Non/partial-rebreather mask bag fails to remain inflated	Insufficient input flow	Increase flowmeter setting
	Tubing disconnect	Ensure that tubing is correctly connected to flowmeter
Patient feels claustrophobic with aerosol mask in use	Confining feeling imposed by mask	Switch to a face tent
Patient has facial injury or burns, but order is for 40% aerosol	Mask may cause irritation or further injury to face	Switch to a face tent
An infant or child receiving 50% O_2 in an isolette must be removed for a special procedure	Infant will breath room air and become hypoxemic	Consider a simple mask that can be easily set up but is not easily dislodged
The Sp_{O_2} of an infant receiving CPAP via nasal prongs drops during episodes of crying	Decrease in F_{IO_2} due to mouth breathing associated with crying	Collaborate with nurse to address reasons for crying (e.g., hunger)
		If crying and decrease in Sp_{O_2} continue, consider an enclosure such as an oxyhood (same F_{IO_2})
Air-entrainment mask delivers higher F_{IO_2} than set	Obstruction of entrainment ports with bedding, clothing, or other items	Remove obstructions and monitor patient

Figure 12-1 is an example of an oxygen therapy protocol algorithm (flowchart) that permits the RT to titrate (or modify) the F_{IO_2} based on a patient's clinical status and in accordance with the preapproved sequence.

Modifying Specialty Gas Therapy

In addition to oxygen therapy, RTs may administer other specialty gases. These gases include helium–oxygen (heliox) and nitric oxide. The NBRC expects you to have a basic understanding of the indications, equipment setup and troubleshooting, and common modifications involved in administering these two gases.

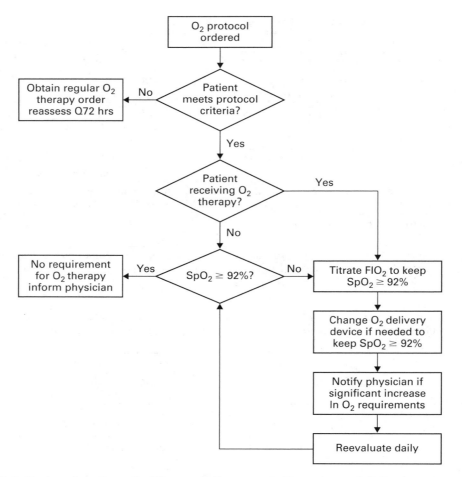

Figure 12-1 Example of an O₂ Therapy Protocol. Note that a full O₂ therapy protocol also would include patient inclusion criteria and specifications for equipment selection.

Helium–Oxygen (Heliox) Therapy

The value of helium in respiratory care is based on its low density. Breathing a helium–oxygen mixture decreases the driving pressure needed in ventilation, particularly in large airways. Hence, heliox can help decrease the work of breathing associated with large airway obstruction. Major indications for this therapy include acute upper airway obstruction, reversible obstructive disorders, postextubation stridor, and croup.

Chapter 4 discusses the equipment and setup needed for applying heliox to spontaneously breathing patients using premixed cylinders of 80%, 70% or 60% He in O₂. For these patients, heliox generally is delivered either via a tight-fitting nonrebreathing mask with the flow sufficient to meet or exceed the patient's minute ventilation and peak inspiratory flow requirements, or via a high-flow nasal cannula. For infants with bronchiolitis, heliox can be administered via an oxyhood. However, the heat loss and hypothermia associated with helium's high thermal conductivity has limited its use for such young patients, with preference now being given to using a high-flow nasal cannula.

Heliox can also be delivered to patients receiving invasive ventilatory support via a cuffed tracheal airway. As specified in Chapter 4, only a ventilator approved by the FDA for heliox delivery should be used for this purpose. At this time, heliox is not recommended for use in conjunction with noninvasive positive-pressure ventilation (NPPV).

Heliox administration also has been combined with jet-nebulized bronchodilator therapy to treat severe acute obstructive disorders such as status asthmaticus, especially when standard therapy fails. Some data indicate that nebulization with heliox improves the delivery and deposition of aerosolized drugs in such patients and results in better clinical improvement compared with using air as the carrier gas. Note that flows need to be increased by 50–100% when using heliox to power drug nebulizers. Moreover, because the inhaled aerosol mass and particle size produced by commonly used SVNs vary substantially, no general guidelines other than using higher flows can be provided for this application.

Irrespective of the delivery method, all patients receiving helium–oxygen mixtures should be closely monitored, and an oxygen analyzer with active alarms should always be used to continuously measure the F_{IO_2} being delivered to the patient. Once heliox is in use, you may need to modify or troubleshoot the therapy. **Table 12-6** summarizes the major situations where such changes may be appropriate.

Inhaled Nitric Oxide Therapy

Inhaled nitric oxide (NO) is a potent pulmonary vasodilator. Because it relaxes the capillary smooth muscle of the pulmonary vessels, this therapy can reduce intrapulmonary shunting, improve arterial oxygenation, and decrease both pulmonary vascular resistance and pulmonary artery pressures.

After several years of testing, inhaled NO was approved for the treatment of term and near-term (more than 34 weeks' gestation) neonates with hypoxemic respiratory failure associated with persistent pulmonary hypertension of the newborn (PPHN). Inhaled NO has also been used in adults to treat pulmonary hypertension associated with acute respiratory distress syndrome (ARDS), although to date no significant improvement in long-term clinical outcomes has been shown in such patients.

Although NO can be administered to spontaneously breathing patients via a nasal cannula or a mask, it is more commonly applied to patients receiving mechanical ventilation. The most common setup is the INOvent (Ikaria) delivery system. The INOvent system includes storage cylinders containing nitric oxide delivered via an injector placed in the inspiratory side of the ventilator circuit, near its outlet. Also included is a sensor that measures the ventilator's inspiratory flow. To achieve the desired NO dose, the injection rate is automatically adjusted in proportion to the measured gas flow. The recommended initial dose of NO is 20 ppm but can often be quickly reduced to 5–6 ppm.

Table 12-6 Common Modifications for Heliox Therapy

Problem/Situation	Possible Cause(s)	Recommended Modification(s)
Patient receiving 80/20 heliox mixture has symptoms of moderate hypoxemia and SpO$_2$ < 90%	Insufficient F_{IO_2} delivery to patient	Analyze the F_{IO_2} to ensure prescribed concentration is being delivered; if confirmed, consider recommending a mixture with a higher F_{IO_2} (e.g., 70/30)
Patient receiving heliox via nonrebreathing mask at 10 L/min, but reservoir bag completely collapses during inspiration	Insufficient input flow	Use a flow adequate to keep bag inflated throughout the breathing cycle; if using standard O$_2$ flowmeter, apply appropriate conversion factor (Chapter 4); consider high-flow cannula administration
Less effective cough and secretion clearance	Lower-density heliox inhibits expulsive phase of coughing	Wash out heliox with air–O$_2$ mixture before coughing
Excessive heat loss and hypothermia for infant receiving heliox via oxyhood	Higher thermal conductivity associated with helium	Warm and humidify gas and closely monitor patient
Variability in medication (bronchodilator) delivery when using heliox	Variability in particle size and deposition due to lower-density gas	Use only nebulizers approved for heliox and monitor patient response to therapy
Patient receiving heliox via invasive ventilation exhibits signs of volume loss or ventilatory insufficiency	Excessive volume loss from insufficient air in ET tube cuff or failure to use conversion factors to adjust ventilator settings	Add air to cuff to ensure an adequate seal (MOV); if airway seal adequate, make sure ventilator is approved for heliox delivery and conversion factors applied to adjust settings
Evidence of lung overdistension ("beaked" pressure–volume graphic) in patient receiving heliox through a ventilator	Excessive volume delivery and lung distension because of failure to account for lower-density gas	Use conversion factors to adjust settings, confirm use of approved ventilator; closely monitor patient

When nitric oxide comes in contact with oxygen, a toxic by-product known as nitrogen dioxide (NO_2) is produced. NO delivery equipment is designed to limit the contact time between these two gases, thereby minimizing the production of NO_2. Nitric oxide, NO_2, and O_2 concentrations are continuously analyzed through a sampling line connected near the distal end of the circuit near the patient's airway. Alarms are used to detect and warn of excessive levels of NO or NO_2, or undesired changes in the F_{IO_2}. NO_2 levels should not exceed 2–3 ppm.

In many cases, the benefits of increased oxygen saturation and decreased pulmonary artery pressure may be seen soon after initiating NO therapy. Treatment may be continued for up to 14 days. Factors to consider when preparing to withdraw therapy are as follows:

- Reduce the NO concentration to the lowest effective dose, ideally 5–6 ppm or less.
- Ensure that the patient is hemodynamically stable.
- Verify patient tolerance of an F_{IO_2} of 40% or less and a PEEP of 5 cm H_2O or less.
- Monitor the patient closely during withdrawal of therapy.
- Prepare to provide hemodynamic support if required.

At the recommended doses, NO has been shown to have minimal toxicity and adverse side effects. Nevertheless, although they remain quite rare, hazards include excessive methemoglobin levels, worsening of congestive heart failure, and rebound effect (reoccurrence of hypoxemia/pulmonary hypertension) soon after withdrawal of therapy. Inhaled NO is also contraindicated in some patients, most notably neonates with certain cardiovascular anomalies such as coarctation of the aorta. **Table 12-7** summarizes instances when modifications to this therapy should be recommended.

Table 12-7 Common Modifications for Inhaled Nitric Oxide Therapy

Problem/Situation	Possible Cause(s)	Recommended Modification(s)
Immediately after initiating NO therapy, NO_2 levels steadily rise above 2–3 ppm	Failure to flush system during setup	Flush system with 100% oxygen before initiating therapy
NO therapy initiated at 20 ppm, but no clinical improvement is seen	Improper equipment setup	Ensure equipment is properly set up and functioning
	Poor or paradoxical response	Recommend alternative (pharmacological) therapy
NO therapy is started with an initial dose of 6 ppm, but no clinical improvement is seen	Initial dose is too low	Recommend an increase in the initial dose, up to 20 ppm, and monitor patient closely
Analyzed nitric oxide (NO) level drops to 0	NO supply tank is empty	Check NO tank pressure and switch or replace NO cylinder
NO, NO_2, and O_2 analyzer readings suddenly drop to 0	Obstructed or disconnected sample line	Check/reconnect gas sampling line, and replace in-line sampling line filter
NO, NO_2, and O_2 analyzer readings altered during bronchodilator therapy via SVN	Alteration of prescribed gas mixture by nebulizer flow	Recommend bronchodilator therapy via MDI or mesh nebulizer (no additional flow)
	Disruption of circuit by nebulizer insertion	Add MDI adaptor to circuit
NO_2 level exceeds 2–3 ppm	NO_2 analyzer malfunction	Check and recalibrate NO_2 analyzer
	Excessive contact time between NO and O_2	Check proper setup of all equipment
During weaning or immediately after withdrawing NO, patient becomes hemodynamically unstable or hypoxemic	Patient not tolerating weaning from NO at this time	If weaning is ongoing, recommend that patient be returned to original NO dosage
	Rebound effect	If NO was recently withdrawn, recommend increased F_{IO_2} and hemodynamic support (vasopressors), consider reinstituting NO therapy, and closely monitor patient

Modifying Bronchial Hygiene Therapy

Bronchial hygiene therapy includes a variety of techniques designed to help mobilize and remove secretions. These techniques include the following:

- Manual and mechanical chest percussion and vibration
- Postural drainage
- Directed coughing
- Positive expiratory pressure (PEP)
- Intrapulmonary percussive ventilation (IPV)
- Mechanical insufflation–exsufflation

These therapies are described in more detail in Chapter 9.

Often, one or more of these techniques can be combined with other therapies to help clear secretions, including bland aerosol administration or inhaled medications (e.g., mucolytics and bronchodilators). When several techniques are employed to clear secretions, the following recommended sequence should generally be followed:

1. Open them up (with bronchodilators)
2. Thin them out (with bland aerosol and/or mucolytic agents)
3. Clear them out (by bronchial hygiene techniques)

While these techniques may be effective in helping clear secretions, in some instances you should modify the position, duration, or technique or recommend a different bronchial hygiene strategy. **Table 12-8** summarizes common problems and situations that may warrant modifying bronchial hygiene therapy, as well as specific changes to consider.

Table 12-8 Common Modifications for Bronchial Hygiene Therapy

Problem/Situation	Possible Cause(s)	Recommended Modification(s)
Patient has pain when you perform directed coughing or percussion	Post abdominal or thoracic surgery or injury (trauma)	Coordinate therapy sessions with pain mediation; assist patient in splinting the operative site; use FET/huff coughing instead of regular cough
Patient cannot generate sufficient cough to clear secretions	Patient has paralysis or neuromuscular weakness	Manually assist exhalation via application of pressure to the thoracic cage or epigastric region (chest compression or "quad cough"*); consider mechanical insufflation–exsufflation (see Chapter 9) or suctioning
Patient coughs violently while in head-down position	Mobilization of secretions or other stimulation of cough mechanism	Discourage strong coughing in head-down position as this can increase ICP; sit patient up until the cough subsides and coach patient in FET/huff coughing
Postural drainage of certain lung segments requires head-down positioning, may not be tolerated, or is contraindicated.	Head-down position may cause vomiting/aspiration, dyspnea, cerebral bleeding, cardiovascular compromise, or worsening of other conditions	Approximate the position as closely as possible; consider lateral decubitus or supine position; consider alternative therapy not requiring positional change, such as mechanical insufflation–exsufflation or PEP; shorten the time interval spent in the position
Patient complains of pain or discomfort during percussion or vibration	Percussion or vibration applied too rigorously or too near an incision or injury site	Reduce percussion/vibration intensity or consider using electric or pneumatic percussor; do not apply too near site of incision or injury; coordinate with pain medication

(continues)

Table 12-8 Common Modifications for Bronchial Hygiene Therapy (*continued*)

Problem/Situation	Possible Cause(s)	Recommended Modification(s)
Patient cannot cooperate with postural drainage or other bronchial hygiene therapy	Patient is aged or confused	Consider alternative therapy not requiring patient cooperation, such as mechanical insufflation–exsufflation
Patient develops excessive secretions in throat and mouth during bronchial hygiene therapy	Secretions being mobilized as a result of therapy	Place patient in upright position, encourage coughing; consider suctioning or mechanical insufflation–exsufflation
Percussion and vibration ordered but potential for bleeding or pain	Recent thoracic surgery or injury	Consider using an electric or pneumatic percussor/vibrator; apply percussion and vibration at a safe distance from incision/injury; coordinate with pain medication
Increased risk of vomiting and/or aspiration	Therapy sessions conflict with mealtime	Schedule therapy at least 30–60 minutes before or after meals
Patient with or at risk for hypoxemia, but for whom bronchial hygiene is indicated	Underlying condition resulting in chronic or acute hypoxemia (e.g., COPD)	Provide additional supplemental O_2 and monitor SpO_2 throughout procedure
	Movement of secretions or mucus plug to larger airways, impeding ventilation	Consider 100% O_2 during therapy for critically ill patients; shorten administration time
Patient on PEP therapy is having difficulty keeping mouthpiece in place	Neuromuscular weakness or difficulty following commands	Coach patient on proper technique, consider PEP via mask or another technique such as postural drainage, percussion, and vibration

* Chest compression or "quad cough" is contraindicated for patients with osteoporosis, patients with flail chest, unconscious patients with unprotected airways, pregnant women, and patients with acute abdominal pathology.

Modifications Relating to the Management of Artificial Airways

Artificial airways are used in clinical practice in a variety of situations. They are primarily indicated for the following reasons:

- To correct impending or actual airway obstruction
- To facilitate ventilation
- To protect the airway
- To remove secretions

Artificial airways (discussed in more detail in Chapter 8) include oropharyngeal and nasopharyngeal airways, laryngeal mask airways (LMA), endotracheal (ET) tubes, and tracheostomy tubes. Once an artificial airway is in place, there may be instances when modifications are in order. **Table 12-9** outlines the most common situations requiring such modifications.

Modifying Suctioning Technique

Suctioning the airway is an effective means of secretion clearance, which can be applied alone or in combination with bronchial hygiene therapy and aerosolized medications. As previously noted in this text, patients should be suctioned with the smallest effective catheter size (less than 50% of the lumen of the ET tube in children and adults, less than 70% of this size in infants), using the lowest suction pressure needed, for not more than 15 seconds. As with other therapies, there are times when you should independently adjust the suctioning technique, as noted in **Table 12-10**.

Modifications in Mechanical Ventilation

Once mechanical ventilation is initiated, it is often necessary to make changes. Changes usually requiring a physician's order include the mode of ventilation, tidal volume, rate, FIO_2, and PEEP.

Table 12-9 Common Modifications When Managing Artificial Airways

Problem/Situation	Possible Cause(s)	Recommended Modification(s)
Nasal discomfort associated with nasopharyngeal airway	Too large a nasopharyngeal airway in use given the patient's size	Use a smaller airway
	Device in place for too long	Switch to the opposite naris; change every 8 hours
Intubated patient has an oropharyngeal airway that is moving excessively	Too small or large an oropharyngeal airway in use	Switch to an appropriately sized airway, measuring from earlobe to corner of mouth (do not tape an oropharyngeal airway in place)
Awake intubated patient with oropharyngeal airway is gagging	Discomfort associated with oropharyngeal airway	Consider removing the airway and using a bite-block device to secure the ET tube
		Recommend sedation (avoid oropharyngeal airway in conscious patients)
Difficult intubation	Glottis is located anteriorly or excessive epiglottic tissue	Reposition patient; consider LMA or fiber-optic intubation
	Incorrect laryngoscope blade/ET tube size	Ensure correct-size ET tube and laryngoscope blade
	Patient agitated or anxious	Recommend sedation, and request that an anesthesiologist perform the procedure
Adult with oral ET tube has absent breath sounds and insufficient chest rise on left side, high peak pressures, and poor oxygenation	Intubation of the right mainstem bronchus likely	Retract ET tube about 2–3 cm; after bilateral breath sounds are heard, resecure tube, monitor patient, and recommend chest x-ray
Gurgling sounds heard around the mouth of an orally intubated, but otherwise stable patient	Most likely insufficient air in ET tube cuff	Add air to cuff to minimal occluding volume and ensure pressure $\leq$ 25 cm H_2O; consider tube with port for aspirating subglottic secretions
	Cuff may be blown or the pilot balloon tubing may have a leak	If cuff does not hold pressure, consider an ET tube exchanger or recommend reintubation
ET tube cuff pressure measured at a pressure in excess of 25 cm H_2O	Excessive air in cuff	Remove air from cuff to achieve pressure $\leq$ 25 cm H_2O but without leak; consider tube with port for aspirating subglottic secretions
	Too small an ET tube	Recommend reintubation (or use ET tube exchanger) with appropriate-sized ET tube
Evidence of mucus plugging or retained/thick secretions for a spontaneously breathing patient with an artificial airway	Humidity deficit due to a bypassed upper airway	Consider continuous or intermittent heated, bland aerosol therapy via tracheostomy collar or T-piece
Evidence of retained or thick secretions for a mechanically ventilated patient with an artificial airway	Humidity deficit due to a bypassed upper airway	If HME or cool humidity system in use, switch to servo-controlled heated humidifier
Patient with an artificial airway has visible secretions, coarse rhonchi, or tactile fremitus over large airways	Excessive secretions	Suction airway using proper-size catheter and vacuum pressures for no more than 10–15 seconds
Redness and excessive green or brown foul-smelling secretions noted around the stoma of a patient's trach	Inflamed/infected stoma	Ensure that stoma is cleaned and inner cannula and dressing changed at least every 8 hours; notify nurse and physician that stoma may be infected
Clinical signs indicate airway obstruction (e.g., high-pressure alarm, little/no expired V_T during mechanical ventilation)	Mucus plug in ET tube	Suction; if problem persists, recommend immediate extubation and reintubation or inner cannula change, if trach

Table 12-10 Common Modifications for Suctioning

Problem/Situation	Possible Cause(s)	Recommended Modification(s)
Catheter does not advance during nasotracheal suctioning	Deviated septum or nasal polyps	Use opposite naris
	Suction catheter too large	Use smaller catheter and more lubricant
Catheter does not advance through an appropriately sized artificial airway	Suction catheter too large	Use a smaller catheter
	Mucus plug obstructing airway	If trach, clean/change inner cannula; if signs of airway obstruction persist, recommend immediate extubation and reintubation
Small amount of blood or streaks noted in secretions	Nasal or airway trauma due to repeated suction attempts	Use smallest effective catheter; use nasal trumpet for repeated nasopharyngeal suctioning; use shallow technique for ET suctioning; consider noninvasive clearance mechanisms (e.g., mechanical insufflation–exsufflation)
Patient becomes hypoxemic during suctioning procedure	Decreased FRC/removal of O_2	Preoxygenate with 100% O_2 (10% greater than baseline in neonates) for 30–60 seconds; limit suction time to 15 seconds; use closed-suction system for patients on ventilators; apply recruitment maneuver to restore FRC
Patient suddenly develops bradycardia during suctioning	Vasovagal response due to suction catheter stimulating airway	Stop suctioning, apply supplemental O_2, monitor patient, and notify nurse and physician; consider shorter suctioning time.
Patient has evidence of loose or mobile secretions that cannot be suctioned	Suction pressure set too low	Increase suction pressure to a maximum of –120 mm Hg (adults) or –80 mm Hg (neonates)
	Suction catheter too small	Use appropriate-size catheter
	Secretions too thick	Ensure adequate humidification, and consider aerosolized mucolytics with bronchodilators
Intubated and mechanically ventilated patient has copious secretions in the left lung	Left-sided bronchitis or pneumonia	Use a Coudé (angled-tip) catheter to aid insertion into the left bronchus
No vacuum pressure	System leak, vacuum off, obstruction or kinking in tubing	Fix system leak, turn vacuum on, fix obstruction or kinked tubing

Normally, as an RT you cannot make these changes independently, unless they are covered under a ventilator management protocol. However, you can and should recommend changes in these parameters when indicated (as discussed in Chapter 13). In most institutions, including the NBRC "hospital," the changes that you can make without a physician's order generally are limited to "secondary" settings such as inspiratory flow, sensitivity, I:E ratio, and alarms.

When modifying ventilator settings, it is generally best to make one change at a time, especially when adjusting either oxygenation (e.g., FIO_2 or PEEP) or ventilation (e.g., tidal volume or respiratory rate). When several changes are implemented simultaneously, it becomes difficult to determine the impact of any single adjustment. Additionally, in cases of patient–ventilator asynchrony or problems with ventilator alarms, it is best to promptly determine whether the origin is related mainly to the patient or to ventilator function. **Table 12-11** summarizes the most common changes that you as an RT can make independently, related to invasive positive-pressure ventilation.

Table 12-11 Common Modifications During Invasive Positive-Pressure Ventilation

Problem/Situation	Possible Cause(s)	Recommended Modification(s)
Patient–ventilator asynchrony (patient origin)	Patient respiratory distress due to excessive secretions, bronchospasm, hypoxemia, or air trapping	Assess patient to help determine whether the problem has a patient or machine origin; if patient related (e.g., mucus, bronchospasm, hypoxemia), address cause (e.g., suction, bronchodilators, increased F_{IO_2}/PEEP), and if not promptly resolved, consider a period of manual ventilation with F_{IO_2} 100%, advise nurse and physician
	Inadequate sedation	Recommend sedation and advise nurse and physician
Patient–ventilator asynchrony (ventilator-setting origin)	Inappropriate trigger sensitivity	Adjust sensitivity: –1 to –2 cm H_2O or 1–3 L/min
	Insufficient inspiratory flow	If using volume control, increase flow to eliminate post-trigger effort or consider using adaptive flow (if available); if using pressure control, adjust rise time to eliminate spiking at plateau (left "dog ear")
	Inadequate expiratory time	Increase inspiratory flow or decrease set rate to achieve an I:E ratio of 1:2 or 1:3
Auto-PEEP, detected (patient origin)	Increase in airway resistance or tachypnea	Suction airway; recommend bronchodilators or sedation, applied external PEEP
Auto-PEEP, detected (machine origin)	Inadequate expiratory time or excessive inspiratory time	Increase inspiratory flow, and consider other measures such as reduction in rate setting or pause time
Insufficient returned tidal volume or sudden decrease in ventilating pressure	Leak in circuit or patient interface	Fix leak in circuit or add air to tube cuff
Patient on mechanical ventilation with HME has thick secretions and increased peak pressure (PIP)	Higher PIP with thick secretions suggests increased airway resistance due to either humidity deficit or partially obstructed HME	Switch to a servo-controlled heated humidifier; suction airway to help remove secretions, particularly once humidifier is replaced
Excessive condensation (rainout) in tubing	Cooling of saturated gas during delivery of breath through ventilator tubing	Use heated-wire circuit or add a water trap
Volume loss from a ventilator circuit for a neonatal or young pediatric patient	Volume loss due to circuit tubing expansion (circuit compliance) and gas compression	Use a low-compliance (stiff) circuit and low-volume innards (humidifier) to minimize volume loss
While weaning, patient develops tachypnea, hypoxemia, and other signs of distress	Patient not tolerating weaning attempt	Place patient back on full ventilator support and monitor closely; recommend changes in settings, such as F_{IO_2}, as appropriate

Chapter 11 provides guidance on procedures for the initial setting of ventilator alarms. **Table 12-12** outlines some of the common problems and situations involving ventilator alarms that are most likely to appear on the NBRC exams, including needed alarm adjustments.

Special mention should be made regarding the use of mechanical deadspace (adding 50–300 mL of extra tubing between the wye connector and the patient's airway) to manage excessive ventilation causing respiratory alkalosis. The addition of mechanical deadspace to the ventilator circuit causes CO_2 rebreathing, and thus should increase the patient's Pa_{CO_2}. However, this result is ensured

Table 12-12 Adjustments to Ventilator Alarms Settings and Monitoring

Problem/Situation	Possible Cause(s)	Recommended Modification(s)
Excessive ventilator alarm activation (primarily patient origin)	*High pressure:* mucus plug, kinked tube, decreased compliance, or bronchospasm	Suction, reposition ET tube, or provide bronchodilator therapy
	Low pressure: disconnect, improved compliance, or leak	Reconnect patient or fix leak (e.g., in nebulizer)
	High rate: patient distress, weaning failure, or agitation	Assess patient, cease weaning attempt, recommend sedation
	High minute volume: hypermetabolic state, hypoxemia, agitation, or brain injury	Recommend ABG, sedation, chemically paralyze patient, add mechanical deadspace
	Low minute volume: leak, hypoventilation, apnea, or weaning failure	Fix leak, place patient back on full ventilator support
Excessive ventilator alarm activation (inappropriate settings)	High-rate alarm set at 20/min is sounding while weaning an adult	Adjust the high-rate alarm to 5–10/min above the actual rate, to a maximum of 30–35/min
	High-pressure alarm for an adult is set at 25 cm H_2O and is sounding	Increase the high-pressure alarm to 5–10 cm H_2O above the actual PIP, subject to a maximum of 45–50 cm H_2O
	Low-minute-ventilation alarm for an adult is set at 2.0 L	Set low-minute-ventilation alarm about 2.0 L/min below the actual minute ventilation, but never below 4.0–5.0 L/min for an adult
	Low-pressure alarm is set at 3 cm H_2O	Set low-pressure alarm about 5–10 cm H_2O below PIP, but never lower than 5 cm H_2O, to ensure that leak or patient disconnect is promptly detected

only in pure control mode ventilation (no patient triggering allowed). In assist/control (A/C) modes, the addition of mechanical deadspace can have untoward effects, such as the patient further increasing the minute ventilation by triggering more breaths. Moreover, in ventilator modes that include spontaneous breathing (such as SIMV) or those protocols that employ low tidal volumes, the addition of mechanical deadspace generally is contraindicated.

Beyond general guidelines for adjusting ventilator alarms, the NBRC expects you to be able to apply these concepts to specific clinical situations. The accompanying box describes several common problems involving ventilator alarm adjustments and discusses the appropriate action in such cases.

Case Summaries: Adjusting and Responding to Ventilator Alarms

Case 1: The Weaning Patient

Problem

An adult patient was recently switched from volume control SIMV (V_T = 550 mL, rate =12/min, FiO_2 = 0.50, PEEP = 5 cm H_2O) to pressure support of 12 cm H_2O and appears to be tolerating weaning well. However, several alarms are sounding, including alarms for low tidal volume (set at 450 mL) and high respiratory rate (set at 25/min).

Discussion

Alarm settings that were appropriate for the original settings may not be appropriate during weaning. In this situation, you should modify alarms to recognize the expected changes in tidal volume and respiratory rate during weaning. In this instance, the low-tidal-volume alarm can be safely decreased to approximately 250–300 mL, and the high respiratory rate can be safely changed to 30–35/min.

Also note that if and when it becomes necessary to switch from pressure support back to full ventilatory support (assist/control) for such reasons as an overnight rest period or failed weaning attempt, it is often necessary to modify the alarms accordingly. In general, the high respiratory rate should be decreased to about 10 above the total respiratory rate (set plus additional), and the low tidal volume should be about 100 mL below the level that is set.

Case 2: Changing Between Pressure Control and Volume Control Ventilation

Problem

An adult patient on pressure control ventilation, with a ΔP (pressure differential) of 20 cm H_2O and +5 cm H_2O PEEP, is switched to volume control A/C (V_T = 550 mL, rate =12/min, F_{IO_2} = 0.50, PEEP = 5 cm H_2O). The high-pressure alarm, which is set at 30 cm H_2O, is sounding, and you see that the PIP on the ventilator is 35 cm H_2O.

Discussion

The high-pressure alarm should be increased to recognize the somewhat higher ventilating pressure of 35 cm H_2O associated with switching to volume ventilation. In this instance, you should increase the high pressure alarm to 5–10 cm H_2O above actual peak airway pressure, subject to a maximum of 45–50 cm H_2O.

Keep in mind that if and when you make the opposite change—that is, if you move this patient from pressure to volume control—the peak airway pressure alarm setting may be too high, given the ventilating pressure of 25 cm H_2O. In such an instance, you should lower the peak airway pressure alarm setting to 30–35 cm H_2O (5–10 cm H_2O above peak airway pressures).

Case 3: Change in Set Volume

Problem

A 5-foot, 10-inch adult patient is initially placed volume control A/C with V_T = 750 mL, rate =12/min, F_{IO_2} = 0.60 and PEEP = 5 cm H_2O. Based on ABG results and a subsequent comprehensive assessment, the V_T is reduced to 550 mL. However, the tidal volume on the apnea (backup) remains at 750 mL. Later, during weaning, the patient becomes apneic, the apnea alarm is activated, and the patient is ventilated at a tidal volume of 750 mL.

Discussion

The tidal volume on the apnea parameters is inappropriately high. Without a reduction in the "apnea" V_T, the patient is at risk for being overventilated and his lungs overdistended, especially if he becomes apneic on a spontaneous or weaning mode. Whenever a significant change is made to the settings, the apnea alarms and settings should be checked and changed, if appropriate, to maximize patient safety. In this instance, the patient's "apnea" tidal volume should be reduced to 550 mL. It is very likely that the low V_T alarm may be need to be adjusted to about 450 mL or 100 mL below the new V_T.

Case 4: Artificial Airway Obstruction

Problem

When caring for a patient on a ventilator, you note that suddenly both the low-V_T and high-pressure-limit alarms are sounding on each inspiration; the patient's SpO_2 is 85% and the heart rate is 148/min.

Discussion

The sudden decrease in V_T and increase in ventilating pressures strongly suggests an acute airway obstruction (e.g., kinked or clogged ET tube). If the patient shows signs of distress and there is a question about the functioning of the ventilator or airway, disconnect the patient from the ventilator and ventilate with 100% O_2 via a manual resuscitator while you troubleshoot the ventilator. If you are still unable to manually ventilate the patient, quickly try to pass a suction catheter; if this is not successful, extubate the patient and manually ventilate with a mask.

Case 5: Remote Alarm Problem

Problem

The ventilator alarm is sounding, but the remote alarm monitor is not activated.

Discussion

This problem appears to be rooted in either disconnection of the remote alarm cable or a remote alarm equipment problem. To identify such problems, remote alarms should be tested during each shift to ensure they are functioning properly. This involves ensuring that the cable is connected and the alarms are functional. Faulty cables or remote alarm units should be immediately replaced or repaired.

Table 12-13 Common Modifications During Noninvasive Positive-Pressure Ventilation

Problem/Situation	Possible Cause	Recommended Modification
Patient's clinical status suggests need for only nocturnal or intermittent ventilation	A variety of conditions resulting in hypoventilation, including neuromuscular conditions and sleep apnea	Consider recommending NPPV
Patient on NPPV objects to discomfort or major leak from nasal mask or other interface	Mask or interface too tight, ill fitting, or otherwise unsuitable	Loosen interface to use minimum pressure to achieve a seal, or consider alternative mask or interface, including nasal pillows
Patient on NPPV complains of extreme airway dryness	Inadequately humidified gas	Consider adding heated humidifier to circuit
Patient is on NPPV with 15 L/min O_2 bleed-in to circuit, but remains mildly hypoxemic	Inability of certain NPPV ventilators to deliver high FIO_2 due to significant dilution with room air	Consider a device capable of delivering high FIO_2s, bleed additional O_2 directly into mask
Patient's mouth is wide open during NPPV via nasal mask, and the pressure fails to reach the set inspiratory pressure	Major leak through the mouth	Consider adding a chin strap or using a full-face mask

In addition to the changes related to invasive positive-pressure ventilation and alarms, you will need to be familiar with the most likely modifications involving noninvasive positive-pressure ventilation. These modifications are described in **Table 12-13**.

Ventilator Waveform Evaluation

In addition to the previously described modifications for mechanically ventilated patients, a review and interpretation of ventilator graphics may help identify the need to make certain changes independently. Following are the most commonly found waveforms that would warrant your independent action.

Patient–Ventilator Asynchrony

Asynchrony between the patient and ventilator can be seen as an irregularly spiked flow or irregular pressure waveform, as depicted in **Figure 12-2**. As discussed in Table 12-11, patient–ventilator asynchrony may originate from either the patient or the ventilator setting. If the asynchrony is patient related, you should independently troubleshoot and address the most common patient

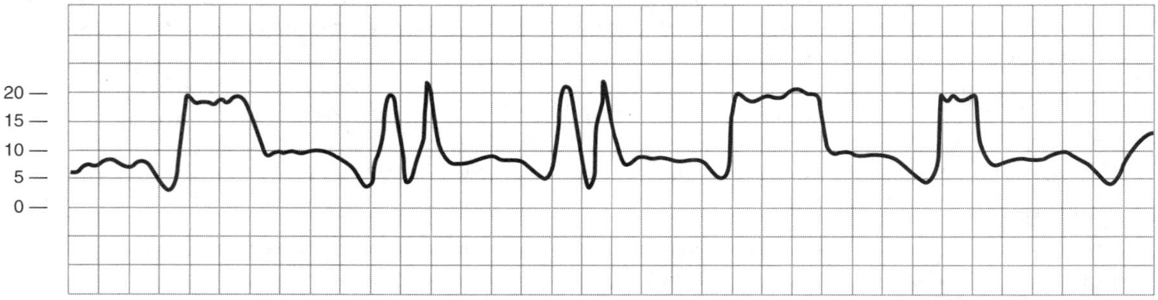

Figure 12-2 A Graphical Display of Patient–Ventilator Asynchrony Showing Irregular Pressure Waveform.

Source: Burns SM, ed. *AACN protocols for practice: noninvasive monitoring* (2nd ed.). Sudbury, MA: Jones and Bartlett Publishers; 2006.

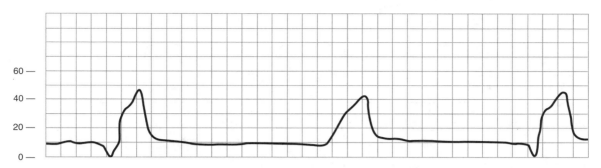

Figure 12-3 Ventilator Graphic Showing Inappropriate Sensitivity. Note that the patient must drop the pressure 10 cm H_2O below baseline to trigger the first and third breaths.

Source: Burns SM, ed. *AACN protocols for practice: noninvasive monitoring* (2nd ed.). Sudbury, MA: Jones and Bartlett Publishers; 2006.

causes, including suctioning a patient with excessive mucus or mucus plugging, recommending bronchodilators for bronchospasm, or recommending sedation for agitated patients. If the problem is related to the ventilator settings, consider inappropriate trigger sensitivity and inadequate inspiratory flow, as they are the most frequent causes of patient–ventilator asynchrony. Usually, increasing the flow or adjusting the sensitivity to a proper level will solve the problem.

Inappropriate Sensitivity

The sensitivity setting is inappropriate when the patient must exert excessive negative pressure or excessive inspiratory flow to initiate a breath, as reflected in **Figure 12-3**. An inappropriate sensitivity setting can impose additional work of breathing on patients and cause patient–ventilator asynchrony. In general, the solution to this problem is to adjust the sensitivity to an appropriate level, usually less than –1 to 2 cm H_2O for a pressure trigger or to 1–3 L/min for a flow trigger.

Volume Loss

Volume loss occurs when the set tidal volume is not delivered to or returned from the patient. The volume–time waveform in **Figure 12-4** reveals this situation in that the exhaled volume does not return to zero. The problem most often involves a leak in the patient–ventilator interface. Leaks usually occur around the artificial airway or a connection in the ventilator circuit. If you determine the leak is due to the artificial airway and the airway is properly positioned, the best fix usually consists of readjusting the cuff pressure to eliminate the leak (see Chapter 8). If you determine that the leak is in the ventilator circuit, either fix the loose connection or replace the circuit.

Auto-PEEP

Auto-PEEP occurs when the patient is still exhaling as the next breath machine is delivered, causing gas to remain trapped in the lungs. Auto-PEEP is most commonly caused by insufficient exhalation

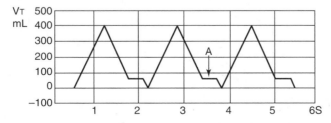

Figure 12-4 Volume–Time Graphic Showing Volume Loss. Note that the expired volume does not return to baseline.

Source: Burns SM, ed. *AACN protocols for practice: noninvasive monitoring* (2nd ed.). Sudbury, MA: Jones and Bartlett Publishers; 2006.

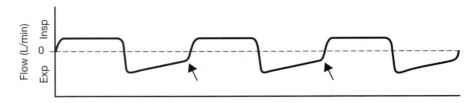

Figure 12-5 Flow–Time Graphic Showing Auto-PEEP. Expiratory flow does not return to zero baseline before the next machine breath, indicating gas-trapping (arrows).

Courtesy of: Strategic Learning Associates, LLC, Little Silver, New Jersey.

time, patient asynchrony, or increased airway resistance. This problem can manifest in several ways, but most commonly takes the form of an expiratory flow waveform that does not return to zero before the next breath, as shown in **Figure 12-5**. To measure the amount of auto-PEEP, you perform an end-expiratory hold maneuver (described in Chapter 11). Once you confirm its presence, you will need to manage this condition according to its cause. If the cause is insufficient exhalation time, you should either increase the inspiratory flow, decrease the inspiratory time, or increase the expiratory time (by decreasing the rate). If auto-PEEP is associated with excessive airway resistance, you can often reduce or eliminate it by suctioning or administering bronchodilators. More details on managing auto-PEEP are provided in Chapter 13.

Overdistension

Excessive ventilatory pressures can cause overdistension of the lung and lead to barotrauma. On a pressure–volume curve, such as that shown in **Figure 12-6**, overdistension becomes apparent when the curve flattens significantly beyond the upper inflection point. Due to its resemblance to a bird, this graphic depiction is sometimes called a "beaked" pressure–volume curve. When you observe this problem, you generally can resolve it by reducing either the set volume or pressure, in accordance with existing protocols. In the absence of a protocol, a change in tidal volume or pressure limit usually requires a physician's orders; thus it would be achieved by recommendation from the RT, rather than independent action.

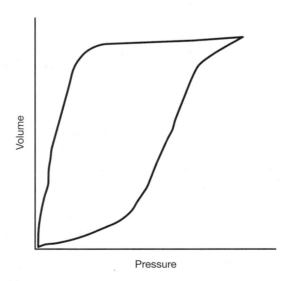

Figure 12-6 Pressure–Volume Loop Indicating Overdistension During a Positive-Pressure Breath. Beyond the upper inflection point, small changes in volume result in very large increases in pressure, making the loop appear like the "beak" of a bird.

Courtesy of: Strategic Learning Associates, LLC, Little Silver, New Jersey.

Weaning from Ventilatory Support

To initiate weaning from ventilatory support, you generally need a physician's order. However, the specific means of weaning often is governed by preapproved protocols, which give you some discretion as to the methods used, including the speed with which the patient may be weaned. Chapter 10 provides details on weaning procedures, including implementation of protocol-based spontaneous breathing trials and weaning ALI/ARDS patients using the NHLBI ARDS protocol.

COMMON ERRORS TO AVOID

You can improve your score by avoiding these mistakes:

- Never continue therapy on a patient who exhibits severe adverse reactions. Instead, if you note adverse reactions, stop the therapy, monitor the patient closely, and notify the physician and nurse.
- Never apply percussion or vibration too close to surgical incisions or chest injury or trauma. Instead, apply the therapy a safe distance (6–12 inches) from incision or injuries.
- Never use incentive spirometry on an uncooperative patient or one who cannot follow commands. Instead, consider recommending IPPB, which can be used to treat or prevent atelectasis regardless of the patient's mental status.
- In general, do not use a standard air-entrainment device to deliver a high F_{IO_2} (greater than 45–50%) to a spontaneously breathing patient. Instead, consider (1) a nonrebreathing mask, (2) a high-flow cannula, (3) two large-volume nebulizers connected in parallel, or (4) a high-output nebulizer.
- Never use an electrically powered (air compressor) device to deliver IPPB therapy to a patient requiring a moderate to high F_{IO_2}. Instead, consider pneumatically powered devices such as the Bird Mark 7 or Bennett PR-II, which can deliver a high F_{IO_2}.
- Never drain tubing condensate back into a nebulizer. Instead, place a water trap in the line to capture the condensate.
- Never use an MDI or a DPI on a patient who is in tachypneic or in severe respiratory distress. Instead, use a small-volume nebulizer.
- Never use a standard nasal cannula on a patient who requires a low F_{IO_2} but who has a high or unstable minute ventilation. Instead, use a high-flow device such as an air-entrainment (Venturi) mask or high-flow nasal cannula.
- During postural drainage, never keep a nauseous patient or a patient who is coughing violently in a head-down position. Instead, sit the patient up, monitor the patient closely, and notify the physician and nurse.
- Never keep a nasopharyngeal airway in place (in the same naris) for more than 1 day.
- Never use a low-flow system, such as a nasal cannula, to administer heliox therapy to spontaneously breathing patients. Instead, administer heliox using either a tight-fitting nonrebreathing mask at a flow of 10–15 L/min or a high-flow nasal cannula.
- Avoid tracheal damage by never inflating endotracheal tube cuffs to pressures above 25 cm H_2O.
- Never keep an undersized ET tube in place for a long time period. Instead, recommend reintubation with an appropriate-size tube.
- Never use excessive suctioning pressure or application time. Instead, suction adult patients with the lowest effective negative pressure for no longer than 10–15 seconds.
- When making changes to ventilator settings, avoid simultaneous changes in parameters affecting either oxygenation (e.g., F_{IO_2} or PEEP) or ventilation (e.g., tidal volume or respiratory rate).
- Never continue using a heat and moisture exchanger for a patient who develops thick, bloody, or copious secretions. In these cases, switch to a heated humidifier.
- Never set the low-minute-ventilation alarm on adults receiving ventilator support below 4.0–5.0 L/min.
- When using a CPAP or BiPAP mask, minimize tissue damage by avoiding too tight a fit.

SURE BETS

In some situations, you can be sure of the right approach to a clinical problem or scenario:

- When you suspect a serious adverse effect of therapy, always stop what you are doing, stabilize the patient, and remain with the patient while notifying the patient's nurse and/or calling for the rapid response team.
- If the adverse effect appears life threatening, initiate a "code blue" (in hospital) or activate the EMS system (in alternative-care sites such as the home).
- Always ensure a good lip seal during IS or IPPB hyperinflation therapy. If a good lip seal is not possible (e.g., owing to neuromuscular weakness) but the patient is at risk for atelectasis, consider IPPB via mask.
- When administering heliox therapy, always use an oxygen analyzer with active alarms to continuously measure the F_{IO_2}.
- Always remember to use the appropriate conversion factor (1.8 for a 80/20 mixture and 1.6 for a 70/30 mixture) when using a standard flowmeter to administer heliox therapy.
- If you suspect insufficient drug delivery with an MDI, always review the patient's technique and consider adding a holding chamber or spacer or adding an actuator assist device for patients who are unable to activate the device.
- Always consider adding humidity for patients on a nasal cannula with flows greater than 4 L/min.
- If the tubing is correctly set up to a nonrebreathing mask and the bag fails to remain at least partially inflated during inspiration, always increase the flow.
- Always preoxygenate and hyperinflate patients with 100% O_2 before suctioning and ensure that the appropriate-size catheter is used.
- Always consider using a Coudé suction catheter when attempting to target the left lung in suctioning.
- Always ensure that the tracheal stoma is cleaned and the inner cannula and dressing are changed at least every 8 hours to minimize the chance of infection.
- To avoid ventilator self-cycling or imposing excessive work on the patient, always ensure that the triggering sensitivity is properly set at –1 to –2 cm H_2O (pressure trigger) or –1 to –3 L/min (flow trigger).
- If the ventilator pressure manometer fluctuates widely during inspiration or if the inspiratory flow waveform is "scalloped," always consider increasing the inspiratory flow.
- When administering nitric oxide (NO) to a mechanically ventilated patient, always ensure that NO, NO_2, and O_2 concentrations are continuously analyzed and are at acceptable levels.
- Always consider increasing the flow if you observe an unintended inverse I:E ratio during volume control ventilation.
- To maximize patient safety and avoid unnecessary alarm activation, always set, check, and adjust ventilator alarms several times during each shift. Pay special attention to low-pressure (disconnect) and low-minute-ventilation alarms.
- Always check and appropriately adjust ventilator alarms when making major ventilator settings changes, such as switching to pressure support to begin weaning.

PRE-TEST ANSWERS AND EXPLANATIONS

Following are this chapter's pre-test answers and explanations. Be sure to review each answer's explanation thoroughly to help you understand why it is correct. If the explanation is still unclear to you, review the chapter content.

12-1. **Correct answer: B.** Stop suctioning and immediately administer oxygen. If you observe any major change in a patient's heart rate or rhythm or other adverse effect, immediately stop the procedure and give oxygen to the patient and provide manual ventilation as necessary.

12-2. **Correct answer: D.** Stop the treatment and stay with the patient until she improves. Should you observe any adverse or untoward effects, immediately stop the treatment and stay at the bedside until the patient is stabilized.

12-3 **Correct answer: A.** Nasal cannula at 4–5 L/min. A simple mask at 5 L/min delivers an F_{IO_2} in the 0.35–0.40 range, as does a nasal cannula at 4–5 L/min. All other choices would result in a substantial change in the F_{IO_2}, and using a mask would not address the issues of confinement and difficulty eating.

12-4. **Correct answer: D.** 1, 2, and 4. Increased expiratory times may be appropriate during the IPPB therapy given to some patients with COPD. This can be achieved by (1) coaching the patient to prolong exhalation, (2) increasing the inspiratory flow, or (3) mechanically retarding exhalation via a flow resistor placed distal to the expiratory port.

12-5. **Correct answer: D.** Decrease total output flow and increase F_{IO_2}. Occlusion of the entrainment port would decrease (or eliminate) air entrainment. Because the entrained air accounts for a significant amount of its output, total flow of the device would drop. The decrease in entrained air would also mean less air diluting the oxygen. Hence, the F_{IO_2} would increase.

12-6. **Correct answer: C.** Administer 100% O_2 through the ventilator for 30–60 seconds prior to suctioning. The best way to prevent hypoxemia during suctioning of adults is preoxygenation with 100% O_2. Whenever possible, avoid disconnecting the patient from the ventilator to do so. For infants, increase the oxygen concentration 10% above the baseline.

12-7. **Correct answer: D.** Lower the cuff pressure to less than 25 cm H_2O and assess for leaks. A pressure of 35 cm H_2O is excessive and could cause tracheal damage. You should first lower the cuff pressure to less than 25 cm H_2O and assess for leakage. If leakage is present at the safer pressure, recommend an ET tube with a port for aspirating subglottic secretions. Replacing the ET tube with a larger size is an alternative.

12-8. **Correct answer: B.** Changing to a heated humidifier. An increase in PIP without an increase in plateau pressure indicates increased airway resistance. Difficulty in suctioning secretions suggests that the increased resistance is caused by retained secretions. Because thick or bloody secretions are contraindications to using an HME, you should switch the patient over to a heated humidifier.

12-9. **Correct answer: A.** Inspiratory flow. During volume control A/C ventilation, I:E ratios normally are maintained in the 1:2 to 1:4 range. An inverse I:E ratio alarm indicates that the I-time exceeds the E-time. This is often due to inadequate inspiratory flow. You should either increase the flow, decrease the volume, or decrease the rate to give more time for exhalation.

12-10. **Correct answer: B.** Increase the flow to 12–15 L/min. Reservoir bag deflation on inspiration is a sign of inadequate flow; increase the flow to prevent room air entrainment and F_{IO_2} reduction.

12-11. **Correct answer: A.** Increase the oxygen flow and reassess the patient. Based on the data given, O_2 has been prescribed per protocol to correct arterial hypoxemia. The initial response indicates that this objective is not being fully met because the Pa_{O_2} is still below the normal range of 80–100 torr. The F_{IO_2} should be gradually increased until the targeted Pa_{O_2} or an Sp_{O_2} greater than 90–92% is achieved.

12-12. **Correct answer: D.** Measuring maximum inspiratory pressure. All of the listed actions except maximum inspiratory pressure (MIP) measurement are indicated in this emergency situation.

12-13. **Correct answer: C.** Change to a simple mask at 5–7 L/min. An Sp_{O_2} of 84% is substantially below normal. However, the nasal O_2 therapy is probably not effective because this patient likely is breathing through his mouth. The O_2 therapy should, therefore, be switched to a mask.

12-14. **Correct answer: B.** Coach the patient to pause before each maneuver. To avoid lightheadedness or dizziness associated with hyperventilation, a patient using incentive spirometry should be coached to perform one or two maneuvers and then to breathe normally for 30–60 seconds before initiating another maneuver.

12-15. **Correct answer: B.** Low-compliance tubing. "Compressed volume" is volume that the patient does not receive due to gas compression and circuit expansion. It is most critical when delivering small volumes to infants and toddlers. To minimize compressed volume loss in these patients, use small-diameter, stiff tubing and humidifiers with low internal volume.

12-16. **Correct answer: D.** Retract the ET tube by 3–4 cm. The most likely problem is right-sided mainstem bronchus intubation, as suggested by the clinical findings, including decreased ventilation to the left chest and a reduction in PaO_2.

12-17. **Correct answer: D.** Change to an aerosol mask. Changing to a mask will eliminate the need for the patient to hold the mouthpiece in place, both benefiting the patient and saving you time.

12-18. **Correct answer: A.** Stop the treatment, stabilize the patient, and inform the physician. Hemoptysis or coughing up blood is a serious side effect of postural drainage, percussion, and vibration. Whenever a severe adverse reaction to therapy occurs, stop what you are doing, stabilize and monitor the patient, and notify the physician.

12-19. **Correct answer: B.** Check and reconnect/replace the gas sampling line and filter. The likely problem is an obstructed or disconnected sample line. To correct this problem, check and reconnect the line, and replace the in-line sampling line filter.

12-20. **Correct answer: C.** Discontinue the treatment and notify the physician. Positive pressure can impair hemodynamic performance. When that outcome occurs, you should stop the treatment, stabilize the patient, and then notify and suggest alternative therapies to the physician.

12-21. **Correct answer: C.** Postpone therapy until you are able to contact the ordering physician. In general, an adrenergic bronchodilator should not be given if a patient already has tachycardia or if the pulse rate increases more than approximately 20 beats/min.

12-22. **Correct answer: A.** Encourage the patient to cough. Rhonchi indicate increased secretions. Patients who develop rhonchi after receiving bland aerosol therapy should be encouraged to cough and clear the secretions.

12-23. **Correct answer: C.** Increase the high-rate alarm to 30–35 /min. During weaning, a modest increase in respiratory rate is common and generally should be tolerated up to a maximum of 30–35/min. for an adult patient.

12-24. **Correct answer: C.** Reconnect the patient to the ventilator with the prior settings. Development of severe agitation, tachypnea, tachycardia/bradycardia, hypotension, asynchronous or paradoxical breathing, angina, or cardiac arrhythmias during weaning usually indicates that ventilatory support should be reinstituted.

12-25. **Correct answer: B.** Stop the treatment, monitor the patient, and notify the doctor. A patient who starts wheezing during an ultrasonic treatment is likely developing bronchospasm in response to the high-density aerosol. In general, when a patient experiences an adverse reaction to therapy, stop the therapy, stabilize and monitor the patient, and then contact the physician.

POST-TEST

To confirm your mastery of this chapter's topical content, you should take the chapter post-test, available online at http://go.jblearning.com/respexamreview. A score of 80% or more indicates that you are adequately prepared for this section of the NBRC written exams. If you score less than 80%, you should continue to review the applicable chapter content. In addition, you may want to access and review the relevant Web links covering this chapter's content (courtesy of RTBoardReview. com), also online at the Jones & Bartlett Learning site.

CHAPTER 13

Recommend Modifications in the Respiratory Care Plan

Albert J. Heuer and Narciso E. Rodriguez

Beyond providing initial respiratory care to patients, you often must recommend modifications to the care plan based on the patient's response and changes in the patient's clinical status. This chapter reviews both the criteria for determining the need for a care plan modification and the implementation of such changes.

OBJECTIVES

In preparing for the shared NBRC exam content, you should demonstrate the knowledge needed to recommend:

1. Procedures such as bronchopulmonary hygiene, patient positioning, fluid/electrolyte therapy, drug therapy, artificial airway management, and weaning from mechanical ventilation
2. Modifications in patient positioning, inhaled drug dosage or concentration, and F_{IO_2}
3. Discontinuation of treatment based on patient response
4. Changes in ventilator modes and techniques

WHAT TO EXPECT ON THIS CATEGORY OF THE NBRC EXAMS

CRT exam: 17 questions; about 15% recall, 60% application, and 25% analysis
WRRT exam: 14 questions; about 10% application and 90% analysis
CSE exam: indeterminate number of questions; however, exam II-G knowledge is a prerequisite to success on CSE Decision-Making sections

PRE-TEST

Carefully respond to each of the following questions. After completing the pre-test, compare your answers with those provided at the end of this chapter. Then, thoroughly review the explanation for each answer to help you understand why it is correct.

13-1. A patient with acute bronchitis is receiving mechanical ventilation. Wheezing is heard over all lung fields, and rhonchi are heard over the central airways. Secretions have been quite thick. The patient's peak pressure is 45 cm H_2O, and plateau pressure is 20 cm H_2O. All of the following would be useful to treat the patient's condition except:
   A. Albuterol (Proventil)
   B. Ipratropium bromide (Atrovent)
   C. Acetylcysteine (Mucomyst)
   D. Pancuronium bromide (Pavulon)

13-2. A 75-year-old female patient with a fractured hip has been bedridden for at least 1 week. The patient has clear breath sounds, but they are diminished slightly in the bases. The patient has normal PFTs based on bedside spirometry. Which of the following should you recommend?

   1. Bronchodilator therapy
   2. Deep suctioning
   3. Incentive spirometry treatments
   4. Coughing and deep breathing

A. 1 and 3 only
B. 2 and 4 only
C. 3 and 4 only
D. 1, 2, and 4 only

13-3. An intubated patient in the ICU needs to undergo bedside bronchoscopy and is in need of short-term moderate sedation. Which of the following agents would you recommend for this procedure?
A. Propofol (Diprivan)
B. Haloperidol (Haldol)
C. Lorazepam (Ativan)
D. Cisatracurium (Nimbex)

13-4. You are assisting a medical resident performing an emergency intubation on a somewhat combative patient. The resident wants to briefly paralyze the patient to facilitate this procedure. Which drug would you recommend for this purpose?
A. Pancuronium (Pavulon)
B. Succinylcholine (Anectine)
C. Vecuronium (Norcuron)
D. Cisatracurium (Nimbex)

13-5. A physician is having difficulty visualizing the airway of an obese patient during an emergency intubation procedure. He asks for your recommendation to quickly secure the airway and provide short-term manual ventilation via a resuscitator. Which measure should you recommend?
A. Performing a cricothyrotomy
B. Inserting an LMA
C. Sedating the patient
D. Using a double-lumen ET tube

13-6. A 90-kg (198 lb) male patient with a flail chest injury is receiving volume control A/C ventilation with an F_{IO_2} of 0.5, a set rate of 18, and a tidal volume of 600 mL. He is involuntarily breathing above the set rate for a total respiratory rate of 28–30/min. Results of an ABG analysis are as follows:

pH	7.52
$Paco_2$	27 torr
HCO_3	21 mEq/L
BE	–2 mEq/L
Pao_2	81 torr
Sao_2	96%

On the basis of these results, which measure would you recommend?

A. Increasing the F_{IO_2}
B. Adding mechanical deadspace
C. Increasing the ventilator rate
D. Increasing the tidal volume

13-7. An 87-year-old nursing home patient is admitted with pneumonia. On assessment, the patient presents with a 103.2°F temperature, dry mucous membranes, urine output of 10 mL/hr for the past 2 hours, mild hypotension, and increased hematocrit on his CBC. You should recommend to the ER physician all of the following *except*:
A. Initiating IV fluids immediately
B. Beginning diuretic therapy
C. Minimizing insensible water loss
D. Documenting fluid intake/output every hour

13-8. A patient with ARDS receiving pressure control ventilation using the NHLBI ARDS protocol remains severely hypoxemic on 90% O_2 and 24 cm H_2O PEEP. Which of the following measures would you consider recommending to further support this patient?
1. Prone positioning
2. High-frequency oscillation ventilation
3. Airway pressure release ventilation
A. 1 only
B. 2 only
C. 1 and 3 only
D. 1, 2, and 3

13-9. A patient with COPD who is receiving volume control A/C ventilation appears to be developing auto-PEEP. Which of the following measures should you recommend to improve this situation?
A. Decreasing the I:E ratio
B. Adding an inspiratory hold
C. Using an inverse I:E ratio
D. Using a decelerating flow pattern

13-10. You are managing a 49-year-old male patient who weighs about 80 kg (175 lb) and is on a mechanical ventilator with the following settings and ABG results:

Ventilator Settings		Blood Gases	
Mode	Vol Ctrl A/C	pH	7.42
V_T	750 mL	$Paco_2$	36 torr
Rate	12/min	Pao_2	58 torr
F_{IO_2}	0.35	HCO_3	23 mEq/L
PEEP	5 cm H_2O		

Which changes should you now recommend to the physician?

A. Increasing the F_{IO_2} to 0.50
B. Changing the mode to SIMV
C. Adding 150 mL of deadspace
D. Increasing the rate to 16/min

13-11. A patient with heart failure is receiving volume control A/C ventilation and has a pulmonary artery catheter in place. The ventilator peak pressure is 45 cm H_2O, and plateau pressure is 25 cm H_2O. The patient's PA pressure is 42/33 mm Hg, and pulmonary artery pressure (PAWP) is 28 mm Hg. Lung sounds indicate dependent crackles and wheezing. Which of the following measures should you recommend?

A. Administering albuterol (Proventil)
B. Decreasing the mean airway pressure
C. Administering furosemide (Lasix)
D. Removing the PA catheter

13-12. A patient is receiving a treatment with 2.5 mg of albuterol and 3 mL of normal saline in the emergency department. The heart rate prior to therapy is 80/min; at the end of therapy, the heart rate is 128/min. Which measure should you recommend?

A. Adding acetylcysteine (Mucomyst) to the treatment
B. Decreasing the dosage of albuterol
C. Increasing the amount of saline per treatment to 5 mL
D. Changing to ipratropium bromide (Atrovent)

13-13. An adult patient who just suffered a cerebral contusion and resulting cerebral edema from an automobile accident is placed on volume control A/C ventilation while in the emergency department. Initial ABG values are as follows:

pH	7.39
$Paco_2$	42 torr
HCO_3	25 mEq/L
BE	0 mEq/L
Pao_2	92 torr
Sao_2	95%

What should you recommend for the management of this patient?

A. Maintaining the current ventilator settings
B. Increasing the patient's minute volume
C. Increasing the inspired O_2 percentage
D. Changing to pressure control ventilation

13-14. Which of the following drugs would be most appropriate to recommend as a substitute for albuterol (Proventil) for a patient who has bronchospasm and whose cardiac rate increases by 50/min with each treatment?

A. Isoetharine (Bronkosol)
B. Isoproterenol (Isuprel)
C. Racemic epinephrine
D. Ipratropium bromide (Atrovent)

13-15. A patient with neuromuscular disease has been on ventilatory support for 4 months via tracheostomy. At this point, she requires only nocturnal ventilator support. Which of the following artificial airways should you recommend?

A. Tracheostomy button
B. Bivona tracheostomy tube
C. Cuffed, fenestrated tracheostomy tube
D. Uncuffed, standard tracheostomy tube

13-16. A physician orders 3 L/min O_2 via simple mask to a 33-year-old postoperative female patient with moderate hypoxemia while breathing room air (Pao_2 = 52 torr). What is the correct action at this time?

A. Carry out the physician's prescription exactly as written
B. Recommend a flow of at least 5 L/min
C. Recommend that the mask be changed to a cannula at 2 L/min
D. Do not apply the oxygen until contacting the medical director

13-17. A patient in combined hypoxemic and hypercapnic respiratory failure due to an acute restrictive disorder is placed on volume control SIMV mode at a rate of 12 /min and a PEEP of 10 cm H_2O. Soon thereafter, she begins to exhibit a paradoxical breathing pattern with intercostal retractions. Which of the following changes should you recommend?

A. Decreasing the PEEP level to 5 cm H_2O
B. Decreasing the rate to 8 breaths/min

C. Switching over to the pure CPAP mode

D. Providing supplemental pressure support

13-18. Which of the following would indicate adequate oxygenation of a patient being considered for weaning from mechanical ventilation?

1. PaO_2/FIO_2 (P/F ratio) < 150
2. $FIO_2 \leq 0.4$–0.5
3. PEEP $\leq$ 5–8 cm H_2O

A. 1 only

B. 2 only

C. 2 and 3 only

D. 1, 2, and 3

13-19. An adult patient who was started on cool mist therapy after extubation begins to develop stridor. Which of the following actions should you recommend?

A. Changing from cool mist to heated aerosol

B. Administering a racemic epinephrine treatment

C. Reintubating the patient immediately

D. Drawing and analyzing an ABG

13-20. An 8-hour-old, 28-week-gestational-age neonate is being maintained in an oxygen hood with an FIO_2 of 0.65. The neonatologist believes that the patient has infant respiratory distress syndrome (IRDS). Based on the following ABG results, what should you recommend?

pH	7.36
$PaCO_2$	44 torr
HCO_3	24 mEq/L
BE	0 mEq/L
PaO_2	52 torr

A. Increasing the O_2 hood concentration to 100%

B. Beginning inhaled nitric oxide (INO) therapy

C. Administering pulmonary surfactant

D. Starting high-frequency ventilation

13-21. A physician asks your recommendation regarding sedation for a mechanically ventilated patient in the ICU. You would consider recommending all of the following to calm this patient *except*:

A. Pentobarbital (Nembutal)

B. Propofol (Diprivan)

C. Lorazepam (Ativan)

D. Cisatracurium (Nimbex)

13-22. A 110-pound female patient in the ICU is receiving volume control A/C ventilation with V_T = 500 mL, rate = 12/min, and FIO_2 = 0.60. The morning x-ray report indicates generalized low lung volumes and developing atelectasis and her SpO_2 has dropped from 91% to 86%. What should you recommend to correct the atelectasis and improve the FRC?

A. Adding 5-10 cm H_2O PEEP

B. Increasing the O_2 concentration

C. Suctioning the patient more frequently

D. Switching to pressure control ventilation

13-23. A 25-year-old patient with asthma has continual symptoms that limit her physical activity. Along with frequent exacerbations of her condition, her FEV_1/FVC is less than 60% of the predicted value. Which of the following drugs should you recommend to help control her condition over the long term?

1. Albuterol (Proventil) MDI 2 puffs 3 times a day
2. Fluticasone (Flovent) MDI 2 puffs 4 times a day
3. Salmeterol (Serevent) 2 puffs 2 times a day

A. 2 only

B. 3 only

C. 2 and 3 only

D. 1 and 2 only

13-24. A patient receiving pressure control A/C ventilation develops sudden respiratory distress. You note decreased chest excursions, decreased breath sounds, and hyperresonance to percussion, all on the left side. Which of the following would you recommend?

1. Obtaining a stat chest x-ray
2. Increasing the FIO_2 to 1.0
3. Decreasing the ventilator PIP

A. 1 only

B. 1 and 2 only

C. 2 and 3 only

D. 1, 2, and 3

13-25. While reviewing the lab chemistry of a patient in metabolic acidosis due to renal failure, which electrolyte would you expect to be abnormally high?

A. Glucose

B. Bicarbonate

C. Chloride

D. Potassium

WHAT YOU NEED TO KNOW: ESSENTIAL CONTENT

Recommending and Modifying Bronchial Hygiene Therapy

The primary indication for bronchial hygiene therapy is to assist patients in clearing retained secretions. The various methods used to aid secretion removal are detailed in Chapter 9. You should recommend the appropriate technique be added to the care plan when clinical findings suggest the presence of retained secretions. Such findings include visible secretions in the airway, coarse breath sounds/rhonchi, ventilator changes indicating increased airway resistance, x-ray changes indicating retained secretions (e.g., atelectasis), ineffective spontaneous coughing, and suspected aspiration of gastric or upper airway secretions.

Chapter 12 covers many of the situations that would warrant modifying bronchial hygiene therapy. In general, modifications may be appropriate in light of preexisting conditions (e.g., increased intracranial pressure), recent procedures (e.g., surgery), patient demographics (e.g., age), or an adverse reaction to the therapy (e.g., hypoxemia). Modifications involve one or more of the following: (1) altering the duration of therapy, (2) altering the positions used, or (3) using a different bronchial hygiene strategy. The accompanying box provides common examples of when to recommend such modifications.

Examples of Bronchial Hygiene Modification

- Shorten the duration of a given postural drainage position for patients who become anxious or otherwise do not tolerate the therapy.

- Discourage strenuous coughing for stroke patients or those otherwise predisposed to increased ICP. Instead, instruct these patients to use a "huff" cough or sit them up until the cough subsides.

- For patients at risk for hypoxemia, provide supplemental O_2 and monitor the Spo_2 throughout the procedure.

- If adverse event (e.g., hypoxemia, bronchospasm, dysrhythmias) occurs, stop the therapy, return patient to original position, administer supplemental O_2, monitor the patient closely, contact the physician, and recommend an alternative strategy.

Recommending Changes in Patient Positioning

Table 13-1 summarizes when it may be appropriate for you to recommend changing a patient's position.

Recommending Insertion or Modifications of Artificial Airways

In some instances, you should recommend the insertion or modification of an artificial airway based on your assessment of the patient. **Table 13-2** summarizes the major indications for insertion of an artificial airway. The various airway equipment used in respiratory care is detailed in Chapter 4. Procedures for inserting artificial airways and the care of such devices are discussed in Chapters 8 and 16.

Chapter 12 discusses the common adjustments in airway management that the RT can perform independently. Other changes involving artificial airways require a physician's order; such changes often relate to the size, type, or other major feature of the artificial airway. **Table 13-3** outlines the most common situations warranting such recommendations.

Recommending Treatment of a Pneumothorax

Pneumothorax is a serious condition that can be life threatening, especially if the gas in the thorax is under pressure (tension pneumothorax). Clinical signs indicating a tension pneumothorax include:

- Sudden respiratory distress/increased work of breathing
- Decreased chest excursion on the affected site

Table 13-1 Recommending Modifications in Patient Position

Clinical Situation	Recommended Position Change
General dyspnea	Semi-Fowler's position (consider recommending other therapy such as supplemental O_2)
Orthopnea (dyspnea while supine) generally associated with CHF	Semi-Fowler's or high Fowler's position (consider recommending other therapy such as supplemental O_2)
Perform postural drainage on a patient with increased ICP or at risk for aspiration	Avoid Trendelenburg (head-down) position; consider rotating the patient laterally to approximate this position
Perform postural drainage on an immobile, bedridden patient	Recommend rotation/vibration bed
Perform IPPB/PEP or oscillation therapy	Semi-Fowler's or Fowler's (avoid slouching); supine is acceptable for patients who are unable to tolerate an upright position
Mechanically ventilated patient with unilateral disease (e.g., consolidation, atelectasis)	Place patient in "good lung down" position
Mechanically ventilated patient with poor oxygenation despite high F_{IO_2} and PEEP	Consider prone positioning or kinetic therapy bed
Chest tube insertion	Involved side should be slightly elevated, with the arm flexed over the head
Thoracentesis	Patient sitting on the edge of the bed, leaning forward over a pillow-draped bedside table, arms crossed, with assistant in front for stability
Immobile patient at risk for bed sores (decubitus ulcers)	Change position (side to side) every 2 hours; use decubitus mattress
Perform CPR on a patient in bed	Place a "compression board" under the patient's back or put bed in "CPR" mode

Table 13-2 Indications for Artificial Airways

Artificial Airway	Indications
Oropharyngeal airway	Stabilize tongue to facilitate ventilation (unconscious patient)
Nasopharyngeal airway	Facilitate frequent nasal suctioning and ventilation
Laryngeal mask airway (LMA)	Facilitate short-term artificial ventilation; an alternative during difficult intubations
Endotracheal tube (oral)	Facilitate airway protection, artificial ventilation (up to 2 weeks), and secretion clearance
Endotracheal tube (nasal)	In the presence of oral or mandibular trauma or pathology, facilitate airway protection, artificial ventilation, and secretion clearance
Tracheostomy tube (cuffed, unfenestrated)	Facilitate long-term airway protection, artificial ventilation, and secretion clearance; improve access for oral care when artificial airway is indicated; potential to improve weaning prospects
Tracheostomy tube (cuffed, fenestrated)	Same indications for standard tracheostomy tube, with the added benefit of permitting phonation (speaking) and testing upper airway patency and control
Tracheostomy tube (uncuffed)	Maintain patent airway (e.g., in obstructive sleep apnea); provide secretion clearance and permit supplemental oxygenation and humidification for a patient with a bypassed upper airway
Tracheostomy button	Maintain patent airway (e.g., in obstructive sleep apnea); provide secretion clearance and permit supplemental oxygenation and humidification for a patient with a bypassed upper airway

Table 13-3 Recommending Modifications for Artificial Airways

Problem/Situation	Possible Cause(s)	Recommendation(s)
Clinical evidence of impending respiratory failure	Inadequate oxygenation (e.g., pneumonia) and/or ventilation (e.g., neuromuscular disease)	Immediate intubation
Clinical evidence of inadequate airway protection	Diminished neurologic function (e.g., drug overdose); airway injury, facial trauma, or burns	Immediate intubation
Difficult intubation	Glottis located anteriorly or excessive epiglottic tissue; incorrect laryngoscope blade/ET tube size; patient agitated or anxious	Repositioning the patient's airway, inserting laryngeal mask airway (LMA), or performing fiberoptic intubation; selecting correct size ET tube and laryngoscope blade or sedating the patient
Excessive ET tube cuff leak despite adequate pilot balloon pressure	Blown ET tube cuff; broken/defective pilot balloon or pilot tube; too small ETT	Reintubation with proper-size tube (e.g., 8.0–9.0 for average adult male)
Intubation indicated in the presence of facial or mandibular trauma or pathology	Oral intubation contraindicated	Nasal intubation or tracheotomy
Oral ETT in place but need for long-term ventilation exists	Failed weaning attempts	Tracheostomy
Trach tube in place but patient with good upper airway control wishes to talk	Improvement in patient condition	Deflate cuff and attach Passy-Muir speaking valve; alternatively, use "talking" trach tube
Need to maintain an airway without an indication for artificial ventilation	Obstructive sleep apnea or upper airway pathology (tumor or scarring); excessive secretion production	Uncuffed trach tube or tracheostomy button
Patient has an artificial airway but a suction catheter cannot be passed	Partial airway obstruction; suction catheter too large	Use smaller catheter; in case of patient compromise, recommend immediate extubation if ET tube being used or change the inner cannula if trach tube being used
Artificial airway no longer indicated	Improvement in patient condition	Extubation
Need for mechanical ventilation in a patient with unilateral lung disease	Unilateral lung infections, localized tumors, lobectomy, pneumonectomy	Double-lumen ET tube

- Decreased or absent breath sounds on the affected site
- Tracheal deviation *away* from the affected site
- Hyperresonant percussion note on the affected side
- Absence of lung markings and radiolucency on the chest x-ray
- Sudden increase in airway pressure (volume control) or decrease in V_T (pressure control) during mechanical ventilation

If you suspect a pneumothorax, you should recommend (1) obtaining a stat chest x-ray and (2) placing the patient on 100% O_2 (helps reabsorb the gas). If the patient is receiving positive-pressure ventilation, you also should recommend changing the settings to minimize peak inspiratory pressures (e.g., decrease PIP or lower V_T). If a *tension* pneumothorax is suspected and the situation appears life threatening, you should recommend either immediate needle decompression or insertion of a chest tube on the appropriate side (see Chapter 15 for details on assisting a physician with chest tube insertion).

Recommending Adjustment in Fluid Balance

As discussed in Chapter 1, the normal fluid intake and output (I/O) for adults is 2–3 liters/day. Maintaining the balance between intake and output is essential to maintain proper metabolic functions. **Table 13-4** lists the signs most commonly associated with alteration of fluid balance and some common management strategies you can recommend.

Recommending Adjustment of Electrolyte Therapy

Monitoring electrolyte concentrations is also very important in critically ill patients and in patients with abnormal fluid balance. For normal electrolyte values, refer to Chapter 1. **Table 13-5** lists the most common causes of abnormal serum levels of the three electrolytes that are typically measured (Na^+, K^+, and Cl^-) and provides some suggested actions you can recommend for their treatment.

Recommending Initiation and Modification of Drug Therapy

Table 13-6 summarizes the most common clinical situations when you should recommend that drug therapy be initiated, and **Table 13-7** indicates those situations in which drug therapy should be modified. See Chapter 15 for indications and recommendations related to ACLS drugs.

Recommending Sedation and Neuromuscular Blockade

Although you cannot independently initiate sedation or muscle relaxant therapy, you may recommend that sedatives, neuroleptics/antipsychotics, analgesics, and paralytics be used. **Table 13-8** includes the major indications for these drugs.

Table 13-4 Common Signs of Fluid Balance Alteration and Management Strategies

Alteration	Common Signs	Recommended Management Strategies
Dehydration (negative I/O)	• Dry mucous membranes • Hypotension • Diminished urine output • ↓ skin turgor • ↑ hematocrit • Thick and tenacious secretions • ↓ central venous pressure (CVP) • ↓ pulmonary artery wedge pressures (PAWP)	• Increase IV fluid intake • Minimize sensible and insensible water loss • If patient receiving mechanical ventilation, provide heated humidification • If thick secretions are present, administer mucolytics • In critically ill patients, insert a CVP or PA catheter to monitor fluid status • Avoid the use of diuretics
Overhydration (positive I/O)	• Pedal edema • Pulmonary edema • Hepatomegaly • Jugular venous distension • ↓ hematocrit • ↑ CVP • ↑ PAWP	• Restrict and closely monitor fluid intake (IV and orally) • Initiate diuretic therapy • Administer inotropic agents if heart failure is suspected • Implement dialysis if renal failure is present • In critically ill patients, insert a CVP or PA catheter to monitor fluid status

Table 13-5 Causes of Abnormal Electrolytes and Recommendations for Their Treatment

Electrolyte	Causes of Low Serum Levels (Hypo)	Causes of High Serum Levels (Hyper)	Recommendation(s)
Sodium	• Diuresis • Overhydration • Antidiuretic hormone abnormalities	• Fluid loss • Diabetes • Antidiuretic hormone abnormalities	• Treat the underlying cause • Monitor fluid balance • Electrolyte replacement therapy
Potassium	• Vomiting • Nasogastric suction • Diarrhea • Diuretics • Renal disease • Metabolic alkalosis	• High-potassium diet • Renal failure • Metabolic acidosis • Red blood cell hemolysis	• Treat the underlying cause • Monitor fluid balance • Electrolyte replacement therapy • If K^+ is low and patient on diuretics, use a "K^+-sparing" agent (e.g., amiloride or spironolactone) • If K^+ is high, administer high-dose aerosolized albuterol or a "K^+-wasting" agent (e.g., Lasix)
Chloride	• Severe vomiting • Chronic respiratory acidosis • Renal disease • Burns • Nasogastric suction • Metabolic alkalosis	• Prolonged diarrhea • Metabolic acidosis • Respiratory alkalosis • Renal disease • Thyroid gland disease	• Treat the underlying cause • Monitor fluid balance • Electrolyte replacement therapy

Sedatives

- These drugs decrease anxiety and produce amnesia, *but they do not alleviate pain*.
- Concerns include long half-lives/drug accumulation (resulting in prolonged effects) and cardiac depression.
- Drug accumulation is a common problem with midazolam (Versed), especially if used for more than 48 hours.
- Cardiac depression is seen mainly with midazolam or propofol (Diprivan).
- Benzodiazepine action can be quickly reversed with flumazenil (Romazicon).
- Propofol (Diprivan) is often the sedative of choice in the ICU for minor invasive procedures. It has a rapid onset and a half-life of less than 30 minutes.
- A single IV dose (2–5 mg) of midazolam (Versed) may be used to facilitate other respiratory procedures such as intubation and bronchoscopy.
- Propofol and midazolam should be used with caution because they often cause hypotension and respiratory depression.

Analgesics

- Analgesics should be prescribed for any patient experiencing pain.
- Morphine is the drug of choice for patients with stable cardiovascular status.
- For patients with unstable cardiovascular status, the histamine-associated hypotension that morphine may cause can be avoided by using fentanyl (Sublimaze) or hydromorphone (Dilaudid).
- Because opioid analgesics can depress respiration, spontaneously breathing patients receiving them should be monitored for the adequacy of ventilation.

Table 13-6 Common Situations in Which to Recommend Drug Therapy

Clinical Situation	Recommendation(s)
Acute airway obstruction associated with asthma or a similar condition	Short-acting adrenergic bronchodilator such as albuterol; consider continuous nebulization, and systemic steroids such as prednisone
Maintenance (prophylactic) medication for asthma management	Any one or a combination of: • An inhaled steroid (e.g., fluticasone) • A long-acting beta-agonist (e.g., Salmeterol) • A leukotriene inhibitor (e.g., montelukast [Singulair]) • A mast cell stabilizer (cromolyn sodium) • Advair (salmeterol and fluticasone)
Chronic airway obstruction associated with COPD	An anticholinergic bronchodilator such as tiotropium bromide, possibly with an adrenergic bronchodilator such as albuterol; plus an inhaled steroid
Retained, thick/tenacious secretions	Acetylcysteine (Mucomyst), dornase alpha (Pulmozyme), or hypertonic saline (6–7%) if cystic fibrosis or bronchiectasis is present
Physician orders acetylcysteine but patient is at risk for bronchospasm	Adding a bronchodilator to prevent bronchospasm
Need to increase the volume of secretions for sputum induction	An aerosolized nebulizer treatment with 3–10% hypertonic saline solution
Postextubation stridor and airway edema	Racemic epinephrine (0.5 mL of 2.25% solution in 3 mL of normal saline)
Need to anesthetize a patient's airway before a bronchoscopy	Lidocaine (1%, 2%, or 4%) or cetacaine via aerosol prior to the procedure
Severe patient agitation or ventilator–patient asynchrony	Sedation with midazolam (Versed) or propofol (Diprivan); if situation requires paralysis, recommend a nondepolarizing agent (e.g., cisatracurium [Nimbex])
Respiratory depression induced by opioids	Opioid antagonist such as naloxone (Narcan) to reverse respiratory depression
Difficult intubation	Sedation with midazolam (Versed) and possibly a short-acting depolarizing paralytic such as succinylcholine (Anectine)
Pulmonary edema associated with CHF and/or peripheral edema due to right heart failure	A quick-acting diuretic such as furosemide (Lasix) and possibly an inotropic medication such as digoxin
Diuretic for a patient with low serum potassium (<3.5 mEq/L)	A potassium-sparing diuretic such as amiloride (Midamor)
Refractory Gram-negative infection of the respiratory tract, especially *Pseudomonas*	Inhaled tobramycin (Tobi), Cayston (Aztreonam), or polymyxin E (Colistin)
Premature newborn having difficulty breathing or with clinical signs of infant respiratory distress syndrome (IRDS)	An exogenous surfactant such as beractant (Survanta), calfactant (Infasurf), or poractant alfa (Curosurf)
Treatment or prevention of influenza	An anti-influenza agent such as oseltamivir (Tamiflu) or zanamivir (Relenza)
Prevention of pneumococcal pneumonia and pneumococcal infections in elderly and immunocompromised patients	Polyvalent pneumococcal vaccine with revaccination every 5 years for very high-risk populations

Table 13-7 Recommending Modifications to Drug Dosage or Concentration

Clinical Situation	Recommendation(s)
Patient heart rate increases by more than 20% of baseline or another unwanted side effect occurs during or after a short-acting beta-agonist broncho-dilator treatment	Stop the treatment, monitor the patient, notify the nurse and doctor, and recommend that either the dose be reduced or a drug with minimal beta$_1$ side effects (e.g., levalbuterol) be considered
A short-acting beta-agonist bronchodilator is pre-scribed and indicated, but the patient has a recent history of uncontrolled atrial fibrillation, significant tachycardia, or other dysrhythmias	Consider a drug with minimal beta$_1$ side effects (e.g., levalbuterol) or an anticholinergic broncho-dilator
A physician orders an incorrect drug dosage (e.g., 25 mg albuterol or 0.5 mL Atrovent) to be given via SVN every 6 hours	Contact the physician immediately for order clari-fications whenever a medication dosage appears incorrect
Prophylactic asthma management in patients aged 2 years or younger	Montelukast (Singulair—the only leukotriene inhibitor approved for young children) or cromolyn sodium (Intal—a mast cell stabilizer)
2 mL of 20% acetylcysteine is ordered, but only 10% acetylcysteine is available	Administer 4 mL (twice the volume) of the more dilute 10% acetylcysteine

Paralytics/Neuromuscular Blocking Agents

- There are two classes of neuromuscular blocking agents: nondepolarizing (inhibit acetylcholine) and depolarizing (prolong depolarization of the postsynaptic receptors).
  - The depolarizing agents such as succinylcholine (Anectine) have a short duration of action and are used for short-term paralysis during intubation.
  - The nondepolarizing agents produce prolonged paralysis and are used for controlled mechanical ventilation. Examples include pancuronium (Pavulon), vecuronium (Norcuron), and cisatracurium (Nimbex).
- Paralytics should never be used unless the patient is receiving full ventilatory support, with properly set disconnect alarms having been tested to confirm their function.
- Paralytics have no sedative or analgesic effects. For this reason, paralytics must always be administered with a sedative and, in the presence of pain, an analgesic.

Neuroleptics/Antipsychotics

- In addition to sedation, neuroleptics and antipsychotics may be given to patients who are experiencing delirium or "ICU psychosis." Symptoms of delirium include disorganized thinking, hallucinations, and disorientation.
- The neuroleptic drug of choice for delirium/psychosis is IV haloperidol (Haldol).

Recommending Changes in Oxygen Therapy

Chapter 4 describes the features and appropriate uses of various O_2 delivery devices. Chapter 12 also contains an example of an O_2 therapy protocol that would allow you to modify therapy inde-pendently based on pre-approved clinical criteria. However, in the absence of such protocols, you may be limited to recommending changes in input flow, delivery device, or FIO_2 to meet the patient's needs. **Table 13-9** outlines some of the common clinical situations that would warrant rec-ommended changes in O_2 therapy.

Recommending Changes in Mechanical Ventilation

During mechanical ventilation, a host of changes may be necessary, many of which require a physician's order. Nevertheless, you should recommend modifications aimed at enhancing oxygenation and ventila-tion, and improving patient synchrony and comfort.

Table 13-8 Indications for Sedatives, Analgesics, Paralytics, and Antipsychotics

Drug Category	Indications
Sedatives	
Barbiturates: • Thiopental (Pentothal) Benzodiazepines: • Diazepam (Valium) • Lorazepam (Ativan) • Midazolam (Versed) Others: • Etomidate (Amidate) • Ketamine (Ketalar) • Propofol (Diprivan)	• Facilitate minor invasive procedures • Facilitate patient–ventilator synchrony • Increase overall patient comfort • Reduce symptoms of "ICU psychosis" • Provide the moderate sedation required in certain ambulatory procedures
Opioid Analgesics	
• Morphine • Codeine • Fentanyl (Sublimaze) • Hydrocodone • Hydromorphone (Dilaudid) • Meperidine (Demerol) • Oxycodone (OxyContin)	• Treatment and management of pain • Any surgical procedures likely to generate pain and suffering • Long-term control of chronic pain • Facilitate patient–ventilator synchrony
Paralytics/Neuromuscular Blocking Agents	
Depolarizing: • Succinylcholine (Anectine) Nondepolarizing: • Cisatracurium (Nimbex) • Pancuronium (Pavulon) • Rocuronium (Zemuron) • Vecuronium (Norcuron)	• Facilitate "control mode" ventilation • Facilitate intubation • Muscle relaxation during surgery • Facilitate patient–ventilator synchrony • Decrease ICP • Reduce oxygen consumption
Neuroleptics/Antipsychotics	
• Haloperidol (Haldol) • Chlorpromazine (Thorazine) • Lithium (Lithobid)	• Hallucinations • ICU psychosis • Dementia

Improving Patient–Ventilator Synchrony

Ideally, all patient respiratory efforts during mechanical ventilation should be in synchrony with applicable machine activity. Whenever this fails to occur, a condition of *patient–ventilator asynchrony* exists. Patient–ventilator asynchrony typically causes patient agitation and respiratory distress. In the most severe cases, the patient may exhibit tachypnea, diaphoresis, accessory muscles use, intercostal retractions, ribcage–abdominal paradox, cardiac arrhythmias, and hypotension.

Patient–ventilator asynchrony can be caused by problems with either the patient or the ventilator. To help differentiate patient-related causes from ventilator-associated causes while at the same time safeguarding the patient, you should disconnect the patient from the ventilator and provide manual ventilation with 100% O_2. If the patient's distress is alleviated by disconnection, the problem likely is related to ventilator function. Conversely, continued patient distress while receiving manual ventilation with 100% O_2 suggests a patient-related cause.

Table 13-9 Recommending Changes in Oxygen Therapy

Clinical Situation	Recommendation(s)
A COPD patient becomes lethargic and disoriented soon after being placed on a nasal cannula at 5 L/min	Recommend that the input flow be reduced to 2 L/min or switch to an air-entrainment mask at 24–28% O_2; continue to closely monitor the patient and notify the nurse
The physician orders oxygen via simple mask with and input flow of 3 L/min for an adult patient	Recommend that the input flow be increased to a minimum of 5 L/min to ensure "washout" of CO_2
A patient on a simple mask at 5 L/min complains that the mask is confining and interferes with his ability to eat	Recommend that the device be switched to a nasal cannula with a flow of 4–6 L/min, which will deliver an equivalent F_{IO_2}
A nasal cannula at 2 L/min is in use on a patient with a high or unstable minute ventilation who requires an F_{IO_2} of 0.28	Recommend a high-flow device such as a 28% air-entrainment mask, which can meet the patient's inspiratory flow needs and maintain a stable F_{IO_2}
A patient on a 40% air-entrainment mask has a Sp_{O_2} of 89%	Recommend that the F_{IO_2} be increased to 0.50 and monitor the patient's response closely
A patient on a simple mask at 10 L/min has a Pa_{O_2} of 212 torr	Recommend a reduction in F_{IO_2}—for example, switching to a nasal cannula at about 5 L/min (F_{IO_2} of about 0.40)
After you switch an adult patient from a simple mask to a nonrebreathing mask, her Sp_{O_2} only increases from 83–87%	Recommend a high-flow nasal cannula at 40 L/min; also consider mask CPAP with high F_{IO_2}
A physician orders a nonrebreathing mask for a "code blue" patient in respiratory arrest	Immediately recommend a BVM that can provide 100% oxygen and can be used to effectively ventilate the patient
A patient in the ER is apparently having a myocardial infarction and is on a nasal cannula at 4 L/min	Recommend a nonrebreathing mask with an input flow sufficient to keep the reservoir bag from collapsing through the breathing cycle
The aerosol mist intermittently disappears from the end of the T-piece of an intubated patient performing a spontaneous breathing trial	Recommend adding a second aerosol nebulizer in tandem or bleeding in supplemental O_2 to increase the total output flow of the system

In either case, you will need to investigate further to identify the likely problem(s) causing asynchrony and distress. Once the specific problem is identified, you should take appropriate corrective action. **Table 13-10** outlines the most common ventilator-associated causes of patient–ventilator asynchrony and the corresponding corrective actions, while **Table 13-11** provides similar guidance for addressing patient-related causes.

Note that auto-PEEP can be either ventilator- or patient-related. Because the management of auto-PEEP differs according to the primary source of the problem, you need to be clear on the cause before implementing your corrective action. The primary ventilator-related cause of auto-PEEP is insufficient expiratory time (discussed subsequently in this chapter). The primary patient-related causes of auto-PEEP that can be corrected are increased secretions and bronchospasm. The only common corrective action is the application of extrinsic PEEP, typically in amounts up to 80% of the measured auto-PEEP level (see Chapter 11 for details on measuring auto-PEEP).

Enhancing Oxygenation

During mechanical ventilation, arterial oxygenation is affected mainly by two parameters—the F_{IO_2} and the PEEP level. The following guidelines apply to adjusting the F_{IO_2} and PEEP level:

- If hyperoxia is present (usually $Pa_{O_2} > 100$ torr), you should lower the parameter (F_{IO_2} or PEEP) that is potentially most dangerous to the patient at that moment.
- If Pa_{O_2} or Sa_{O_2} is low (< 60 torr or < 90%), hypoxemia is present.
  - Increase the F_{IO_2} if it is less than 0.60.
  - Increase PEEP if the $F_{IO_2} \geq 0.60$.

Table 13-10 Causes of and Corrective Actions for Ventilator-Associated Asynchrony

Cause	Corrective Action
Improper trigger sensitivity	Adjust pressure trigger level to –1 to –2 cm H_2O or recommend a flow trigger at 1–3 L/min
Inadequate FIO_2 or PEEP	Increase FIO_2 up to 0.60 to achieve target SpO_2 of 90–92%; consider recommending PEEP $\geq$ 10 cm H_2O if there is an inadequate response to high FIO_2
Flow problems	Adjust flow or use flow waveform (volume control); use pressure control or a mode that provides flow compensation; adjust rise time and/or flow termination criteria (pressure control)
Rate problems	If using an A/C mode, set the rate to ensure an adequate expiratory time; if using SIMV, increase the mandatory rate or pressure support until the spontaneous rate is acceptable (< 25/min)
Inappropriate tidal volume or pressure limit	Ensure an appropriate V_T setting or DP to achieve tidal volume in the 4–10 mL/kg range; inspect the pressure–volume curve for overdistension (see Chapter 12)
Inadequate minute ventilation	Ensure a minimum $\dot{V}_E$ of at least 4–6 L/min, or higher if appropriate
Mode problems	Give preference to pressure control modes or those providing flow compensation; place the patient back on the previous mode if the change was not tolerated
Auto-PEEP	Decrease the mandatory rate, increase the inspiratory flow, decrease V_T or $\dot{V}_E$, allow spontaneous breathing (SIMV), or apply extrinsic PEEP

Table 13-11 Causes of and Corrective Actions for Patient-Related Asynchrony

Cause	Recommended Action(s)
Partial or complete airway obstruction	Attempt to pass a suction catheter or otherwise clear occlusion; if using a trach tube, remove/replace the inner cannula; recommend extubation/reintubation
Auto-PEEP	Keep the airway clear or remove secretions; administer bronchodilator therapy; replace a small tracheal airway with a larger one; apply extrinsic PEEP
Pneumothorax likely	Obtain a stat chest x-ray; perform needle decompression or recommend insertion of a chest tube
Bronchospasm	Administer prescribed bronchodilators, or recommend them if they have not been prescribed
Increased secretions	Suction the airway and recommend mucolytics as appropriate
Pain	Pain medication (e.g., morphine)
Anxiety	Sedatives or anxiolytics (e.g., Versed)
Seizures	Antiseizure medication (e.g., Dilantin)
ICU psychosis or delirium	Antipsychotics (e.g., Haldol)

According to these guidelines, if a patient on 10 cm H_2O PEEP and 75% O_2 has a PaO_2 of 175 torr, the high FIO_2 is of most concern (O_2 toxicity) and should be lowered. In contrast, if a patient receiving 18 cm H_2O PEEP and 45% oxygen has a PaO_2 of 150 torr, the high PEEP level is of most concern (barotrauma) and should be lowered.

Likewise, the parameter you choose to raise depends on the cause of the hypoxemia. To decide between adding PEEP or increasing FIO_2, you should follow the "60-60 rule" to determine the cause and treatment of hypoxemia:

- If PaO_2 > 60 torr on FIO_2 < 0.6, the problem is mainly a V/Q imbalance that will respond to a simple increase in FIO_2.
- If PaO_2 < 60 torr on FIO_2 > 0.6, the problem is shunting and PEEP/ CPAP must be added or increased.

Methods to determine the "best" or optimal PEEP levels are discussed in detail in Chapter 10.

Improving Alveolar Ventilation

You can confirm the presence of abnormal alveolar ventilation via an ABG report showing an abnormal pH due to an abnormal $PaCO_2$. A low $PaCO_2$ can be normalized by decreasing the $\dot{V}E$. Conversely, a high $PaCO_2$ can be restored to normal levels by increasing the $\dot{V}E$. To estimate how much you should increase or decrease the $\dot{V}E$, use the following formula:

$$\text{new } \dot{V}E = \text{current } \dot{V}E = x \frac{\text{current } PaCO_2}{\text{desired } PaCO_2}$$

In applying this formula, you must be careful in specifying the desired $PaCO_2$. *The goal should be the $PaCO_2$ that normalizes the pH.* Although in the majority of situations this means a normal $PaCO_2$ of 40 torr, this may not always be the case. For example, in a patient with COPD who develops ventilatory failure "on top" of a compensated respiratory acidosis, the desired $PaCO_2$ could be substantially higher than normal.

You can change the minute ventilation by changing either the rate or the delivered tidal volume. Exactly how you change $\dot{V}E$ depends on the mode of ventilation in use. Refer to Table 10-6 in Chapter 10 for detailed guidance on how to increase or decrease $\dot{V}E$ for the most common modes of ventilation. Note that as long as the patient's VT is properly set up (4–10 mL/kg PBW with a plateau pressure less than 30 cm H_2O), rate changes are the preferred method to alter $\dot{V}E$.

Adjusting the Inspiratory to Expiratory Time Ratio (I:E Ratio)

As the parameter name makes clear, the I:E ratio is simply the ratio of the inspiratory time (I-time) to expiratory time (E-time). For ease of understanding, the numerator of this ratio (the I-time) usually is expressed as 1 (e.g., 1:1, 1:2, 1:3). Normal I:E ratios during spontaneous breathing typically range between 1:2 and 1:3. However, in patients with expiratory airflow obstruction (e.g., patients with COPD), the E-time is prolonged, resulting in *lower* I:E ratios such as 1:4 or 1:5.

During mechanical ventilation in the A/C modes, the I:E ratio can be controlled and altered. Precise control is possible only in the pure control mode (no patient triggering allowed), but adjustments also can be made when some machine breaths are patient triggered.

Factors affecting the I:E ratio during A/C ventilation include any parameter that alters either the I-time or E-time. During volume control A/C, I-time is a function of the set flow and volume—that is, I-time = volume (L) ÷ flow (L/sec). During pressure control A/C, the I-time usually is set by the clinician. In both modes, the E-time is simply the time remaining between each breath cycle and is determined by the I-time and frequency (f) of machine breaths. **Table 13-12** provides example I:E ratio computations for both volume and pressure control A/C. Appendix B provides more detail on time-related computations that you may see on the NBRC exams.

Note that on some ventilators and in some modes, the time parameter set or monitored is the %I-time (also called the *duty cycle*). %I-time is computed as follows:

$$\%\text{I-time} = \frac{\text{I-time}}{\text{I-time} + \text{E-time}} \times 100$$

Based on this formula, example I:E ratios and their %I-time equivalents are shown here:

Table 13-12 Example I:E Ratio Computations

Mode	Ventilator Settings	Inspiratory Time (I-time)	Breath Cycle Time (60 ÷ f)	Expiratory Time (E-time)	I:E Ratio
Volume control A/C	V_T = 500 mL Flow = 60 L/min (1.0 L/sec) Rate (f) = 20/min	0. 5 L ÷ 1.0 L/sec = 0.5 sec	60 ÷ 20 = 3.0 sec	3.0 − 0.5 = 2.5 sec	0.5 ÷ 2.5 = 1:5
Pressure control A/C	PIP = 30 cm H_2O I-time = 2.0 sec Rate (f) = 10/min	Set = 2.0 sec	60 ÷ 10 = 6.0 sec	6.0 − 2.0 = 4.0 sec	2.0 ÷ 4.0 = 1:2

I:E Ratio	%I-time
1:4	20%
1:3	25%
1:2	33%
1:1	50%
2:1	67%

Knowing the %I-time allows quick computation of the needed inspiratory flow during volume control ventilation using the following formula:

$$\text{Needed flow} = \frac{\text{minute volume (L)}}{\text{\%I-time (decimal)}}$$

See the accompanying box for an example of this computation.

Determination of Inspiratory Flow Setting During Volume Control Ventilation

Example: An apneic patient receiving volume control A/C ventilation at a rate of 15/min has a V_T of 600 mL. The physician orders an I:E ratio of 1:4. Which inspiratory flow should you set to achieve these parameters?

First, compute the minute volume:

$\dot{V}_E = 15 \times 600 = 9,000$ mL/min = 9.0 L/min

Next, convert the I:E ratio into percent inspiratory time:

%I-time = I-time ÷ (I-time + E-time) = 1 ÷ (1 + 4) = 20%

Last, compute the inspiratory flow needed (be sure to use the decimal equivalent for %I-time):

Needed flow = 9.0 ÷ 0.20 = 45 L/min

Note also that increasing the %I-time is equivalent to increasing the I:E ratio, whereas decreasing the %I-time is equivalent to decreasing the I:E ratio. On some ventilators, you can increase the %I-time to exceed 50% (equivalent to I:E ratios greater than 1:1). Mechanical ventilation with I:E ratios greater than 1:1 is called *inverse ratio ventilation (IRV)*. In the past, IRV has been applied as salvage therapy for severe ARDS. However, due to its significant risks and unproven benefits, IRV is no longer recommended for this purpose.

More frequently, you will need to *decrease or lower* a patient's I:E ratio. This situation occurs commonly when providing mechanical ventilation to patients with severe expiratory airflow obstruction. As previously discussed, during spontaneous breathing these patients typically exhibit prolonged E-times and *low* I:E ratios, such as 1:4 or 1:5. If similar ratios are not provided during mechanical ventilation, air trapping or auto-PEEP will occur. If auto-PEEP is present and the I:E ratio is high (e.g., 1:1 or 1:2), the first step usually is to adjust the settings to allow sufficient time for complete exhalation. To do so requires decreasing the I:E ratio to a value more normal for these patients, such as 1:4

or 1:5. You can decrease the I:E ratio by increasing the E-time and/or decreasing the I-time. Methods to do so are summarized in **Table 13-13**.

Modifying Ventilator Modes and Techniques

Chapter 10 covers the initiation of mechanical ventilation, including the various modes of ventilation. In many situations a change in ventilator mode may be required. **Table 13-14** summarizes the most common situations warranting such changes.

Table 13-13 Methods for Decreasing the I:E Ratio During A/C Ventilation

Goal	Volume Control	Pressure Control
Increase E-time	• Decrease set respiratory rate • Switch to low-rate SIMV	• Decrease set respiratory rate • Switch to low-rate SIMV
Decrease I-time	• Increase inspiratory flow • Decrease tidal volume	• Decrease I-time and %I-time

Table 13-14 Ventilator Mode/Mode Changes

Clinical Situation	Recommended Mode or Change
Full ventilatory support is needed, but rate and/or breathing pattern must be controlled (e.g., hyperventilation syndrome)	Volume or pressure control A/C with sedative and/or paralytic
Full ventilatory support upon ventilator initiation; failed weaning attempt	Volume or pressure control A/C mode or normal-rate SIMV
Full ventilator support is needed, but total respiratory rate results in hyperventilation (respiratory alkalosis) on A/C mode	Switch to volume or pressure control normal-rate SIMV
To provide incremental lowering of ventilatory support, such as during weaning or to improve spontaneous tidal volume	Volume or pressure control normal-rate SIMV with pressure support
To overcome the imposed work of breathing caused by artificial airways or ventilator circuit	Add/increment pressure support level or implement automatic tube compensation (if available)
To boost spontaneous tidal volume in patients with muscle weakness in SIMV or spontaneous modes	Add/increment pressure support level
To overcome tachypnea or low tidal volume during SIMV with signs of increased work of breathing	Add/increment pressure support level
To reduce airway pressures (plateau pressure) in patients with low lung compliance (ARDS) on volume control A/C	Switch to pressure control A/C with maximum PIP = 30 cm H_2O
To support ventilation and oxygenation in patients with ARDS if NHLBI protocol fails	Consider high-frequency oscillation ventilation (HFOV) or airway pressure release ventilation (APRV)
To avoid intubation of patients requiring short-term ventilatory support due to exacerbations of COPD	Provide noninvasive positive-pressure ventilation (NPPV)
To avoid reintubation of patients who develop mild to moderate hypercapnia after extubation	Provide NPPV
To avoid or minimize atelectasis associated with low-volume lung protection strategies	Switch to APRV or apply lung recruitment maneuvers

Monitoring and Adjusting Alarm Settings

Chapter 11 describes the procedures for setting ventilator alarm limits. **Table 13-15** summarizes common alarm scenarios and the recommended actions.

The first rule in monitoring and responding to ventilator alarms is to ensure patient safety. As when patient–ventilator asynchrony or distress occurs, this means removing the patient from the ventilator and providing manual ventilation and oxygenation while the situation is being evaluated. Another important consideration regarding ventilator alarms is to ensure a functional remote monitoring system is in place wherever clinicians might be out of "sight and sound" range of the patient.

Adjusting Ventilator Settings Based on Graphics

Chapter 12 describes situations in which you should independently modify ventilator settings based on waveform assessment. In addition to remedies that you may independently initiate, such as correcting inappropriate sensitivity, there are other changes that you may only recommend to the physician, such as initiating sedation for asynchrony. **Table 13-16** summarizes the most common of these situations, along with their recommended solutions.

Changing the Type of Ventilator or Breathing Circuit

Chapter 4 provides general criteria for selecting ventilators based on patient variables, application settings, and needed capabilities as well as guidance on the use of ventilator circuits. The most common changes in ventilator circuitry likely to appear on the NBRC exams include the following:

- Using low-compliance circuit for neonates and young pediatric patients to minimize volume loss

Table 13-15 Common Ventilator Alarms and Recommended Adjustments or Actions

Ventilator Alarm Activated	Recommended Action(s)*
Ventilator inoperative/loss of power	Manually ventilate patient and troubleshoot ventilator; replace ventilator if necessary
Low pressure, low PEEP/CPAP	Check for and fix circuit or airway leaks or disconnections
Low exhaled minute ventilation	Check and fix leaks or disconnections; consider failed weaning attempt
High pressure limit	If *sudden* rise in PIP, suction secretions, alleviate mucus plug, place bite block, recommend sedation (if patient is agitated), and assess for pneumothorax; if *gradual* rise in PIP, consider bronchodilators (if due to increased resistance) or recommend pressure control ventilation (if due to decreased compliance)
High exhaled minute ventilation	If using A/C, consider switching to SIMV or sedating the patient; if A/C mode with respiratory alkalosis consider adding mechanical deadspace
High respiratory rate	Assess for pain/anxiety or any other cause of respiratory distress; during weaning attempts, consider failure to wean and return to previous settings or add pressure support if on SIMV
F_{IO_2}	Analyze F_{IO_2} with separate O_2 analyzer; if a discrepancy is noted, calibrate the ventilator analyzer and/or replace its sensor
Temperature	Check settings, water feed, and temperature sensors, and replace heater, circuit, and sensors
Apnea	Recommend return to A/C mode, if weaning is in progress, or reduction in sedation, if warranted

*The recommended action anticipates that with any ventilator alarm activation that either exceeds approximately 30–60 seconds or is accompanied by patient distress, you will conduct a quick but thorough assessment of the patient–ventilator interface before taking any of the proposed actions.

Table 13-16 Recommending Adjustment of Ventilator Settings Based on Graphics

Clinical Situation	Recommended Action(s)
Patient–ventilator asynchrony: Seen on graphical waveform as irregularly spiked flow or irregular pressure waveform (see Figure 12-2)	Differentiate ventilator-related causes from patient-related causes; see Table 13-10 for correcting ventilator-associated causes and Table 13-11 for correcting patient-related causes
Auto-PEEP: Manifested in several ways on ventilator graphics, including an expiratory flow waveform that does not return to baseline before the next breath (see Figure 12-5)	Differentiate ventilator-related causes from patient-related causes; see Table 13-10 for correcting ventilator-associated auto-PEEP and Table 13-11 for correcting patient-associated auto-PEEP
Overdistension: Evidenced on the waveform graphic by a "beak" at the upper inflection point in the volume/pressure loop (see Figure 12-6)	Reduce the set volume (volume control) or pressure limit (pressure control) in accordance with existing protocols or recommend the reduction needed to eliminate "beaking"
Airway leaks: Seen as a failure of the expiratory volume waveform to return to baseline (see Figure 12-4)	Check for leaks and/or disconnections on the patient–ventilator system; if a chest tube is present, check for a water-seal chamber leak and consider bronchopulmonary fistula

- Changing or modifying a single-limb circuit by adding PEEP capabilities to the exhalation valve
- Adding mechanical deadspace to the circuit to raise the $Paco_2$ and manage acute respiratory alkalosis (generally limited to A/C modes)

Other Recommendations Related to Ventilator Settings

Other ventilator modifications that you may recommend involve those designed to minimize ventilator-induced lung injury. Chapter 10 details the most common ventilator strategies as applied to patients with acute respiratory failure. Other related lung-protective strategies you may recommend include the following:

- Volume control ventilation with low tidal volumes (4–6 mL/kg of PBW)
- Volume control ventilation with low plateau pressures (< 30 cm H_2O)
- Pressure control ventilation with PIP < 30 cm H_2O
- "Dual-mode" ventilation (e.g., pressure-regulated volume control [PRVC])
- Airway pressure release ventilation (APRV)

You may recommend these techniques in conjunction with *permissive hypercapnia*. Permissive hypercapnia is a ventilation strategy in which a higher than normal $Paco_2$ is accepted in exchange for the lower risk of lung injury associated with smaller VT or PIPs. In general, you can accept hypercapnia/respiratory acidosis until the pH falls below 7.25–7.30, at which point you would recommend either an increase in rate or administration of sodium bicarbonate.

A final area in which you might recommend special ventilator settings involves specific clinical conditions. Patients with a clinically significant bronchopulmonary fistula who do not ventilate or oxygenate well on other settings may respond well to high-frequency oscillation ventilation. Likewise, patients on a ventilator who are particularly at risk for developing atelectasis may be candidates for "open-lung" techniques such as recruitment maneuvers involving periodic use of PEEP levels as high as 20–30 cm H_2O for a short period of time.

Recommending Weaning from Mechanical Ventilation

Once mechanical ventilation is initiated, your treatment plan should aim to successfully remove the patient from ventilatory support as soon as possible. Chapter 2 outlines and describes the traditional bedside parameters used in assessing ventilation and ventilatory mechanics, such as vital capacity and NIF/MIP. Although those measures are still taught and used in some settings to assess a patient's readiness to wean, recent evidence-based guidelines now recommend different criteria. According to these guidelines, patients on mechanical ventilation should undergo weaning assessment whenever the following criteria are met:

- Evidence indicating at least some reversal of the underlying cause of respiratory failure
- Adequate oxygenation (e.g., $Pao_2/Fio_2 \geq 150–200$, PEEP $\leq 5–8$ cm H_2O, and $Fio_2 \leq 0.4–0.5$)
- pH ≥ 7.25
- Hemodynamic stability (no myocardial ischemia or significant hypotension)
- The ability to initiate an inspiratory effort

Once these criteria are met, weaning assessment should begin, usually with an initial short period of spontaneous breathing during which you assess the patient's respiratory pattern (rate, V_T, RSBI), adequacy of gas exchange (Spo_2, ABGs, capnography), hemodynamic stability, and subjective comfort. Patients who tolerate a 30- to 120-minute trial of spontaneous breathing should be considered for removal of ventilatory support and extubation.

Recommending Extubation

The decision to extubate a patient who successfully completes a spontaneous breathing trial should be made separately from the weaning assessment. A patient is ready for extubation if (1) the upper airway is patent and can be adequately protected, and (2) secretions can be effectively cleared. Airway patency and the potential for postextubation obstruction can be assessed by performing the cuff leak test (as described in Chapter 8). A positive gag reflex and the ability of the patient to raise his or her head off the bed indicate adequate airway protection. In addition, the ability to clear secretions is evident if the patient is alert, coughs deeply on suctioning, and can generate a MEP/PE_{max} greater than 60 cm H_2O. More in depth assessment of both airway patency and protection in patients with tracheostomy tubes can be provided using a fenestrated tube.

COMMON ERRORS TO AVOID

You can improve your score by avoiding these mistakes:

- When performing postural drainage, avoid head-down positions for patients with increased ICP.
- Never recommend sedatives to relieve pain; sedatives can decrease anxiety but do not alleviate pain.
- Never recommend weaning a patient from mechanical ventilation if the patient is hemodynamically compromised, has unstable vital signs, or requires Fio_2 greater than 0.50–0.60 or PEEP greater than 10 cm H_2O.
- Never recommend prophylactic drugs (e.g., cromolyn sodium) or long-acting beta-agonists such as salmeterol for patients experiencing an acute asthmatic episode.
- Never initiate low inspiratory flows or short expiratory times on ventilator patients who are at risk for air trapping and auto-PEEP.
- Never recommend sedation for patient–ventilator asynchrony before ruling out other patient causes such as bronchospasm, airway obstruction, and pneumothorax, as well as ventilator-related causes such as insufficient inspiratory flow or pressure support.
- Never set a low-pressure (disconnect) alarm much lower than 5–8 cm H_2O.

SURE BETS

In some situations, you can be sure of the right approach to a clinical problem or scenario:

- Always stop postural drainage in the head-down position if the patient begins coughing vigorously. Sit the patient up and stabilize the situation before continuing with therapy.
- To facilitate a difficult intubation, always consider recommending a rapid-acting/short-duration depolarizing paralytic such as succinylcholine (Anectine).
- Always recommend rapid-sequence intubation for patients with clinical signs of impending respiratory failure or inadequate airway protection.

- Always consider a laryngeal mask airway as an alternative to intubation in the presence of a difficult airway.
- To avoid excessive ET tube cuff leak after intubation, always recommend inserting the correct-size ET tube.
- Always recommend placing a spontaneous-breathing patient who is dyspneic in Fowler's or high Fowler's position, to help promote chest excursion/lung expansion.
- Always recommend a fast-acting adrenergic bronchodilator for a patient with severe bronchospasm associated with asthma or a similar condition.
- For patients with unstable or high minute ventilation who need a low to moderate FIO_2 (0.24–0.50), always recommend a high-flow device such as an air-entrainment mask.
- For patient–ventilator asynchrony, always consider and recommend measures to address both patient-related causes, such as airway obstruction and anxiety, and machine-related causes, such as inappropriate trigger sensitivity or inspiratory flow.
- Always recommend increasing PEEP above 5–10 cm H_2O for patients on a ventilator who are hemodynamically stable but hypoxemic despite an FIO_2 greater than 0.50–0.60.
- Always recommend increasing either the ΔP (IPAP – EPAP) or the respiratory rate when seeking to increase the $\dot{V}E$ for a patient on noninvasive ventilatory support.
- Always ensure there is appropriate full ventilatory support backup before recommending that a patient be placed on a weaning mode, such as CPAP or pressure support.
- Always consider recommending a pressure-targeted or dual mode of ventilation when attempting to reduce a patient's peak, plateau, or mean airway pressure.
- When a patient in ARDS does not respond well to conventional volume and pressure modes of ventilation, consider recommending high-frequency oscillation ventilation.
- When responding to a ventilator alarm, always start by checking patient causes such as disconnect or airway leak (low pressure) or bronchospasm or secretions (high pressure).
- Always disconnect a patient from the ventilator and initiate manual ventilation with 100% oxygen if the patient is in distress or an alarm situation cannot immediately be rectified.

PRE-TEST ANSWERS AND EXPLANATIONS

Following are this chapter's pre-test answers and explanations. Be sure to review each answer's explanation thoroughly to help you understand why it is correct. If the explanation is still unclear to you, review the chapter content.

13-1. **Correct answer: D.** Pancuronium bromide (Pavulon). Based on the clinical presentation, the immediate problem appears to be bronchospasm (wheezing) and thick secretions (rhonchi) causing an increase in airway resistance (increased PIP – plateau pressure). A bronchodilator (albuterol or ipratropium) *and* a mucolytic (acetylcysteine) are indicated to treat this situation. Pancuronium bromide (Pavulon) is a nondepolarizing neuromuscular blocking agent that will not achieve bronchodilation or clear the airways.

13-2. **Correct answer: C.** 3 and 4 only. At this point, the patient is at high risk for developing atelectasis due to retained secretions and immobility. An initial regimen of incentive spirometry and deep breathing and coughing may well prevent atelectasis and aid secretion clearance.

13-3. **Correct answer: A.** Propofol (Diprivan). Propofol is the agent of choice for rapid sedation of patients undergoing minor invasive procedures because it has a quick action and short half-life (less than 30 minutes).

13-4. **Correct answer: B.** Succinylcholine (Anectine). For relatively short-term paralysis during procedures such as endotracheal intubation, a depolarizing agent such as succinylcholine (Anectine) is recommended. Nondepolarizing agents such as pancuronium (Pavulon), vecuronium (Norcuron), and cisatracurium (Nimbex) produce prolonged paralysis and are generally used for long-term management of mechanically ventilated patients.

13-5. **Correct answer: B.** Inserting an LMA. A laryngeal mask airway is an alternative way to quickly secure a patient's airway when ET intubation is difficult, such as when the RT is unable to properly visualize the vocal cords.

13-6. **Correct answer: B.** Adding mechanical deadspace. Adding mechanical deadspace will cause rebreathing of CO_2, so that $PaCO_2$ will increase. Another potential solution would have been to switch to the SIMV mode or to sedate the patient, but these options are not available.

13-7. **Correct answer: B.** Beginning diuretic therapy. The clinical picture indicates dehydration. IV fluids should be started immediately, with I/O carefully documented. Also, efforts should be made to minimize insensible water loss. Diuretics are contraindicated in dehydrated patients.

13-8. **Correct answer: D.** 1, 2, and 3. In a mechanically ventilated patient with poor oxygenation despite high FIO_2 and PEEP, prone positioning may help reduce shunting and improve oxygenation. Consideration can also be given to alternative modes of ventilation such as high-frequency oscillation ventilation (HFOV) or airway pressure release ventilation (APRV).

13-9. **Correct answer: A.** Decreasing the I:E ratio. Due to their high expiratory flow resistance, COPD patients are more likely to develop auto-PEEP during mechanical ventilation. If this problem is associated with bronchospasm, you should recommend a bronchodilator. If not, you can recommend decreasing the I:E ratio by (1) shortening inspiration (by using higher flows, reducing %I-time, and/or lower tidal volumes) or (2) lengthening the expiratory time by using lower rates or switching to SIMV. Another alternative is to apply external PEEP up to approximately 80% of the measured auto-PEEP.

13-10. **Correct answer: A.** Increasing the FIO_2 to 0.50. The blood gas analysis indicates normal ventilation and acid–base balance with moderate hypoxemia. With an FIO_2 below 0.50, the hypoxemia is most likely due to a V/Q imbalance. In this instance, you should increase the FIO_2 to 0.50. If this step does not adequately address the problem, you may need to consider an increase in PEEP.

13-11. **Correct answer: C.** Administering furosemide (Lasix). The diagnosis of heart failure and the increased PA and PAWP suggest that this patient is in congestive heart failure. To alleviate the accumulation of fluid in the patient's lungs, the therapy plan should generally include a rapid-acting diuretic such as furosemide (Lasix) as well as positive inotropic agents as digoxin and dopamine.

13-12. **Correct answer: B.** Decreasing the dosage of albuterol. The significant increase in heart rate (more than 20 from baseline) indicates that the albuterol dosage is provoking systemic side effects in this patient. Before considering a different drug, you should recommend trying a reduced dosage of albuterol and monitor the patient carefully for both desired effects and side effects.

13-13. **Correct answer: B.** Increasing the minute volume on the ventilator. Although the ABG values are within normal limits, deliberate hyperventilation of patients with closed-head trauma may be beneficial during the early hours of their management. Hyperventilation promotes cerebral vasoconstriction (low $PaCO_2$) and decrease the intracranial pressure (ICP). Typically, the $PaCO_2$ is maintained in the 30–35 mm Hg range. Note that the effect of hyperventilation wanes after several hours and that this technique is not recommended for ongoing management. Other therapies, including osmotic diuresis, draining of CSF fluid, and sedation are used for ongoing management.

13-14. **Correct answer: D.** Ipratropium bromide (Atrovent). Most sympathetic bronchodilators will result in some β1 stimulation, causing an increase in heart rate. In this instance, a therapist might recommend an anticholinergic bronchodilator such as ipratropium bromide (Atrovent).

13-15. **Correct answer: C.** Cuffed, fenestrated tracheostomy tube. For a patient with a tracheotomy on long-term mechanical ventilation who still requires intermittent support, recommend a cuffed, fenestrated trach tube. With the inner cannula in place and the cuff inflated, a fenestrated tube can be used for positive-pressure ventilation. However, because these tubes have openings in the posterior curvature of their outer cannula, air can move through the tube when the inner cannula is removed. This allows phonation (talking). In addition, by removing the tube's inner cannula, plugging the outer cannula, and deflating its cuff, you can test the patient's ability to maintain normal upper airway function.

13-16. Correct answer: B. Recommend a flow of at least 5 L/min. With this level of hypoxemia, this patient should immediately receive a moderate FIO_2, as available by a simple mask. However, a simple mask requires a flow of at least 5 L/min to prevent CO_2 rebreathing.

13-17. Correct answer: D. Providing supplemental pressure support. SIMV with PEEP is an appropriate choice for a patient in combined hypoxemic and hypercapnic respiratory failure due to an acute restrictive disorder. Coexisting respiratory muscle fatigue in these patients may necessitate the addition of pressure support ventilation to supplement the spontaneous breaths during SIMV or overcome the resistance imposed by the artificial airway.

13-18. Correct answer: C. 2 and 3 only. The oxygenation of a patient being considered for weaning from mechanical ventilation is considered adequate if (1) $PaO_2/FIO_2 \geq 150-200$, (2) PEEP $\leq 5-8$ cm H_2O, and (3) the patient's $FIO_2 \leq 0.4-0.5$.

13-19. Correct answer: B. Administering a racemic epinephrine treatment. The development of stridor after extubation indicates glottic or soft-tissue edema. When you hear stridor, you should be wary of the development of additional problems, as the swelling can dramatically worsen. If stridor is present, a racemic epinephrine treatment may be given to lessen the swelling. In children, postextubation edema is often subglottic and may require reinsertion of the airway.

13-20. Correct answer: C. Administering pulmonary surfactant. The acid–base balance for this infant is within the normal range; hence mechanical ventilation is not warranted. However, the patient has refractory hypoxemia ($PaO_2 < 60$ with $FIO_2 \geq 0.60$), probably due to shunting from the IRDS. Because normal surfactant production is lacking in premature babies and is thought to contribute to IRDS, exogenous surfactant administration is indicated for these infants. Increasing the FIO_2 to 100% is not warranted at this time, and this step may increase the risk of retinopathy of prematurity (ROP). INO therapy is indicated only for persistent pulmonary hypotension of the newborn (PPHN).

13-21. Correct answer: D. Cisatracurium (Nimbex). Sedatives commonly used to calm patients in the ICU include benzodiazepines such as lorazepam (Ativan), barbiturates such as pentobarbital (Nembutal), and propofol (Diprivan). Cisatracurium (Nimbex) is a neuromuscular blocking agent, not a sedative.

13-22. Correct answer: A. Adding 5–10 cm H_2O PEEP. In mechanically ventilated patients with atelectasis and significant hypoxemia, PEEP is indicated. PEEP increases the FRC by recruiting collapsed alveoli, which improves oxygenation by decreasing shunting. Increasing the patient's tidal volume might be an additional consideration, except that it already is at the upper limit of the recommend range (4–10 mL/kg).

13-23. Correct answer: C. 2 and 3 only. Based on the symptoms and PFT results, the patient has severe persistent asthma. Long-term control of severe persistent asthma is best achieved by combining both an inhaled corticosteroid (e.g., fluticasone) and a long-acting adrenergic bronchodilator (e.g., salmeterol). Short-acting inhaled beta-agonists such as albuterol are also prescribed but are indicated for quick relief of exacerbations, not long-term control.

13-24 Correct answer: D. 1, 2, and 3. If you suspect a pneumothorax, you should recommend (1) obtaining a stat chest x-ray and (2) placing the patient on 100% O_2 (helps reabsorb the gas). If the patient is on mechanical ventilation, you also should recommend decreasing the PIP or V_T. If a *tension* pneumothorax is suspected and the situation appears life threatening, you should recommend either immediate needle decompression or insertion of a chest tube on the appropriate side.

13-25. **Correct answer: D.** Potassium. Metabolic acidosis increases H^+ levels outside the cells. In an effort to buffer this acidosis, intracellular K^+ ions are exchanged with extracellular H^+, producing hyperkalemia in the blood/serum. Correcting the metabolic acidosis usually corrects the hyperkalemia.

POST-TEST

To confirm your mastery of this chapter's topical content, you should take the chapter post-test, available online at http://go.jblearning.com/respexamreview. A score of 80% or more indicates that you are adequately prepared for this section of the NBRC written exams. If you score less than 80%, you should continue to review the applicable chapter content. In addition, you may want to access and review the relevant Web links covering this chapter's content (courtesy of RTBoardReview.com), also online at the Jones & Bartlett Learning site.

Determine Appropriateness of the Prescribed Respiratory Care Plan and Recommend Modifications

Craig L. Scanlan and Albert J. Heuer
(previous version authored by Louis M. Sinopoli)

The ability to determine appropriate therapy and recommend modifications requires integration of the basics, such as indications and treatment options, with analysis and decision making. To be successful in this section of the NBRC exams, you must focus on (1) collecting and analyzing patient data, and (2) selecting the appropriate course of therapy.

OBJECTIVES

In preparing for the shared NBRC exam content, you should demonstrate the knowledge needed to:

1. Analyze available information to determine the patient's pathophysiological state
2. Determine the appropriateness of prescribed therapy and goals for the identified pathophysiological state
3. Recommend changes in the therapeutic plan when indicated
4. Develop and perform respiratory care quality assurance activities, and monitor their outcomes
5. Develop and apply respiratory care protocols, and monitor their outcomes

WHAT TO EXPECT ON THIS CATEGORY OF THE NBRC EXAMS

CRT exam: 4 questions; typically 25% recall and 75% application
WRRT exam: 6 questions; typically one-third application and two-thirds analysis
CSE exam: indeterminate number of questions; however, exam III-H knowledge is a prerequisite to success on both CSE Information Gathering and Decision-Making sections

PRE-TEST

Carefully respond to each of the following questions. After completing the pre-test, compare your answers to those provided at the end of this chapter. Then thoroughly review each answer's explanation to help understand why it is correct.

14-1. A patient who is breathing room air and in a coma as a result of acute carbon monoxide poisoning has a Pao_2 of 95 torr and a $Paco_2$ of 30 torr. Which of the following changes in the treatment plan would you recommend?
   A. Administer high concentrations of oxygen
   B. Initiate mechanical ventilation
   C. Initiate chest percussion and postural drainage
   D. Administer mask CPAP

14-2. IPPB treatments are sometimes given to patients with emphysema to:
   A. Lower the diaphragm
   B. Abolish the cough reflex
   C. Improve alveolar ventilation
   D. Increase FRC

14-3. Which of the following conditions is an indication for the use of CPAP?
   A. Tension pneumothorax
   B. Pulmonary embolism
   C. Pulmonary edema
   D. Asthma

14-4. What is the primary aim in treating cardiogenic pulmonary edema?
   A. Increase venous return to the heart
   B. Decrease right heart and systemic venous pressures
   C. Decrease left heart and pulmonary vascular pressures
   D. Increase pulmonary fluid and blood volume

14-5. Despite an intensive regimen of incentive spirometry, chest percussion, and nasotracheal suctioning, a postoperative patient continues to exhibit clinical manifestations of atelectasis due to large airway obstruction. What is the best treatment approach in this case?
   A. Intubation and mechanical ventilation
   B. Bedside therapeutic bronchoscopy
   C. Transtracheal aspiration
   D. Aerosol therapy with acetylcysteine

14-6. You would initiate O_2 therapy in all of the following cases *except*:
   A. Treating carbon monoxide poisoning
   B. Decreasing myocardial work
   C. Treating absorption atelectasis
   D. Treating arterial hypoxemia

14-7. Volume control A/C ventilation is initiated on a patient who just suffered a severe closed head injury. Which of the following goals would you recommend for the early hours of ventilatory support?
   A. Allow as much spontaneous breathing as possible (SIMV)
   B. Maintain a $Paco_2$ of 50–60 torr (deliberate hypoventilation)
   C. Maintain a high mean pressure using 10–15 cm H_2O PEEP
   D. Maintain a $Paco_2$ of 30–35 torr (deliberate hyperventilation)

14-8. You are reviewing a postoperative patient's care plan. The attending physician has changed a medical resident's order for the patient from albuterol via SVN to IPPB therapy. Which goal is the most likely justification for this change?

   A To enhance mucociliary clearance
   B. To increase arterial oxygen content
   C. To compensate for developing CO_2 retention
   D. To improve lung expansion/prevent atelectasis

14-9. Which of the following would you recommend for a patient who has emphysema with chronic $Paco_2$ retention and who experiences hypoxemia at rest?
   A. CPAP
   B. Incentive spirometry
   C. Oxygen via nonrebreathing mask
   D. Low-flow oxygen

14-10. A patient with a history of CHF is admitted to the ED with dyspnea and pink, watery, frothy secretions. Which of the following would you recommend for his care?
   A. Bronchodilator therapy
   B. BiPAP with 100% O_2
   C. Bronchial hygiene therapy
   D. Directed coughing

14-11. Which of the following is the first step in respiratory care protocol application?
   A. Observe universal precautions at all times
   B. Review medical records
   C. Check the physician order for the respiratory care protocol
   D. Perform initial patient evaluation

14-12. All of the following are potential sources of data for identifying patient care–related problems in a comprehensive quality improvement program *except*:
   A. Analysis of department budgeting
   B. Audit of patient medical records
   C. Examination of incident reports
   D. Review of patient ratings and complaints

14-13. Which of the following could be used as quality assurance outcome criteria to assess the effectiveness of bronchial hygiene therapy?
   1. Change in sputum production
   2. Change in chest x-ray
   3. Patient subjective response to therapy
   4. Change in ABG values or Spo_2

A. 1 and 2 only
B. 2 and 4 only
C. 1, 3, and 4
D. 1, 2, 3, and 4

14-14. As part of your department's quality improvement program, you identify an infection control problem. Which of the following should be investigated as potential causes of this problem?
   1. Lack of proper training
   2. Equipment or supply deficiencies
   3. Failure to follow set procedures
   A. 2 only
   B. 3 only
   C. 1 and 3 only
   D. 1, 2, and 3

14-15. Which of the following mechanisms is the best way to objectively assess the effectiveness of therapy in a quality assurance program?
   A. Assess the post-treatment status of patients on one or more predefined criteria
   B. Survey a sample of patients who received the therapy to determine their satisfaction
   C. Compare pre- and post-treatment patient status on one or more predefined criteria
   D. Analyze morbidity and mortality statistics for patients receiving the specified therapy

WHAT YOU NEED TO KNOW: ESSENTIAL CONTENT

Analyzing Available Data to Determine Pathophysiological State

A good respiratory care plan begins with careful identification and assessment of the patient's condition. Once you identify the patient's problem(s), you should plan on providing or recommending the most appropriate therapies. For example, if assessment indicates that wheezing and a reduced FEV_1 would respond to bronchodilator therapy, your plan should include aerosolized beta-agonists. **Table 14-1** summarizes common findings in patients undergoing respiratory care ("Findings"), the problem or problems that these findings usually indicate ("Assessment"), and the types of therapy that should be provided or recommended ("Considerations for Care Plan").

Reviewing Prescribed Therapy to Establish a Therapeutic Plan

In reviewing prescribed therapy, it is important to pay attention to the specifications in the order as well as the logical use of the therapy given the patient's problem. A typical plan should specify:

- Therapeutic objectives
- Specifics of equipment type and settings
- Drug names, dosages, and frequency of administration
- Relevant cautions or protocols to follow

In addition, interdisciplinary and family plans should specify:

- Interdisciplinary requirements, conflicts, and solutions
- Family requirements for education, communication, and monitoring

Determining the Appropriateness of Prescribed Therapy and Goals

On the NBRC exams, you must first identify specific information about the patient's pathophysiological state, such as respiratory failure (Table 14-1). Then, you must analyze the data provided to determine the appropriate course of action. For example, if a patient suffering from a drug overdose is in ventilatory failure, then mechanical ventilation to address hypoventilation will be needed. However, if the problem is hypoxemia caused by shunting (as in ARDS), then mechanical ventilation with PEEP and a focus on oxygenation is appropriate.

Table 14-1 Common Findings, Assessment, and Planning in Respiratory Care Patients

Findings	Assessment	Considerations for Care Plan
Airways		
Wheezing	Bronchospasm and inflammation	Bronchodilator therapy; inhaled corticosteroids
	Congestive heart failure (CHF)	Diuretic (e.g., Lasix*)
Stridor	Laryngeal edema	Cool, bland aerosol/racemic epinephrine
	Tumor/mass	Bronchoscopy*
Rhonchi/tactile fremitus	Secretions in large airways	Directed coughing; PEP/vibratory PEP therapy; mechanical insufflation–exsufflation (MI-E); suctioning
Cough		
Weak cough	Poor secretion clearance	Directed coughing; MI-E; suctioning
Secretions		
More than 30 mL/day	Excessive secretions	Bronchial hygiene therapy; systemic hydration; bland aerosol therapy; suctioning
Mucopurulent (yellow/thick) sputum	Acute airway infection	Treat underlying cause*; antibiotic therapy*
Pink, watery, frothy secretions	Pulmonary edema	Treat underlying cause* (e.g., CHF); CPAP or BiPAP with oxygen
Lungs		
Dull percussion note, bronchial breath sounds	Infiltrates, atelectasis, consolidation	Incentive spirometry, IPPB, PAP, O_2 therapy; consider therapeutic bronchoscopy* for atelectasis due to large airway obstruction
Opacity on chest x-ray	Infiltrates, atelectasis, consolidation	Incentive spirometry, IPPB, PAP, O_2 therapy; consider therapeutic bronchoscopy* for atelectasis due to large airway obstruction
Pleural Space		
Hyperresonant percussion	Pneumothorax	Evacuate air*; lung-expansion therapy
Dull percussion	Pleural effusion	Evacuate fluid*; lung-expansion therapy
Acid–Base Disorders		
Acute respiratory acidosis	Acute ventilatory failure	Mechanical ventilation (consider NPPV initially)*
Compensated respiratory acidosis	Chronic ventilatory failure	Low-flow O_2; bronchial hygiene therapy
Metabolic alkalosis	Hypokalemia	Treat underlying cause*; give potassium*
	Hypochloremia	Treat underlying cause*; give chloride*
Metabolic acidosis	Shock/lactic acidosis	O_2 therapy; restore circulation; administer $NaHCO_3$*
	Ketoacidosis (diabetes)	Treat underlying cause*; administer $NaHCO_3$*; hyperventilate
	Renal failure	Treat underlying cause*; dialysis*
Oxygenation		
$Pa_{O_2} > 60$ torr $F_{I_{O_2}} < 0.60$	Moderate hypoxemia; V/Q imbalance	O_2 therapy; treat underlying cause
$Pa_{O_2} < 60$ torr $F_{I_{O_2}} > 0.60$	Severe hypoxemia; shunting	PEEP/CPAP, oxygen

*Physician ordered.

Adapted from: Des Jardins T, Burton GG, Tietsort J. *Respiratory care case studies: The therapist driven protocol approach.* St. Louis, MO: Mosby-Yearbook; 1997.

Recommending Changes in the Therapeutic Plan When Indicated Based on Data

If the data indicate the therapeutic plan is not meeting the desired objectives, then you should recommend appropriate changes. For example, if a patient with a weak cough is having problems with secretion clearance and the problem persists after a regimen of directed coughing, you should recommend either mechanical insufflation–exsufflation or nasotracheal suctioning (Table 14-1).

Performing Respiratory Care Quality Assurance

Respiratory care quality improvement activities usually focus on identifying and resolving problems related to patient care and clinical performance. According to the AARC, the goals of a respiratory care quality improvement plan should include at least the following:

- Provide ongoing monitoring of both the quality and appropriateness of respiratory care
- Ensure that respiratory care methods and procedures are cost-efficient
- Ensure that respiratory care methods and procedures are effective
- Identify, rank, and resolve patient care–related problems

Nine key steps are needed to systematically implement a quality improvement plan. As depicted in **Figure 14-1**, these steps include (1) identification of problems, (2) determination of problem causes, (3) ranking of problems, (4) development of strategies for problem resolution, (5) development of appropriate measures, (6) implementation of problem resolution strategies, (7) compilation of results, (8) evaluation of outcomes, and (9) reporting of results.

Successful implementation of the quality improvement plan demands that the respiratory care service develop criteria addressing the therapeutic goals, appropriateness, and means of evaluating the effectiveness of each specific high-utilization and high-risk procedure. What follows is an example of a quality improvement protocol for oxygen therapy, with the applicable criteria summarized in the accompanying box.

Identifying Problems

Using the quality improvement process just described, various data sources, including patients' medical records, would be used to determine the extent to which oxygen-therapy services are being

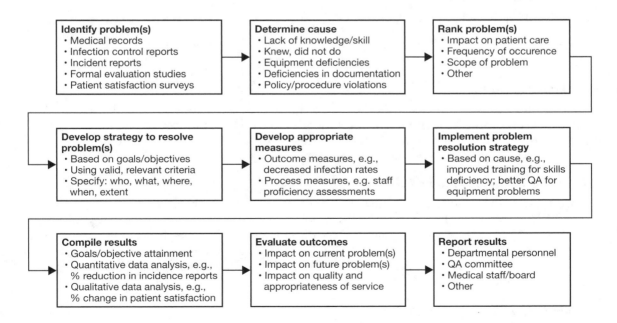

Figure 14-1 Respiratory Care Quality Assurance Flowchart.

Modified from: Hastings D. The AARC's model quality assurance plan. *AARC Times*. 1988;12(2), 25.

appropriately used. Normally, an objective problem indicator, such as "90% of all patients receiving oxygen therapy will meet the appropriateness of care criteria," is helpful in problem identification. If the indicator is not being met (e.g., if only 70% of the patients meet the appropriateness of therapy criteria), a problem exists.

Quality Assurance Criteria for Oxygen Therapy

(a) Therapeutic Goals

1. To prevent or reverse hypoxemia and tissue hypoxia

2. To decrease myocardial work

3. To decrease the work of breathing

(b) Appropriateness of Care

1. The patient must be diagnosed as having or being at risk of developing hypoxemia and/or tissue hypoxia; or

2. The patient must be diagnosed as having suffered a myocardial infarction within the last 72 hours; and

3. Dosing and mode of therapy will follow the criteria specified in the Respiratory Care Procedure Manual.

(c) Evaluation of the Effectiveness of Therapy

Effectiveness of therapy is evaluated by comparing the pre-treatment and post-treatment status of the patient according to the following criteria. To be considered effective, at least one item from the following list must apply:

- Achievement of a satisfactory Pao_2 (> 60 torr) or Spo_2 (> 90-92%)
- Reversal or absence of cyanosis
- Decrease in heart rate
- Decrease in blood pressure
- Resolution of cardiac dysrhythmias
- Decrease in respiratory rate
- Increase in level of consciousness
- Decrease in %HbCO
- Relief of dyspnea

Source: Adapted from Larson K. The well-defined quality assurance plan. *AARC Times*. 1988;12(2):1524.

Determining Causes

Once a problem has been identified, its cause must be determined. For example, if only 70% of the patients receiving oxygen therapy meet the specified criteria, this can be due to several factors, including the ordering physicians' lack of knowledge of the criteria, their failure to follow known criteria, or their failure to discontinue therapy when indicated.

Resolving Identified Problems

Once the underlying cause is identified, a strategy to resolve the problem must be developed, implemented, and evaluated. For example, if the problem with oxygen therapy use is based on the new medical residents' failure to follow the criteria, proper education may be needed. Once implemented, the impact of the selected strategy on the desired outcome should be assessed. For example, we would want to know whether the in-service education program for the medical residents resulted in better compliance with the oxygen therapy criteria.

Reporting and Ongoing Monitoring

Problem identification and resolution activities, including the relative success of intervention strategies, must be documented and reported regularly. Moreover, even successful interventions must be monitored over time to ensure a given problem does not recur.

Developing, Monitoring, and Applying Respiratory Care Protocols

The NBRC exams require that candidates be proficient in applying treatment protocols. Physicians have traditionally written orders for respiratory care services that were specific and allowed no variation by the therapist providing the treatment. Protocols allow properly trained respiratory therapists to independently initiate and adjust therapy, within guidelines previously established by the medical staff. Key elements required in a medically acceptable respiratory care protocol include the following:

- Clearly stated objectives
- Outline of the protocol, including a decision tree or algorithm
- Description of alternative choices at decision and action points
- Description of potential complications and corrections
- Description of end points and decision points where the physician must be contacted

Major steps in the application of a respiratory care protocol are as follows:

1. Check/confirm physician protocol order
2. Conduct chart review (e.g., admitting diagnosis, history & physical, diagnostic test results)
3. Assess patient (e.g., vital signs, breath sounds, SpO_2, ABGs, spirometry)
4. Confirm appropriateness of protocol (e.g., indications, contraindications, objectives, therapy selection)
5. Collaborate with other providers to integrate protocol into overall patient management
6. Implement protocol
   a. Provide essential patient/family education
   b. Initiate selected therapy
   c. Monitor patient response
   d. Assess therapy outcomes
   e. Adjust or alter therapy as allowed to optimize outcomes
   f. Reassess patient with each treatment or at a pre-established frequency
   g. Discontinue protocol/notify physician if
      I. a serious adverse response occurs or
      II. a protocol limit or boundary rule takes effect or
      III. the therapy objectives are achieved
7. Document protocol application, modification and discontinuation in medical record

Examples of Protocol Algorithms

NBRC exam candidates should be familiar with the protocols most commonly used in respiratory care. A good place to start is the "Resources" section of the American Association for Respiratory Care's website at www.aarc.org (access limited to members). There you will find examples of nationally developed protocols covering the areas of general adult acute care, adult mechanical ventilation, general pediatric acute care, and pediatric intensive care. Other respiratory care-related protocols can be found in professional journals or by conducting online searches. As an example, **Figure 14-2** provides the basic algorithm for a protocol to initiate and adjust invasive mechanical ventilation on adult patients.

Protocol Monitoring and Quality Assurance

Successful implementation of respiratory care protocols requires ongoing quality monitoring to assess their effectiveness. Elements of protocol implementation that should be monitored include therapist competency, medical and therapist compliance, protocol outcomes, participant feedback, and patient satisfaction. Relevant protocol outcome measures can include the following:

- Appropriateness of physician protocol orders
- Comparison of protocol patients to those receiving care by standard order (e.g., by diagnosis-related group [DRG], case-mix index, or some other criterion)

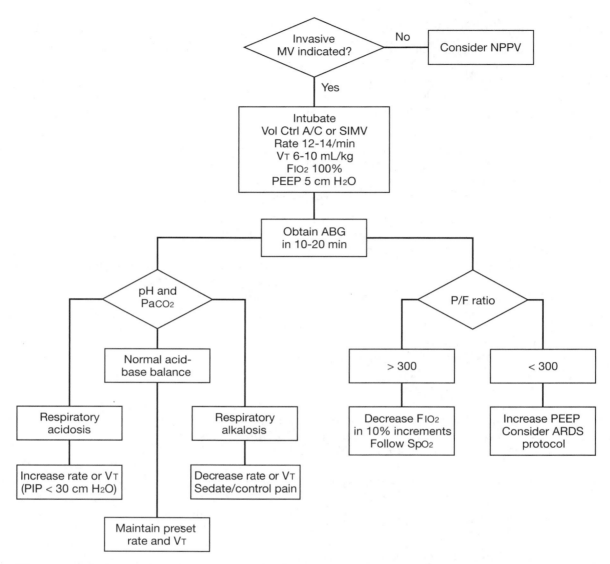

Figure 14-2 Example Algorithm of Protocol for Initial Application and Adjustment of Adult Invasive Mechanical Ventilation.

Courtesy of: Strategic Learning Associates, LLC, Little Silver, New Jersey

- Costs (direct costs, number of procedures, duration of treatment, missed treatments)
- Clinical outcomes (changes in physiologic measures such as SpO_2 or $FEV_1\%$; adverse responses; length of stay; readmissions)
- Effect on staff (productivity, satisfaction)
- Miscellaneous (percentage of protocol patients versus percentage of physician-directed patients)
- Number of patients on protocols by DRG, case-mix index or severity score, assessment scoring system for severity of respiratory illness, and patient satisfaction scores

COMMON ERRORS TO AVOID

You can improve your score by avoiding these mistakes:

- Never assume that all wheezing is due to bronchospasm or asthma; congestive heart failure can cause similar symptoms but requires different treatment (e.g., a diuretic and inotropic medication).

- Never recommend mechanical ventilation for the initial management of chronic ventilatory failure (blood gas results indicate compensated respiratory acidosis); instead, recommend conservative management (e.g., low-flow O_2) and careful monitoring.
- Never rely on high FIO_2s (> 0.60) in the presence of severe hypoxemia due to shunting (can cause O_2 toxicity and worsen the problem); instead, recommend adding PEEP/CPAP.
- Never proceed with a protocol beyond a defined limit or boundary or when a notification criterion requires you to contact the physician.

SURE BETS

In some situations, you can be sure of the right approach to a clinical problem or scenario:

- Always assess the patient's pathophysiological state before recommending any course of action.
- Always differentiate atelectasis/consolidation from pleural effusion before recommending the appropriate treatment.
- Always recommend oxygen and circulatory support when metabolic acidosis is due to shock.
- Always recommend CPAP/PEEP in the presence of severe hypoxemia due to shunting (PaO_2 < 60 torr on FIO_2 > 0.60).
- Whenever evaluation data indicate that a care plan is not meeting the desired objectives, always consider or recommend appropriate changes.
- When formulating care plans, always consider family education and communication.
- In quality assurance, always try to identify the cause(s) of problems before developing corrective strategies.
- Always conduct a comprehensive initial patient evaluation before developing a respiratory care plan or implementing a protocol.
- Always include multiple methods to assess the efficacy of therapy (patient outcomes) in your care plans.
- Always document any adjustments in therapy (including reasons for change) in the patient record.

PRE-TEST ANSWERS AND EXPLANATIONS

Following are this chapter's pre-test answers and explanations. Be sure to review each answer's explanation thoroughly to help you understand why it is correct. If the explanation is still unclear to you, review the chapter content.

14-1. **Correct answer: A.** Administer high concentrations of oxygen. In this case, the PaO_2 is misleading because it represents only dissolved oxygen (CO alters oxyhemoglobin saturation but not PaO_2). The immediate history and finding of coma are a sufficient basis to recommend a high FIO_2 level to help eliminate the carbon monoxide.

14-2. **Correct answer: C.** Improve alveolar ventilation. IPPB is used on patients who cannot (due to the increased work of breathing) or will not take a deep breath. Its primary function is to increase alveolar ventilation by taking over the work of breathing.

14-3. **Correct answer: C.** Pulmonary edema. CPAP can help overcome the shunting and hypoxemia common in both cardiogenic and noncardiogenic pulmonary edema. In cardiogenic pulmonary edema, CPAP can help decrease venous return, thereby decreasing pulmonary blood flows and pressures. In noncardiogenic pulmonary edema (e.g., ARDS), CPAP (or PEEP) opens collapsed alveoli and decreases shunting.

14-4. **Correct answer: C.** Decrease left heart and pulmonary vascular pressures. The primary aim in treating cardiogenic pulmonary edema is to decrease left heart and pulmonary vascular pressures. Note that one key to the correct answer is to identify the therapeutic goal for a patient with the given condition.

14-5. **Correct answer: B.** Bedside therapeutic bronchoscopy. Should conservative measures fail in treating atelectasis due to large airway obstruction, therapeutic bronchoscopy is indicated. This procedure can usually be performed at the bedside with conscious sedation. Note that data are collected and analyzed in this question, and you are expected to pick the plan that best matches the data and analysis provided.

14-6. **Correct answer: C.** Treating absorption atelectasis. Indications for O_2 therapy include documented hypoxemia, acute care situations in which hypoxemia is common (e.g., shock, trauma, CO poisoning), acute myocardial infarction, and short-term therapy for patients likely to develop hypoxemia (e.g., during postanesthesia recovery). Absorption atelectasis is a potential hazard of supplemental O_2.

14-7. **Correct answer: D.** Maintain a $Paco_2$ of 30–35 torr (deliberate hyperventilation). Hyperventilation is sometimes used immediately after head trauma or surgery in order to promote cerebral vasoconstriction (low $Paco_2$) and decrease the intracranial pressure (ICP). Typically, the low $Paco_2$ is maintained in the 30–35 mm Hg range. Note that the effect of hyperventilation wanes after several hours and that this technique is not recommended for ongoing management. Other therapies, including osmotic diuresis, draining of CSF fluid, and sedation are used for ongoing management.

14-8. **Correct answer: D.** Improve lung expansion/prevent atelectasis. IPPB is used instead of incentive spirometry when a patient cannot (physically) or will not take a deep breath. The only goal that fits this application is to improve lung expansion/prevent atelectasis.

14-9. **Correct answer: D.** Low-flow oxygen. Patients with emphysema may hypoventilate when given moderate to high concentrations of O_2 (due to elimination of their hypoxic drive). It is therefore recommended that the Pao_2 of hypoxemic COPD patients be titrated to the 55–60 torr range (88–90% saturation). Normally, this goal can be achieved using low-flow (1–2 L/min) oxygen or a 24% or 28% air entrainment mask.

14-10. **Correct answer: B.** BiPAP with 100% O_2. Based on the history and clinical findings, the patient likely is suffering from acute pulmonary edema due to heart failure. The respiratory care plan should include positive pressure therapy (e.g., BiPAP) with 100% O_2. (see Table 14-1).

14-11. **Correct answer: C.** Check the physician order for the respiratory care protocol. See the major steps in applying respiratory care protocols outlined in this chapter.

14-12. **Correct answer: A.** Analysis of department budgeting. The department's budget should not receive much consideration when investigating the causes of patient care–related issues.

14-13. **Correct answer: D.** 1, 2, 3, and 4. All of these data could be used as quality assurance outcome criteria. Remember—outcome criteria for quality assurance fall into one of two categories: subjective or objective. If objective data support improvement but the patient's subjective feelings suggest otherwise, that must also be considered in the analysis and plan.

14-14. **Correct answer: D.** 1, 2, and 3. All three items in this list should be investigated as potential causes of an infection control problem. Training can affect how procedures are carried out, supply deficiencies can make therapists not change equipment as often as recommended, and failure to follow set infection control procedures for whatever reason will result in a failed quality assurance program.

14-15. **Correct answer: C.** Compare pre- and post-treatment patient status on one or more predefined criteria. Comparison of pre- and post-treatment status on pre-defined criteria ensures that you do not jump to therapeutic conclusions without the data to support such conclusions.

POST-TEST

To confirm your mastery of this chapter's topical content, you should take the chapter post-test, available online at http://go.jblearning.com/respexamreview. A score of 80% or more indicates that you are adequately prepared for this section of the NBRC written exams. If you score less than 80%, you should continue to review the applicable chapter content. In addition, you may want to access and review the relevant Web links covering this chapter's content (courtesy of RTBoardReview. com), also online at the Jones & Bartlett Learning site.

Initiate, Conduct, or Modify Respiratory Care Techniques in an Emergency Setting

CHAPTER 15

Albert J. Heuer

Respiratory therapists play a vital role in providing prompt and appropriate care in emergency settings. For this reason, the NBRC assesses your knowledge on providing emergency care on all of its exams. Although only a small number of questions are involved, the scope of required knowledge is very broad, demanding a significant portion of your preparation time.

OBJECTIVES

In preparing for the shared NBRC exam content, you should demonstrate the knowledge needed to:

1. Treat cardiopulmonary collapse by being able to:
   a. Recognize cardiopulmonary emergencies
   b. Initiate appropriate respiratory care in emergency settings
   c. Apply basic and advanced life support protocols
   d. Assist in the diagnosis and treatment of a tension pneumothorax
2. Participate in safe and effective intrahospital and external patient transport
3. Participate as a member of the medical emergency team (MET)
4. Prepare for and assist with disaster management

WHAT TO EXPECT ON THIS CATEGORY OF THE CRT EXAM

CRT exam: 3 questions; typically one-third each recall, application, and analysis
WRRT exam: 3 questions; generally one-third application and two-thirds analysis
CSE exam: indeterminate number of questions; however, exam III-I knowledge is a prerequisite to success on CSE Information Gathering and Decision-Making sections

PRE-TEST

Carefully respond to each of the following questions. After completing the pre-test, compare your answers with those provided at the end of this chapter. Then thoroughly review each answer's explanation to help understand why it is correct.

15-1. During a "code blue" or other medical emergency, a physician is having trouble starting an intravenous line. Which of the following drugs can be placed down an endotracheal tube during emergency life support?
1. Naloxone
2. Lidocaine
3. Atropine
4. Epinephrine
A. 2 and 4 only
B. 1, 2, and 3
C. 3 and 4 only
D. 1, 2, 3, and 4

15-2. Which site is most preferred when checking the pulse of an unresponsive adult?
A. Brachial artery
B. Jugular vein
C. Carotid artery
D. Radial artery

15-3. At the onset of adult mouth-to-mouth or mouth-to-mask ventilation for an adult, which type of breathing should you provide?
A. Two normal breaths
B. Four fast, shallow breaths

C. Four slow, deep breaths
D. One very slow breath

15-4. After two attempts of ventilating an infant in respiratory arrest, you still cannot deliver breaths. At this point, what should you do?
  A. Apply back blows, followed by chest thrusts
  B. Try to ventilate again with smaller puffs
  C. Apply 6–10 strong abdominal thrusts
  D. Provide external cardiac compressions

15-5. What is the ideal ratio of chest compressions to rescue breaths that should be given by a single rescuer during a cardiopulmonary resuscitation (CPR) attempt on an adult?
  A. 5:1
  B. 15:2
  C. 2:15
  D. 30:2

15-6. When transporting critically ill patients in unpressurized aircraft, it is often necessary to make which adjustment to maintain adequate oxygenation?
  A. Increase the F_{IO_2}
  B. Decrease the minute volume
  C. Decrease the F_{IO_2}
  D. Increase the minute volume

15-7. What are the proper rate and depth of external chest compressions for an adult?
  A. 80–100/min with a depth of 1 inch
  B. 70–80/min with a depth of 1–1½ inches

C. At least 100/min with a depth of at least 2 inches
D. 60–80/min with a depth of 1½ to 2 inches

15-8. What is the initial energy range for biphasic defibrillation of ventricular fibrillation?
  A. 120–200 joules
  B. 200–280 joules
  C. 280–360 joules
  D. 360–440 joules

15-9. All of the following monitoring equipment is *mandatory* when transporting a critically ill patient within or outside of the hospital *except*:
  A. End-tidal CO_2 monitor
  B. Oxygen source/delivery device
  C. Blrtood pressure monitor/cuff
  D. Cardiac monitor/defibrillator

15-10. If the number of ICU ventilators needed to support patients in respiratory failure after a chemical disaster is insufficient to meet the need, what should your *initial* response be?
  A. Contact other local facilities and arrange for patient transfers
  B. Call and order additional backup ventilators from the vendor
  C. Use available in-house anesthesia and/ or transport ventilators
  D. Assign patients without equipment to triage priority "black"

WHAT YOU NEED TO KNOW: ESSENTIAL CONTENT

Basic Life Support

Basic life support (BLS) is the foundation for most emergency care. You should expect that concepts related to BLS will be included on all NBRC exams, but especially the CRT exam.

   BLS can help restore ventilation and circulation to victims without the use of specialized equipment. These procedures should be applied until the victim is revived or until advanced life support equipment and personnel are available. In sequence, the key steps in BLS are as follows (note the change from the former airway–breathing-circulation pattern, or A-B-C to C-A-B):

1. Assess the victim for unresponsiveness ("tap and shout") and *look* for normal or abnormal breathing.
2. Activate the emergency medical system and secure either an automated external defibrillator (AED) or standard defibrillator.
3. In adults and children, check for a carotid artery pulse; in infants check for a brachial artery pulse.
4. If there is no pulse, begin compressions (at least 100 per minute for adults) for 2 minutes (C).

5. If the patient is not breathing, open the airway using the head tilt–chin lift or jaw-thrust maneuver (A).
6. Give two normal breaths, each lasting 1 second (B).
7. If a breath does not make the patient's chest rise, reposition the head and try again.
8. Continue CPR with cycles of 30 chest compression and two breaths for 2 minutes (five cycles); reassess after every five cycles.

Table 15-1 outlines the key differences in these basic life support steps as applied to adults, children (1–8 years old), and infants (less than 1 year old).

Advanced Cardiac Life Support (ACLS)

In addition to demonstrating competency in basic life support, the NBRC expects that you will be able to treat cardiopulmonary collapse according to the American Heart Association (AHA) ACLS

Table 15-1 Summary of Basic Life Support

BLS Element	Adult/Older Child (> 8 years)	Child (1–8 years)	Infant (< 1 year)
When to activate EMS/call a "code blue" after assessing unresponsiveness	Call immediately and get a defibrillator.	In case of a witnessed sudden collapse and if you are alone, call immediately and get a defibrillator. If no a sudden collapse, administer CPR for 2 minutes before activation.	Call after providing 2 minutes of care, if alone.
Pulse check (maximum: 10 seconds)	Carotid/femoral	Carotid/femoral	Brachial
Compression location	Two hands on breastbone between nipples	One or two hands on breastbone between nipples	Two fingers on breastbone just below the nipple line; use two-thumb technique for neonates
Compression depth	At least 2 inches	At least one-third the depth of chest or about 2 inches	At least one-third the depth of chest or about 1½ inches
Compression:breath ratio (single provider)	30:2	30:2	30:2
Compression:breath ratio (two providers)	30:2[a]	15:2	15:2
Compression rate	At least 100/minute		
Breathing method	Lay personnel: mouth-to-mouth (barrier device if available) Healthcare provider: bag-valve--mask ventilation and O_2 ASAP	Same as adult	Same as adult
Foreign body airway obstruction in a responsive victim	Abdominal thrusts (Heimlich maneuver)	Abdominal thrusts (Heimlich maneuver)	Alternate five back blows with five chest thrusts
Automated external defibrillator (AED) use	Yes	Yes; if child pads are not available, use adult pads	Yes; if child pads are not available, use adult pads
	Deliver one shock, followed immediately by 2 minutes of CPR, then reassess		

[a] Once an advanced airway is in place, give on breath every 8 seconds simultaneously with compressions.

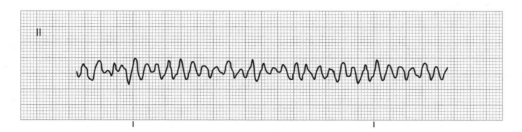

Figure 15-1 Example of Ventricular Fibrillation.

Source: Garcia T, Miller GT. *Arrhythmia recognition: the art of interpretation.* Sudbury, MA: Jones and Bartlett Publishers; 2004.

protocols. These protocols are summarized in clinical algorithms for specific cardiopulmonary emergencies.

Adult Resuscitation Protocols

The most common adult cardiopulmonary emergencies stem from one of four cardiac dysrhythmias that produce pulselessness. These rhythms include ventricular fibrillation (VF), rapid ventricular tachycardia (VT), pulseless electrical activity (PEA), and asystole. Example ECG tracings for VF and VT are depicted in **Figure 15-1** and **Figure 15-2**, respectively.

In addition, the ACLS algorithm for responding to adult cardiac arrest is shown in **Figure 15-3**. For the NBRC exams, you should first be able to quickly recognize these lethal rhythms and then promptly apply the appropriate steps in this algorithm.

ACLS Drugs

ACLS also involves the use of an array of medications. NBRC exam candidates are expected to have good general knowledge of the key emergency medications. **Table 15-2** summarizes the most common IV ACLS drugs administered to adults. In the absence of IV access, some medications may be instilled through an ET tube, as noted in the table.

Equipment

To succeed on this section of the NBRC exams, you should be familiar with the key equipment used in emergencies, including resuscitation devices and artificial airways (Chapter 4). You also will be expected to know how to properly apply both AEDs and standard defibrillators. This knowledge includes selecting the initial and subsequent defibrillator energy levels or doses to apply to both adult and pediatric patients with shockable rhythms (ventricular fibrillation and pulseless or polymorphic ventricular tachycardia), as outlined in **Table 15-3**.

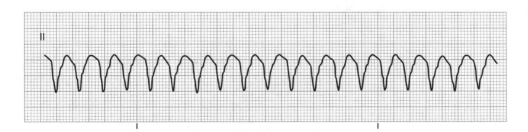

Figure 15-2 Example of Ventricular Tachycardia.

Source: Garcia T, Miller GT. *Arrhythmia recognition: the art of interpretation.* Sudbury, MA: Jones and Bartlett Publishers; 2004.

Table 15-2 ACLS Medication Summary

Medication	Initial Adult IV Dosage	Classification/Indication
Epinephrine*	1 mg every 3–5 minutes	Vasoconstrictor; may improve cerebral perfusion
Vasopressin (ADH)	40 units × 1	Vasoconstrictor; may improve cerebral perfusion
Atropine*	0.5 mg every 3–5 minutes, up to a maximum of 3 mg/kg	Cardiac stimulant (anticholinergic) used for selected bradycardias
Amiodarone (Cordarone)	300 mg rapid infusion followed by 150 mg in 3–5 minutes and every 10 minutes, up to 2.2 g/day	Antiarrhythmic for VF and VT
Lidocaine*	Initial dose of 1.0–1.5 mg/kg, with additional doses of 0.5–0.75 mg/kg every 5–10 minutes, up to 3 mg/kg	Antiarrhythmic for VF and VT, primarily as an alternative to amiodarone

*Denotes a medication that may be instilled via ET tube if IV access is not established. In such cases, it is recommended that the dose be doubled and that it be followed with the instillation of 10 mL normal saline.

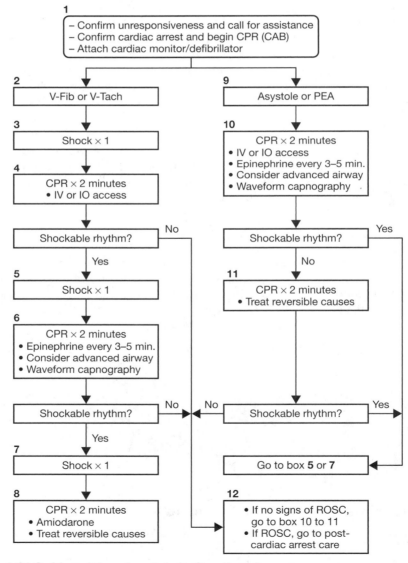

Figure 15-3 ACLS Algorithm for Adult Cardiac Arrest.

Table 15-3 Defibrillation Doses For Shockable Rhythms

Patient	Initial Dose*	Subsequent Doses
Adult	120-200 J or as recommended by the manufacturer	Same as initial dose (higher energy levels may be considered)
Child	2 J/kg	At least 4 J/kg (higher energy levels may be considered)
*The above doses are for modern biphasic defibrillators. For older monophasic devices, apply an initial dose of 360 J to adults and 2 J/kg to children.		

Monitoring and Assessment

You are expected to know the major ways in which a patient should be assessed during CPR and immediately following a successful resuscitation. This may range from periodic pulse and breathing checks, generally after five cycles of CPR, to more advanced assessment methods, including electrocardiography, pulse oximetry, arterial blood gas monitoring, and intra-arterial blood pressure measurement (if available). Candidates should note that due to its ability to assess both the adequacy of ventilation and the effectiveness of cardiac compressions, *waveform capnography is now recommended as a standard of care during resuscitation efforts*. These monitoring and assessment methods are covered in more detail in Chapter 11.

Pediatric and Neonatal Emergencies

For the NBRC exams, you need to have sound general knowledge of pediatric and neonatal emergency care. Variations of BLS techniques for children and infants are detailed in Table 15-1. When treating children, the NBRC will expect that you can follow the key pediatric advanced life support (PALS) and neonatal resuscitation protocols.

Pediatric Resuscitation

The most likely NBRC exam scenarios involving pediatric advanced life support are those for pulseless arrest. As depicted in **Figure 15-4**, the PALS algorithm for pulseless arrest is similar to the algorithm for adults, with the exception that the defibrillation shock and medications dosages vary by patient weight. One of the most common medical emergencies associated with pediatric patients is airway obstruction by foreign body; consequently, you should be familiar with practices for responding to obstructed airways in both conscious and unconscious pediatric patients (see Table 15-1).

Neonatal Resuscitation

In addition to pediatric resuscitation, you must be familiar with the resuscitation protocol for neonates, as shown in **Figure 15-5**. Babies who are flaccid, cyanotic, or apneic in the delivery room normally require stimulation and supplemental O_2. If color, heart rate, and breathing are not restored within 30 seconds, you should provide manual positive-pressure ventilation via face mask. *A heart rate less than 60 always requires chest compressions in a neonate*. If the infant does not respond to these measures, epinephrine should be administered and intubation and mechanical ventilation considered.

Treat a Tension Pneumothorax

A cardiopulmonary emergency likely to appear in some form on the NBRC exams is tension pneumothorax. You should be familiar with the most common signs and symptoms, as well as emergency treatment, of this potentially life-threatening disorder.

A pneumothorax occurs when a tear or rupture in lung tissue permits air to escape into the pleural space. A simple pneumothorax may occur spontaneously (e.g., during vigorous coughing) and can go unnoticed at the time, eventually resolving without treatment. A *tension* pneumothorax, in contrast, occurs when air under pressure enters the pleural space. This condition is even more serious for patients receiving positive-pressure ventilation, which invariably causes a rapid buildup

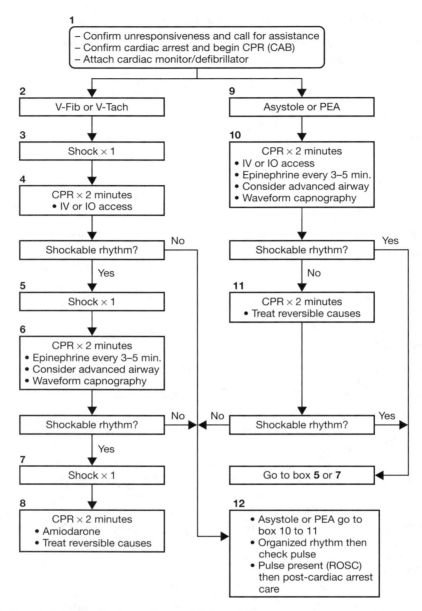

Figure 15-4 Pediatric Pulseless Arrest Algorithm.

of pleural pressure, which compresses the heart, lungs, and great vessels. Patients experiencing a tension pneumothorax can deteriorate quite rapidly. For this reason, prompt detection and treatment are essential.

Factors that may predispose patients to a tension pneumothorax include mechanical ventilation with high airway pressures (more than 40–45 cm H_2O), chest trauma, and conditions associated with excessively high compliance such as advanced emphysema. When any of these factors is coupled with a rapid decline in clinical status, you should consider the possibility of a tension pneumothorax. While such a diagnosis is generally confirmed via a chest x-ray, you should be mindful of the following clinical manifestations:

- Rapid decline in cardiopulmonary status (hypotension, hypoxemia)
- Decreased or absent breath sounds on the affected side
- Hyperresonance to percussion of the affected side

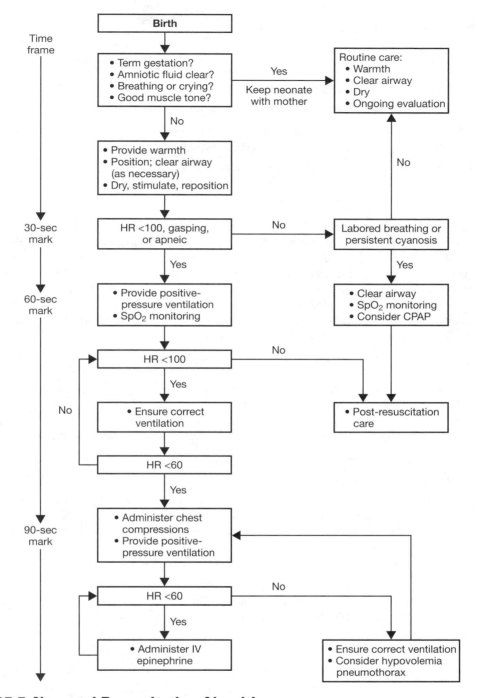

Figure 15-5 Neonatal Resuscitation Algorithm.

- Tracheal shift *away from* the affected side (severe cases)
- Rapid increase in ventilator pressures during volume control ventilation
- Shock or PEA (severe, untreated cases)

A chest x-ray confirming the diagnosis of a tension pneumothorax will typically show hyperlucency and a collapsed lung, flattening of the diaphragm, and expansion of the rib spaces—all on the affected side. In addition, a mediastinal shift to the opposite side is typically observed.

Basic Procedure for Needle Thoracostomy

1. Place patient in an upright position, if tolerated.

2. Locate puncture site (second intercostal space in the midclavicular line).

3. Prepare site with Betadine and/or alcohol scrubs.

4. Insert angiocath over the top of the third rib until the catheter hub is against the chest wall.

5. Listen for a rush of air and observe the patient's cardiorespiratory status.

6. Remove the needle and secure the angiocath and attach a flutter (Heimlich valve).

7. Immediately prepare for tube thoracostomy (chest tube insertion)

Once a tension pneumothorax is confirmed, the treatment is emergency decompression of the chest, also known as *needle thoracostomy*. As outlined in the accompanying box, needle thoracostomy involves insertion of a large-bore angiocath (14 gauge for adults, 18 or 20 gauge for infants) into the second intercostal space over the top of the third rib in the midclavicular line. This procedure should be done using sterile technique, and proper placement should elicit a rush of air through the catheter, often followed by rapid improvement in cardiovascular status. Because needle thoracostomy simply converts a tension pneumothorax into a simple pneumothorax, full resolution of the problem usually requires the insertion of a conventional chest tube, as discussed in Chapter 16.

Patient Transport

The NBRC expects you to be competent in transporting critically ill patients, both within the hospital complex and externally via land or air transport. The main focus is on ensuring patient safety during transport, through proper planning and execution. Concepts covered elsewhere in this text, including airway management and O_2 cylinder duration of flow, may be included in this portion of the exams.

Intra-hospital Patient Transport

Most transports take place within a hospital or healthcare facility. The first step in planning for transport is to assess whether the patient is stable enough to be moved. This assessment should include measurement of vital signs, hemodynamic parameters, oxygenation, ventilation, and any other relevant clinical indicators associated with patient stability. According to the AARC, a patient should not be moved if any of the following criteria cannot be reasonably ensured during transport:

- Provision of adequate oxygenation and ventilation
- Maintenance of acceptable hemodynamic performance
- Adequate monitoring of the patient's cardiopulmonary status
- Maintenance of airway control

In most cases, critically ill patients are transported by a team consisting of a critical care nurse and respiratory therapist, with an ACLS-trained physician also accompanying unstable patients. The transport team should communicate in advance with the receiving team to confirm readiness to receive the patient, including any specialized equipment needed at the receiving site. As with all patient interventions, the transport should be well documented in the record, to include the physician's order and patient status throughout the transition period.

The minimum monitoring needed during transport consists of heart and respiratory rate monitoring, pulse oximetry, and noninvasive blood pressure monitoring (all usually provided via a multichannel portable monitor). Body temperature should be monitored in those patients at risk for hypothermia. Invasive blood pressure monitoring is recommended for patients already having an A-line in place who are under treatment with vasoactive drugs or who are hemodynamically unstable. ICP should continue to be monitored during transport of neurology patients.

Basic support equipment includes a drug kit (e.g., IV supplies, ACLS drugs, sedatives, analgesics), an O_2 source with sufficient duration of flow (plus a 30-minute reserve), and a fully charged battery-operated infusion pump and defibrillator (often incorporated into the portable monitor). Additional equipment needed to transport intubated patients requiring mechanical ventilation includes a transport ventilator with backup manual resuscitator with PEEP valve and mask, an intubation kit, and a battery-powered suction pump with suction supplies. A capnograph (which may be incorporated into multichannel monitor) is recommended for patients requiring strict control of P_{CO_2} levels, such as those with neurological disorders.

During transport of pediatric patients, a complete kit comprising resuscitation equipment and drugs for children must accompany the patient, particularly a self-inflating bag, a face mask, and an intubation kit adapted to the age of the child, as well as an intraosseous catheterization kit.

Ideally, the ventilator used for transport should be a high-performance portable device capable of delivering the same level and type of support as that provided to the patient in ICU. If possible, simple single-limb circuits with a HEPA filter and HME for humidification should be used. If the patient requires a function that available portable ventilators cannot provide, you should determine *prior to actual transport* if adequate support can be delivered by the less capable device. Patients receiving noninvasive positive-pressure ventilation (NPPV) should continue to be supported in this mode with a high-performance portable NPPV device. Whether designed for invasive or noninvasive use, the portable ventilator's interface should not allow for any accidental changes to the settings. Parameters that must be monitored include airway pressures (PIP, PEEP) and expired V_T, with mandatory alarms for high pressure, patient disconnection, interruption of the gas or electricity supply, and ventilator failure.

For transport of pediatric patients, all equipment and supplies (including drugs) must be appropriate to the age of the child, with an intraosseous catheterization kit included should IV access not be available. For children weighing less than 15 kg (33 lb), the transport ventilator must be certified for pediatric use and be able to accurately deliver the smaller tidal volumes and higher rates required by these patients.

Basic quality assurance demands that all equipment be checked for proper operation prior to transport. Electric supply and recharging capabilities of all electrically powered devices (monitor, infusion and suction pumps, ventilator) must be compatible with use at all times, with sufficient battery power ensured for the full duration of the transport. To confirm proper operation and patient tolerance, the transport ventilator should be connected to the patient 5–10 minutes before leaving the patient's room. Likewise, the function of the portable suction pump should checked, as well as the laryngoscope light source in the intubation kit.

After confirming equipment operation, the patient should be prepared for transport. Key aspects of patient preparation that the RT member of the team should address include the following:

- Before transport, document the patient's respiratory status and ventilator settings in the record (a transport form may be used for this purpose).
- Check and confirm all connections between the equipment and the patient before beginning transport.
- Place the patient in the same position as that maintained in ICU.
- Verify the ET tube cuff pressure before (and after) transport.
- For patients requiring strict control of Pa_{CO_2}, obtain an arterial sample before transport and record the Pa_{CO_2}–$P_{ET}CO_2$ gradient.

During transport, each time the patient is mobilized, you should conduct a thorough verification of all equipment–patient connections. Should any problems with the patient–ventilator interface arise, you should immediately switch to manual ventilation with 100% O_2 and (if required) PEEP.

External Transport

Special considerations pertain to transporting critically ill patients outside the hospital include the following:

- Choosing the mode of transport (ground versus air)
- Managing increased patient movement and stimulation
- Accommodating the need for special personnel and equipment
- Addressing the effects of altitude on Pa_{O_2} and closed air spaces

Factors affecting the choice of transport mode include the distance to be traveled, the patient's condition, the availability of ambulance or aircraft, and the weather. **Table 15-4** summarizes the major advantages and disadvantages of transporting patients via ground, helicopter, and fixed-wing aircraft.

Once the transport mode is selected, it is important to secure the patient and all equipment to prevent unwanted movement. You also should be aware that patient overstimulation and stress can occur during transportation, due to vehicle movement, noise, vibration, or insufficient temperature control. These problems are particularly serious when transporting infants and children, who are most vulnerable to such stimuli. For these reasons, all patients being externally transported should be properly positioned and secured, with appropriate sound protection and temperature control being implemented.

In terms of monitoring, high background noise (especially in aircraft) may necessitate using an automated noninvasive system to monitor blood pressure and an amplified stethoscope to assess breath sounds. Moreover, because most audible medical equipment alarms cannot be heard in noisy aircraft, you should depend on good patient assessment and monitoring visual alarms.

Equipment needs for air and land transport are essentially the same as those for intrahospital transport. Ideally, the transport ventilator should function using either 110-volt AC power (supplied by a generator or inverter in the ambulance or aircraft) or 12-volt DC power (the typical voltage provided by a vehicle battery/alternator). If the ventilator is to be used for air transport, ensure that its volume, pressure, and flow settings can be adjusted either manually or automatically for variations in altitude/barometric pressure. In addition, include a calibrated O_2 analyzer and a SVN with applicable drugs for inhalation (e.g., bronchodilators, racemic epinephrine), should they be needed.

For air transport, you must understand the effects of altitude on oxygenation. As the aircraft climbs to cruising altitude, atmospheric and cabin pressures decrease. As demonstrated in **Table 15-5**, in unpressurized cabins this creates a *hypobaric* condition, which lowers the inspired, alveolar, and arterial P_{O_2}. At altitudes greater than 5,000 to 8,000 feet, even a patient with normal lung function can suffer mild hypoxemia without supplemental O_2.

Table 15-4 Advantages and Disadvantages of Patient Transport via Ground and Air

Mode	Advantages	Disadvantages
Ground/ambulance	1. Generally most efficient within a 100-mile distance 2. Often usable in inclement weather or when landing sites are not available 3. Provides more work area for the transport team 4. Less vibration and noise than helicopter	1. Generally slower than air travel 2. Not practical in difficult terrain
Helicopter	1. Most efficient for distances between 100 and 250 miles 2. Faster than ground methods 3. May be faster for short distances in difficult terrain 4. Can often land near the hospital	1. High noise and vibration resulting in overstimulation 2. May be grounded in inclement weather 3. Small work area 4. Expensive to maintain and operate 5. Hypobaric effects
Fixed-wing aircraft	1. Fastest and most efficient for distances in excess of 250 miles 2. Less vibration and noise than helicopter 3. Able to travel at high altitudes, perhaps over inclement weather	1. May be grounded in inclement weather 2. Must be landed at an airport 3. Small work area 4. Expensive to maintain and operate 5. Hypobaric effects

Table 15-5 Effect of Altitude on Oxygenation with FIO_2 = 0.21

Altitude (ft)	PB^a	PIO_2	PAO_2	PaO_2^b
0	760	160	100	95
2,000	706	148	88	83
5,000	632	133	73	68
8,000	565	119	59	54
10,000	523	110	50	45
[a] All pressures in torr/mm Hg.				
[b] Assumes a $P(A-a)O_2$ of 5 torr and no compensation.				

To compute a patient's equivalent FIO_2 needs at altitude compared with sea level, you should apply the following formula:

$$FIO_2 \text{ at altitude} = FIO_2 \text{ at sea level} \times \frac{760}{PB \text{ altitude}}$$

where "PB altitude" equals the barometric pressure in torr at the cruising altitude used for transport. For example, assume you are transporting a patient receiving 50% oxygen at sea level in an airplane cruising at 8,000 feet (PB = 565 torr). You would compute the needed FIO_2 as follows:

$$FIO_2 \text{ at altitude} = 0.50 \times \frac{760}{565}\ 0.67$$

Note that at 8,000 ft or higher, you cannot provide an FIO_2 equivalent to 0.80 or more at sea level. For this reason, patients requiring 80% or more O_2 at sea level will likely have to either be placed on PEEP/CPAP or have their PEEP levels raised to ensure adequate oxygenation.

Some transport aircraft provide pressurized cabins. Depending on the aircraft, cabin pressures may range from those equivalent to altitudes between 5,000 and 8,000 feet. In these cases, you still need to compute an equivalent FIO_2, but you should substitute the known cabin pressure for the PB at altitude.

Of course, the goal of O_2 supplementation should generally be to achieve a SpO_2 of 90% or greater, regardless of FIO_2 or altitude. Fortunately, pulse oximetry readings are not affected by altitude and are the best way to judge the adequacy of oxygenation during transport.

Another factor to consider during air transport is the relationship between gas volume and pressure. According to Boyle's law, as altitude increases and atmospheric pressure drops, gas volume increases, and vice versa. Such changes in gas volume can affect tracheal tube cuff pressures and ventilator function.

In terms of cuff pressures, as altitude increases, so, too, does the volume of gas in the cuff. Because the tube cuff is restricted in its ability to expand within the trachea, even small increases in volume can result in large increases in pressure. The only good way to accommodate these changes (and those associated with descent from altitude) is to readjust the cuff pressure when the altitude is changing.

In terms of ventilator function, different devices perform differently at altitude. For example, volume control ventilators that use turbines or blowers will tend to deliver *lower* than set volumes at altitude, whereas those using differential pressure transducers to measure and regulate flow will tend to deliver *higher* than set volumes at altitude. One solution used with microprocessor-controlled ventilators is to temporarily disconnect the patient (while manually providing support) and recalibrate the device once you reach cruising altitude. Another solution is to follow the ventilator manufacturer's recommendation for adjusting settings at various altitudes. Alternatively, you can empirically adjust VT or PIP according to end-tidal CO_2 levels as monitored by capnography. Unfortunately, capnometers also are affected by altitude, with the $PETCO_2$ reading being falsely low at altitude. This error can be overcome by recalibrating the device's high reading at the cruising altitude with a precision gas mixture (usually 5% CO_2).

Other complications are associated with "trapped" gas volume changes—that is, gas in an enclosed space that cannot equilibrate with the ambient pressure. This is a common problem in patients with a pneumothorax or excessive gas in the stomach or bowel. Such problems should be identified and managed prior to transport—for example, via insertion of a chest or nasogastric tube. Finally, if a patient suffering from decompression sickness (the "bends") has to be transported to a hyperbaric facility, you should try to ensure that the cabin pressure is maintained at or near sea level because lower ambient pressure worsens this condition.

Medical Emergency Teams

Today, most hospitals have established medical emergency teams (METs), also known as *rapid response teams*. Their purpose is to intervene and help stabilize patients who are rapidly deteriorating outside of the ICU setting. The team is often composed of an ICU nurse, a physician or physician assistant, and a respiratory therapist.

The MET is generally activated when a patient exhibits signs and symptoms of physiologic instability prior to cardiopulmonary arrest. For adults, the specific criteria for doing so often include one or more of the following:

- Acute change in mental status or overall clinical appearance
- Heart rate < 40 or > 130, or respiratory rate < 8/min or > 30/min
- Systolic blood pressure < 90 mm Hg
- SpO_2 < 90%, especially with supplemental O_2
- Acute change in urinary output to less than 50 mL over 4 hours

The most common MET interventions performed or assisted by respiratory therapists include suctioning, adjusting the FIO_2, providing noninvasive ventilation, administering bronchodilators, and intubating. Once the MET has responded, the event should be recorded in the patient's medical record. In general, the documentation should reflect the time and duration of care, the patient's vital signs and clinical status (before, during, and after the event), any interventions and procedures applied, the clinical outcome (transferred to ICU or step-down unit), and the names and disciplines of the team members who responded.

Disaster Management

NBRC exams can contain questions on the broad topic of disaster management and response. The NBRC is most likely to focus on hospital and respiratory care department preparedness for meeting the surge capacity needs associated with mass-casualty events, as well as the implementation of triage and decontamination/isolation procedures.

In terms of preparedness, all healthcare facilities are expected to have in place disaster management plans. Such plans must take into account how to care for a surge of critically ill/injured patients after a mass-casualty event. For most hospitals, this means being able to triple their capacity to support critically ill/injured patients for at least 10 days without external assistance. Additionally, hospitals need to plan for how the facility itself can manage direct damage or loss of resources, as might occur during natural catastrophes such as floods or earthquakes or as the result of hostile actions such as a nuclear bomb attack.

For the respiratory care department, preparedness planning involves consideration of at least the following elements:

- Estimating the number of surge patients who may require
  - Ventilatory support
  - Medical gas therapy (O_2 or air)
  - Suction (vacuum)
- Assessing personnel needs and resources
  - Number of staff required to meet patient needs during the surge
  - Call-back procedures to obtain additional staff
  - Plan to augment staffing with nonrespiratory personnel
- Planning for equipment needs
  - Inventory and plan for using *all* available ventilators that could support the critically ill/injured (including anesthesia, transport, MRI, and NPPV ventilators)

- ○ Mechanism to acquire additional ventilators (e.g., from vendors, other hospitals, or the Strategic National Stockpile)
  - ○ Plan to temporarily support and transfer patients if backup equipment unavailable (e.g., using manual resuscitators)
  - ○ Plan to address failure of gas supply system, including deployment of backup gas sources

In terms of the ventilator equipment to meet surge capacity, these devices ideally should (1) be able to support pediatric and adult patients with either significant airflow obstruction or ARDS, (2) function *without* high-pressure medical gas (use low-flow O_2 to regulate FIO_2), (3) ensure delivery of a set minute volume to apneic patients, and (4) have apnea, circuit disconnect, low gas source, low battery, and high peak airway pressure alarms. Although anesthesia, transport, MRI, and NPPV ventilators may not meet all of these expectations, they can and should be enlisted for use until more capable equipment is available.

In regard to augmenting staffing, nonrespiratory personnel could be assigned to assist with selected respiratory procedures such as suctioning or vital signs/SpO_2 monitoring (e.g., EMTs if available) or aerosol drug therapy (e.g., physical therapists). Evidence indicates that just-in-time training for such personnel is sufficient to allow them to safely perform these duties, which can free up the respiratory staff for managing patients receiving ventilatory support.

Based on the departmental plan and likely use of facilities other than the ICU to support a patient surge, respiratory therapists should additionally be prepared to perform the following tasks:

- Transport critically ill patients within and outside the facility
- Support increased medical emergency team activity, especially on wards "converted" to ICUs
- Assist in discharge/transfer of noncritically ill ICU patients
- Supervise general respiratory care provided by nonrespiratory personnel
- Obtain and put in use in-house anesthesia, transport, MRI, and NPPV ventilators
- Be prepared to receive ventilators from the Strategic National Stockpile
- Direct logistic resupply for ventilators, oxygen, and other respiratory support equipment

As outlined in **Table 15-6**, the specific role of respiratory therapists in responding to disasters also varies somewhat depending on the type of event.

Table 15-6 Role of the Respiratory Therapist in Disaster Response

Category	Resulting Patient Conditions	Respiratory Therapist Roles (in Addition to Patient Monitoring)
Natural catastrophe (e.g., earthquake, flood, fire, tornado)	Trauma (chest/head), near-drowning, thermal burns, hypovolemic or septic shock, dehydration	Initial assessment/triage, infection control, cleaning, disinfection, sterilization, barrier and isolation, PPE
Chemical (e.g., chlorine gas)	Inhalation injury, ventilatory/ oxygenation respiratory failure, chemical burns, pneumonia, sepsis, ARDS	Prompt recognition and initial assessment, triage and decontamination, airway management, ventilation and oxygenation, common antidote therapy (e.g., atropine for nerve agents)
Biological (natural [e.g., SARS] or bioterrorist [e.g., anthrax])	Inhalation injury, ventilatory/ oxygenation respiratory failure, pneumonia, sepsis, ARDS	Prompt recognition and initial assessment, triage, airway management, ventilation and oxygenation, infection control, isolation techniques, antimicrobial therapy
Radiologic/nuclear	Trauma, blast injuries, profound thermal burns, inhalation injury, radiation poisoning, dehydration	Prompt recognition and initial assessment, triage and decontamination, airway management, ventilation and oxygenation, isolation, and barrier techniques specific to ionizing radiation

Table 15-7 Disaster Triage Priorities

Triage Priority	Description	Action (After Decontamination If CBRN Incident)
Green/minor	Patients with minor injuries that can wait for appropriate treatment; the "walking wounded"	Move to waiting area or discharge
Yellow/delayed	Patients with potentially serious injuries, but whose status is not expected to deteriorate significantly over several hours	Move to ED
Red/immediate	Patients with life-threatening but treatable injuries requiring rapid medical attention (within 60 minutes); includes compromise to the patient's airway, breathing, or circulation	Move to ED or ICU or converted tertiary care area
Black/expectant	Deceased patients or victims who are unlikely to survive given the severity of their injuries, level of available care, or both; palliative care and pain relief should be provided	Leave in receiving area or (if deceased) move to morgue

Due to the large number and variable type of casualties that may present to a healthcare facility after a disaster, rapid triage is essential. Personnel assigned to triage responsibilities must evaluate each patient and quickly prioritize the various patients' management, using a scheme like that outlined in **Table 15-7**. If the disaster involves a suspected chemical, biological, radiological, or nuclear (CBRN) incident, triage takes place *outside the facility* and is conducted in conjunction with decontamination.

If the surge of patients needing critical care (triage category "red/immediate") exceeds the capacity of the facility, care expectation may need to be modified. Under extreme surge conditions, critical care support may be limited to provision of mechanical ventilation, IV fluid resuscitation, vasopressor administration, specific antidote or antimicrobial administration, and sedation and analgesia.

In addition, if the surge capacity is exhausted, some patients may need to be excluded from receiving even this basic level of critical care or even withdrawn from support in favor of those in greater need. The primary criterion used to make these judgments is the patient's risk of death, with the tool most commonly employed for this purpose being the Sequential Organ Failure Assessment

---

Criteria for Excluding Patients from Critical Care When Surge Capacity Is Exhausted (Any One)

- SOFA score indicating mortality risk of 80% or greater
- Multiple organ failure
- Severe acute disorder with low probability of survival (e.g., severe trauma or burns)
- Cardiac arrest (unwitnessed or witnessed but not responsive to electrical therapy)
- Advanced untreatable neuromuscular disease
- Metastatic malignant disease
- Advanced and irreversible neurologic event or condition
- End-stage organ failure
  - New York Heart Association Class III or IV heart failure
  - Stage IV COPD ($FEV_1 < 30\%$ predicted, dyspnea at rest)
- Severe baseline cognitive impairment
- Age of 85 years or older

(SOFA) score. A patient's SOFA score combines measures of the P/F ratio, platelet count, bilirubin level, creatinine level or urine output, severity of hypotension, and Glasgow Coma Scale score. A computed SOFA score indicating a mortality risk of 80% or greater is the primary basis for excluding patients under extreme surge conditions from receiving critical care. Other exclusion criteria that may be considered are summarized in the accompanying box.

For CBRN mass-casualty events, triage, decontamination, and treatment usually proceed in sequence through specific "zones," each requiring a different level of personal protective equipment (PPE) for healthcare personnel. Given its potentially high risk of hazardous contamination, the initial triage area is termed the "hot zone," in which National Institute for Occupational Safety and Health (NIOSH)–approved self-contained breathing apparatus (SCBA) should be employed. Decontamination occurs in the "warm zone," where NIOSH-approved hooded powered air-purifying respirators (PAPR) with FR57 filters are recommended. All RT departments should have protocols in place for providing respiratory support to patients in the warm zone. After decontamination, patients are received in the treatment area, where standard PPE precautions are normally satisfactory. In some cases, decontamination and initial medical treatment may occur simultaneously. For these reasons, you should be proficient in the use of all types and levels of personal protective equipment.

In terms of managing large outbreaks of respiratory infections, the following considerations apply:

1. All persons with signs or symptoms of a respiratory infection (e.g., cough, labored breathing) should be instructed to maintain good respiratory hygiene/cough etiquette:
   a. Cover the nose and mouth when coughing or sneezing.
   b. Use tissues to contain respiratory secretions.
   c. Dispose of tissues in the nearest waste receptacle after use.
   d. Wash hands after contact with respiratory secretions and contaminated objects and materials.
2. Healthcare facilities should ensure that tissues, hands-free receptacles, and hand hygiene facilities are provided to patients and visitors.
3. Healthcare facilities should offer surgical masks to persons who are coughing and encourage them to sit at least 3 feet away from others.
4. Healthcare workers should practice droplet precautions, in addition to standard precautions, when examining a patient with symptoms of a respiratory infection.
5. Once a likely infectious agent is suspected, appropriate infection control measures need to be activated:
   a. Placement of the patient in a negative-pressure isolation room (where available)
   b. Use of standard, contact, and droplet precautions
   c. Use of airborne precautions (including N95 respirators for all persons entering the room)
   d. Restriction of patient movement (and use of a surgical mask for transport)
   e. Avoiding droplet-producing procedures (e.g., nebulizers, chest physiotherapy, bronchoscopy)

COMMON ERRORS TO AVOID

You can improve your score by avoiding these mistakes:

- Avoid compressions in excess of ½ to 1 inch during infant CPR to help prevent injury to the patient.
- *Don't treat the monitor!* If the monitor shows asystole but the patient appears awake, alert, and in no apparent distress, do not begin CPR.
- Never treat a pneumothorax until the diagnosis has been confirmed with a chest x-ray.
- Never forget to include a manual resuscitator *and mask* for backup ventilation when you are transporting an intubated patient on a transport ventilator.
- Never use an adult manual resuscitator to ventilate a neonate. Use the appropriate age-specific equipment.
- Don't forget that during air transport, pressure changes may necessitate adjustments in F_{IO_2}, ventilator settings, and ET cuff pressures.

- Never wait for a physician to arrive to begin assessing a patient as part of a medical emergency team.
- During management of respiratory epidemics, avoid droplet-producing procedures (e.g., nebulizers on patients with suspected infections).

SURE BETS

In some situations, you can be sure of the right approach to a clinical problem or scenario:

- Always remember the CAB (circulation–airway–breathing) of CPR, and always call for a defibrillator.
- Always assess the patient before starting CPR; the individual may simply be sleeping!
- Always give a compression-to-breath ratio of 30:2 in single-rescuer CPR, regardless of the victim's age.
- Always give compressions at a depth of at least 2 inches for adults.
- If the chest doesn't rise with the first breath in CPR, don't panic—always reposition the head and try again!
- Always suspect a tension pneumothorax when a patient is rapidly deteriorating and exhibits a unilateral decrease in breath sounds and chest expansion, hyperresonance to percussion on the affected side, and shift of the trachea away from the affected side.
- When assisting a physician with a needle thoracostomy for the emergency treatment of a tension pneumothorax, always recommend that the needle be placed in the second intercostal space (above the third rib), in the midclavicular line.
- Always apply chest compressions to a neonate whose heart rate is less than 60/min.
- When assisting in the transport of a critically ill patient, always ensure that you have an adequate oxygen supply, as well as all required age-appropriate respiratory equipment.
- Always practice droplet precautions, in addition to standard precautions, when examining a patient with symptoms of a respiratory infection.

PRE-TEST ANSWERS AND EXPLANATIONS

Following are this chapter's pre-test answers and explanations. Be sure to review each answer's explanation thoroughly to help you understand why it is correct. If the explanation is still unclear to you, review the chapter content.

15-1. **Correct answer: D.** 1, 2, 3, and 4. Lidocaine, epinephrine, atropine, and naloxone (L-E-A-N) all can be administered via the ET tube during emergency life support.

15-2. **Correct answer: D.** Carotid artery. The carotid artery is the best site to check the pulse of an unresponsive adult.

15-3. **Correct answer: A.** Two normal breaths. According to the American Heart Association guidelines, after assessing for a pulse and giving about 2 minutes of compressions, if appropriate, you should give two normal breaths, each lasting about 1 second.

15-4. **Correct answer: A.** Apply back blows, followed by chest thrusts. After two failed attempts to ventilate an infant in respiratory arrest, airway obstruction is the most likely culprit. To overcome the obstruction, combine back blows with chest thrusts.

15-5. **Correct answer: D.** 30:2. In accordance with AHA guidelines, in one- and two-rescuer CPR for adults, the ratio for chest compressions to breaths is 30 compressions to every two breaths, with a reassessment after five cycles.

15-6. **Correct answer: A.** Increase the F_{IO_2}. According to Dalton's law, the ambient P_{O_2} drops as the altitude increases, due to the fall in P_B. For example, a patient breathing room air would need an F_{IO_2} of approximately 31% to maintain the same Pa_{O_2} at 10,000 feet altitude. For this reason, you often must increase a patient's F_{IO_2} during air transport.

15-7. **Correct answer: C.** At least 100/min with a depth of at least 2 inches. For adult resuscitation, use a chest compression rate of at least 100/min with a depth of at least 2 inches.

15-8. **Correct answer: A.** 120–200 joules. The initial energy level for defibrillation using the typical biphasic device is 120–200 joules or as per the manufacturer's recommendations (if an older monophasic defibrillator uses 360 joules). If the recommended device dosage is unknown, apply the maximum. Subsequent shocks are given after each 2-minute cycle with equivalent dosage (high doses can be considered if available).

15-9. **Correct answer: A.** End-tidal CO_2 monitor. A blood pressure monitor (or standard blood pressure cuff), an oxygen source and delivery device, and a cardiac monitor/defibrillator should accompany every critically ill patient on transport. A CO_2 monitor is preferred, but is not required.

15-10. **Correct answer: C.** Use available in-house anesthesia and/or transport ventilators. Should a patient surge exhaust the ICU ventilator inventory, the first step should be to obtain and put into use any available in-house anesthesia, transport, MRI, or NPPV ventilators that could meet individual patient needs. This can buy time until more capable equipment can be obtained.

POST-TEST

To confirm your mastery of this chapter's topical content, you should take the chapter post-test, available online at http://go.jblearning.com/respexamreview. A score of 80% or more indicates that you are adequately prepared for this section of the NBRC written exams. If you score less than 80%, you should continue to review the applicable chapter content. In addition, you may want to access and review the relevant Web links covering this chapter's content (courtesy of RTBoardReview.com), also online at the Jones & Bartlett Learning site.

Act as an Assistant to the Physician Performing Special Procedures

CHAPTER 16

Albert J. Heuer

In addition to directly providing respiratory care to patients, respiratory therapists (RTs) often assist physicians with a variety of special procedures. The NBRC expects exam candidates to be especially proficient in assisting physicians with intubation and bronchoscopy, and have a good understanding of how to support several other common bedside interventions. As with emergency care, only a few questions are included in this section of the written exams. However, because the scope of covered knowledge is broad and because not all RTs have experience with all these procedures, you need to devote a good portion of your time to reviewing this essential content.

OBJECTIVES

In preparing for the shared NBRC exam content, you should demonstrate the knowledge needed to act as an assistant to the physician performing the following special procedures:

1. Intubation
2. Bronchoscopy
3. Thoracentesis
4. Tracheostomy
5. Chest tube insertion
6. Cardioversion
7. Moderate (conscious) sedation
8. Insertion of venous or arterial catheters

In preparing for the RRT-specific NBRC exam content, you should demonstrate the knowledge needed to act as an assistant to the physician performing:

9. Insertion of venous or arterial catheters

WHAT TO EXPECT ON THIS CATEGORY OF THE NBRC EXAMS

CRT exam: 2 questions; 50% recall and 50% application
WRRT exam: 2 questions; 100% analysis
CSE exam: indeterminate number of questions; however, exam III-J knowledge is a prerequisite to success on CSE Information Gathering and Decision-Making sections.

PRE-TEST

Carefully respond to each of the following questions. After completing the pre-test, compare your answers with those provided at the end of each chapter. Then, thoroughly review the explanation for each answer to help you understand why it is correct.

16-1. You are assisting in performing a bronchoscopy on a spontaneously breathing patient who is alert, awake, and anxious. Which of the following medications should you recommend for the patient's anxiety prior to the procedure?
   A. Lidocaine HCl (Xylocaine)
   B. Vecuronium bromide (Norcuron)
   C. Epinephrine (Adrenaline)
   D. Midazolam HCl (Versed)

16-2. While the physician is performing a fiberoptic bronchoscopy on a spontaneously breathing patient, a patient's SpO_2 drops from 91% to 84%. Which of the following actions would be appropriate?
   1. Applying suction through the scope's open channel
   2. Delivering O_2 through the scope's open channel
   3. Increasing the cannula or mask O_2 flow
   A. 1 and 2
   B. 2 and 3
   C. 1 and 3
   D. 1, 2, and 3

16-3. Which initial energy level would you recommend to a physician preparing to perform cardioversion on a patient in atrial flutter?
   A. 50–100 joules
   B. 150–200 joules
   C. 200–250 joules
   D. 250–300 joules

16-4. In which position should you place a mobile, conscious patient to facilitate a thoracentesis procedure?
   A. Lying flat, supine, head on pillow
   B. Lying flat, prone, feet raised 12 inches
   C. Sitting up, leaning slightly forward, and supported in front
   D. Semi-Fowler's with knees raised

16-5. You are assisting a physician who is intubating an adult patient. Three attempts to pass the tube have been unsuccessful, but you can still ventilate the patient between attempts with a manual resuscitator and mask. Which of the following actions would you recommend at this time?
   A. Perform an emergency cricothyrotomy
   B. Place an intubating laryngeal mask airway
   C. Initiate transtracheal jet ventilation
   D. Paralyze the patient and continue manual ventilation

16-6. You are caring for a mechanically ventilated patient who has been orally intubated for 2 weeks and has failed multiple weaning attempts over the past 2 days. What should you recommend at this time?
   A. Immediate extubation
   B. Placing a smaller oral ET tube
   C. Performing a tracheotomy
   D. Placing a nasopharyngeal airway

16-7. While assisting a physician who is inserting a pulmonary artery catheter, you note a change-over on the monitor from pulsatile pressures of about 25/5 mm Hg to pulsatile pressures of 25/15 mm Hg. Which of the following has occurred?
   A. The catheter has advanced from the right atrium to the right ventricle
   B. The catheter has moved from the right ventricle to the pulmonary artery
   C. The catheter has advanced into the pulmonary wedge position
   D. The catheter has moved from the vena cava into the right atrium

16-8. The physician asks for your input regarding chest tube placement for a patient with a pneumothorax. In which anatomic location should you recommend the tube be inserted?
   A. The second intercostal space at the midaxillary line
   B. The second or third intercostal space at the anterior axillary line
   C. The fourth or fifth intercostal space at the midclavicular line
   D. The fourth or fifth intercostal space at the anterior axillary line

16-9. A physician is about to perform cardioversion on a patient with unstable atrial flutter who is receiving O_2 via a nonrebreather mask. After the initial shock has been delivered, the patient's SpO_2 drops to 85%, respirations become slow and shallow, and heart rate drops to 82/min with normal sinus rhythm. What should the next immediate action be?
   A. Open the airway and provide manual ventilation with 100% O_2
   B. Administer 2 mg of naloxone (Narcan)
   C. Quickly deliver another synchronized shock
   D. Intubate and place on mechanical ventilation

16-10. You are assisting a physician with an elective intubation. In addition to auscultation, which methods should you recommend to confirm proper tube placement?
1. Waveform capnometry
2. Chest x-ray
3. Co-oximetry
4. CO_2 colorimetry
A. 1, 2, and 4
B. 2, 3, and 4
C. 1 and 3 only
D. 1, 2, 3, and 4

WHAT YOU NEED TO KNOW: ESSENTIAL CONTENT

Common Elements of Each Procedure

The procedures outlined in this chapter all have common elements that you will need to follow before, during, and after implementation. Rather than repeat these steps in the description of each procedure in this chapter, they are noted as follows:

Before Each Procedure

- Verify, interpret, and evaluate the physician's order or protocol
- Review the medical record for contraindications, hazards, and informed consent, if appropriate
- Wash hands and apply standard transmission-based precautions
- Gather all equipment
- Identify the patient
- Take a preprocedure time-out, if appropriate (e.g., bronchoscopy)

During Each Procedure

- Assess the patient and ensure that monitoring equipment is functioning properly
- Respond to any adverse reactions

After Each Procedure

- Remove, properly dispose of, and process all equipment
- Reassess the patient's clinical status
- Respond to any adverse reactions
- Document the procedure, the patient's tolerance of it, and any other relevant details

Assisting with Endotracheal Intubation

Outside the operating room, endotracheal (ET) intubation generally is performed as a lifesaving measure by either properly trained RTs or physicians. Chapter 8 outlines the procedure as performed by RTs. Here the focus is on your role when assisting a physician with intubation.

Primary indications for ET intubation include respiratory or cardiac arrest, airway compromise or other need to protect the lower airway, and invasive ventilatory support. The only absolute contraindication against intubation is a documented do not resuscitate (DNR)/do not intubate (DNI) order. Relative contraindications include the following:

1. Severe airway trauma or obstruction that does not permit safe passage of an ET tube
2. Head/neck injuries requiring immobilization of the cervical spine
3. Mallampati Class 4 airway (Chapter 2) or other indicators of difficult intubation

Table 16-1 summarizes the RT's role in assisting with a standard bedside intubation.

Chapter 8 details the equipment and supplies needed for routine ET intubation. **Table 16-2** outlines the equipment that may be used to support difficult airway protocols. Although such protocols vary by institution, they are all meant to guide action whenever a trained professional

Table 16-1 Respiratory Therapist Role When Assisting with Intubation

Therapist's Function	Purpose
Before the Procedure	
Confirm that no contraindications or DNR or DNI orders exist	To ensure the patient's or family's advance directives are upheld
Gather and check operation of all equipment (Chapter 8)	To minimize delays and to ensure patient well-being
Confirm that suction (oral and tracheal) is available	To ensure secretion clearance and better visualization of the glottis
Inflate ET tube cuff, check it for leaks, then fully deflate	To confirm ET tube cuff integrity, prepare for insertion
Lubricate the ET tube and prepare stylet (Chapter 8)	To aid tube insertion
Inspect/assess airway (Chapter 2)	To determine if difficult intubation is likely or special procedures/equipment will be needed
Remove dentures or dental appliances (e.g., bridges) if present	To facilitate laryngoscopy, avoid aspiration of appliances
During the Procedure	
Place patient in the sniffing position, unless contraindicated (e.g., cervical spine injury)	To facilitate visualization of the glottis
Anesthetize the airway, if appropriate	To minimize the gag reflex and patient discomfort
Preoxygenate patient with F_{IO_2} of 100%	To prevent procedural hypoxemia
Monitor the patient's vital signs and clinical status, including response to moderate sedation, if given	To ensure patient safety and detect adverse response(s)
Assist with oral suctioning, laryngoscope insertion, application of cricoid pressure, and other measures	To help ensure a prompt and safe intubation
Inflate the cuff, manually secure ET tube, ventilate and oxygenate the patient via manual resuscitator/BVM	To provide/restore ventilation and oxygenation and protect the lower airway
Assess tube placement via auscultation and CO_2 detection (Chapter 8)	To ensure tube placement and patient safety
If tube placement is in question, deflate cuff, reposition tube, and reattempt manual ventilation	To ensure patient safety
If three unsuccessful intubation attempts, recommend proceeding with the difficult airway protocol (varies by institution)	To ensure patient safety
After the Procedure	
Note and mark the ET tube insertion depth and secure it in place	To ensure proper tube placement and patient safety
Ensure a chest x-ray is obtained and the tube repositioned as needed	To confirm tube placement and ensure patient safety
Reassess patient's clinical status	To ensure patient safety
Suction patient if necessary	To maintain airway patency
Ensure appropriate humidification, ventilation, and oxygenation	To ensure patient safety
Verify that intubation and any follow-up orders (e.g., ventilator settings) have been documented in the chart	To meet legal record keeping requirements

experiences difficulty with mask ventilation or cannot quickly insert an ET tube using conventional laryngoscopy in three or fewer attempts.

Positioning the Patient and Preparing the Airway

When assisting with an intubation, you may need to pull the patient to the head of the bed. Unless a cervical spine injury is suspected, you should then place the patient in the "sniffing" position

Table 16-2 Equipment Commonly Used to Support Difficult Airway Protocols

Equipment or Supplies	Use
A supraglottic airway (e.g., LMA, Combitube, or cuffed oropharyngeal airway [COPA])	Generally the first option in establishing an airway if ET intubation fails; can be inserted with the patient's head/neck in neutral position; *contraindicated if high risk of aspiration*
Intubating LMA (e.g., Fastrach)	An LMA with a large-diameter tube that allows passage of an ET tube; once the ET tube is placed, the LMA is carefully removed
Fiberoptic bronchoscope	Inserted into the ET tube and used to visually guide intubation through the vocal cords; can be performed through an intubating LMA
Standard "gum elastic Bougie" or ventilating tracheal tube introducer	Long, narrow flexible plastic rod with angled tip that is inserted via laryngoscopy into trachea, with its position confirmed visually or via a "clicking" feel as the tip moves over tracheal rings; the ET tube is inserted over the introducer, which is then withdrawn; ventilating introducers are hollow, allowing ventilation without an ET tube via either 15-mm or jet adapters
Videolaryngoscope (e.g., Glidescope, C-Mac, Airtraq)	Laryngoscope with either a small video screen or remote video monitor used during direct laryngoscopy to enhance visualization and tube insertion
Lighted stylet/lightwand	Stylet with a light bulb at tip; inserted into ET tube with bulb at the tube bevel and the tube angled to about 120° before insertion ("hockey stick" bend); *inserted blindly*; tracheal position confirmed by midline glow below thyroid cartilage (may require decreased room lighting)
Fiberoptic stylet (e.g., Levitan, Bonfil, Shikani, Foley)	Equivalent in concept and use to fiberoptic bronchoscope, but smaller, shorter, and typically portable (battery powered); can be used with direct laryngoscopy or inserted blindly
Percutaneous cricothyrotomy kit (e.g., Nu-Trake, QuickTrach, Pertrach)	Puncture of cricothyroid membrane and dilation of the opening until large enough to place an ET or trach tube; patients generally must be at least 5 years old
Jet ventilation setup (50-psi hose, adjustable regulator, jet control valve, 13- to 14-gauge angiocath or ventilating stylet)	Manually triggered ventilation with 100% O_2 provided via either ventilating stylet inserted orally or 13- to 14-gauge angiocath inserted percutaneously into trachea; surgical airway of choice for children younger than 12 years due to their small tracheal diameter and the resulting hazard of cricothyrotomy
Retrograde intubation kit (syringe with angiocath needle, guidewire, introducing catheter, forceps, ventilator adapters)	Puncture of cricothyroid membrane using Seldinger method with a guidewire inserted toward head; wire is pulled from mouth with forceps; introducing catheter is threaded over wire into trachea, then the wire is removed, the ET tube is inserted over the catheter, and the catheter removed; the catheter can provide ventilation without an ET tube

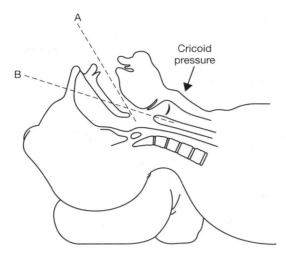

Figure 16-1 Sniffing Position for Intubation. The neck is slightly flexed, and the head is extended. Place a pillow or towels under the head and neck, but not under the shoulders. Compared to the angle with no flexion or extension (A), this position provides a straighter line of vision from the mouth to the vocal cords (B). External pressure applied to the cricoid cartilage (Sellick maneuver) can provide even better alignment of the anatomic structures for intubation.

Courtesy of: Strategic Learning Associates, LLC, Little Silver, New Jersey.

(**Figure 16-1**). Once the patient is positioned properly, you may need to clear secretions or vomitus from the pharynx using a Yankauer tip. In addition, spraying the pharynx with a local anesthetic such as 2% tetracaine (Cetacaine) aids intubation in conscious patients, by blocking the gag reflex. For elective intubation, you can nebulize a 4% lidocaine solution via SVN.

To minimize risks when intubating a patient with a suspected cervical spine injury, the RT should try to ensure the least cervical spine movement possible. This is usually accomplished via a procedure called manual in-line *stabilization* (MILS). As depicted in **Figure 16-2**, to implement MILS when assisting a physician with intubation, you normally stand at the side of the bed, cradle the patient's mastoids, and grasp the occiput with your fingers (a similar technique also can be performed from the head of the bed). Once stabilized, the head and neck should be maintained in a

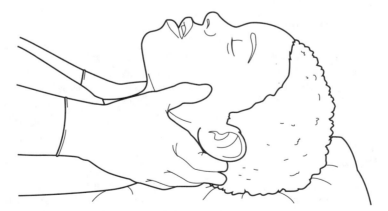

Figure 16-2 Manual In-Line Stabilization. Technique used from the side of the bed to immobilize the head and neck during intubation of a patient with suspected cervical spine injury (a similar method can be used when positioned at the head of the bed).

neutral position throughout the procedure. If a cervical collar is in use, you may need to remove the front portion to implement MILS. Upon successful intubation, you then promptly resecure the collar.

If difficulty persists with standard direct laryngoscopy using MILS, the physician may decide to use a fiberoptic stylet, videolaryngoscope, fiberoptic bronchoscope, or lightwand, all of which can facilitate intubation while still maintaining a neutral head/neck position.

Monitoring the Patient

The patient's vital signs and SpO_2 should be monitored before, during, and immediately following intubation. In addition, heart rate and rhythm should be assessed (via ECG) throughout the procedure. For sedated patients, special attention should be paid to adverse drug reactions, including nausea, hypotension, and respiratory depression. You should frequently communicate the patient's vital signs and clinical status to the physician who is performing the intubation, especially if any deterioration occurs.

Assisting with Tube Insertion

As an RT, you can take several measures to help the physician promptly insert the ET tube. First, you should ensure the proper size ET tube is selected (Chapter 8). For oral intubation, you also can suggest using a standard intubating stylet. Alternatively, if the patient is deemed to have a difficult airway or has suffered cervical trauma, you should suggest a fiberoptic stylet or lightwand, if available. *To prevent trauma during intubation, stylet tips must never extend beyond the ET tube tip.*

During laryngoscopy, the physician may ask you to perform the Sellick maneuver (Figure 16-1). It involves application of moderate downward pressure on the cricoid cartilage, which can help the physician better visualize the glottis.

In the rare circumstance when a physician chooses the nasal route, ensure that Magill forceps are available. The ET tube should also be well lubricated to aid passage through the nose. *Do not use a stylet for nasal intubation!* Once the tube tip is in the oropharynx, you may help open the mouth so the physician can insert the laryngoscope. The physician will then use the forceps to direct the tube between the cords.

In general, each intubation attempt should not exceed 30 seconds, and you should keep the physician informed of the elapsed time. Once the ET tube is positioned in the trachea, you should inflate the cuff with approximately 10 mL of air, temporarily secure the tube with your hand or tape, and then immediately begin manual ventilation with 100% O_2.

If the physician has initial difficulty with intubation, you should be prepared to perform the following tasks:

- Resume ventilating the patient with the manual resuscitator and 100% O_2
- Suction the oral pharynx or airway
- Have at least one smaller-size ET tube readily available

After three unsuccessful intubation attempts, you should suggest proceeding with an appropriate difficult airway option, usually defined by your institution's protocol. Typically, if the patient can be manually ventilated but not intubated using direct laryngoscopy (the "can ventilate, can't intubate" scenario), you should suggest insertion of either an LMA or an intubating LMA, followed by fiberoptic–assisted ET intubation. If it is clear that the patient cannot be manually ventilated or intubated (the "can't ventilate, can't intubate" scenario), and hypoxemia is present and worsening, you should suggest immediately proceeding with invasive airway access, via either cricothyrotomy or percutaneous jet ventilation.

Assessing Tube Placement

Immediately following intubation and manual ventilation, you should assess ET tube placement via auscultation and patient observation. Additional assurance of tube placement in the trachea is provided using either a disposable colorimetric CO_2 detector or capnograph. Two colorimetric detectors are available: one for patients weighing more than 15 kg (33 lb) and one for those weighing less than 15 kg. You place the detector *between* the patient's ET tube and manual resuscitator. If the ET tube is in the trachea, the device will change color from purple (less than 0.5% CO_2) to tan/

yellow (2% or more CO_2) with each exhalation. Note that during cardiac arrest—even with good tube placement and adequate ventilation—a patient's CO_2 levels may remain near zero due to poor pulmonary blood flow, yielding a false-negative result. Generally, expired CO_2 levels increase with the return of spontaneous circulation (ROSC). Unfortunately, CO_2 analysis cannot detect mainstem bronchial intubation.

After preliminary assessment of placement and while awaiting x-ray results, you should temporarily secure the tube and record its insertion depth to the incisors using its centimeter markings. After confirming proper placement via chest x-ray, you should consider securing the tube using a commercially available device designed for this purpose.

Rapid-Sequence Intubation

Certain situations may warrant a special procedure called *rapid-sequence intubation* (RSI). RSI is the preferred method for intubating conscious patients who have not fasted and are at high risk for aspiration. As depicted in **Figure 16-3**, to facilitate intubation, the patient is immediately rendered

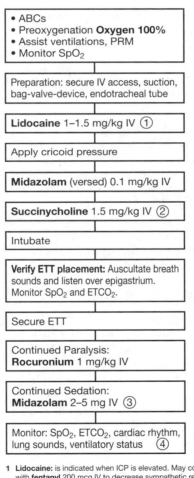

- ABCs
- Preoxygenation **Oxygen 100%**
- Assist ventilations, PRM
- Monitor SpO_2

Preparation: secure IV access, suction, bag-valve-device, endotracheal tube

Lidocaine 1–1.5 mg/kg IV ①

Apply cricoid pressure

Midazolam (versed) 0.1 mg/kg IV

Succinycholine 1.5 mg/kg IV ②

Intubate

Verify ETT placement: Auscultate breath sounds and listen over epigastrium. Monitor SpO_2 and $ETCO_2$.

Secure ETT

Continued Paralysis: **Rocuronium** 1 mg/kg IV

Continued Sedation: **Midazolam** 2–5 mg IV ③

Monitor: SpO_2, $ETCO_2$, cardiac rhythm, lung sounds, ventilatory status ④

1 **Lidocaine:** is indicated when ICP is elevated. May consider premedicating with **fentanyl** 200 mcg IV to decrease sympathetic response.
2 **Succinylcholine:** obtain history. **Do not give succinylcholine if family history of malignant hyperthermia is noted. Succinylcholine is contraindicated in penetrating eye injury, severe burns or crush injuries that are 2–5 days old, or in the presence of hyperkalemia or in patients with chronic muscular conditions (i.e., muscular dystrophy).** The onset of **succinylcholine** is 30–60 seconds; duration is 8–10 minutes.
3 **Consider pain control measures. Neither paralytics nor sedatives provide pain control.**
4 **Keep the patient warm.** Paralyzed patients lose much of their ability to generate body heat.

Figure 16-3 Rapid-Sequence Intubation Algorithm.

Source: Porter W. *Porter's pocket guide to emergency and critical care.* Sudbury, MA: Jones and Bartlett Publishers; 2007.

unconscious using a short-acting anesthetic, such as etomidate, and is paralyzed using either succinylcholine or a nondepolarizing neuromuscular blocker such as rocuronium. The goal is to rapidly intubate the patient without having to provide manual ventilation. Note that RSI generally is not to be used for "crash" airway management of unconscious patients. In these cases, you should proceed with or recommend immediate manual ventilation and intubation without anesthesia induction or paralysis.

Assisting with Bronchoscopy

Therapeutic indications for bronchoscopy include removal of secretions, mucus plugs, obstructing tissues, or foreign bodies. As previously discussed, fiberoptic bronchoscopy also can be used to facilitate intubation. Diagnostic use includes airway visualization to assess for injuries (e.g., smoke inhalation, tracheoesophageal [TE] fistula) or the anatomic causes of abnormalities such as hemoptysis or stridor. In addition, diagnostic bronchoscopy is used to obtain fluid or tissue specimens for microbiologic or cytologic assessment via bronchial washings, brush biopsy, bronchoalveolar lavage, and endobronchial and transbronchial biopsy. Contraindications to performing fiberoptic bronchoscopy are summarized in **Table 16-3**. It is imperative that all patients for whom a bronchoscopy is planned be prescreened for these contraindications.

Role of the Respiratory Therapist

Table 16-4 summarizes the potential functions you may fulfill when assisting physicians performing bronchoscopy, followed by some elaboration of the key supporting activities.

Patient Preparation

You should ensure that the patient takes nothing by mouth (NPO) at least 8 hours in advance of the procedure. Routine oral medications (especially asthma drugs) may be taken. Routine lab work, including measurement of clotting times, CBC, and platelet count, is essential to exclude a bleeding disorder—especially if a biopsy is to be performed. Preprocedural ABGs, pulse oximetry, and spirometry may be considered to assess for risk of hypoxemia. Also measure pulmonary reserves and document airway hyperactivity. Moderate sedation (described later in this chapter) is provided 15–30 minutes before the procedure. Atropine is given as a vagolytic agent at the same time unless contraindicated by the presence of dysrhythmias, glaucoma, or urinary retention.

Table 16-3 Contraindications to Bronchoscopy

Absolute	Relative
• Absence of patient consent (except in emergencies)	• Lack of patient cooperation
• Absence of an experienced clinician to perform the procedure	• Recent MI or unstable angina
	• Partial tracheal obstruction
• Lack of resources to manage complications such as cardiopulmonary arrest, pneumothorax, or bleeding	• Moderate-to-severe hypoxemia or hypercapnea
	• Uremia and pulmonary hypertension
• Inability to adequately oxygenate the patient during the procedure	• Lung abscess
	• Superior vena cava obstructions
• Coagulopathy or uncontrolled bleeding	• Debility, malnutrition
• Severe obstructive airway disease	• Respiratory failure requiring mechanical ventilation
• Severe refractory hypoxemia	
• Unstable hemodynamic status, including dysrhythmias	• Disorders requiring large or multiple transbronchial biopsies
	• Known or suspected pregnancy (if radiation exposure)

Table 16-4 Respiratory Therapist Role When Assisting with Bronchoscopy

Therapist's Function	Purpose
Before the Procedure	
Help identify the potential need for a bronchoscopy such as retained secretions or foreign body removal	To determine which patients may benefit from the procedure to maximize clinical outcomes
Prepare and ensure proper function of equipment, including bronchoscope, light source, video monitor and recorder, medications, and specimen traps	To minimize unnecessary delay and likelihood of patient harm from the procedure
Prepare the patient, providing patient education and premedication	To minimize untoward delays and maximize patient well-being
During the Procedure	
Monitor patient's vital signs and clinical status, including response to moderate sedation, if given	To ensure patient safety and detect adverse response(s)
Assist physician in obtaining specimens; help with medication preparation (e.g., epinephrine)	To minimize unnecessary delay and likelihood of patient harm from the procedure
After the Procedure	
Reassess patient's clinical status/confirm stability	To ensure patient safety
Ensure specimens are properly labeled and sent to lab	To help ensure accurate diagnosis and treatment
Verify that the procedure and any follow-up orders have been documented in the chart	To meet legal record keeping requirements
Clean and disinfect/sterilize equipment; ensure its proper storage (Chapter 5)	To minimize nosocomial infection risk and potential damage to equipment

Equipment

A fiberoptic bronchoscope (**Figure 16-4**) and light source are needed for this procedure. The bronchoscope is equipped with a thumb lever that allows angulation of the distal end of the instrument. A 2- to 2.6-mm channel runs the length of the scope. This channel is used to (1) inject medications or lavage fluid, (2) aspirate secretions, and (3) obtain fluid or tissue specimens. Tissue specimens are obtained using specialized instruments, such as bronchial brushes and forceps.

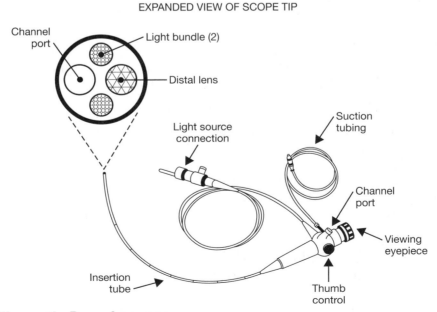

Figure 16-4 Fiberoptic Bronchoscope.

Courtesy of: Strategic Learning Associates, LLC, Little Silver, New Jersey.

Chapter 4 provides details on the care and maintenance of bronchoscopes, including disinfection methods.

Procedure

Bronchoscopy may be performed with the patient in a supine or sitting position. In mechanically ventilated patients, bronchoscopy is performed through the ET or tracheostomy tube using a special adaptor that allows insertion of the scope without disconnecting the ventilator. This approach provides for continued ventilation and maintenance of inspired oxygen and PEEP levels during the procedure.

If the patient is not intubated, the upper airway should be anesthetized in the same manner as recommended for ET intubation. In addition, the bronchoscope tip is lubricated with Xylocaine jelly before passage through the nose or mouth (the latter requires a bite block). Next, 2% lidocaine is injected through the bronchoscopic channel to anesthetize the vocal cords and lower airway. Once adequate anesthesia has been obtained, a detailed examination is performed. Subsequently, other procedures such as biopsies, washings, and brushings can be carried out.

Patient Monitoring, Sample Collection, and Postprocedural Care

The patient's vital signs and SpO_2 must be closely monitored before, during, and after bronchoscopy. As with ET intubation, the ECG also should be monitored, especially in high-risk patients. Patients with asthma or hyperreactive airways are prone to bronchospasm and laryngospasm, so they require especially careful preparation and monitoring. Because the PaO_2 typically falls during bronchoscopy, supplemental O_2 should always be given, either via a nasal cannula (for the oral route) or a mask modified to allow passage of the scope through the nose. If the patient is intubated, the FIO_2 should be increased by 10% or more during the procedure. If the SpO_2 drops below 90% during bronchoscopy, immediately increase the FIO_2, or else halt the procedure and give O_2 through the bronchoscope's open channel.

When assisting with sample collection, you typically place tissue specimens in a fixing agent such as formalin. Mucus and lavage fluids are aspirated into empty sterile collection bottles for additional analysis. After proper labeling, tissue specimens and fluids are then transported to the applicable lab according to your institution's infection control protocol.

After the procedure, the patient should remain NPO for at least 2 hours or until the gag reflex is restored. Due to medication effects, outpatients should not be allowed to drive until the following day. Transient fever and mild hemoptysis may be noted for the next 24 hours, with bleeding most common after biopsy procedures.

Assisting with Tracheotomy

Tracheotomy is indicated to bypass partial or complete upper airway obstruction, to facilitate prolonged mechanical ventilation, or to provide access for frequent secretion clearance. There are no absolute contraindications for this procedure. However, because it can cause bleeding, elective tracheotomy should not be performed until severe coagulopathies are corrected. In addition, critically ill patients should be stabilized as much as possible beforehand.

Equipment

Bedside tracheotomy may be performed via traditional surgical incision or by using the percutaneous dilator method. The necessary equipment is provided via a tracheotomy tray or kit. Equipment you will need to assist with this procedure includes the following:
- PPE (gown and gloves, mask, and cap)
- Extra trach tubes (one size smaller and one size larger)
- 10-mL syringe, for adding or removing air in cuffs
- Scissors for removing tape or another securing device
- Manual resuscitator (BVM)
- Flowmeter and O_2 source

Role of the Respiratory Therapist

In general, the physician performing the tracheotomy will be assisted by a second clinician with surgical training. However, as outlined in **Table 16-5**, the RT also can assume a vital role, especially when the procedure is performed to replace an ET tube. For details on ongoing care of a patient with an established tracheostomy, see Chapter 8.

Potential complications include adverse reactions to sedation, tissue trauma at the incision site, airway compromise or loss of a patent airway, excessive bleeding, hypoxemia, and aspiration. Should you note or suspect any of these problems during the procedure, be sure to immediately communicate your concern to the physician.

Assisting with Thoracentesis

Thoracentesis involves inserting a needle or catheter into the pleural space to remove accumulated fluid (pleural effusion). A lateral chest x-ray can help identify the presence and amount of pleural fluid. In addition, ultrasonography can help ascertain fluid location and guide needle insertion during the procedure.

Therapeutically, thoracentesis is performed whenever excessive pleural fluid interferes with lung expansion. Diagnostically, pleural fluid obtained via thoracentesis is analyzed to help determine the presence of underlying conditions such as infection, malignancy, CHF, or cirrhosis. There are no absolute contraindications for thoracentesis. Relative contraindications include the following:

- An uncooperative patient
- Severe uncorrected bleeding disorder
- Severe bullous lung disease

Table 16-5 Respiratory Therapist Role When Assisting with Tracheotomy

Therapist's Function	Purpose
Before the Procedure	
Ensure that a crash cart and intubation equipment are readily available	To enhance patient safety and address potentially life-threatening responses to this procedure
Ensure that trach tubes one size smaller and one size larger than that being inserted are available	To ensure availability of the equipment necessary to remove the old ET tube, monitor the patient, and oxygenate/ventilate the patient
Patient/caregiver education	To ensure that the patient and/or caregiver(s) understand the procedure
During the Procedure	
Ensure adequate airway at all times	To ensure patient safety
Monitor patient's vital signs and clinical status, including response to moderate sedation, if given	To ensure patient safety and detect complications and adverse response(s)
Per the physician's instructions, deflate the ET tube cuff, remove tape, and slowly withdraw tube (ET tube should be removed *just before* insertion of trach tube)	To ensure an adequate airway and transition to tracheostomy tube
Ensure proper placement of trach tube via breath sounds and CO_2 detection	To ensure patient ventilation and safety
Secure trach tube and continue ventilating through it	To ensure an adequate airway and prevent accidental decannulation
After the Procedure	
Make sure a chest x-ray is ordered	To ensure proper tube placement and lack of any major tissue trauma

Equipment

All needed equipment used for thoracentesis usually is included in a sterilized kit, with the key component being the fluid removal device, typically consisting of an 8 French angiocath over a long (7.5-inch) 18-gauge needle with a three-way stopcock and self-sealing valve, and a 50–60 mL collection syringe. For sample collection, either a large-volume sterile drainage bottle/bag (therapeutic thoracentesis) or sterile specimen or blood vials (diagnostic thoracentesis) are needed. Supplies include PPE, sterile surgical draping, chlorhexidine solution for skin asepsis, and adhesive dressings/gauze pads. Drugs include an anxiolytic and sedative (for premedication), as well as a local anesthetic (1% or 2% lidocaine) for pain. In addition to procedure-specific equipment, you will want to gather and set up the apparatus needed to monitor vital signs and SpO_2, and provide supplemental O_2. It is also wise to have ready the equipment needed to insert a chest tube.

Role of the Respiratory Therapist

As an RT, you may assist the physician before, during, and immediately following thoracentesis. Prior to the procedure, your assessment of the patient may actually indicate the presence of an effusion, by findings such as localized gravity-dependent dullness to percussion and decreased breath sounds. When such findings are combined with the presence of predisposing factors such as malignancy, CHF, or respiratory infection, you should inform the nurse and physician.

Once the decision is made to proceed with thoracentesis, you can assist by confirming the physician's order and signed informed consent, helping gather needed equipment, and positioning the patient. You may also want to recommend premedication with a cough suppressant because coughing during the procedure can cause lung or pleural trauma. Conscious patients who can be mobilized generally should be positioned sitting up and leaning slightly forward, supported in front by an adjustable bedside table. Immobile or unconscious patients should be placed with the affected side down on the very edge of the bed, slighted rotated from supine (toward the bed edge), with the ipsilateral arm behind the head and the mid-/posterior axillary line accessible for needle insertion (elevating the head of the bed to 30° may help).

During the procedure, you should ensure that the patient remains as still as possible and avoids coughing. In addition, you should perform the following tasks:

- Support the patient verbally and describe the steps of the procedure as needed
- Monitor vital signs and SpO_2
- Observe for signs of distress, such as dyspnea, pallor, and coughing
- Provide supplemental O_2 to maintain the SpO_2 at 90% or greater

After the procedure, you should ensure that all fluid specimens are properly labeled and processed, and that the results are documented in the patient record. You also should continuing monitoring and documenting the patient's vital signs and SpO_2 and observing for changes in cough, sputum production, breathing pattern, and breath sounds, as well as the occurrence of any chest pain or hemoptysis. If dyspnea, hypotension, chest pain, or hemoptysis develops, you should immediately contact the physician. Last, where indicated or required by institutional protocol, you should ensure that a postprocedural imaging study (x-ray or ultrasound) is performed to rule out a pneumothorax.

Assisting with Chest Tube Insertion (Tube Thoracostomy)

Chapter 15 describes needle thoracostomy for emergency treatment of tension pneumothorax. For ongoing management of pneumothorax or for removal of pleural fluid, blood, or pus (empyema), a chest tube needs to be inserted. As with thoracentesis, relative contraindications include an uncooperative patient and severe coagulopathy.

Equipment

When assisting the physician with chest tube insertion, one of your primary roles may be to gather equipment. As with thoracentesis, the procedure-specific equipment is provided in a sterile kit, and includes a selection of chest tubes (24–36 Fr), surgical instruments (scalpels, Mayo scissors, tissue forceps, Kelly clamps), a suture set, sterile draping, chlorhexidine sponges for skin asepsis, syringes, hypodermic needles, and local anesthetic. A chest tube drainage system needs to be obtained separately and set up in advance of the procedure.

After establishing access via surgical incision, the physician inserts the tube into the pleural space. For pneumothorax, the tube typically is placed into the fourth or fifth intercostal space at the anterior axillary line, while for fluid drainage more gravity-dependent locations are used. Once secured, the tube is connected to the drainage system, to which 15–20 cm H_2O of suction is applied. Chapter 4 provides details on the setup, maintenance, and troubleshooting of chest tube drainage systems.

Role of the Respiratory Therapist

In addition to helping gather needed equipment (including in some settings proper setup of the chest tube drainage system), your role as RT when assisting with chest tube insertion mainly involves monitoring the patient, as well as helping identify and respond to any adverse reactions, both during and after the procedure. Note that serious adverse responses such as excessive bleeding or hemodynamic instability may require special measures or even resuscitative efforts.

The chest tube is removed once the condition that led to its insertion has resolved. During the first day or two after its removal, you should help monitor the patient's status with particular emphasis on the recurrence of the pneumothorax or underlying pathology, as well as any other adverse response. *Crepitus at the site of insertion always suggests recurrence of air leakage into the pleural space.*

Assisting with Cardioversion

Synchronized cardioversion involves the application of an electrical shock to the heart that is synchronized to occur with the R wave of an ECG. Synchronization avoids shocking the heart during its relative refractory period, when a shock could cause ventricular fibrillation (V-fib). Cardioversion is indicated primarily to treat supraventricular tachycardia (SVT) due to atrial fibrillation and flutter. This procedure also is used to treat monomorphic ventricular tachycardia (V-tach) with pulses. It should not be used to treat multifocal atrial or junctional tachycardia. Cardioversion must never be used to treat *V-fib, pulseless V-tach, or polymorphic (irregular) V-tach, all of which require unsynchronized defibrillation* (Chapter 15). **Table 16-6** lists the dysrhythmias that can be treated with cardioversion, along with the recommended biphasic energy levels for adult patients. In general, immediate cardioversion is needed if the ventricular rate exceeds 150/min despite efforts to control it with appropriate drugs.

Role of the Respiratory Therapist

Your role in cardioversion primarily involves monitoring the patient and ensuring adequate oxygenation via the appropriate O_2 therapy modality. ACLS-trained RTs also may be responsible for applying the paddles and initiating the shock. Because in rare instances patients receiving cardioversion may worsen and require resuscitation, you also should ensure that an intubation tray, suction equipment, and a manual resuscitator and mask (BVM) are available. Key elements in the cardioversion procedure are outlined in the accompanying box.

Table 16-6 Energy Levels for Synchronized Cardioversion of Adults

Dysrhythmia	Adult Energy Levels (Joules, Biphasic)[a]
Atrial fibrillation	120–200 J; increase in stepwise fashion if not successful[b]
Atrial flutter	50–100 J; increase in stepwise fashion if not successful
Monomorphic V-tach with pulse (if stable)	100 J; increase in stepwise fashion if not successful
[a] For children, the recommended starting dose is 0.5–1 J/kg; if not successful, increment up to 2 J/kg.	
[b] Start with 200 J if using an older monophasic device.	

Key Elements of the Cardioversion Procedure

1. Ensure proper patient premedication with a sedative (e.g., Versed) and, optionally, analgesia (e.g., fentanyl).

2. Turn defibrillator/cardioverter on.

3. Set the device to *Sync* mode.

4. Using paddles or chest leads, confirm R-wave recognition indicating synchronization.

5. Select appropriate energy level for the identified dysrhythmia (Table 16-6).

6. Position conductor pads on patient (or apply gel to paddles).

7. Position paddles on patient.*

8. Announce to team members, "Charging defibrillator—stand clear!" and then press *Charge* button.

9. Forcefully voice the final clearing command or sequence (varies by institutional protocol).

10. Apply about 25 lbs of pressure on both paddles and press the *Shock* button(s).

11. Check the monitor; if tachycardia persists, increase the energy level in stepwise fashion.

12. Be sure to reactivate *Sync* mode after each attempt.

*There are two common paddle positions: anterolateral (A-L) and anteroposterior (A-P). In the A-L position, one paddle is positioned on the left midaxillary line at the fourth or fifth intercostal space, with the other placed over the second or third intercostal space just to the right of the sternum. In the A-P position, one paddle is placed next to the sternum (as with A-L placement), with the other placed on the patient's back between the tip of the left scapula and spine. A-P placement is more effective than A-L positioning for converting persistent atrial fibrillation and is less likely to damage an implanted pacemaker.

Assisting with Moderate (Conscious) Sedation

Without some form of sedation, many of the procedures described in this chapter would be uncomfortable or even intolerable for the patient. For this reason, selected medications may be administered to patients to induce a state of consciousness known as *moderate or conscious sedation*.

When moderately sedated, the patient should be arousable with an intact respiratory drive. Once the sedation is administered, your assessment of the patient should include vital signs, cardiopulmonary and airway status, SpO_2, and any adverse side effects from the procedure or the medications. Hence, it is imperative that you are familiar with the most common medications used to provide moderate sedation, their major side effects, and reversing agents (**Table 16-7**).

Note that the respiratory depressant effects of propofol are potentiated by the benzodiazepines. For this reason, propofol should be administered only where appropriate monitoring tools and ACLS trained staff are available, as well as the equipment and supplies needed to provide supplemental O_2, airway management, artificial ventilation, and cardiopulmonary resuscitation.

Table 16-7 Moderate Sedation Medications

Drug	Classification	Key Side Effects	Reversing Agent (Antagonist)
Midazolam (Versed)	Benzodiazepine	Hypotension, sleepiness and confusion, impaired reflexes	Flumazenil (Romazicon)
Lorazepam (Ativan)	Benzodiazepine	Same as midazolam	Flumazenil (Romazicon)
Diazepam (Valium)	Benzodiazepine	Same as midazolam	Flumazenil (Romazicon)
Propofol (Diprivan)	Sedative/hypnotic/ general anesthetic	Hypotension, transient apnea, respiratory depression	None (however, a single dose lasts only minutes)
Fentanyl (Fentanyl citrate)	Opioid narcotic analgesic	Respiratory depression, confusion, nausea	Naloxone (Narcan)
Meperidine (Demerol)	Opioid narcotic analgesic	Confusion, hypotension, histamine release, nausea	Naloxone (Narcan)

Assisting with Pulmonary Artery Catheterization (RRT-Specific Content)

As with most special procedures, your presence at the bedside may involve helping monitor and support patients undergoing pulmonary artery (PA) catheterization, as well as assisting with selected components of the procedure itself. Preparation, monitoring, and patient support during PA catheterization are essentially the same as for the other special procedures discussed in this chapter—namely, equipment setup, patient premedication, vital signs/SpO_2 monitoring, and observing for adverse effects, among other tasks.

The basic equipment needed for PA catheterization is similar to that described in Chapter 11 for arterial line insertion—that is, a pressurized IV system, a continuous flush device, and a pressure transducer connected to a bedside monitor displaying the pressure waveform. Because in some institutions (including the NBRC hospital) RTs may be responsible for setup and maintenance of this equipment, you should familiarize yourself with the proper use of indwelling catheters (Chapter 2), their troubleshooting (Chapter 4), and the CDC's central-line infection control bundle (Chapter 5).

The procedure for inserting a PA catheter also is similar to that described in Chapter 11 for an arterial line, but is performed only by a physician or an approved physician assistant/nurse practitioner. Key differences include the catheter itself, the transducer and monitor setup, and the insertion location and method.

A typical adult PA catheter (also known as a "Swan-Ganz" catheter) is 7 to 8 Fr in diameter and approximately 110 cm long. A small balloon located near the tip is used to "float" the catheter into the pulmonary artery and obtain wedge pressure measurements. All PA catheters have at least three lumens/ports: a CVP/atrial (proximal) lumen, a distal PA lumen, and a lumen for balloon inflation/deflation. Externally, the proximal lumen port is used to aspirate blood, measure CVP, and inject drugs. The distal PA lumen port is used to measure PA and PA wedge pressures, obtain mixed venous blood samples, and inject drugs. Other connectors may include those for a cardiac output (CO) computer, pacemaker wires, and an $S\overline{v}O_2$ sensor. PA catheters used for CO measurement have a thermistor near the tip that measures temperature changes when a bolus of cool fluid is injected into the proximal port (CO is inversely proportional to the area under the computer's time–temperature curve).

In terms of monitoring equipment, because PA catheters are placed in the low-pressure venous side of the circulation, the selected transducer must provide accurate measurement in the appropriate pressure range (typically 0 to 50 mm Hg) and the monitor pressure display range must be toggled to low. As with A-lines, before insertion the transducers should be calibrated and zero balanced, all lines and catheter ports flushed, and the balloon inflated to test for leaks (*using only the 1.0- or 1.5-mL syringe that comes with the catheter*).

PA catheters typically are introduced percutaneously via either the right internal jugular vein (the shortest and straightest path to the heart) or the left subclavian vein. When assisting with subclavian vein access, you should be on guard for pneumothorax as a potential complication. Once the catheter is in the superior vena cava, the physician may have you inflate the balloon (again only to the recommended 1.0- to 1.5-mL volume) to aid flotation of the catheter through the heart and into the pulmonary artery. As indicated in **Figure 16-5**, as the catheter advances, distinct pressure changes occur that indicate its position. Initially CVP/RA (right atrial) pressure is displayed. As the catheter passes through the tricuspid valve into the right ventricle (RV), systolic pressures rise sharply due to RV contraction. As the catheter passes through the pulmonary valve into the pulmonary artery (PA), the diastolic pressures rise and a dicrotic notch appears, corresponding to pulmonary valve closure. As the catheter eventually "wedges" into a small pulmonary artery, pulse pressure variations disappear. This pressure is the pulmonary arterial wedge pressure (PAWP, also known as pulmonary "capillary" wedge pressure). PAWP reflects left atrial pressure, which in turn normally equals left ventricular end-diastolic pressure or LV preload. Once the catheter is confirmed to be in the wedge position, it is slightly withdrawn until PA pressures are restored and then the balloon is fully deflated. Thereafter, measurement of PAWP is obtained by inflating the balloon, which has the same effect as actual wedging.

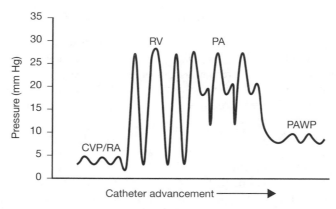

Figure 16-5 Display of Typical Vascular Pressures During Insertion of a Pulmonary Artery Catheter. CVP/RA = central venous pressure/right atrium; RV = right ventricle; PA = pulmonary artery; PAWP = pulmonary artery wedge pressure.

Courtesy of: Strategic Learning Associates, LLC, Little Silver, New Jersey.

Should the physician ask you to obtain either PA or PAWP pressure measurements, follow the guidance provided in Chapter 2. To ensure accurate measurements, you may first need to confirm the responsiveness of the system via a flush test. As indicated in **Figure 16-6**, when flushed, a responsive system rapidly produces a rectangular waveform. Once flushing ends, the pressure immediately drops straight down to below the baseline. A brief and oscillation then occurs, followed by quick return of a well-defined PA pressure waveform. If you do not observe the brief oscillations when flushing ends, or if the pressure waveform returns only slowly and lacks a well-defined dicrotic notch, the system is dampened and will not provide accurate measurements until corrected. See Chapter 4 for information on how to correct a dampened pressure waveform.

The physician also may ask you to obtain a mixed venous blood sample from a PA catheter, either to assess tissue oxygenation or to calculate cardiac output using the Fick method. Good guidance on properly obtaining such samples is provided in Chapter 11.

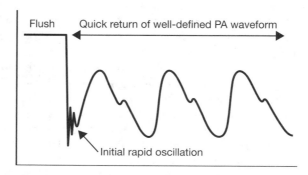

Figure 16-6 Flush Test for a PA Catheter System.

Courtesy of: Strategic Learning Associates, LLC, Little Silver, New Jersey.

COMMON ERRORS TO AVOID

You can improve your score by avoiding these mistakes:

- To minimize tissue trauma, never permit the tip of a stylet to extend beyond the end of an ET tube.
- Never attempt to assist with ET intubation unless a complete intubation tray, suction source and catheter(s), and a CO_2 detection device (capnograph or colorimeter) are available.
- Never use only one means to verify ET tube placement. Instead, confirm tube position with at least two methods, including auscultation, capnography or CO_2 colorimetry, and chest x-ray.
- Never place a patient with suspected cervical spine injury in a "sniffing position" for intubation.
- Never use a stylet for nasal intubation.
- Never recommend proceeding with bronchoscopy in the presence of absolute contraindications such as refractory hypoxemia, hemodynamic instability, or inability to oxygenate the patient.
- When assisting with a tracheostomy, do not remove the ET tube until just before insertion of the trach tube.
- Never recommend synchronized cardioversion to treat ventricular fibrillation, pulseless V-tach, or polymorphic (irregular) V-tach; instead, recommend defibrillation.
- Never inflate a PA catheter balloon to more than the recommended maximum volume (usually 1.0 to 1.5 mL).

SURE BETS

In some situations, you can be sure of the right approach to a clinical problem or scenario:

- Always forcefully voice a final *clear* command and verify that no one is in contact with the patient before delivering a shock.
- When positioning patients for a thoracentesis procedure, always ensure they are adequately supported in front to help prevent them from falling.
- Always confirm proper functioning of the ET tube cuff, pilot balloon, and valve prior to intubation.
- After each attempt at cardioversion, always activate Sync mode again, in addition to selecting the appropriate energy level.
- Always recommend a tracheostomy when prolonged invasive mechanical ventilation is expected.
- Always recommend immediate chest tube insertion or needle decompression for a patient with a confirmed tension pneumothorax.
- Always suggest diagnostic ultrasound to help identify the best site for thoracentesis and guide needle insertion.
- Always closely monitor a patient's vital signs, SpO_2, and other relevant clinical indicators when assisting with special procedures; if necessary, administer supplemental O_2 to prevent or reverse hypoxemia.
- Always ensure that a manual resuscitator with mask and O_2 source are nearby in case a patient experiences major adverse effects during special procedures.
- Always make sure the patient is NPO for at least 8 hours prior to bronchoscopy (to minimize aspiration risk).
- Always recommend an x-ray after to confirm tube position after ET intubation and chest tube insertion.
- Always consider that air leakage might be occurring at a chest tube insertion site when you detect localized crepitus.
- Always be prepared to support ventilation and manage the airway of patients undergoing moderate sedation, especially when propofol (Diprivan) is used.
- When assisting with insertion of a PA catheter via subclavian vein access, always be on guard for pneumothorax as a potential complication.

PRE-TEST ANSWERS AND EXPLANATIONS

Following are this chapter's pre-test answers and explanations. Be sure to review each answer's explanation thoroughly to help you understand why it is correct. If the explanation is still unclear to you, review the chapter content or the references and/or refer to this chapter's supplemental resources on the CD.

16-1. **Correct answer: D.** Midazolam HCl (Versed). Benzodiazepines such as midazolam (Versed) are usually recommended to provide moderate sedation and reduce anxiety during special procedures. The effects of benzodiazepines can be reversed with flumazenil.

16-2. **Correct answer: B.** 2 and 3. During bronchoscopy, the patient's oxygenation should be monitored continuously via pulse oximetry. If desaturation occurs, the F_{IO_2} should be increased, or the procedure can be halted and O_2 can be given through the bronchoscope's open channel.

16-3. **Correct answer: A.** 50–100 joules. In accordance with AHA guidelines, the initial biphasic energy level for performing cardioversion for a patient in atrial flutter should be 50 to 100 joules. Energy levels can be increased in a stepwise fashion if initial attempts are unsuccessful.

16-4. **Correct answer: C.** Sitting up, leaning slightly forward, and supported in front. When positioning conscious mobile patients for thoracentesis, you should sit them up, have them lean slightly forward, and provide an adjustable bedside table on which they can place their arms for support.

16-5. **Correct answer: B.** Place an intubating laryngeal mask airway. After three unsuccessful intubation attempts, if the patient still can be manually ventilated (the "can ventilate, can't intubate" scenario), suggest inserting an LMA or an intubating LMA, followed by fiberoptic intubation. If the patient cannot be manually ventilated or intubated (the "can't ventilate, can't intubate" scenario) and is hypoxemic, you should suggest immediately invasive airway access, via either cricothyrotomy or percutaneous jet ventilation.

16-6. **Correct answer: C.** Performing a tracheotomy. A tracheotomy should be performed because recent weaning has been unsuccessful and it is likely that the patient will require mechanical ventilation for some time. In addition, tracheostomy tubes may actually facilitate weaning because they are much shorter and, therefore, impose less flow resistance.

16-7. **Correct answer: B.** The catheter has moved from the right ventricle to the pulmonary artery. During insertion of a PA catheter, pressure waveforms indicate its position. In the RA, pressures are less than 8–10 mm Hg and barely pulsatile. As the catheter moves into the RV, a change-over to pulsatile pressures of about 25/5 mm Hg occurs. As the catheter passes into the PA, pulsatile pressures continue, but with a raised diastolic baseline (about 25/12 mm Hg).

16-8. **Correct answer: D.** The fourth or fifth intercostal space at the anterior axillary line. In most instances, a chest tube is generally inserted through the fourth or fifth intercostal space at the anterior axillary line.

16-9. **Correct answer: A.** Open the airway and provide manual ventilation with 100% O_2. The next immediate action should be to open the patient's airway and provide oxygenation and ventilation, as the patient's airway might have become obstructed due to oversedation or the patient's own anatomy.

16-10. **Correct answer: A.** 1, 2, and 4. Besides auscultation of the chest and stomach, other methods such as observation of chest movement, tube length (centimeters to the teeth), capnometry, colorimetry, and fiberoptic laryngoscopy can be used to confirm ET tube position at bedside. In addition, a chest x-ray should be ordered to determine proper tube placement.

POST-TEST

To confirm your mastery of this chapter's topical content, you should take the chapter post-test, available online at http://go.jblearning.com/respexamreview. A score of 80% or more indicates that you are adequately prepared for this section of the NBRC written exams. If you score less than 80%, you should continue to review the applicable chapter content. In addition, you may want to access and review the relevant Web links covering this chapter's content (courtesy of RTBoardReview. com), also online at the Jones & Bartlett Learning site.

Initiate and Conduct Pulmonary Rehabilitation and Home Care

CHAPTER 17

Albert J. Heuer
(prior version co-authored with Kenneth A. Wyka)

Pulmonary rehabilitation and home care are important respiratory care specialties. However, because RTs' practice in these areas is limited, the NBRC includes only a small number of related test items. Fortunately, most questions on these topics can be answered based on your general clinical knowledge. Here we focus on specific skills unique to these settings that will help you do well on this section of the exams.

OBJECTIVES

In preparing for the shared NBRC exam content, you should demonstrate the knowledge needed to:

1. Explain planned therapy and goals of pulmonary rehabilitation and home care to patients and their family
2. Educate the patient and family in health management and smoking cessation (covered in Chapter 7)
3. Monitor and maintain home respiratory equipment
4. Modify respiratory care procedures for home use
5. Instruct the patient and family to ensure safety and infection control
6. Interact with a case manager
7. Properly document pulmonary rehabilitation and home care plan and outcomes

In preparing for the RRT-specific NBRC exam content, you should demonstrate the knowledge needed to:

1. Initiate and adjust apnea monitors
2. Initiate treatment for sleep disorders (e.g., CPAP)

WHAT TO EXPECT ON THIS CATEGORY OF THE NBRC EXAMS

CRT exam: 2 questions; 50% recall and 50% application
WRRT exam: 2 questions; 50% application and 50% analysis
CSE exam: indeterminate number of questions; however, exam II-K knowledge is included as a potential case management area (under COPD)

PRE-TEST

Carefully respond to each of the following questions. After completing the pre-test, compare your answers with those provided at the end of this chapter. Then thoroughly review each answer's explanation to help understand why it is correct.

17-1. The essential goals of pulmonary rehabilitation include all of the following *except*:
   A. Improving exercise tolerance
   B. Reducing perceived dyspnea
   C. Improving health-related quality of life
   D. Reversing lung damage

17-2. To return rehabilitation patients to the highest level of functional capacity, all of the following approaches should be used *except*:
   A. Multidisciplinary team approach
   B. Disease management education
   C. Mandated participation
   D. Smoking cessation and counseling

17-3. To maximize cardiovascular benefit, patients in pulmonary rehabilitation programs should exercise to what range of their predicted maximum heart rate?
   A. 45–60%
   B. 60–75%
   C. 75–90%
   D. 90–100%

17-4. What is the primary purpose of patient record keeping in pulmonary rehabilitation?
   A. Document patient involvement and outcomes
   B. Justify third-party insurance reimbursement
   C. Provide data to support rehabilitation research
   D. Avoid potential legal issues or questions

17-5. When educating patients on proper use of home O_2 therapy, they should be instructed to do which of the following if they suspect an equipment problem?
   A. Call the home care company and 911
   B. Switch to a backup supply of O_2 at an equivalent liter flow
   C. Disassemble, clean, and reassemble the equipment
   D. Refer to the equipment user's manual

17-6. Emergency situations that home mechanical ventilation caregivers must be trained to recognize and manage include all of the following *except:*
   A. Ventilator or power failure
   B. Tension pneumothorax
   C. Artificial airway obstruction
   D. Ventilator circuit problems

17-7. You have been asked to organize a patient/family education program as part of a discharge plan for a patient requiring home mechanical ventilation. Which of the following methods would be best for training the family in operation of the chosen ventilator?
   A. Put the patient on the selected device while still hospitalized
   B. Set up and review the ventilator after the patient gets home
   C. Show the family the ventilator in a full-day session
   D. Give the family the operating manual for the ventilator

17-8. Which of the following are acceptable indicators of hypoxemia for purposes of justifying home oxygen therapy reimbursement under Medicare?
   1. A resting Pao_2 of 55 torr (room air)
   2. A nocturnal fall in Spo_2 from 95% to 91%
   3. A resting arterial Spo_2 of 84% (room air)
   A. 1 and 2 only
   B. 2 and 3 only
   C. 1 and 3 only
   D. 1, 2, and 3

17-9. When training the parents of an infant prescribed home apnea monitoring how to respond to a low respiratory rate alarm, you would instruct them to *first*:
   A. Check the electrode connections
   B. Quickly assess the infant
   C. Silence the applicable alarm
   D. Stimulate the infant to breathe

17-10. All of the following solutions are acceptable for the disinfection of reusable semicritical home care equipment, *except*:
   A. 1:50 dilution of sodium hypochlorite
   B. 70% isopropyl alcohol
   C. 1:1 solution of vinegar and water
   D. 3% hydrogen peroxide

WHAT YOU NEED TO KNOW: ESSENTIAL CONTENT

Pulmonary Rehabilitation

Aspects of pulmonary rehabilitation that all NBRC candidates should familiarize themselves with include the purpose and goals, patient selection, program components, and proper documentation. Essential goals for pulmonary rehabilitation include the following:

- Improving a patient's exercise tolerance
- Reducing the level of perceived dyspnea
- Improving health-related quality of life
- Reducing ED visits and hospital admissions
- Reducing the costs of health care

Consistent with these goals, the primary benefits to rehabilitation participants are improvements in activities of daily living (ADLs) capabilities, sense of well-being, and decreased frequency of exacerbations and hospitalizations. *However, rehabilitation cannot reverse the disease process.* To meet these goals and return patients to the highest possible level of functional capacity, rehabilitation programs use the following strategies:

- Multidisciplinary approach, including respiratory care
- Active medical direction and involvement
- Disease management education and related counseling (Chapter 7)
- Multiple forms of treatment, including breathing retraining and physical conditioning
- Flexible specific approaches to meet individual needs

Patient Selection

Candidates for pulmonary rehabilitation include patients with COPD, asthma, bronchiectasis, cystic fibrosis, and interstitial lung diseases (e.g., pulmonary fibrosis, sarcoidosis), and those for whom lung volume reduction surgery is planned or has been completed. Applicable candidates are then screened to verify that they are motivated to participate and (for smokers) willing to pursue a smoking cessation plan. Where appropriate, patients also should be evaluated for practical issues such as health insurance coverage and transportation needs. Additional medical screening generally includes the following elements:

- Complete history and physical exam (see Chapter 2)
- Laboratory testing (CBC, chem profile, alpha$_1$ antitrypsin titer)
- Electrocardiogram
- Arterial blood gas analysis
- Pulmonary function testing
- Chest x-ray

Either a simple exercise tolerance test (e.g., 6MWD) or comprehensive exercise capacity evaluation (Chapter 2) also may be prescribed. These tests are used to (1) screen patients for enrollment, (2) establish their baseline performance, (3) monitor their progress, and (4) measure improvement after program completion. Comprehensive exercise test results justifying inclusion in a rehabilitation program include a Vo_{2max} that is less than 75% of the predicted value and a breathing reserve of less than 30% (Chapter 2).

Program Components

Smoking Cessation

Most rehabilitation programs require that smokers enroll in a smoking cessation program, a key element in health management education. Details on health management and smoking cessation education are provided in Chapter 7.

Table 17-1 Educational Topics for a Pulmonary Rehabilitation Program

Topic	Key Points
Program purpose and the need for patient's active participation	Return the patient to the highest functional level and tolerance for ADLs
Cardiopulmonary anatomy, physiology, and pathophysiology	Structure of the heart and lungs, including how they normally work and how disease alters their structure and function
Breathing techniques and retraining	Diaphragmatic and pursed-lip breathing techniques, inspiratory resistance breathing
Stress management and relaxation	Ways to cope with stress, proper breathing techniques, and avoidance of panic breathing
Physical reconditioning	Exercises to promote agility, strength, and endurance
Cardiopulmonary pharmacology	Major cardiopulmonary medications, including their effects on the body and proper usage
Home care equipment	Use and maintenance of O_2 and other respiratory care devices, including small-volume nebulizers
Bronchopulmonary hygiene	Postural drainage positions and other airway clearance methods
Nutrition and diet	Key elements of good nutrition, weight control, and proper hydration
Specific strategies for maximizing ADLs	Vocational counseling focusing on activities that promote a more active and productive lifestyle

Patient Education

Table 17-1 lists educational topics commonly covered in pulmonary rehabilitation programs.

In terms of instructional strategies for rehabilitation participants, we recommend the following steps:

- Create a comfortable learning environment that encourages family/caregiver participation.
- Break sessions down into brief segments.
- Use lay terminology and supplemental materials appropriate to each patient's educational level.
- Appeal to varied learning styles (e.g., visual, hands-on).
- Reinforce key concepts and follow-up.

Breathing Techniques and Exercises

Breathing techniques used in rehabilitation include pursed-lip breathing, diaphragmatic or abdominal breathing, coughing techniques (e.g., "huff coughing"), and use of inspiratory resistance and positive expiratory pressure (PEP) devices. **Table 17-2** briefly describes the rationale for these various techniques and exercises as used in pulmonary rehabilitation. More details are provided in Chapters 4, 9, and 10.

Physical Reconditioning Exercises

Exercises used in rehabilitation fall into three general categories. First are warm-up/stretch activities, conducted before other exercises. These exercises are low stress and intended to increase blood flow and range of motion and help prevent injury. Second are aerobic activities such as walking and cycling. These exercises build up a participant's endurance to perform sustained ADLs. Last are strength-building exercises such as weight lifting and calisthenics, which can increase a participant's ability to hold a given position and lift objects.

Table 17-2 Types of Breathing Techniques and Exercises for Pulmonary Rehabilitation

Breathing Exercise	Rationale
Pursed-lip breathing	Encourages a slower exhalation while creating back-pressure to prevent airway collapse and air trapping
Diaphragmatic breathing	Promotes diaphragmatic excursion and effective ventilation, which reduces accessory muscle use
Inspiratory resistance breathing	Strengthens ventilatory muscles by creating inspiratory flow or threshold resistance
Positive expiratory pressure (PEP) therapy	Improves distribution of ventilation and assists in airway clearance
Glossopharyngeal or "frog" breathing	Uses glossopharyngeal muscles to capture and swallow air, which improves spontaneous ventilation (patients with neuromuscular diseases)

Monitoring

During exercise, patients' Spo_2, heart rate, respiratory rate, and blood pressure should be monitored, as well as their overall appearance. To achieve optimal cardiovascular benefit, patients' targeted heart rate should be at least 60% but no higher than 75% of their predicted maximum (= 220 – age). Patients who demonstrated desaturation during activity should receive supplemental O_2 as needed. You should terminate exercise and closely monitor any patient who experiences angina, muscle cramps, severe fatigue, or excessive dyspnea, or who exhibits other signs of distress. If the situation appears life-threatening, you should activate the available emergency response system.

Documenting Patient Progress

Rehabilitation records must be maintained by both program personnel and patients. These records should document all patient activities performed, responses to these activities (favorable or adverse), and overall progress. Progress during each session normally is documented in either the *Progress Notes* section of the patient record or (where applicable) a separate *Rehabilitation* section. You should also encourage patients to maintain a log of all exercise activities performed at home, both for progress monitoring and as a motivational tool. All documentation should be kept on file for both medical and legal reasons and for insurance reimbursement purposes.

Respiratory Home Care

Prescribed respiratory home care services include, but are not limited to, the following:

- Patient assessment and monitoring
- Diagnostic and therapeutic services
- Patient/caregiver disease management education
- Patient follow-up

All services require a physician's order and must be provided under appropriate law, regulation, and medical direction. Following is a review of the most common respiratory care modalities delivered in the home, as likely to be assessed on NBRC exams.

Home O_2 Therapy

O_2 therapy is the respiratory modality most commonly used at home. General concepts related to O_2 therapy are discussed in Chapter 4 and elsewhere throughout this text. Here we focus on the unique aspects of home O_2 therapy.

In addition to receiving a physician's order for this therapy, the patient must qualify for Medicare or private insurance reimbursement by meeting diagnostic and blood O_2 level criteria. For patients with COPD or other chronic pulmonary disorders to qualify, their Spo_2 must be 88% or less, or their

Pa_{O_2} must be 55 torr or less on room air. Patients with COPD having a secondary diagnosis such as cor pulmonale can qualify with slightly higher blood O_2 content—that is, with an Sp_{O_2} of 89% or less, or a Pa_{O_2} between 56 and 59 torr.

Home O_2 therapy also differs in the types of storage and delivery systems used. These systems include O_2 concentrators, liquid O_2 (LOX) systems, and high-pressure gaseous O_2 cylinders. What follows are the essential details on the use of these systems.

Concentrators

An O_2 concentrator is an electrically powered device that physically separates the O_2 in room air from nitrogen. Most concentrators use sodium-aluminum silicate pellets to absorb nitrogen, CO_2, and water vapor and produce about 90–95% O_2 at flows up to 10 L/min. O_2 concentrators are the most cost-efficient supply method for patients in alternative settings who need continuous low-flow O_2.

Portable O_2 concentrators (POCs) are smaller versions of standard home concentrators, powered by household AC, 12-volt DC (available in cars, RVs, and motor homes), or batteries. The typical battery life is 1 to 4 hours, with some models having optional battery packs that can extend use time to more than 6 hours.

Most POCs deliver O_2 only in the pulse-dose mode, which is sufficient for those with low O_2 needs (30% or less O_2). Some units also can operate in a continuous-flow mode. In general, only continuous-flow units can provide more than 30% O_2, which is needed to provide adequate F_{IO_2} at altitude (e.g., in airliner cabins). Unfortunately, most continuous-flow POCs are bigger and heavier than pulse-dose-only units and, therefore, are less portable.

The basic procedure for start-up and operation of a POC is as follows:

1. Before operation, make sure the air intake filter is clean and positioned correctly.
2. Locate and position the unit in a well-ventilated area with the air inlets and outlets unobstructed; in a small room or car, keep a window open.
3. Connect the unit to the best available power source (AC first, auto-DC next, battery last).
4. Connect a nasal cannula to the O_2 outlet.
5. Turn the unit on, confirm power-up status, and set the prescribed flow.
6. Confirm that the unit is sensing inhalation (flashing indicator with pulse sound).
7. After start-up, the unit should reach its maximum O_2 output in approximately 1–2 minutes.

POCs generally are simple to operate and reliable. To deal with common problems or service needs, most have indicators to warn the user of malfunction. **Table 17-3** summarizes common POC indicator warnings and the appropriate action the patient should be trained to take when the indicator is activated.

Table 17-3 Portable O₂ Concentrator Warning Indicators and Corrective Actions

Indicator	Recommended Action
Low battery	• Immediately switch to AC/DC power; then charge the battery • If no alternative power is available, switch to a backup O_2 supply
Cannula disconnect	• Check the cannula connections • Ensure that you are breathing through your nose • If alarm persists, switch to backup O_2 supply and contact the home care provider
Capacity exceeded	• Reduce activity and/or switch to backup O_2 supply • If alarm persists, contact the home care provider
General malfunction	• Turn the unit off and switch to backup O_2 supply • Contact the home care provider
Service needed or low O_2 concentration	• Contact the home care provider to arrange for inspection and service and provision of a replacement unit

Liquid O₂ Systems

Home LOX is stored below its critical temperature (at approximately –300°F) in small thermos-like cylinders that require no refrigeration. Because 1 L of liquid O_2 vaporizes into 860 L of gaseous O_2, LOX systems are the most efficient way to store supplemental O_2. When flow is turned on, the LOX passes through a vaporizing coil, where exposure to ambient temperatures warms and converts it to a gas. It then leaves the system through a flow-metering control valve.

Depending on the model, a stationary home storage cylinder (the "base" unit) holds between 45 and 100 pounds of LOX. To calculate duration of flow, you first must convert the LOX weight in pounds to the equivalent volume of gaseous O_2 in liters. At normal operating pressures, 1 pound of LOX equals approximately 344 liters of gaseous O_2. To determine how long the contents will last in minutes, you simply divide the total available gaseous O_2, by the prescribed flow (L/min).

Portable LOX systems are used in conjunction with a stationary base unit, from which they are filled as needed. When full, the typical portable unit holds about 1 liter of LOX and weighs less than 6 pounds. When used with a demand-flow delivery device (described subsequently), these systems can provide 8 or more hours of supplemental O_2.

Basic steps for filling/using a portable LOX system include the following:

1. To prevent icing, remove any moisture from the connectors on both the reservoir and the portable unit with a clean, lint-free cloth.
2. Check the reservoir to make sure it has enough LOX and is at the proper operating pressure (usually 24 psig).
3. Turn the portable unit's flow control knob off.
4. Align the portable unit and reservoir connectors; press down firmly until they engage.
5. Open the reservoir vent valve (a hissing noise confirms filling).
6. Close the reservoir vent valve after observing the portable unit venting excess O_2.
7. Press the release on the reservoir and gently pull the portable unit off the reservoir.
8. Inspect the portable unit indicator to verify that it is full.
9. Connect the delivery cannula to the portable unit, making sure it is firmly attached to the pulse-dose controller.
10. Adjust the flow control to the prescribed setting and confirm that the unit is pulsing during breathing (see the subsequent section on low-flow O_2 therapy devices).

To prevent frostbite burns, users must avoid touching LOX or parts of the unit in contact with LOX. It is normal for both stationary reservoirs and portable units to intermittently vent to the atmosphere. Because a continuously venting LOX unit suggests a malfunction and represents a potential fire hazard, nearby flame sources should immediately be shut off and the area should be cleared of all but essential personnel and well ventilated.

Compressed (Gaseous) O₂ Cylinders

Compressed O_2 cylinders are used in home care primarily as a backup to liquid or concentrator systems or for ambulation. In addition to the cylinder gas, a pressure-reducing valve with a metering device is needed to deliver O_2 at the prescribed flow. Because flows typically range from 0.25 to 4.0 L/min for home care patients, a low-flow metering device should be used.

For ambulation, small portable gaseous cylinders are used, typically the M-6/B, M-9/C, D, or E sizes. **Table 17-4** provides the factors needed to compute the duration of flow for these cylinders, as well as example calculations for various flows.

Oxygen Appliances

The appliances of choice for home O_2 therapy are either simple low-flow devices or O_2-conserving systems. High-flow systems are used as well, but primarily for bland aerosol delivery (covered later in this chapter).

The low-flow device most commonly used at home is the nasal cannula. In the home settings, cannulas generally are used at flows of 4 L/min or less for adults and 2 L/min or less for infants. At these flows, supplemental humidification generally is not needed. However, consideration should

Table 17-4 Duration of Flow in Hours for Portable O$_2$ Cylinders

| L/min | Cylinder (Factor) | | | |
	M-6/B (0.07)	M-9/C (0.11)	D (0.16)	E (0.28)
9.5	5.5	8.2	13.8	22.7
0.75	3.6	5.5	9.2	15.2
1.0	2.7	4.1	6.9	11.4
1.5	1.8	2.8	4.6	7.6
2.0	1.4	2.1	3.5	5.7
2.5	1.1	0.7	2.8	4.5
3.0	0.9	1.4	2.3	3.8
3.5	0.8	1.2	2.0	3.2
4.0	0.7	1.0	1.7	2.8

be given to providing supplemental humidification for any patient who complains of nasal dryness or experiences related symptoms.

Transtracheal catheters have been used as alternative low-flow devices. However, because their insertion requires a surgical incision and is associated with potential problems of pain, bleeding, infection, and obstruction, these devices are rarely used today.

To increase duration of flow, most portable O$_2$ systems incorporate a gas-conserving system. As described in Chapter 4, O$_2$-conserving systems use a trigger mechanism to sense the user's breathing effort and deliver O$_2$ only during inspiration (demand flow or "pulse dose" delivery). Due to performance variations, the appropriate flow setting for patients using these systems must be determined empirically—that is, by adjusting the flow until the desired SpO$_2$ is achieved. For troubleshooting these systems, you should teach patients who suspect a problem to always switch to a backup supply of continuous O$_2$ via nasal cannula at the equivalent liter flow (usually 2 to 3 times the demand-flow setting or 2–4 L/min) until technical support can be provided.

Recommending, Troubleshooting, and Modifying Home O$_2$ Systems

Certain clinical scenarios regarding home O$_2$ systems commonly appear on the NBRC exams. For example, you should remember that a patient with restricted activity may need only an O$_2$ concentrator and a gaseous cylinder for backup. In contrast, you should always recommend a portable source (portable concentrator, LOX unit, or small cylinder) for ambulatory patients. For patients who are especially active or mobile or who need an extended duration of flow, be sure the system incorporates an O$_2$-conserving device.

Another important aspect of home O$_2$ therapy involves equipment troubleshooting and modification. As such, related questions may appear in some form on the NBRC exams. **Table 17-5** summarizes the problems most commonly encountered with home O$_2$ systems, as well as the recommended corrective actions or modifications.

Bland Aerosol Therapy

Bland aerosols may be used at home to help overcome a humidity deficit (e.g., in patients with trach tubes) and as an adjunct to bronchial hygiene therapy (e.g., in patients with cystic fibrosis). The aerosol can be produced by either an ultrasonic or a jet nebulizer. If using a jet nebulizer, a 50-psi air compressor is required. Supplemental O$_2$ may be "bled in" from a concentrator or LOX system. The major problem with bland aerosol therapy is infection control. To reduce the incidence of infection, equipment and patient delivery systems must be cleaned and disinfected, as described later in this chapter.

Aerosol Drug Administration

As in the acute care setting, the inhalation route can be used for drug administration to home care patients. Most inhaled drugs are available in either metered-dose inhaler (MDI) or dry-powder

Table 17-5 Basic Home Oxygen Troubleshooting

O₂ System	Problem	Corrective Action/Modification
Concentrator	Machine will not turn on	Check electric power source, including plug and circuit breaker; if power source is working, place patient on backup gaseous system, as appropriate, and replace the concentrator.
	Analyzed F$_{IO_2}$ is less than 85–90% of manufacturer's specifications	The sodium-aluminum pellets are likely exhausted. Place patient on backup gaseous system, as appropriate, and replace the concentrator.
	Patient on nasal cannula at 4 L/min or more complains of nasal dryness	Add a bubble humidifier.
Liquid	Liquid tank is making a slight intermittent hissing sound	Occasional hissing of stationary liquid O₂ systems occurs with normal venting; it is likely that no action is needed, except to keep the tank upright.
	Tank is making a very loud and constant hissing sound, and/or a steady stream of "mist" can be seen coming from the tank	Loud and constant hissing suggests a problem with liquid systems; place the patient on backup O₂ and replace the liquid system.
Gaseous tanks	O₂ regulator is turned on, but no oxygen is coming out	Either the tank has not been turned on or it is empty; if no flow occurs with both tank and regulator turned on, replace tank.

inhaler (DPI) form, with their effectiveness depending on proper training and use (see Chapter 4). If these delivery methods are not feasible, the caregiver can use a small-volume nebulizer (SVN) powered by a low-output compressor or a portable electronic (ultrasonic or mesh) nebulizer.

Airway Care and Secretion Clearance

Home care patients with trach tubes require both daily stoma care and suctioning. Tracheostomy care can be provided by most trained caregivers, but tube changes should be performed only by the patient's nurse, physician, or respiratory therapist.

As described in Chapters 4 and 9, tracheobronchial suctioning in the home is accomplished using a portable suction pump with collection bottle and suction tubing. Although some patients can be taught to suction themselves, it is more common to train caregivers on the proper procedure. Daily maintenance and cleaning are a must. To help control home care supply costs, it is not uncommon for a single suction catheter to be used for 24 hours and then discarded. To prevent bacterial growth, catheters are placed in a disinfecting solution such as hydrogen peroxide between suctioning attempts.

Airway clearance methods available for patients with intact upper airways are described in Chapter 9. These methods, which can be taught to home care patients and their caregivers, include directed coughing and postural drainage, percussion, and vibration. Additional assistance with secretion clearance, which is particularly useful for patients living alone, can be provided by mechanical adjuncts such as PEP devices and high-frequency chest compression vest systems. Cough-assist devices such as the mechanical in-exsufflator also are gaining more widespread acceptance at home.

Home Mechanical Ventilation

While most patients are weaned from mechanical ventilation in an acute care facility, some ventilator-dependent patients are discharged to the home setting. Many of these patients have underlying cardiopulmonary conditions such as COPD, whereas others may have been diagnosed with neuromuscular diseases or have spinal cord trauma. General goals of home mechanical ventilation include the following:

- Sustaining and extending life
- Enhancing the quality of life
- Reducing morbidity

- Improving or sustaining physical and psychological function
- Enhancing growth and development (children)
- Providing cost-effective care

Patients being considered for discharge to the home with mechanical ventilation should meet the following criteria:

- Be clinically stable for at least 2 weeks and have desire to go home
- Have been on continuous ventilation for at least 30 days without successful weaning
- Not require cardiac monitoring
- Have a tracheostomy tube in place (unless using noninvasive ventilation)
- Demonstrate control of any seizure activity with the prescribed medication protocol
- Not require acute care IV medications such as vasodilators
- Have family members and/or caregivers willing and capable of taking on support responsibilities
- Have undergone a complete medical and financial assessment by the case manager (post acute care)

In general, patients should *not* be considered for home ventilatory support in these circumstances:

- They require more than 40% O_2 or more than 10 cm H_2O PEEP.
- They need continuous invasive monitoring.
- The home physical environment is deemed unsafe by the discharge team.

Home environmental issues include fire, health, or safety hazards; unsanitary conditions; and inadequate heating, ventilation, or electrical service.

The choice of home care ventilator is based on a patient's clinical needs and available resources. Ideally, the patient should be placed on the ventilator that will be used in the home setting *before discharge*. When this approach is used, caregivers can be oriented to the equipment and their role and responsibilities in a well-controlled setting with full medical support.

The key patient factor in ventilator selection is type of airway—that is, tracheostomy versus intact upper airway. For patients with trach tubes requiring continuous support, the common choice is an electrically powered, volume-controlled ventilator using a single-limb circuit (Chapter 4). For patients with an intact upper airway who need only intermittent support (e.g., at night), electrically powered, pressure-limited ventilators with noninvasive interfaces are popular choices. Patients who would otherwise be suited for noninvasive positive-pressure ventilation but object to mask or mouthpiece interfaces may be considered candidates for negative-pressure ventilation, usually via a chest cuirass or "pneumosuit."

Positive-pressure ventilators for home use should meet the following criteria:

- Be electrically powered with battery backup
- Be simple, easy to use, and reliable
- Provide a wide range of respiratory rates
- Ensure accurate delivery of tidal volumes or pressures
- Provide a range of modes, including A/C, SIMV, CPAP, and pressure support
- Provide adequate humidification of inspired gas
- Have variable flow capability
- Allow variable F_{IO_2} (generally via an adjustable bleed-in port)
- Incorporate appropriate alarms:
  - Mandatory disconnect (low-pressure or low-volume) and high-pressure alarms
  - Remote and secondary (e.g., apnea monitor) disconnect alarms for high-risk patients

Additional considerations for home care ventilation include the following:

- A backup ventilator should be available for patients who:
  - Cannot maintain spontaneous ventilation for 4 or more hours
  - Live in an area where a replacement ventilator cannot be provided within 2 hours
- Caring for a ventilator-dependent patient in the home is labor intensive and involves extensive education and training for the family and/or caregivers, including infection control measures.

Table 17-6 Home Ventilator Troubleshooting

Problem	Corrective Action/Modification
Machine will not turn on	Ensure adequate ventilation and use a backup ventilator or manual resuscitator, as appropriate; then check power source such as the plug and circuit breaker
Ventilator-dependent patient lives in a rural area that experiences frequent power outages	Ensure that the utility company is notified in writing of the patient's needs and that a backup power source such as a generator is in place
Caregiver cannot immediately fix an alarm and patient appears to be in distress	Remove patient from ventilator, use a backup ventilator or manual resuscitator as needed, and call 911; consider CPR as appropriate
Patient with a trach tube is in distress; when off the ventilator, extreme resistance is felt when bagging	Call 911, attempt to pass a suction catheter, and then resume manual ventilation with 100% F_{IO_2}; consider CPR as appropriate
Patient on pressure-limited ventilation objects to the discomfort of the nasal mask	Consider a different interface such as nasal pillows or recommend a negative-pressure ventilator

- Additional equipment needed may include a hospital bed, supplemental O_2, suction equipment, and related supplies.
- Arrangements must be in place for emergency situations, including power outages.

The NBRC also expects candidates be able to address problems frequently encountered during home mechanical ventilation. While aspects of ventilator troubleshooting are covered elsewhere in this text, the most common problems and corrective actions or modifications specific to home mechanical ventilation are summarized in **Table 17-6**.

Treatment of Sleep Disorders (RRT-Specific Content)

Sleep-disordered breathing and apnea–hypopnea syndrome are disorders characterized by either complete cessation of breathing (apnea) or notable reduction in ventilation (hypopnea) during sleep. Physiologic causes include airway obstruction due to relaxation or collapse of the upper airway tissues (*obstructive sleep apnea* [OSA]) or a failure of the respiratory center to activate the respiratory muscles (*central sleep apnea* [CSA]). Diagnosis of sleep disorders, including use of the *polysomnography exam* (PSG), is discussed in Chapter 1. **Table 17-7** summarizes the treatments typically used for obstructive and central sleep apnea.

Nasal CPAP remains the most widely used home treatment for OSA. With proper use, CPAP can dramatically lessen or resolve the many problems associated with OSA, such as morning headaches, daytime hypersomnolence, and cognitive impairment. As a result, this therapy can enhance the patient's quality of life and may also lessen the incidence of more severe complications, such as systemic and pulmonary hypertension.

A CPAP setup consists of a flow generator, breathing circuit, patient interface (e.g., nasal mask, nasal pillows), and headgear. Most systems provide pressures up to 20–30 cm H_2O. As discussed in Chapter 2, the optimal CPAP pressure normally is determined by a titration study, which is conducted either in conjunction with a polysomnography exam in the sleep lab or at home using an auto-titrating device. Many units now have a ramp feature that gradually raises the pressure to the prescribed level over a time interval. This gradual elevation helps some patients fall asleep and may increase therapy compliance.

Whereas CPAP applies a constant airway pressure, the separate inspiratory and expiratory pressure settings available with BiPAP systems make this mode a better choice to support patients needing enhanced ventilation, such as those with central sleep apnea or neuromuscular weakness. BiPAP also may increase patient comfort and, therefore, improve patient compliance, even among those patients with OSA.

Table 17-7 Treatments for Obstructive and Central Sleep Apnea

Obstructive Sleep Apnea	Central Sleep Apnea
Weight reduction—essential for obese patients with OSA.	Treatment of the underlying disorder (e.g., if CSA is due to heart failure, optimize cardiac function).
Alteration in sleep posture—sleeping in either a side-lying or head-up position can benefit some patients.	CPAP—may improve cardiac function with congestive heart failure.
Avoidance of alcohol and drugs that depress the central nervous system (e.g., sedatives/hypnotics).	Bilevel positive airway pressure (BiPAP)—provides supplemental ventilation.
CPAP—the most frequently prescribed and generally most effective treatment for OSA. The optimal CPAP level is determined by titration study. BiPAP, may also be used as a more tolerable alternative to CPAP.	Adaptive servo ventilation (ASV)—the treatment for most forms of CSA. It should be prescribed based on PSG exam.
Oral appliances—optimally position the tongue and mandible to help overcome or prevent obstruction.	Acetazolamide (Diamox)—increases excretion of HCO_3, which causes metabolic acidosis and presumably shifts the apneic threshold of Pa_{CO_2} to a lower level.
Uvulopalatopharyngoplasty—surgical removal of portions of the soft palate, uvula, and tonsils, and suturing together of the palatoglossal and palatopharyngeal arches.	Theophylline—a phosphodiesterase inhibitor with respiratory stimulant properties.
Tracheostomy—a last resort for patients with severe OSA whose problem persists despite common medical or surgical interventions.	Sedative-hypnotics (e.g., temazepam))—minimize ventilation instability caused by sleep–wake transitions.

Although CPAP is an effective treatment for sleep apnea, several problems associated with this therapy may warrant corrective action or modification, as summarized in **Table 17-8**.

Home Apnea Monitoring (RRT-Specific Content)

Recently born infants who exhibit frequent apnea spells generally are not discharged until these episodes resolve or become less severe. However, in certain instances, home apnea monitoring remains a viable option for warning caregivers of babies at risk for certain life-threatening events. Apnea monitoring equipment and procedures and the basic interpretation of signaled events are covered in Chapter 2. The only key difference in equipment is that any apnea monitor used in the home should include an event recorder.

The primary indication for home apnea monitoring is for infants at risk for recurrent apnea, bradycardia, and hypoxemia after hospital discharge. Home apnea monitoring also may be indicated for infants who are technology dependent (e.g., on a ventilator or CPAP), have unstable airways,

Table 17-8 Problems Associated with CPAP and Corrective Action

Problem	Corrective Action/Modification
Patient complains of overall discomfort from excessive flow and noise	Use ramp feature to gradually build up to prescribed pressure
Skin irritation or facial soreness from excessive mask pressure	Use different interface (e.g., nasal pillows), add supplemental cushioning, adjust straps on headgear, ensure proper cleaning of interface
Conjunctivitis	Adjust interface to eliminate leak around eyes
Epistaxis (nosebleed) or excessive nasal dryness	Add a circuit humidifier or ensure adequate household humidity
Inability to maintain adequate pressure	Check circuit connections for leak, use a chin strap to prevent pressure loss through mouth, use a different interface

have conditions affecting control of breathing, or have chronic lung disease. *Home apnea monitoring should not be prescribed or recommended to prevent sudden infant death syndrome (SIDS).*

A good home apnea monitoring program involves a multidisciplinary team effort that integrates medical, educational, technical, psychosocial, and community support. Ideally, a conference should be held with the family/caregivers *before discharge*. The conference should be primarily educational in focus, and attend to the following topics:

- Emergency procedures, including CPR
- Monitor setup and alarm settings (Chapter 2)
- Alarm evaluation and response
- Monitor troubleshooting
- Psychosocial support, including social services involvement, as appropriate
- Phone, text, and email contact information for technical help/support

You will need to confirm caregiver competencies through return demonstration and reinforcement, as necessary. Specific procedural elements that need to be emphasized include the following:

- Displaying CPR guidelines near the crib and emergency numbers near the phone
- Ensuring there is an extra set of electrodes and lead wires
- Avoiding use of extension cords
- Positioning the baby on the side or back on a firm, flat surface
- Keeping the baby on the monitor at all times, except as instructed (e.g., during bathing)
- Responding to all monitor alarms by:
  - Initially assessing the infant
  - Determining if the alarm is real or false
  - Responding to a real alarm as appropriate (initially by stimulating the baby)
  - Responding to a false alarm by troubleshooting electrodes and connections
- Avoiding alteration of alarm settings to reduce noise
- Keeping the monitor plugged in and using the battery only when needed (e.g., for travel or power outage)
- Repositioning the electrode belt daily or electrodes every 2 days
- Avoiding application of oils or lotions near the electrodes
- Basic equipment troubleshooting

The local electric company and EMS system should be notified of the infant's location and needs so that care can be provided in the event of a power outage or medical emergency. Follow-up visits may be more frequent at first, but are needed less often as the family becomes skilled with the equipment and alarm responses. Apnea monitoring usually is discontinued when the infant reaches 43 weeks' postmenstrual age or after the recorder data logs indicate cessation of major events, whichever comes last. To provide absolute confirmation of event cessation, some physicians will prescribe an overnight pneumocardiogram, which in addition to chest motion and heart rate measures SpO_2 and air flow.

Education of the Home Care Patient and Caregivers

Regardless of the type of equipment used, patients and caregivers must be educated on its safe application and maintenance, basic troubleshooting, and cleaning and disinfection. In providing this instruction, you should follow the general principles previously noted in the rehabilitation section of this chapter. In addition, the following education strategies apply in the home setting:

- Limit educational sessions to about 1 hour or less to avoid "information overload."
- Thoroughly demonstrate all procedure(s) and require caregivers to provide return demonstrations.
- Ensure that emergency procedures, such as power outages and patient emergencies, are adequately covered.
- Leave printed "EZ read" information about the procedures.
- Document all aspects of the education session(s) in the patient record.
- Follow up to reinforce material, as appropriate.

Table 17-9 Instructional Topics for Respiratory Home Care

Modality	Topic
General	• Safe and effective use of equipment • Basic equipment troubleshooting • Equipment cleaning and disinfection • Emergency procedures • How to order supplies • How to contact the home care company
Home O$_2$ therapy	• Posting "No Smoking" signs and ensuring that smoking is not allowed where O$_2$ is in use • Avoiding trip/fall hazards from O$_2$ extension tubing • Proper placement, securing, and use of O$_2$ cylinders
Home mechanical ventilation	• Basic response to ventilator alarms • Basic airway clearance and maintenance (if a trach tube is in place) • Use of the backup ventilator and manual resuscitator
CPAP and BiPAP	• Adjusting the mask, nasal pillows, or other interface to ensure a proper fit and comfort • Application of measures to improve patient tolerance, such as humidification and a "ramp" feature
Apnea monitors	• Responding to monitor alarms and troubleshooting • CPR and emergency procedures

Beyond general educational strategies and principles, a variety of topics should be covered as part of family and caregivers education. **Table 17-9** lists general home educational topics for which you should provide patient and caregiver instruction, as well as examples of specific topics for the most commonly used home care modalities, including oxygen, mechanical ventilation, CPAP therapy, and apnea monitoring.

Infection Control

Chapter 5 covers the main infection control principles in respiratory therapy. As previously indicated, you as the RT are responsible for educating home care patients and caregivers regarding infection control procedures, including hand hygiene, proper cleaning, disinfection, and safe storage of equipment. Specific guidance you should provide includes the following:

- Friends or relatives with respiratory infections should be discouraged from visiting the patient.
- Proper hand washing or disinfecting lotions should be applied to the hands before and after handling patients or respiratory equipment.
- Standard and transmission-based precautions should be used as appropriate.
- Wherever practical, disposable equipment (e.g., ventilator circuits) should be used.
- Sterile water should be used in nebulizers, although distilled water is acceptable for humidifiers.
- Noncritical reusable items such as blood pressure cuffs can be cleaned with a household detergent.
- Prior to disinfection, all reusable, semicritical objects such as nebulizers, breathing circuits, and tracheal airway components should be scrubbed in detergent to remove organic material, then thoroughly washed, rinsed, and allowed to air-dry in a clean location.
- After cleaning, reusable semicritical objects should be disinfected by immersion in either an EPA-registered intermediate-level disinfectant or one of the following solutions:

- 70% isopropyl alcohol for 5 minutes
- 3% hydrogen peroxide for 30 minutes
- 1:50 dilution of household bleach (sodium hypochlorite) for 5 minutes

- Household products other than bleach (e.g., ammonia, vinegar, Borax, liquid detergents) should *not* be used to disinfect reusable semicritical equipment because they are ineffective against *Staphylococcus aureus*.
- Cleaned and disinfected equipment should be stored in a separate "clean" area.
- In the unlikely scenario where a reusable critical home care item requires sterilization, use a chemical sterilant or boiling (according to the manufacturer's recommendations).

Interacting with the Case Manager

The intricacies of today's healthcare system and the complexities of care often dictate involvement of a case manager. The case manager typically is a clinician working for a healthcare facility or insurance provider who assumes overall responsibility for coordinating care plan implementation and avoiding unnecessary delays or costs in care delivery. To effectively interact with the case manager and other members of the home care team, you need to possess the following attributes:

- Professional appearance and attitude
- Effective communication skills
- Outstanding clinical and technical skills
- A strong team orientation
- Effective organizational skills
- Good follow-up abilities

In addition, several themes are often the focus of communication between you and the case manager. You can optimize your interaction with the case manager and contribute to achieving optimal healthcare outcomes by being as knowledgeable as possible about the patient's condition and by anticipating specific topics that may arise during such encounters. These topics may include:

- The patient's diagnoses and chief complaints
- Initial therapy and clinical indications
- Modifications to therapy (and their justifications)
- Ethical, cultural, and religious considerations
- Resuscitation status (full code versus DNR)
- The patient's readiness for discharge
- Barriers to discharge, such as caregiver limitations
- The most suitable setting to which the patient should be discharged
- Equipment and modalities the patient will need
- Needed patient and caregiver training/education
- Reimbursement for equipment and procedures

Documentation

The documentation for home care is similar to that in other settings, in that a physician's order must be verified and a care plan should be devised (in conjunction with the interdisciplinary team and the case manager, as appropriate). In addition, all therapy, diagnostic procedures, and educational efforts should be recorded, along with the patient's response to them. Typically this information is noted in the *Progress Notes* or similar section of the patient record. Proper judgment should be used in communicating the appropriate clinical information to other members of the care team.

In addition to these general considerations, following are some unique aspects of documentation that apply to home care patients:

- *Home care treatment plan*: documents the assessment; outlines goals and therapies.
- *Ongoing assessment form*: provides a regular summary regarding the patient's clinical status, equipment functioning, and cleanliness, as well as modifications to goals and therapies.

- *Certificate of medical necessity*: documents that a patient has met the qualifications for reimbursement of home oxygen, as previously mentioned in this chapter.
- *Patient education checklists*: may be used both as teaching tools and to document that the patient was properly instructed on all respiratory modalities.
- *Assignment of benefits form*: patient authorization for the home care company to receive direct reimbursement from third-party insurance payers for equipment and services.
- *Discharge summary*: describes the course of therapy and final status of goal attainment.

COMMON ERRORS TO AVOID

You can improve your score by avoiding these mistakes:

- Never use using technical or "textbook" terms when communicating with rehabilitation or home care patients.
- Never suggest to patients that rehabilitation will reverse the underlying disease process.
- Never have rehabilitation patients limit their participation to simply attending classes; they need to actively engage in their own self-care, such as through regular exercise, good nutrition, and record maintenance.
- Never limit a mobile home care patient to a stationary O_2 delivery system; instead, always recommend an appropriate portable source.
- Unless detailed in the doctor's order (e.g., higher flow for exercise), never instruct a home care patient to change the prescribed O_2 liter flow.
- Do not recommend home apnea monitoring to prevent SIDS.
- Do not recommend household products other than bleach for disinfecting reusable home care equipment.

SURE BETS

In some situations, you can be sure of the right approach to a clinical problem or scenario:

- Always recommend an exercise tolerance test to help screen patients for pulmonary rehabilitation.
- Always recommend that rehabilitation patients who smoke enroll in a smoking cessation program as a condition of participation.
- The physical reconditioning component of rehabilitation should always include both aerobic and strength-training exercises.
- Always have rehabilitation patients warm up before performing strengthening and aerobic activities.
- Patients with an SpO_2 of less than 88% or a PaO_2 of less than 55 torr on room air will generally always qualify for home O_2 therapy reimbursement through Medicare and most other health payers.
- Always supply a backup system for home O_2 and ventilator-dependent patients.
- Always ensure that a prescribed home apnea monitor has event recording capability.
- During a home visit, always check the equipment's functioning and cleanliness, determine the patient's compliance with therapy, assess the patient, and modify goals as necessary.
- Always recommend a polysomnography study for a patient suspected of having a sleep disorder; if a diagnosis of OSA is confirmed, recommend CPAP or BiPAP therapy.
- Always educate home care patients and caregivers to properly clean and disinfect equipment according to CDC recommendations.

PRE-TEST ANSWERS AND EXPLANATIONS

Following are this chapter's pre-test answers and explanations. Be sure to review each answer's explanation thoroughly to help you understand why it is correct. If the explanation is still unclear to you, review the chapter content.

17-1. **Correct answer: D.** Reversing lung damage. The goals of pulmonary rehabilitation include improving exercise tolerance, enhancing health-related quality of life, and reducing perceived dyspnea in participants. The goals do not include reversing lung damage.

17-2. **Correct answer: C.** Mandated participation. To achieve the goals of pulmonary rehabilitation requires a multidisciplinary team approach, effective disease management education, and smoking cessation support.

17-3. **Correct answer: B.** 60–75%. To maximize cardiovascular benefit during physical reconditioning, patients should exercise to between 60% and 75% of their predicted maximum heart rates. Lower levels have minimum cardiovascular benefit, whereas higher levels place patients at risk for cardiovascular events.

17-4. **Correct answer: A.** Document patient involvement and outcomes. The other responses are valid but not the primary reason for documenting patient activity and response.

17-5. **Correct answer: B.** Switch to a backup O_2 supply at the equivalent liter flow. When home care patients on O_2 initially suspect an equipment problem, they should be instructed to switch to their backup supply (usually cylinder gas) at the equivalent liter flow. They should call for help only after ensuring continuity of therapy.

17-6. **Correct answer: B.** Tension pneumothorax. Emergency situations that caregivers must be trained to recognize and properly deal with include ventilator or power failure, ventilator circuit problems, airway emergencies, and cardiac arrest.

17-7. **Correct answer: A.** Put the patient on the selected device while still hospitalized. Ideally, the patient should be placed on the actual ventilator that will be used in the home setting before discharge.

17-8. **Correct answer: C.** 1 and 3 only. The threshold to qualify for home O_2 therapy reimbursement under Medicare is a resting PaO_2 of 55 torr or less or an SpO_2 of 88% or less for a single pulmonary diagnosis (COPD), or a PaO_2 between 56 and 59 torr or an SpO_2 of 89% with a secondary diagnosis, such as COPD with cor pulmonale.

17-9. **Correct answer: B.** The first step in responding to a home apnea monitor alarm is to quickly assess the infant. This helps determine if the alarm is real or false and will direct the appropriate response (real alarm: stimulate the baby; false alarm: check equipment and connections).

17-10. **Correct answer: C.** 1:1 solution of vinegar and water. Household products *other than bleach* (e.g., ammonia, vinegar, Borax, liquid detergents) should not be used to disinfect reusable semicritical home care items because they are ineffective against *Staphylococcus aureus*.

POST-TEST

To confirm your mastery of this chapter's topical content, you should take the chapter post-test, available online at http://go.jblearning.com/respexamreview. A score of 80% or more indicates that you are adequately prepared for this section of the NBRC written exams. If you score less than 80%, you should continue to review the applicable chapter content. In addition, you may want to access and review the relevant Web links covering this chapter's content (courtesy of RTBoardReview.com), also online at the Jones & Bartlett Learning site.

SECTION II

Clinical Simulation Exam (CSE) Preparation

CHAPTER 18

Preparing for the Clinical Simulation Exam

Craig L. Scanlan

Your path to registry includes taking and passing the NBRC Clinical Simulation Exam (CSE). Besides being the most costly exam in that pathway, it is also the most difficult. First-time pass rates for the CSE have historically averaged between 50-60%, *the lowest of any NBRC exam.* Thus, if you want to avoid the high reapplication fee and achieve the RRT credential on your first attempt, you will want to be well prepared for this unique exam.

In our experience, the "difficulty" of the CSE and the resultant high failure rate experienced by RRT candidates are due more to poor or ill-informed preparation than to the level or complexity of the test itself. Yes, the CSE has a unique structure, and yes, correctly navigating through a problem's sections requires skill in application and analysis. However, knowing these simple facts should guide you to take a different approach when preparing for the CSE.

To properly prepare for the CSE, we recommend that you treat your experience like any good general going to war. The first rule of war is to know your enemy. In this case, that means becoming fully familiar with both the content and structure of the CSE *and* recognizing how that knowledge can help guide your exam preparation.

CSE CONTENT

Whereas the CRT and WRRT exams are organized exclusively by topical content, the NBRC organizes the CSE by both topical content and disease category. With this knowledge of the enemy in hand, you should then prepare for your looming "battle" by focusing on *both* the exam's topical coverage *and* on disease management.

CSE Topical Coverage

As with the NBRC CRT and WRRT exams, knowing your enemy means knowing exactly which topics are covered on the CSE. Most of this information is provided to you via the CSE detailed content outline in the current NBRC candidate handbook.

The CSE topical content covers the same three major categories covered on both the CRT and WRRT exams—that is, Patient Data, Equipment, and Therapeutic Procedures. A more in depth analysis of the CSE Examination Matrix reveals another simple but very important fact: the topics covered on the CSE represent the *combined content* of the CRT and WRRT multiple-choice exams.

How is this understanding important when planning your topical content review for the CSE? First, knowing that the simulation exam content spans the scope of *all topics* included on CRT and WRRT means that if you recently took and passed both of these tests, you are already fairly well prepared for the CSE's topical content. Related to this conclusion is our strong recommendation *against* taking the WRRT and CSE on the same day (with the single combined CRT+RRT written exam introduced in 2015 this will not be possible). Instead, we advise candidates to divide their RRT testing into two stages, taking *and passing* the WRRT exam first, followed by scheduling and taking the CSE. Following this approach, you can use your WRRT scores to help prepare for the CSE and, therefore, increase your odds of passing it. Combine this with the fact that 6 hours of testing on the same day (2 hours for the WRRT and 4 hours for the CSE) likely will cause fatigue and negatively affect your performance, and the choice should be clear. If you are concerned about costs, be aware that the fees for scheduling the WRRT and CSE on separate days currently are no higher than the fees you would pay to take them together.

The second important tip you can glean from knowing that the CSE covers all CRT and WRRT topics relates to using this text. Obviously, all essential topical content for both the CRT and WRRT exams is covered in Chapters 1–17, corresponding to the 17 major NBRC exam topics. Thus a topical content review for the CSE should include review of all prior chapters in this text.

However, to better focus your topical review for the CSE, we recommend you first carefully assess your CRT and WRRT exam score reports and use that information to prioritize your CSE topic-oriented preparation time. This, of course, assumes that you have followed our advice and already taken and passed both the CRT and WRRT exams.

First, simply compare your overall scaled score between exams. If there is a large difference in your scaled scores, you should prioritize reviewing the content corresponding to the *lowest* of the two exam scores. For example, if your scaled score on the CRT is 83 and your scaled score on the WRRT is 75, your topical review for the CSE should prioritize RRT-specific content. This text makes that job a bit easier by clearly delineating the NBRC content that is shared across its certification and registry exams and the content that is specific to the RRT level (i.e., the WRRT and CSE exams). Although this important distinction is provided via each chapter's objectives, for easy access we have collated the current NBRC RRT-specific topical content in the accompanying box.

To refine your topical review even further, we recommend you convert each of your 17 topical scores for both the CRT and WRRT to percent scores and either record them in a table like **Table 18-1** or use a spreadsheet program to semi-automate the process. Then, using 75% as the "cut score" for each topic, apply the following guidelines to your CSE topical preparation:

Current RRT-Specific Topical Content

- Exam Section I-A (Text Chapter 1)
  - Review and assess data relating to the diagnosis and treatment of sleep disorders
- Exam Section I-B (Text Chapter 2)
  - Review a chest radiograph to determine the quality of imaging
  - Perform and interpret the results of exhaled nitric oxide measurement
  - Select, obtain, and interpret ventilator graphics
  - Detect auto-PEEP
- Exam Section I-C (Text Chapter 3)
  - Recommend blood tests
  - Recommend insertion of monitoring catheters
  - Recommend thoracentesis
- Exam Section II-A (Text Chapter 4)
  - Manipulate portable oxygen systems
  - Manipulate incubators/isolettes
  - Manipulate He/O_2 delivery systems
  - Manipulate high-frequency chest-wall oscillators
  - Manipulate high-frequency ventilators
  - Manipulate hemodynamic monitoring devices
- Exam Section III-H (also *shared* Exam Section III-A content, so it is covered in Chapter 7)
  - Conduct health management education
- Exam Section III-J (Text Chapter 16)
  - Assist with inserting venous (CVP/PA) and arterial catheters
- Exam Section III-K (Text Chapter 17)
  - Initiate and adjust apnea monitors
  - Initiate treatment for sleep disorders (e.g., CPAP)

Table 18-1 Self-Assessment of Written Exam Topical Scores (CRT and WRRT Exams)

Topic	CRT	WRRT
I. Patient Data Evaluation and Recommendations		
A. Review Data in the Patient Record		
B. Collect and Evaluate Additional Pertinent Clinical Information		
C. Recommend Procedures to Obtain Additional Data		
II. Equipment Manipulation, Infection Control, and Quality Control		
A. Manipulate Equipment by Order or Protocol		
B. Ensure Infection Control		
C. Perform Quality Control Procedures		
III. Initiation and Modification of Therapeutic Procedures		
A. Maintain Records and Communicate Information		
B. Maintain a Patent Airway Including the Care of Artificial Airways		
C. Remove Bronchopulmonary Secretions		
D. Achieve Adequate Respiratory Support		
E. Evaluate and Monitor the Patient's Responses to Respiratory Care		
F. Independently Modify Therapeutic Procedures		
G. Recommend Modifications in the Respiratory Care Plan		
H. Determine the Appropriateness of Care Plan and Recommend Modifications		
I. Initiate, Conduct, or Modify Techniques in an Emergency Setting		
J. Act as an Assistant to the Physician Performing Special Procedures		
K. Initiate and Conduct Pulmonary Rehabilitation and Home Care		

- *High priority* for review: *both* CRT and WRRT topic scores < 75%
- *Moderate priority* for review: either CRT or WRRT topic score < 75%
- *Low priority* for review: both CRT and WRRT topic scores > 75%

CSE Content by Disease Category

What most candidates miss—and, in our opinion, why many fail the CSE—is that this exam's content also is organized by disease category. Currently the CSE includes 10 cases or problems (plus two test cases), selected from seven disease management categories.* **Table 18-2** outlines these categories, the number of cases likely to appear on the current CSE, and specific case examples cited by the NBRC for each category.

We recommend that you spend the majority of your CSE prep time focusing on disease management by case. Specifically, your preparation for the CSE should include review of assessment and problem identification, procedures, skills, and treatment plans/protocols related to these seven disease management categories *and* the example cases identified by the NBRC. Preparation by case is the key to CSE success!

How should you prepare for disease management by case? Differently! Topical content is relatively easy to specify and is well covered here (Chapters 1–17) and in many comprehensive respiratory care textbooks. However, disease management by case is not as well defined, so it requires a different preparatory approach. In our experience, the best strategy is to use appropriate resource materials to review the pathophysiology and the medical, surgical, and respiratory management of each of the common disorders identified by the NBRC.

---

*Beginning in 2015, the NBRC CSE exam will include a larger number of shorter problems. Visit http://go.jblearning.com/respexamreview for details on the 2015 changes to the NBRC exams and suggestions on how these changes should influence your preparation.

Table 18-2 Disease Management Categories and Cases Likely to Appear on the CSE

Disease Management Category	Likely Number of Cases	Examples of Cases That May Appear
Adults with COPD	2	Preoperative/postoperative evaluation Critical care management Mechanical ventilation PFT evaluation Home care/rehabilitation Infection control
Adults with trauma	1–2	Chest/head/skeletal injury Burns Smoke inhalation Hypothermia
Adults with cardiovascular disease	1–2	Congestive heart failure Coronary artery disease Valvular heart disease Cardiac surgery
Adults with neurologic/neuromuscular disorders	1–2	Myasthenia gravis Guillain-Barré syndrome Tetanus Muscular dystrophy Drug overdose
Pediatric patients	1	Epiglottitis Croup Bronchiolitis Asthma Cystic fibrosis Foreign body aspiration Toxic substance ingestion Bronchopulmonary dysplasia
Neonatal patients	1	Delivery room management Resuscitation Infant apnea Meconium aspiration Respiratory distress syndrome Congenital heart defect
Adults with other problems	1	Thoracic surgery Head and neck surgery Carbon monoxide poisoning Obesity-hypoventilation AIDS

What are appropriate resource materials? We recommend that you access whatever textbook resources were used in your respiratory or cardiopulmonary pathophysiology course(s) in school. These materials may include focused pathophysiology and disease management texts written for respiratory therapists or relevant disease-oriented chapters in more comprehensive texts. However, because pathophysiology-focused texts are organized by disease category and emphasize both diagnosis and management, they are a better choice for CSE preparation than most comprehensive texts.

Either way, you should extract and summarize in writing at least the following basic information about each of the common disorders identified by the NBRC:

- Definition and causes (etiology)
- Pathophysiology (how the disorder alters structure or function)
- Clinical manifestations (signs and symptoms)
- Test results used to confirm diagnosis (e.g., lab results, PFT, imaging studies)
- Differential diagnosis (including which findings distinguish this condition)

Cystic fibrosis	
Etiology: Inherited disorder causing abnormal exocrine glands function	
Pathophysiology: Chronic resp infections, GI problems, decreased pancreatic enzymes	
Clinical S&S: Chronic cough + sputum; frequent respiratory infections; nasal polyps and sinusitis; clubbing; steatorrhea (fatty stool); failure to thrive	
Dx tests: Genetic testing; patient history; clinical S&S; sweat Cl >60 mmols/L; X-ray: hyperinflation, peribronchial thickening, bronchiectasis, infiltrates, atelectasis, RV hypertrophy; PFT: progressive ↓ FEV₁; ↑ RV/TLC ratio (air trapping); microorganism: P. aeruginosa most common, also H. infuenzae, S. aureus, burkholderia cepacia	
Differential Dx: Asthma, bronchiectasis, bronchiolitis, ciliary dyskinesia	
General med/surg Rx: Treat airway obstruction/respiratory infection, provide nutritional support and patient/family education, regular follow-up	
Resp mgmt: Inhaled bronchodilator, pulmozyme (dornase alfa), hypertonic saline, antibiotics e.g., TOBI (tobramycin), colistin (polymyxin E) or cayston (aztreonam); airway clearance therapy, exercise. Assess: SpO₂/PaO₂, sputum production, breath sounds, x-ray, FEV₁ Patient education re: meds, airway clearance techniques, aerosols delivery devices, infection control	

Figure 18-1 Example Disease Management Case Summary: Cystic Fibrosis.

Courtesy of: Strategic Learning Associates, LLC, Little Silver, New Jersey.

- General medical/surgical treatment
- Respiratory management (therapy and assessment)
- Common complications and their management

Figure 18-1 provides an example of a good summary extraction for cystic fibrosis, as it might appear on an index card. In fact, because many RT programs require it, you may already have a collection of index cards or page forms like this one covering most of the common disorders you need to review for the CSE exam. And now you know why! To facilitate your CSE review, we have encapsulated much of this information for you in Chapter 20 as "Clinical Simulation Exam Case Management Pearls."

We also recommend you copy the clinical manifestations and the test results used to confirm diagnosis to the back of each summary card or sheet. In this manner, you turn each summary into a "flashcard" that you can use to assess and enhance your diagnostic acumen—for example, given these findings, what is the most likely disorder? The importance of building your diagnostic skills in preparing for the CSE is discussed in more detail subsequently.

In addition to these resources, you will want to gather and review selected clinical practice guidelines. A good place to start is with the AARC Clinical Practice Guidelines, a complete listing of which is provided in Appendix C (Selected Sources) and all of which are available online at the *Respiratory Care* journal site (www.rcjournal.com/cpgs/). The AARC guidelines are an invaluable source of information with which all therapists should be familiar and from which the NBRC draws essential content. You should pay particular attention to the newer evidence-based guidelines published in *Respiratory Care*.

Although the AARC guidelines provide excellent procedural guidance (especially in regard to assessing respiratory care interventions), you will want to supplement this knowledge with current disease management guidelines, as provided mainly by professional medical organizations. Disease management guidelines covering most of the cases likely to appear on the CSE are readily available online and easily found using the U.S. Department of Health and Human Services' National Guideline Clearinghouse (http://guideline.gov). **Figure 18-2** provides a partial screenshot of a search for bronchiolitis guidelines on this site. Here, as in many cases, multiple guidelines were retrieved on the prevention, diagnosis, and treatment of this disorder. In such cases, the National Guideline Clearinghouse often provides very useful short syntheses of the available guidelines. Knowing that the NBRC cases selected for inclusion on the CSE generally abide by professional organization guidelines should provide sufficient motivation to obtain and review them when preparing for this exam.

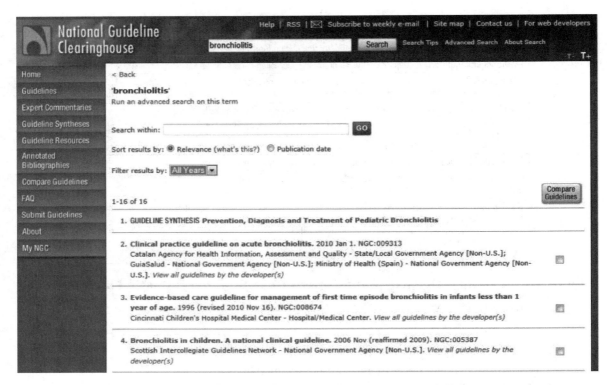

Figure 18-2 National Guideline Clearinghouse Search Results for Bronchiolitis Guidelines.

Also available to you through Jones & Bartlett Learning (and courtesy of RTBoardReview) is a regularly updated compilation of Web-based disease management resources, organized according to the seven disease management categories covered on the CSE. To access these resources, visit the companion website for this book at http://go.jblearning.com/respexamreview.

CSE STRUCTURE

In addition to understanding its unique content, as part of your preparation for your upcoming "battle" with the CSE, you need to take into account the exam's unique structure, which differs substantially from the NBRC written exams. Your success on the CSE requires that you fully understand this structure and know how to apply this information when preparing for this exam.

Overall Structure and Sections

As previously discussed, rather than using single-concept, multiple-choice items, the CSE takes you through a set of clinical cases or patient management problems. Each case consists of a variable number of sections (averaging 8–12 sections on the current CSE) in which you assess the patient's status and recommend or take appropriate actions as the situation evolves over time. Sections in which you collect and evaluate information are termed *Information Gathering* (IG) sections, whereas sections in which you recommend or implement interventions are called *Decision-Making* (DM) sections.

Figure 18-3 provides an example "map" showing the structure of a hypothetical simulation of a case involving a 57-year-old patient who has recently undergone coronary artery bypass (CABG) surgery and has worsening respiratory status. This problem includes 11 sections—that is, three IG sections and 8 DM sections. As with most CSE problems, there is an ideal pathway through the case, along with one or more "branches." In this example, Section 6 is a branch off the idea path that provides the opportunity to correct a wrong decision (a corrective branch). Branching may also occur to allow for equivalent decisions—for example, initiating full ventilatory support with assist/control ventilation or normal rate SIMV.

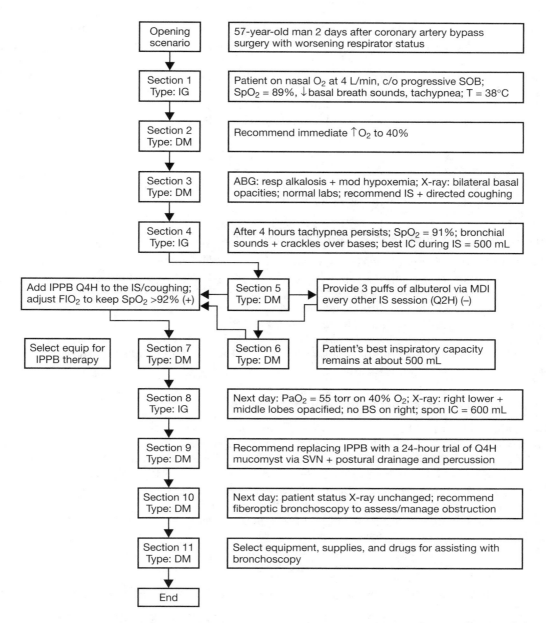

Figure 18-3 Map of Hypothetical Simulation for a 57-Year-Old Man Post CABG Surgery.

Courtesy of: Strategic Learning Associates, LLC, Little Silver, New Jersey.

Currently IG and DM sections are graded separately, with each section's score based on the sum of the individually weighted options you select within that section. For each section, NBRC content experts set a minimum pass level. The overall IG or DM passing score for a given problem is simply the sum of all the applicable section minimum pass levels. Beginning in 2015, separate scoring of IG and DM sections will end, with a single combined minimum pass level used to determine if you pass or fail the CSE.

Relationship Between Information Gathering and Decision Making

Section 1 in Figure 18-3 is an example of an IG section in which a proper assessment would reveal that the patient is on 4 L/min nasal cannula with an SpO_2 of 89%, is complaining of progressive shortness of breath (SOB) and is tachypneic, and has decreased breath sounds at the bases and a slightly elevated temperature. Section 2 is an example of a DM section, in which the correct initial action (one among many choices) is to increase the F_{IO_2} to 40%. Note this correct action or decision (like all actions in a CSE case) depends on the prior collection *and proper evaluation* of the relevant information—in this case, the evidence indicating hypoxemia and the suggestion that the patient has developed or is developing postoperative atelectasis.

Understanding this linkage between IG and DM sections is critical to your CSE preparation. Key pointers related to this understanding include the following:

1. You need to know which information to gather.
2. You need to know what the information means.
3. Your decisions always must be made in context.
4. The context usually involves a *presumptive* diagnosis.

Relationship Between NBRC Topics and CSE Skills

The good news is that your *topical preparation* for the CSE (and for the CRT and WRRT exams) will help you address these important points. As indicated in **Table 18-3**, simulation exam IG sections assess knowledge and skills similar to those emphasized in Section I of the topical content outlines (which information you need to know *and* what it means). Likewise, the skills required to do well on simulation exam DM sections are emphasized in Sections III-E through III-H. Knowing these parallels in coverage and emphasis can be extremely helpful in planning your preparation. That is not to say you should disregard other topics—just that CSE information gathering and decision-making skills best correlate with these particular areas of content.

Disease Management and Diagnostic Reasoning

Given these close parallels between topical content and CSE skills, why is disease management preparation so important? Because your decision making always must be made in context (pointer 3), and that context usually involves making a diagnosis (pointer 4). In our example problem (Figure 18-3), it never is stated that the patient has developed or is developing postoperative atelectasis. Instead, you must *presume* this to be the case—that is, you make a presumptive diagnosis. To make a presumptive diagnosis, you must carefully interpret the information you gather. Only by knowing the problem you are dealing with can you make good management decisions. *Thus making correct decisions requires making a correct diagnosis.*

Table 18-3 Relationship Between CSE Section Skills and NBRC Major Topics

CSE Sections	Related Major Topics
Information Gathering	**I. *Patient Data Evaluation and Recommendations (Chapters 1–3)***
	A. Review Data in the Patient Record
	B. Collect/Evaluate Additional Clinical Information
	C. Recommend Procedures to Obtain Additional Data
Decision Making	***III. Initiation and Modification of Procedures (Chapters 11–14)***
	E. Evaluate/Monitor the Patient's Objective and Subjective Responses to Respiratory Care
	F. Independently Modify Therapeutic Procedures Based on the Patient's Response
	G. Recommend Modifications in the Care Plan Based on the Patient's Response
	H. Determine the Appropriateness of the Care Plan and Recommend Modifications When Indicated

But you are not a physician and disease diagnosis is not specified in the NBRC exam topical outlines! Well, yes and no. You are not a physician, but "buried" in major topic H of the NBRC topical outlines (Determine the Appropriateness of the Care Plan and Recommend Modifications) are the following two skills:

- Analyze the available information to determine the pathophysiological state (H-1).
- Determine the appropriateness of prescribed therapy and goals for the identified pathophysiological state (H-3).

This is exactly what is meant by making your decisions in context. First, determining the pathophysiological state means determining a presumptive diagnosis. Second, determining the appropriate therapy and goals for the identified pathophysiological state means taking actions or making recommendations with good knowledge of what is wrong with the patient at the time the decision must be made.

Based on our experience, it is in these areas that candidates have the most difficulty on the CSE, which explains why low DM scores are the most common reason for exam failure. To overcome this problem, we recommend you apply a technique called *reciprocal reasoning*. What is reciprocal reasoning? It simply means that instead of thinking from disease or disorder to clinical findings (a common approach when studying for pathophysiology exams), you *reverse this reasoning* and think from clinical findings back to likely disorder (the process used by physicians in making diagnoses). For example:

Instead of Asking	Ask
What are the clinical findings that a patient suffering from postoperative atelectasis would exhibit?	What is the likely problem in a postoperative thoracic surgery patient who exhibits progressive hypoxemia, dyspnea, decreased breath sounds, mild fever, dull percussion note, and a chest x-ray indicating areas of opacification?

Of course, many disorders share at least some clinical findings. In our example (Figure 18-3), the initial information is also at least partially consistent with a diagnosis of pneumonia. This, of course, is why we recommend that your disease management preparation include identifying the common differential diagnoses for each condition and understanding what distinguishes the given diagnosis from those with similar findings. Returning to our example, a sputum C&S would be one test that could help distinguish atelectasis from pneumonia and, therefore, would be one element to include in your information-gathering strategy. The bottom line is that you should not link a diagnosis to findings without consideration of other possible causes; instead, you should become familiar with common differential diagnoses and know what distinguishes each from the others.

SUMMARY OF CSE PREPARATION DO'S AND DON'TS

In summary, some strategies used to prepare for the CSE are similar to those used to study for the CRT or WRRT exams. At the same time, the unique content and structure of this exam demand a different approach. The following "Do's and Don'ts" summarize the approach we recommend to maximize your odds of passing the CSE.

Do's

- Do schedule your CSE separately from *and only after passing* the WRRT.
- Do focus on *both* the exam's topical coverage and disease management.
- Do prioritize your topical content review by assessing your CRT and WRRT scores.
- For your topical review, do emphasize topics I-A through I-C (Chapters 1–3 in this text) and topics III-E through III-H (Chapters 11–14 in this text).
- Do spend the majority of your CSE preparation on disease management by case.
- Do use pathophysiology-focused texts for CSE disease management preparation.
- Do access and review current clinical practice and disease management guidelines.

- Do prepare written summaries covering the basic information about each common disorder you are likely to see on the CSE.
- Do be familiar with common differential diagnoses for a given disorder and know what distinguishes each from the others.

Don'ts

- Don't schedule your CSE on the same day as you take the WRRT; your WRRT scores can help you prepare for the CSE.
- Don't prepare for the CSE by focusing solely on topical content.
- Don't prepare for the CSE by thinking from disorder to clinical findings; instead, reverse this reasoning and think from clinical findings back to likely disorder.
- Don't link a diagnosis to findings without considering other possible causes (e.g., differential diagnoses).

CHAPTER 19

Taking the Clinical Simulation Exam

Craig L. Scanlan

To pass the NBRC Clinical Simulation Exam (CSE), you obviously need to master the relevant content, as detailed in Chapter 18. However, your success on the CSE also requires that you fully understand its structure and format, and be able to use this information to become more proficient in taking this unique exam. Specifically, the CSE requires a different set of skills from those needed to succeed on multiple-choice exams (the test-taking tips covered in Appendix A). The intent of this chapter is to provide you with those skills, thereby increasing your likelihood of passing this portion of your boards.

CSE COMPUTER TESTING FORMAT AND OPTION SCORING

Rather than asking a large number of single-concept multiple-choice questions, the NBRC CSE has you progress through a set of patient cases. Currently, the CSE includes as many as 12 cases, 10 of which are graded and 1 or 2 of which are being "pre-tested" and are ungraded. Because the ungraded cases are not identified, you need to treat all problems as counting toward your CSE scores. You have 4 hours to complete all cases.*

As described in Chapter 18, each case involves, on average, 8 to 12 response sections. In *Information Gathering (IG) sections*, you gather and assess the patient's status and/or response to interventions; in *Decision-Making (DM) sections*, you take actions or make recommendations.

As depicted in **Figure 19-1**, the computer presents each section of the case in three scrolling windows: the scenario window, the option window, and the history window. The scenario window provides current information about the patient or evolving situation. The options window contains all the choices available to you in a given section. The history window displays the options you chose and their results for either the current section or case as a whole. A button allows you to "toggle" back and forth between these two different information views. A digital clock to help track elapsed time also can be toggled on/off, and a help screen can be activated anytime during the exam.

Section scenarios also direct you to either "CHOOSE ONLY ONE" or to "SELECT AS MANY" of the responses provided in the options window. For IG sections, you always can select as many items as you consider necessary to assess the patient's current status. In most DM sections, you are directed to select the single best action or recommendation. Occasionally DM sections permit selection of multiple actions.

This response format differs significantly from the CRT/WRRT multiple-choice format in several respects. First, some CSE sections allow you to select multiple options. Second, *once you check a CSE option, you cannot change your response.* Third, each individual CSE response is graded on a 6-point scale, rather than as simply right or wrong. Finally, every response you select provides feedback.

We provide guidance on selecting multiple options later in this chapter. In regard to not being able to change responses, you obviously want to be as certain as possible about selecting an option before checking it. However, due to the unique way options are scored and the allowance for corrective action, only infrequently will a given choice cause serious or permanent "damage" from which you cannot recover.

---

*Starting in 2015, the CSE will include a larger number of shorter problems, but retain the 4-hour time limit. For updates on the NBRC's 2015 credentialing exam changes, be sure to visit this text's accompanying Jones & Bartlett Learning website at http://go.jblearning. com/respexamreview (described in Appendix D).

Table 19-1 Illustrative CSE Options Scoring Scale

Score	General Meaning (*not official NBRC scaling*)
+3*	Critically necessary in identifying or resolving the problem
+2	Strongly facilitative in identifying or resolving the problem
+1	Somewhat facilitative in identifying or resolving the problem
−1	Uninformative or potentially harmful in identifying or resolving the problem
−2	Wastes critical time in identifying the problem or causes some patient harm
−3*	Unnecessarily invasive, gravely harmful, or illegal action
*+3 or −3 scoring is rare; the majority of options are scored in the +2 to −2 range.	

Part of the reason that a "wrong" choice may not seriously affect your overall CSE grade is that your responses are scored on a variable scale like that depicted in **Table 19-1**. What this example scale makes clear is that some responses are "less wrong" than others (and some "more right" than others). Thus, if you must make an error in responding, you want it to be a minor error (−1) as opposed to a serious one (−2 to −3).

But how do you know if a given choice is in error or how serious the error might be? Technically, you do not know. However, every option in a CSE case provides some sort of feedback.

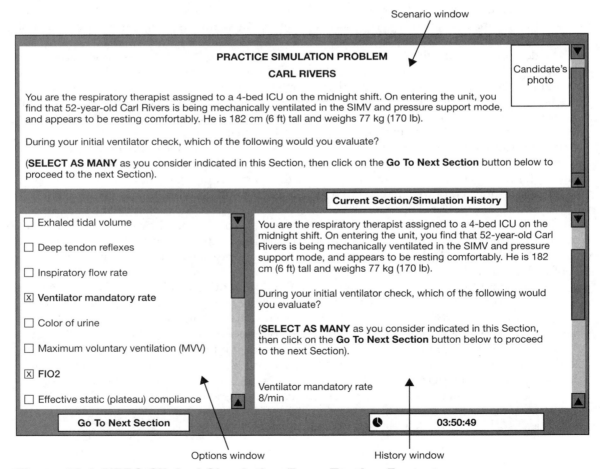

Figure 19-1 NBRC Clinical Simulation Exam Testing Format.

Source: NBRC Candidate Handbook and Application, Figure 4 (p. 15). © 2013 The National Board for Respiratory Care, Inc.

For IG options, this typically includes either the requested patient data or feedback such as "Results pending" or "Sample sent to laboratory" or "Not performed" or "Physician disagrees." Likewise, for DM sections, feedback may include new patient status information or "Done" or "Ordered" or "Not done—make another selection in this section" or "Physician disagrees—make another selection in this section." Although none of this feedback definitively indicates that a right or wrong choice has been made, when considered in context you usually can deduce the impact and take appropriate corrective action.

For IG sections, feedback such as "Not performed" or "Physician disagrees" suggests that your choice may be wasting time, may cause harm to the patient, or may be unnecessarily invasive. If you receive this type of feedback and remaining unselected options could provide equivalent information but are quicker, easier to obtain, less harmful, or less invasive, be sure to select them. In this manner, you will likely be able to "cancel out" a negatively weighted response with a positive one.

For DM sections, the "Not done" or "Physician disagrees" feedback that directs you to make another selection may or may not indicate an error. In some cases, this feedback is used to force a choice (without penalty) that guides you to the next programmed section of the case. However, the same type of feedback may indicate that you have made an error. This is usually apparent if after making a decision you are directed to a section indicating a worsening of the patient's status. If so, do not fret over what may have been an incorrect action or recommendation. Instead, realize that likely you are being given the opportunity to correct your initial error. Such "corrective branches" in a case never allow you to completely recoup any lost points, but they do allow you to mitigate the impact of a prior bad decision. For example, if a DM choice scored as −2 provides a corrective branch. likely the best remedial action will be scored −1, with the net result being still negative, *but less so*. In these situations, the key is to use the feedback provided in the case to recognize the potential error and correct it forthwith.

SCENARIO GUIDANCE

Typically the opening scenario describes the setting, your role, and basic patient information. As the case evolves, subsequent scenarios provide additional patient information, including response to therapy. **Table 19-2** provides our general guidance regarding CSE scenarios as a series of basic "Do's and Don'ts."

If the scenario indicates an emergency situation:

- Gather only essential or quick-to-obtain information; do not waste time performing or recommending complex or lengthy assessment procedures.
- Once the problem at hand is clear, immediately proceed with the applicable emergency protocol.

Also, from the opening scenario onward, you should be building your list of potential problems and figuring out how to distinguish among those with common signs and symptoms—that is, performing a *differential diagnosis*. **Table 19-3** lists examples of differential diagnoses that often crop up on the CSE, along with some of the diagnostic tools that can help distinguish between them. This is important because *depending on the diagnosis/problem at hand, treatments can be very different*.

Table 19-2 Scenario Do's and Don'ts

Do's	Don'ts
Do decide if the situation is an emergency and begin "differential diagnosis" early on.	Don't make assumptions about the scenario—consider only the facts presented to you.
Do identify and assess all key patient data (objective/subjective), including any information indicating changes in patient status.	Don't worry if the setting (e.g., PFT lab or patient's home) or situation is unfamiliar to you. Your basic knowledge of respiratory care will always apply, regardless of setting or situation.

Table 19-3 Examples of Clinical Simulation Exam Differential Diagnoses

Example Differential Diagnoses	Key Information to Seek
Adult	
Reversible obstruction (asthma) versus COPD	Pre/post bronchodilator
Myasthenia gravis versus Guillain-Barré syndrome	Tensilon test, AChR, CSF fluid
Congestive heart failure versus ARDS	History; pulmonary artery wedge pressure
CO poisoning versus alcohol/drug overdose	History (CO exposure), HbCO
Pediatric/Neonatal	
Epiglottitis versus laryngotracheobronchitis (croup)	Symptoms + neck x-rays (AP and lateral)
Childhood asthma versus foreign body aspiration	Chest/neck x-rays, CT scan
Infant pulmonary hypertension versus RDS	Pre/post ductal SpO_2, chest x-ray

INFORMATION GATHERING GUIDANCE

Do's and Don'ts

You determine the diagnosis or problem at hand as well as the patient's response to therapy primarily via the IG sections of the case. As with CSE scenarios, important Do's and Don'ts apply to selecting options in IG sections, as outlined in **Table 19-4**.

In regard to reviewing and considering all IG options, it is important to note that the CSE options window usually must be scrolled to reveal all choices. Don't miss out on possible good choices by failing to reveal all the options available to you!

The most important criterion to consider in selecting available IG options is their *relevance*—that is, will the information be helpful in identifying the problem or resolving the situation at hand? For example, if the patient likely has a progressive neuromuscular disorder or is being considered for weaning from ventilatory support, a vital capacity measurement may be relevant and, therefore, would be indicated. However, the same measure would not provide useful information (and would waste time) when caring for a patient with an acute myocardial infarction in the Emergency Department.

We also recommend selecting IG options in logical order, from basic to advanced. For example, if the patient's pulse is irregular, consider selecting the ECG, if available, for the additional information it may provide. In this manner, selection of one option may indicate the need to choose another.

"Always Select" Choices

Although you probably have been taught that there are few, if any, absolutes in patient management, when taking the CSE a few generally do apply. Typically this information is vital, quick to

Table 19-4 Information Gathering Do's and Don'ts

Do's	Don'ts
Do review and *consider* all options.	Don't be too curious about unfamiliar options—if you have never heard of it, it likely is there to distract you.
Do prioritize options yielding data that can identify the problem or resolve *the situation at hand*.	Don't skimp on choices—trying to figure out the problem with the least amount of data is a mistake that will cost you points.
Do select options in logical order, from basic to advanced.	Don't select all options—usually at least some of the choices carry a penalty.

Table 19-5 Selecting Respiratory-Related Information

Information	Select To
Arterial blood gas	Assess acid–base balance, ventilation, or oxygenation
Tracheal position	Identify pneumothorax (shift away) or atelectasis (shift toward)
Percussion	Identify pneumothorax (high pitch) or consolidation /pneumonia (dull note)
MIP/NIF	Assess respiratory muscle strength (neuromuscular disorders, weaning)
Vital capacity (VC)	Assess inspiratory/expiratory muscle function (neuromuscular disorders, weaning)
$\dot{V}_E$, RR, RSBI	Evaluate adequacy of ventilation (need for ventilatory support/weaning)
Sputum production	Assess for infection or secretion clearance problems

obtain, and almost always helpful in identifying the problem at hand or the patient's response to therapy. Information in the "Always Select" category includes the following:

- General appearance (e.g., color)
- Vital signs
  - ○ Respiratory rate—always
  - ○ Heat rate—always
  - ○ Pulse oximetry Spo_2 (*obtain Sao_2 via CO-oximetry if the patient has experienced smoke inhalation*)
  - ○ Blood pressure—if the patient has a cardiovascular problem
  - ○ Body temperature—if infection/hypothermia is likely
- Level of consciousness
  - ○ *Basic*: sensorium assessment (e.g., "oriented × 3")
  - ○ *Advanced*: Glasgow Coma Scale score (e.g., for patients who are unconscious or brain-injured)
- Breath sounds
- History of present illness (if readily available)

Selecting Respiratory-Related Information

As described in **Table 19-5**, additional respiratory-related information that you may want to consider will depend on the situation at hand. For example, an arterial blood gas is needed only if knowledge of the patient's acid–base balance, ventilation, or oxygenation is required to identify the problem or make a decision. Likewise, other common respiratory-related information will be relevant in some situations, but not in others.

Selecting Pulmonary Function and Exercise Test Information

In a similar manner, you should be sensible in seeking PFT or exercise test information. For example, not every patient situation calls for a diffusing capacity study or comprehensive exercise evaluation. You can help eliminate some of these unnecessary choices by asking yourself a simple question: "If I had this information in this situation, what would I do with it?" **Table 19-6** provides additional guidance on selecting PFT or exercise test data in CSE IG sections.

Table 19-6 Selecting Pulmonary Function and Exercise Test Information

Test	Select To
Spirometry (FEV)	Assess surgical risk, detect obstruction/reversibility
FRC, RV, TLC	Differentiate between obstructive and restrictive conditions
Bronchoprovocation	Assess for airway hyperresponsiveness and inflammation
Diffusing capacity (DLco)	Identify the cause of restrictive disorders, assess feasibility of lung reduction surgery
Exercise testing	Evaluate tolerance for exertion (e.g., for pulmonary rehabilitation), diagnose coronary artery disease, differentiate cardiac versus pulmonary limits to exercise capacity

Table 19-7 Selecting Laboratory Tests

Information	Select It
Hb, Hct, RBCs	Evaluate O_2 carrying capacity; assess for anemia, hemodilution, or hemoconcentration
WBCs, differential	Assess for presence of bacterial/viral infections
Platelets, INR, PT	Evaluate blood clotting (ABGs) and bleeding abnormalities
Electrolytes	Determine type of metabolic acid–base imbalance (anion gap); identify causes of selected cardiac arrhythmias and neuromuscular abnormalities
BUN, creatinine	Assess renal function and metabolic acid–base imbalances
Lactate/lactic acid	Determine presence of tissue hypoxia (e.g., shock, ARDS, CN poisoning)
Total protein, albumin	Assess for malnutrition, weaning difficulties, or liver disease
Cardiac enzymes (CK, troponin, BNP)	Assess for myocardial damage (MI)/CHF

Of course, PFT information also serves as a good illustration of testing that should be deferred in emergency situations. For example, you would *not* recommend obtaining bedside spirometry data for a patient in the Emergency Department who is currently being treated for a severe exacerbation of asthma.

Selecting Laboratory Tests

Laboratory tests also appear as common options in IG sections of the CSE exam. Listed in **Table 19-7** are the lab tests that most frequently appear on the CSE exam, along with their common use. As with PFTs, selection of lab data is situation specific. For example, although cardiac enzymes would be a good choice when assessing an adult patient with acute chest pain, they would not be needed to evaluate a child with metabolic acidosis due to renal failure.

Selecting Imaging Studies

The other common diagnostic procedures that often appear in IG sections are various imaging modalities. As with lab tests, not all imaging tests apply to all situations. As outlined in **Table 19-8**, you should select the test only if it is indicated and can provide information needed to identify or resolve the problem at hand. In terms of emergency situations, you should note that chest and neck x-rays, CT scans, and thoracic ultrasound are all standard tools in emergency medicine and may be indicated in selected situations, especially head or chest trauma.

Table 19-8 Selecting Imaging Studies

Information	Select To
Chest x-ray	Assess for atelectasis, consolidation, pneumothorax, and tube and catheter positions
Neck x-rays	Differentiate causes of stridor (croup versus epiglottis); to detect foreign body aspiration
CT/MRI	*Thoracic*: Detect tumors, aortic aneurysm, and chest trauma *Head/neck*: Evaluate for traumatic brain, neck, or spine injury
CT angiography	Identify presence and extent of pulmonary embolism
Thoracic ultrasound	Detect fluid in thorax, pneumothorax, or chest trauma; to guide thoracentesis
PET scan	Identify malignant tumors

Table 19-9 Selecting Cardiovascular-Related Information

Information	Select To
Peripheral pulses	Assess rate/rhythm
Arterial blood pressure	To assess cardiac function/adequacy of perfusion
Urine output	To assess for shock or effect of diuretics
CVP/PA pressures	To assess fluid balance
PA wedge pressure (PAWP)	To assess for left ventricular failure
Cardiac output/index	To assess for shock and its treatment
Ejection fraction	To assess left ventricular function and its treatment
Mixed venous O_2	To assess tissue oxygenation

Information Needs in Cases Involving a Cardiovascular Disorder

The current CSE can include as many as two cases involving patients with cardiovascular disorders. For this reason, you will want to select carefully among the available options provided for these patients. In most cases, the patient's peripheral pulse and blood pressure are "Always" choices, with urine output also a good option if available. The more advanced tests in **Table 19-9** should be selected only if a CVP or pulmonary artery (PA) catheter is or will be in place and *only if the information is essential in patient management*. For example, if the doctor is trying to differentiate between CHF and ARDS in a patient with hypoxemia and bilateral infiltrates on x-ray, the pulmonary artery wedge pressure (PAWP) would provide essential information. However, this is one of the few current indications for PA catheter measurements. Were the case to involve basic management of a patient with systemic hypertension, a request for PA catheter data would be considered unnecessarily invasive and potentially harmful.

Information Needs in Cases Involving a Neurologic or Neuromuscular Disorder

Because the CSE also may include as many as two cases involving patients with neurologic or neuromuscular disorders and a separate head injury case (under the trauma category), you will likewise want to select sensibly among the choices given to you. **Table 19-10** summarizes our guidance on selecting information in managing these cases. Assessing a patient's level of consciousness was already described as an "Always Select" option, with obtaining the Glasgow Coma Scale score being important if the patient is unconscious. The gag reflex and ability to swallow are both important as is assessing upper airway protection, while more sophisticated tests such as EEGs and ICP measurements have narrower indications.

Table 19-10 Selecting Neurologic or Neuromuscular-Related Information

Information	Select To
Muscle tone	Differentiate lower motor neuron disorders (hypotonia) from upper neuron disorders (hypertonia)
Deep tendon reflex	Assess for peripheral neuropathy, polymyositis, muscular dystrophy, or paralysis
Gag reflex	Assess level of consciousness/anesthesia or upper airway control
Ability to swallow	Assess upper airway control/aspiration risk
Glasgow Coma Scale score	Determine the level/depth of coma and mortality risk
Babinski reflex	Assess for brain damage
EEG	Stage sleep or confirm brain death
EMG/nerve conduction	Test neuromusclar function in disorders such as ALS, myasthenia gravis, and muscular dystrophy
ICP	Monitor patients with traumatic brain injury

ANALYSIS: THE MISSING LINK BETWEEN INFORMATION GATHERING AND DECISION MAKING

In our experience, many candidates who fail the CSE do so not because they select the wrong information, but rather because they do not apply the information to the situation at hand. This problem is usually evident when the candidate has a high IG score but a low DM score.

The problem in these cases is failing to understand that information gathering involves not one but *two* key steps:

1. You must select the right information.
2. Once the information is in hand, you need to analyze what it means.

Based on our prior guidance, selecting the right information should not be overly difficult. The more challenging task is analyzing what the selected information means and what to do with it. As indicated in **Figure 19-2**, *analysis* represents the missing link between gathering the needed information and making the correct decisions.

Of course, to correctly analyze patient information, you first must know what constitutes "normal" for each and every data element. Tables of normal values and reference ranges are provided for all essential patient data throughout Section I of this text (Chapters 1–17). However, beyond "knowing your normal," you need to recognize what an abnormal result means, in terms of both altered function *and* treatment options. A simple example would be a fall in SpO_2 from 93% to 88% in an adult on 2 L/min nasal O_2 who recently underwent upper abdominal surgery. You would rightfully conclude that this result is below normal and requires an increase in FIO_2 or O_2 flow. However, you should also consider that this finding may indicate a developing atelectasis, which could require some form of lung expansion therapy. As previously discussed, this simple finding should also provoke consideration of other more advanced information, such as the patient's most recent chest x-ray.

DECISION-MAKING GUIDANCE

After information gathering, you normally will be presented with one or more DM sections. These sections typically provide you with options for managing the problem, usually in the form of taking an action or making a recommendation.

Do's and Don'ts

As with IG sections and as delineated in **Table 19-11**, there are "Do's and Don'ts" that apply to selecting options in DM sections.

The first "Do" is the most critical—that is, selecting the best action based on your analysis of the information you have gathered. Although there are hundreds of different patient situations that you might encounter, only a limited number of decision-making actions apply to the most common clinical findings seen on the simulation exam.

Decision Making Based on Physical Assessment Findings

As shown in **Table 19-12**, several common physical findings can help you identify the most likely problem and, therefore, the most appropriate action. For example, if you hear wheezing on auscultation, the most likely problems are bronchospasm and congestive heart failure. If other data such

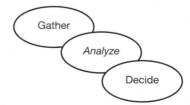

Figure 19-2 Analysis: The Critical Link Between Information Gathering and Decision Making.

Table 19-11 Decision Making Do's and Don'ts

Do's	Don'ts
Do select the best action based on your analysis of the prior information.	Don't worry if your favorite action is missing.
Do think about your choice before making a selection.	Don't select more than one choice unless directed to do so.
Do read all responses carefully (e.g., "Physician disagrees," "Action taken").	Don't select unfamiliar actions.

as the patient's history indicate bronchospasm, the most appropriate action would be bronchodilator administration. Conversely, if the problem appears to be congestive heart failure, diuresis and administration of a positive inotropic agent should be recommended.

Decision Making Based on Problems with Secretions and/or Airway Clearance

Similar guidance applies if the information given indicates potential problems with secretions or airway clearance (**Table 19-13**). Again, the findings suggest the problem, and the problem establishes the action or actions needed to resolve it. This is the basic sequence of reasoning that must guide you in linking information and action.

Decision Making Based on Problems Involving Acid–Base Imbalances

Because a substantial number of CSE cases usually involve disturbances in acid–base balance, you need to be proficient both in blood gas interpretation and in the management of these disturbances. **Table 19-14** provides a basic summary of the problems and appropriate actions indicated for the most common acid–base imbalances you will see on the CSE. For example, besides identifying the presence of an acute metabolic acidosis in a patient with shock-like symptoms, you would need to know that this condition likely is a lactic acidosis and that measures to improve tissue oxygenation need to be implemented, including providing a high F_{IO_2} and improving cardiac output.

Decision Making Based on Problems Involving Disturbances of Oxygenation

When responding to blood gas data, we strongly recommend that you assess oxygenation separately from acid–base balance and ventilation. In this regard, recognizing the presence of hypoxemia represents only part of the needed task in a CSE case. You must then identify the basic pathophysiologic cause of the low P_{O_2} or saturation and treat it accordingly, as outlined in **Table 19-15**. To

Table 19-12 Basic Decision Making Based on Physical Assessment Findings

Information Gathering	Analysis (Likely Problems)	Decision Making/Action
Wheezing	Bronchospasm	Bronchodilator therapy
	CHF	Diuretics, positive inotropes*
Inspiratory stridor	Laryngeal edema	Cool mist/racemic epinephrine
	Tumor/mass	Bronchoscopy*
Rhonchi/tactile fremitus	Secretions in large airways	Bronchial hygiene therapy, suctioning
Dull percussion note, bronchial breath sounds	Infiltrates, atelectasis, consolidation	Lung expansion therapy, O_2 therapy
Opacity on chest x-ray	Infiltrates, atelectasis, consolidation	Lung expansion therapy, O_2 therapy
Hyperresonant percussion	Pneumothorax	Evacuate air*/lung expansion therapy
Dull percussion	Pleural effusion	Evacuate fluid*/lung expansion therapy
*Actions you would recommend.		

Table 19-13 Basic Decision Making for Problems with Secretions or Airway Clearance

Information Gathering	Analysis (Likely Problems)	Decision Making/Action
Weak cough	Poor secretion clearance	Bronchial hygiene therapy, suctioning
Amount: more than 30 mL/day	Excessive secretions	Bronchial hygiene therapy, suctioning
Yellow/opaque sputum	Acute airway infection	Treat underlying cause, antibiotic therapy*
Frothy secretions	Pulmonary edema	Treat underlying cause (CHF*), PAP therapy (CPAP/BiPAP), O_2 therapy
*Actions you would recommend.		

Table 19-14 Basic Decision Making for Acid–Base Imbalance

Information Gathering	Analysis (Likely Problems)	Decision Making/Action
$\downarrow pH = \dfrac{\rightarrow HCO_3^-}{\uparrow PaCO_2}$	Acute ventilatory failure (acute respiratory acidosis)	Mechanical ventilation*
$\rightarrow pH = \dfrac{\uparrow HCO_3^-}{\uparrow PaCO_2}$	Chronic ventilatory failure (compensated respiratory acidosis, as in COPD)	Low-flow O_2, bronchial hygiene therapy; if worsens $\Rightarrow$ NPPV*; avoid intubation if possible
$\uparrow pH = \dfrac{\uparrow HCO_3^-}{\rightarrow PaCO_2}$	Acute metabolic alkalosis	Hypokalemia $\Rightarrow$ give potassium* Hypochloremia $\Rightarrow$ give chloride*
$\downarrow pH = \dfrac{\downarrow HCO_3^-}{\rightarrow PaCO_2}$	Acute metabolic acidosis	Increase ventilation (temporary); if lactic acidosis $\Rightarrow$ give O_2 and restore perfusion; treat underlying cause*
$\uparrow$ = increased; $\downarrow$ = decreased; $\rightarrow$ normal/unchanged.		
*Actions you would recommend.		

Table 19-15 Basic Decision Making for Oxygenation Disturbances

Information Gathering	Analysis (Likely Problems)	Decision Making/Action
$Pa_{O_2} > 60$ torr $F_{IO_2} < 0.60$	Moderate hypoxemia (V/Q imbalance)	O_2 therapy Treat underlying cause*
$Pa_{O_2} < 60$ torr $F_{IO_2} > 0.60$	Severe hypoxemia (pulmonary shunting)	O_2 therapy, PEEP/CPAP Treat underlying cause*
*Actions you would recommend.		

that end greater we teach the 60/60 rule: If the Pao_2 is greater than 60 torr on less than 60% O_2, the likely problem is a V/Q imbalance, which usually responds well to simple O_2 therapy. In contrast, if the arterial Po_2 is less than 60 torr on more than 60% O_2, the likely problem is a physiologic shunt, which in addition to supplemental O_2 will require either PEEP or CPAP.

PACING YOURSELF WHEN TAKING THE CSE

Our last suggestion is the simplest: You need to pace yourself to ensure that you can complete all of CSE cases in the available time. In our experience, candidates who do not complete all CSE problems are destined to fail. Based on the number of problems (11–12) currently included on the CSE and the exam time limit of 4 hours, you should spend, on average, no more than 20 minutes on each problem. However, because problems vary in complexity, our best advice for the current CSE is to ensure completion of at least three problems every hour.[*]

SUMMARY GUIDANCE AND NEXT STEPS

To succeed on the NBRC CSE exam, you need to be proficient in the management of a broad variety of cases that RTs can encounter in clinical practice. In addition to good knowledge of disease management, you need to apply a consistent reasoning process as you progress through each section of your CSE problems:

1. *Gather* the information most consistent with the situation at hand.
2. *Analyze* the information to identify the likely problem and current patient status.
3. *Decide* on the action(s) most likely to resolve the identified problem.

Consistent application of this process will help boost both your scores, increasing your likelihood of passing the CSE and obtaining your RRT credential.

Your next steps? Apply what you have learned here by completing the seven practice problems available online at the accompanying Jones & Bartlett Learning website (see Appendix D for details). These practice problems are designed to give you experience with the CSE format and to help you apply the case management and CSE test-taking skills reviewed here and in Chapter 18. If your score poorly on any individual practice problem or consistently have difficulty with either information gathering or decision making, we recommend you review this chapter's guidance and the corresponding disease management "pearls" provided in Chapter 20. In addition, you may want to access and review the supplemental disease management resources we provide, also accessible via the Jones & Bartlett Learning website. Then retake the applicable practice problem until you achieve passing scores for both information gathering and decision making. Only after gaining confidence with the CSE format and demonstrating good disease management and case-reasoning skills should you schedule your CSE session.

---

[*]With the larger number of problems being included on the CSE starting in 2015, you will likely need to maintain a pace of about *five cases per hour* to ensure exam completion within the 4-hour time limit.

CHAPTER 20

Clinical Simulation Exam Case Management Pearls

Craig L. Scanlan, Narciso E. Rodriguez, and Albert J. Heuer

As emphasized in Chapters 18 and 19, success on the NBRC Clinical Simulation Examination (CSE) requires proficiency in case management. In the NBRC "hospital," respiratory therapists (RTs) are expected to be broadly experienced in managing a large variety of disorders, including those affecting various organ systems and patient age categories, as well as different levels of acuity.

Although it is impossible to cover every disorder that RTs might encounter on the CSE, this chapter aims to assist candidates in reviewing management of the most common problems. We do so using the basic NBRC CSE disease categories as the organizing principle. In each category, we present those disorders we believe are most likely to appear on the CSE. For each disorder, we then provide "pearls" or valuable pointers covering both the essential elements of assessment and information gathering needed to evaluate the typical case and the currently recommended treatments or decisions required to achieve successful outcomes.

Careful review of these management pearls, in combination with applicable online resources accompanying this book, will provide a strong foundation for your success on the CSE.

CHRONIC OBSTRUCTIVE PULMONARY DISEASE

Chronic obstructive pulmonary disease (COPD) encompasses several disease entities, all characterized by chronic, progressive airway obstruction that is not fully reversible with treatment. Airway obstruction is caused by inflammation due to inhalation of noxious particles or gases, especially tobacco smoke.

Assessment/Information Gathering

The primary disease entities categorized as COPD are emphysema and chronic bronchitis. Emphysema is defined in pathologic terms as irreversible destruction of the alveolar walls causing enlargement of the distal air spaces, collapse of the small airways, air trapping, and hyperinflation. Chronic bronchitis is defined by its symptoms—that is, a productive cough for at least 3 months per year for at least 2 years. Although most patients with COPD exhibit elements of both disorders, some key characteristics differentiate patients with a primary diagnosis of emphysema from those suffering mainly from chronic bronchitis (**Table 20-1**).

Treatment/Decision Making

Because the underlying disease process cannot be reversed, treatment of stable COPD aims to increase patients' life expectancy and quality of life, while also decreasing complications and exacerbations requiring hospitalization. To do so requires a comprehensive approach that includes disease management education and smoking cessation (Chapter 7), pulmonary rehabilitation (Chapter 17), and avoidance of recurrent infections via immunization against influenza and pneumococcal pneumonia. As indicated in **Table 20-2**, additional treatment is "stepped up" according to the stage of disease progression and the worsening of symptoms. Note that neither mucolytics nor routine use of antibiotics are recommended to manage stable COPD, even in its advanced stages.

Screening criteria for lung volume reduction surgery (LVRS) in advanced-stage emphysema include the following:
* Severe disability despite maximal medical treatment
* Primary upper lobe involvement (confirmed by CT scan)

- $FEV_1 \leq 45\%$ predicted, RV $\geq 150\%$ predicted, DLco > 20% predicted
- $Paco_2$ < 60 torr and Pao_2 > 45 torr (room air)
- $Spo_2 \geq 90\%$ on < 6 L/min O_2
- 6MWD < 140 m (Chapter 2)
- Absence of significant cardiovascular comorbidities

Table 20-1 Emphysema Versus Chronic Bronchitis

Characteristic	Emphysema	Chronic Bronchitis
Age	More than 50 years old	More than 35 years old
Cough	Late; scanty sputum	Early; copious mucopurulent sputum
Dyspnea	Severe, early	Mild, late
Appearance	Thin and cachectic; barrel chest (elevated ribs), accessory muscle use at rest	Normal weight or obese; cyanotic, peripheral edema, jugular venous distension
Chest exam	↓ breath sounds, hyperresonant to percussion, ↓ diaphragm excursion	Rhonchi, wheezing
X-ray	Hyperinflation, small heart, flattened diaphragm, ↑ A-P diameter on lateral film	Prominent vessels, large heart (↑ CT ratio)
Spirometry	FEV_1/FVC ($FEV_1\%$) < 70% after bronchodilator therapy	FEV_1/FVC ($FEV_1\%$) < 70% after bronchodilator therapy
Lung volumes	Increased RV, TLC	Increased RV
Airway resistance	Increased (small airways)	Increased (large airways)
Compliance	Increased	Normal
DLco	Decreased	Normal
Arterial blood gases	Mild hypoxemia; may have normal $Paco_2$	Chronic respiratory acidosis with moderate hypoxemia
Other lab tests	Decreased α_1-antitrypsin*	Polycythemia

*Evident in less than 1% of COPD patients; should be assessed if emphysema appears at a young age (45 years or younger) or without history of smoking.

Table 20-2 COPD Treatment Approaches by Severity Stage

Stage I: Mild	Stage II: Moderate	Stage III: Severe	Stage IV: Very Severe
Diagnostic/Prognostic Criteria			
• FEV_1/FVC < 70% • FEV1 ≥ 80% predicted	• FEV1/FVC < 70% • FEV1 = 50–79% predicted • SOB on exertion	• FEV_1/FVC < 70% • FEV_1 = 30–49% predicted • SOB on exertion • Frequent exacerbations	• FEV_1/FVC < 70% • FEV_1 < 30% predicted *or* • FEV_1 < 50% predicted + chronic respiratory failure
"Stepped" Treatment Approaches *(All stages should include disease management education, smoking cessation, pulmonary rehabilitation, and influenza and pneumococcal vaccination)*			
• SABA or inhaled anticholinergic (e.g., tiotropium) PRN	• Regular use of LABA • Consider combined LABA + long-acting anticholinergic	• Add inhaled steroids if frequent exacerbations • Consider combining steroid + LABA (e.g., fluticasone + salmeterol)	• Add long-term O_2 therapy (Chapter 17) if justified • Consider lung volume reduction surgery (emphysema only)

SABA = short-acting β-agonist; LABA = long-acting β-agonist.

In the event of a patient requiring emergency treatment for an acute exacerbation of COPD, the following guidelines apply:

- Provide supplemental O_2 to maintain Pao_2 at 60–65 torr or Spo_2 at 88–92%
- Recommend increasing the beta-agonist dose
- Recommend adding an inhaled anticholinergic (if not already prescribed)
- Recommend initiating IV aminophylline if there is an inadequate response to inhaled agents
- Recommend systemic steroids
- Recommend antibiotic therapy if secretions are copious and purulent
- Recommend noninvasive ventilation (NPPV) if the patient deteriorates despite aggressive management and exhibits worsening respiratory acidosis with decreased level of consciousness

TRAUMA

Regardless of the specific injury, all trauma management begins with efforts to secure the airway and restore and maintain adequate perfusion, ventilation, and oxygenation using the appropriate basic and advanced life support protocols. All trauma patients initially should receive 100% O_2 via nonrebreathing mask, bag-valve-mask, or advanced airway. Simultaneous rapid assessment of the victim should quickly reveal the specific type of injuries sustained and direct the additional management needed beyond the initial resuscitation stage.

Chest Trauma

Chest trauma may result from either penetrating or blunt injury. Penetrating chest trauma most commonly is due to knife or gunshot wounds. In penetrating trauma, injury can occur to *any* thoracic structure. In addition to specific structural damage, bleeding can cause hemothorax or hemopericardium, and air leakage can result in pneumothorax or pneumopericardium. "Sucking" chest wounds initially should be covered with an occlusive dressing (e.g., Vaseline gauze pad) to permit adequate ventilation and help prevent tension pneumothorax. Definitive treatment of penetrating chest trauma always involves surgical repair.

Most blunt chest trauma occurs in motor vehicle accidents (MVAs). Other causes of blunt chest trauma include falls, sports injuries, crush injuries, and explosions. The injuries seen in blunt chest trauma are caused primarily by the rapid deceleration that occurs with direct impact or blow to the thorax. **Table 20-3** summarizes the various ribcage, pulmonary, and cardiac injuries that can occur with blunt chest trauma, their key clinical findings, primary diagnostic tests, and basic treatment options.

As outlined in Table 20-3, the general management of blunt chest trauma varies according to the type of injury. Respiratory management pearls follow.

Assessment/Information Gathering

- Because the full effects of pulmonary contusion may not be apparent for 24–48 hours, patients should be admitted and closely monitored, especially for worsening hypoxemia (approximately 50% of these patients develop ARDS).
- Recommend diagnostic tests according to type of trauma (Table 20-3); in addition, recommend CBC, hemoglobin, hematocrit (to assess for blood loss or hemodilution), coagulation tests, and ABGs.
- *Do not* recommend an initial chest x-ray or CT scan if there are clear signs of tension pneumothorax; instead, recommend immediate treatment via needle decompression or tube thoracostomy (Chapter 16). Then and only then should the patient undergo imaging.
- Fractures of the lower "floating" ribs (11–12) may be associated with diaphragmatic tears and trauma to the liver or spleen; recommend abdominal ultrasound (for hemoperitoneum) and CT scan (to assess organ damage).

Treatment/Decision Making

- Indications for ET intubation in chest trauma patients include apnea, profound shock, and inadequate ventilation.

Table 20-3 Summary of Blunt Chest Trauma

Injury	Clinical Findings	Diagnosis	Treatment
Ribcage Injuries			
Fractured ribs, sternum	Pain, tenderness, and crepitus at fracture sites; inspiratory pain	CXR	Epidural analgesia
Flail chest (flail segment)	Fracture site/inspiratory pain, paradoxical chest motion (in with inspiration/out with expiration); dyspnea, tachypnea	CXR	Epidural analgesia, surgical fixation
Airway/Pulmonary Injuries			
Laryngeal or tracheal crush injury/fractures	Severe respiratory distress with stridor, inability to speak	Bronchoscopy	Cricothyrotomy, tracheotomy, surgical repair
Pulmonary contusion	Dyspnea, tachypnea, tachycardia, crackles, hypoxemia (may be delayed)	CXR, CT scan	Supplemental O_2, PEEP/CPAP
Pneumothorax	Dyspnea, inspiratory pain *If tension*: cyanosis, tachypnea, tachycardia, hypotension, pulsus paradoxus, ↓ breath sounds and hyperresonance on affected side; mediastinal shift *away* from affected side	Clinical findings, CXR, CT scan (imaging to follow treatment if tension pneumothorax)	Needle decompression, tube thoracostomy (chest tubes)
Hemothorax	↓ breath sounds and dullness to percussion on affected side; signs of shock	CXR, thoracic US	Tube thoracostomy (chest tubes)
Cardiac Injuries			
Myocardial contusion	Dysrhythmias (e.g., tachycardia); accumulation of pericardial fluid	CXR, 12-lead ECG, serum troponin, cardiac echo	Antiarrhythmic agents, pericardial drainage, surgery
Pericardial tamponade	Hypotension, ↓ heart sounds, and distended jugular veins (Beck's triad); tachycardia	CXR, 12-lead ECG, serum troponin, cardiac echo, thoracic US	Pericardiocentesis, IV fluids, inotropic agents; *avoid positive-pressure ventilation*
Aortic tear	Shock; skin above nipple line is normal, but below is pale, cold, or clammy; carotid/radial pulses stronger than femoral pulse	CXR, CT scan, cardiac echo	Surgical repair
Ruptured myocardium	Profound shock	CXR, cardiac echo	Surgical repair
Commotio cordis	Sudden cardiac arrest due to blow to the precordial region	History	Early CPR and rapid defibrillation
CT = computed tomography; CXR = chest x-ray; ECG = electrocardiogram; US = ultrasound.			

- Recommend epidural analgesia for ribcage fracture pain; epidurals allow painless deep breathing and coughing without depressing respiration.
- Adjunctive measures to recommend in the care of patients with chest trauma include early mobilization and aggressive bronchial hygiene therapy (to prevent pneumonia).
- *Do not* recommend steroids for treatment of pulmonary contusion.
- Only recommend mechanical ventilation to correct abnormal gas exchange (with pulmonary contusion)—*not* to treat chest wall instability (flail chest).
  - Intubation and A/C or SIMV with PEEP is the standard approach.
  - Recommend a trial of mask CPAP or BiPAP for the alert, compliant patient with marginal respiratory status.

○ Apply NHLBI ARDS protocol if ALI/ARDS develops (Chapter 10).
○ Recommend HFOV for patients failing A/C or SIMV with PEEP (Chapter 10).
○ Recommend independent lung ventilation for patients with severe unilateral contusion if (1) severe shunting persists or (2) "cross-over" bleeding is affecting the good lung.

Head Trauma (Traumatic Brain Injury)

Trauma to the brain causes hemorrhage and edema. In "closed head" traumatic brain injury (TBI), tissue swelling and blood pooling increase intracranial pressure (ICP). When the ICP rises above 15 to 20 mm Hg, cerebral blood flow can decrease, resulting in a secondary ischemia. Prolonged cerebral ischemia causes brain death. The general goal in managing head trauma, therefore, is to avoid secondary injury by preserving cerebral blood flow. Respiratory management pearls follow.

Assessment/Information Gathering

- Your initial assessment should include airway patency, SpO_2, level of consciousness, ability to communicate, and pupil size and reactivity.
- To help avoid hypercapnia, continuous capnography (expired CO_2) monitoring should be implemented if available.
- Use the Glasgow Coma Scale (Chapter 2) to categorize the injury as being mild (score 14 or 15), moderate (9 to 13), or severe (8 or less).
- Assess for other related injuries (see the sections on chest and spinal cord injuries) and hemodynamic stability/shock.
- Note that Cheyne-Stokes breathing and slow/irregular respirations are common in TBI.
- Recognize the signs of a potentially life-threatening hematoma: hemiparesis or aphasia, unequal and/or sluggish pupillary responses, progressive decline in mental status, and coma.

Treatment/Decision Making

- Initial emergency management
  ○ Recommend that a cervical collar be kept in place until the patient is evaluated for spinal cord damage.
  ○ Initially provide 100% O_2 via nonrebreathing mask, bag-valve-mask, or advanced airway to keep SpO_2 above 95%, *while maintaining the patient's head and neck in a neutral position.*
  ○ If providing ventilation, initially aim to keep the $PaCO_2$ between 35 and 40 torr (normocapnia).
  ○ Recommend fluid resuscitation and vasopressors to keep mean arterial pressure (MAP) greater than 75 mm Hg.
  ○ Recommend IV mannitol or hypertonic saline if the patient exhibits posturing and unequal or nonreactive pupils.
  ○ If the Glasgow Coma Scale score is 8 or less, or if the patient is unable to protect the airway, recommend rapid-sequence intubation (Chapter 16); if oral/nasal intubation is not possible due to airway trauma, recommend cricothyrotomy or tracheotomy.
  ○ If life-threatening hematoma is likely, recommend its surgical removal.
- Ongoing management/monitoring
  ○ Recommend continuous monitoring of arterial BP (via A-line), ICP, and SpO_2; the goal is to keep ICP less than 20 mm Hg and cerebral perfusion pressure (CPP) at 60 mm Hg or higher (CPP = MAP − ICP).
  ○ Recommend vasopressors (e.g., norepinephrine) to maintain MAP/CPP as needed.
  ○ To help lower ICP, recommend:
    - Elevating the head of the bed 30–40°
    - Sedating the patient with a benzodiazepine or propofol (Chapter 16)
  ○ Recommend osmotherapy (mannitol/hypertonic saline) and/or ventricular drainage to decrease ICP.
  ○ Recommend an anticonvulsant (e.g., phenytoin) if seizures are a problem.

- ○ Recommend neuromuscular blockade, high-dose barbiturate coma, or decompressive craniectomy if ICP remains high.
- ○ Do *not* recommend high-dose steroids (they do not improve survival).
- If mechanical ventilation is required:
  - ○ Aim to achieve $Paco_2$ of 35–40 torr, PIP ≤ 30 cm H_2O, Spo_2 > 95%, and good patient–ventilator synchrony.
  - ○ Avoid hypercapnia (causes cerebral vasodilation and increases ICP).
  - ○ Avoid high levels of PEEP (can decrease MAP, increase ICP, and decrease CPP).
  - ○ Avoid prophylactic/routine hyperventilation (lowers ICP but can cause cerebral ischemia). Consider only in the following circumstances:
    - To lessen ICP increases prior to procedures such as suctioning
    - In the presence of confirmed cerebral herniation
    - As salvage therapy when high ICP does not respond to standard treatment
  - ○ If neuromuscular blockade has been implemented, implement a strict management protocol to ensure support should ventilator disconnection or failure occur.

Spinal Cord Injuries

Spinal cord injury (SCI) is seen most often in motor vehicle accidents, falls, gunshot wounds, and sporting mishaps. Cord neurons may suffer destruction from direct trauma; compression by bone fragments, disk material, edema, or hematoma; or ischemia from interruption of blood flow.

There are two broad classes of SCI: tetraplegia and paraplegia. Tetraplegia involves injury to the cord's cervical segments (C1–C7) and partial or complete loss of muscle function in all four extremities. Injuries resulting in paraplegia occur lower in the cord (thoracic, lumbar, or sacral segments), causing loss of motor and/or sensory function in the lower limbs and trunk. Tetraplegia and paraplegia can be further classified as being complete (no sensory or motor function below the injury) or incomplete (preservation of some sensory or motor function).

In general, the higher the level of injury, the greater its effect on respiration. Patients with injuries above the C3 level suffer damage to the nerves innervating the respiratory muscles and, therefore, typically require some form of artificial ventilatory support. Mid-cervical injuries (C3–C5) may leave some nerves intact and allow the patient to breathe without ventilatory support, at least some of the time. Patients suffering injuries below the C5 level may be able to breathe on their own, but can experience a reduced vital capacity and inability to effectively cough and clear secretions. Cervical cord injuries also can cause loss of autonomic function, resulting in *neurogenic shock* and the accompanying signs of hypotension, vasodilation, bradycardia, and hypothermia.

The full impact of a SCI may not be immediately apparent. After the initial insult, edema, bleeding, or ischemia can gradually cause worsening of the injury, in some cases progressing in severity from incomplete to complete. Such secondary damage (if not treated) also can cause the injury level to rise one or two cervical segments in the hours to days following the initial trauma.

As with all trauma management, initial efforts require rapid stabilization of the patient with concurrent assessment for the specific type and extent of injury. Additional respiratory management pearls follow.

Assessment/Information Gathering

- Conduct assessment only when you are sure the patient's head, neck, and spine are immobilized and maintained in a neutral position.
- Continuous pulse oximetry *and* end-tidal CO_2 (capnometry) monitoring should be implemented for all patients having severe SCI.
- Carefully evaluate airway patency, respiratory rate, chest and abdominal movement, and presence of chest wall or head injuries (approximately 1 in 4 patients with SCI also has head trauma). *If apnea is present, assume complete high cervical injury and immediately initiate manual ventilation.*
- Determine by recent history and observation if the patient was under the influence of drugs or intoxicated with alcohol (can mimic SCI or mask some neurologic findings).

- Recommend measurement of pulse, blood pressure, and core temperature to detect hypotension and differentiate among causes of shock:
  - Shock is likely *neurogenic* if the patient has an injury above T6 with bradycardia and hypothermia (the patient's skin may also be flushed, warm, and dry due to vasodilation).
  - Shock is likely *hemorrhagic* if the patient has an injury at or below T6 with tachycardia and normal core temperature (extremities may be cold and clammy with pallor or acrocyanosis evident).
- Recommend ABG, CBC, hemoglobin and/or hematocrit (for blood loss); chemistry panel, coagulation profile, blood lactate and base deficit (to assess for shock); and toxicology screen (to differentiate drug-related CNS effects).
- For any patient with cervical pain or neurologic deficit (and in all elderly patients admitted with suspected neck injury), recommend CT scan or standard AP, lateral, and *odontoid* neck x-rays (the odontoid beam is directed through the open mouth to assess the C1 area).
- Recommend MRI (1) if CT/x-ray is negative but the clinical picture supports cord damage or (2) to assess for soft-tissue "non-osseous" injuries such as hemorrhage and hematoma.
- Recommend bladder catheterization and I/O monitoring to help assess the patient's circulatory status and relieve the complications of urinary retention (often seen in neurogenic shock).
- After any needed resuscitation, recommend evaluation of the patient's sensory response (to touch + pin prick) and motor strength (limb flexor/extensor muscles) using a standardized assessment tool.
- After stabilization, if the patient is conscious and exhibits spontaneous respirations, recommend assessment of respiratory muscle function via measurement of VC and MIP/NIF.

Treatment/Decision Making

Treatment of SCI involves at least two phases: the immediate acute postinjury phase (typically in the ED and ICU) and a subsequent chronic phase of lifelong care.

Acute Phase

- The patient initially should be immobilized and treated in the supine position; if repositioning is needed (e.g., to avoid aspiration), the patient should be carefully "log-rolled" so that the head, neck, and torso are turned as a unit.
- To further help avoid aspiration, recommend insertion of an NG tube.
- Initially provide 100% O_2 via nonrebreathing mask or manual resuscitator to keep SpO_2 above 95%, *while maintaining the patient's head and neck in a neutral position.*
- If the patient is agitated, combative, or fighting against restraints, recommend either a short-acting sedative/hypnotic (e.g., midazolam) or an antipsychotic (e.g., haloperidol or droperidol).
- Airway management:
  - Maintain the cervical spine in neutral alignment at all times.
  - To maintain airway patency and prevent aspiration, keep the oropharynx clear of secretions; however, avoid vigorous suctioning that could cause gagging, retching, or bradycardia.
  - If ET intubation is indicated, recommend either fiberoptic intubation or rapid-sequence orotracheal intubation with manual in-line stabilization (Chapter 16).
  - Be prepared for severe bradycardia from unopposed vagal stimulation during intubation; preoxygenation and IV atropine or topical lidocaine spray can minimize this response.
- If the patient is likely to remain ventilator-dependent, recommend a tracheotomy early in the hospitalization period.
- Because patients with SCI are at high risk for aspiration and pneumonia, initiate a rigorous VAP protocol for those receiving mechanical ventilation (Chapter 5).
- Management of shock:
  - Recommend fluid resuscitation and vasopressors, with the goal being a systolic BP greater than 85–90 mm Hg with a normal heat rate (60–100/min) and rhythm.
  - Recommend atropine to treat significant bradycardia.

- ° For a patient in neurogenic shock, recommend vasopressors that include beta stimulation such as dopamine or norepinephrine (pure α-adrenergic agents such as phenylephrine can worsen bradycardia).
- Recommend external rewarming or warm, humidified O_2 to treat hypothermia.
- In some SCI protocols, administration of high doses of methylprednisolone within 8 hours of the initial injury is considered an option; if this choice is offered as a recommendation on the CSE, select it.

Chronic Phase

In the chronic phase of SCI management, the goals are to prevent atelectasis and pneumonia, liberate the patient from full-time ventilatory support, and enhance the quality of life. The following chronic phase guidelines apply mainly to those patients who retain some respiratory muscle function:

- Ensure that a comprehensive discharge plan addresses needed home modifications, caregiver training, medical equipment and assistive technologies, emergency provisions (e.g., backup generator), transportation needs, avocational and recreational activities, and supportive community resources.
- For ventilator-dependent SCI patients, recommend large tidal volumes (up to 1.0 L) to relieve the common sensation of dyspnea that these patients experience.
- To facilitate speech for a ventilator-dependent patient with a trach who has good secretion control, deflate the cuff and either attach a one-way speaking valve (Chapter 4) or increase the tidal volume.
- For patients likely to require long-term ventilatory support, recommend a trial of noninvasive ventilation (positive or negative pressure) or diaphragmatic pacing.
- To help avoid atelectasis and promote at least part-time liberation from mechanical ventilation, implement inspiratory muscle training (Chapter 10).
- Recommend an abdominal binder to improve diaphragmatic function (properly positioned binders facilitate chest expansion by increasing the zone of apposition between the diaphragm and ribcage).
- Teach patients with an intact upper airway glossopharyngeal or "frog" breathing (breathing by repetitive swallowing of mouthfuls of air).
- To facilitate coughing and secretion removal, implement or teach caregivers to apply the "quad cough" technique or use mechanical insufflation–exsufflation (Chapter 9).
- Because sleep-disordered breathing is a common complication of SCI, recommend either an in-home or laboratory polysomnography exam for symptomatic patients.

Burns/Smoke Inhalation

Burns are among the most devastating and complex forms of trauma. Most burns are due to flame exposure, with burns due to hot liquids (scalding) being the next most common. Less common are burns caused by electrical current and chemicals.

The severity of a burn and the patient's likelihood of survival are determined by the percentage of body surface area (BSA) affected and the burn depth. Percent BSA is estimated using either the standardized Lund and Browder chart or the "Rule of Nines" (adult head 9%, each arm 9%, each leg 18%, front and rear torso 18% each). Burn depth can be either partial thickness (not extending through all skin layers) or full thickness (extending through all skin layers into the subcutaneous tissues). Partial-thickness burns are further categorized as superficial (affecting the epidermis only), superficial dermal (extending into the upper dermal layers), or deep dermal (extending deeper into the dermal layers, but not completely through the skin).

In general, a severe burn is one extending into or through the dermis and covering more than 25–30% BSA. In patients who experience such burns, the release of cytokines and other inflammatory mediators from the burn site can cause body-wide/systemic effects. Cardiovascular changes include increased capillary permeability, with massive loss of both fluid and protein into the interstitial space. Vasoconstriction occurs in both the peripheral circulation and the gut, along with a decrease in heart contractility. If not immediately treated, these changes can result in "burn shock" and multiorgan failure.

In addition to these serious cardiovascular effects, major burns can increase the patient's metabolic rate by as much as threefold. Burns also impair a patient's immune response, increasing the likelihood of infection. Last, the body's release of pro-inflammatory mediators in a severe burn can indirectly affect the lungs, causing bronchoconstriction, pulmonary edema, and—in the worst case—ALI/ARDS.

Compounding this problem are *direct* inhalation injuries, which occur in as many as one-third of all serious burns. Inhalation injuries can include one or more of the following: (1) direct thermal damage to the upper airway from inhaling hot gases (thermal injury below the larynx is rare); (2) chemical injury to the lungs due to inhalation of toxic by-products of combustion found in smoke; and (3) damage to O_2 delivery and cellular O_2 utilization through exposure to carbon monoxide or hydrogen cyanide gas. Inhalation injuries significantly increase mortality over that predicted from cutaneous burns alone. Indeed, some estimates suggest that as many as 3 out of 4 deaths following major burns are due to inhalation injury.

Management of major burns proceeds through several phases, here referred to as the "four R's": resuscitation, resurfacing, rehabilitation, and reconstruction. Typically the full range of needed support throughout these four phases is provided in specialized burn centers. Most respiratory management occurs during the resuscitation phase, in which essential support is provided to vital organ systems to help ensure patient survival. Key management pearls during this phase follow.

Assessment/Information Gathering

- Recommend CBC, electrolytes, lactate, ABG, CO-oximetry, and a coagulation profile.
- Assess sensorium and coma level (Glasgow Coma Scale) if the patient is unresponsive.
- Recommend chest x-ray (may be negative early on).
- Monitor Spo_2, and watch for signs and symptoms of hypoxemia.
- Assess for signs of inhalation injury: facial/neck burns, singed nasal hairs, sooty sputum, dyspnea, cyanosis, hoarseness, coughing, and stridor (closed-space fire victims are most prone to inhalation injuries).
- Assess for signs and symptoms of cyanide (CN) poisoning: headache; confusion, seizures or coma, chest tightness, nausea/vomiting, mydriasis; dyspnea, tachypnea, hyperpnea, and either hypertension (early) or hypotension (late). Note also that blood lactate is typically high (≥ 8 mmol/L), indicating tissue hypoxia/anaerobic metabolism.
- Reevaluate the patient's airway and oxygenation status frequently (inhalation injuries may take several hours to develop).
- Because chest x-rays may not detect inhalation injuries, recommend fiberoptic bronchoscopy to assess airway damage.

Treatment/Decision Making

- Recommend covering the patient to prevent heat and fluid loss.
- Immediately administer as high an O_2 concentration as possible (via nonrebreathing mask or high-flow cannula) to all patients suspected of inhalation injury; thereafter titrate the oxygen level to maintain the Spo_2 above 90%.
- Recommend immediate IV access and fluid and electrolyte replacement therapy (a 70-kg patient may need 8–10 L or more over the first 24 hours following injury).
- Recommend urinary catheterization to help monitor fluid balance (the output goal is approximately 1.0 mL/kg/hr).
- Recommend morphine analgesia for severe pain; be on guard for respiratory depression.
- If the patient has electrical burns, recommend a 12-lead ECG and cardiac biomarkers.
- Circumferential full-thickness burns of the thorax greatly reduce chest-wall compliance; recommend prompt escharotomy (incision/removal of the charred dead tissue) to allow for effective ventilation.
- Patients with smoke inhalation should be admitted if they are hypoxemic ($Pao_2 < 60$ torr), have an HbCO greater than 15%, have metabolic acidosis, or are experiencing bronchospasm and/or painful or difficult swallowing.
- If %HbCO is greater than 25% with signs of neurologic or cardiac impairment, recommend hyperbaric oxygenation (at 3 ATA) if available.

- If cyanide poisoning is suspected, recommend immediate treatment with either hydroxocobalamin (also known as vitamin B_{12a} or "cyanokit") or sulfanegen TEA.
- If bronchospasm is present, recommend aerosolized bronchodilators, *N*-acetylcysteine (Mucomyst), and heparin (to prevent plugging from fibrin clots and cellular debris); accompany aerosol therapy with bronchial hygiene/airway clearance therapy appropriate to the patient's condition.
- Do *not* recommend prophylactic steroids or antibiotics for inhalation injuries (antibiotics should be used only when respiratory tract infection is suspected or confirmed).
- Patients should be referred to a burn center in the following circumstances:
  - Partial-thickness burns exceeding 10% BSA, full-thickness burns exceeding 5% BSA, or circumferential burns
  - Burns with associated inhalation injury
- Airway management
  - If airway injury is confirmed, recommend ET intubation; if the vocal cords are damaged or the patient is likely to require mechanical ventilation for more than 10–12 days, recommend tracheotomy.
  - In patients with neck/facial burns and airway edema, reintubation after accidental extubation can be very difficult. To avoid this problem:
    - Recommend adequate patient sedation to prevent self-extubation.
    - Properly secure the ET tube (may require stapling the tape to the patient's skin).
    - Be prepared with backup methods to secure the airway (e.g., LMA, cricothyrotomy).
  - To prevent acute ET tube obstruction from endobronchial debris, provide BTPS humidification and implement a rigorous bronchial hygiene/airway clearance protocol.
- Mechanical ventilation
  - Consider an initial trial of noninvasive ventilation for the burn patient with mild-to-moderate respiratory distress but no major inhalation injury or facial burns.
  - Apply active humidification (*not* an HME) to minimize insensible water loss and prevent tube occlusion.
  - Use high minute volumes to accommodate high metabolic rates (best achieved via high rates as opposed to high VT); accept mild-to-moderate respiratory acidosis to prevent compounding the pulmonary injury.
  - If acute hypoxemic respiratory failure develops (P/F ratio < 300 and bilateral diffuse infiltrates on x-ray consistent with pulmonary edema), apply the NHLBI ARDS protocol for ventilator management (Chapter 10).
  - Rigorously apply the VAP protocol to minimize the likelihood of pneumonia (acute bacterial invasion peaks at 2–3 days after inhalation injury).
- Weaning/extubation
  - Recognize that staged excisions and skin grafting procedures can delay weaning for days or weeks.
  - Recommend inhaled racemic epinephrine for patients who develop mild stridor after extubation; if stridor is more severe, consider noninvasive ventilation or heliox therapy.

Hypothermia

Hypothermia occurs whenever exposure to cold causes a drop in core body temperature to less than 35°C (95°F). Although classically associated with outdoor activities occurring in winter months, nearly half of all hypothermia deaths occur in the elderly, with homeless people, drug/alcohol abusers, and mentally ill individuals also being at high risk.

Depending on core body temperature, hypothermia can be classified as being mild, moderate, or severe. **Table 20-4** differentiates among these levels of hypothermia and their typical clinical findings.

Key management pearls for patients admitted with accidental hypothermia follow.

Assessment/Information Gathering

- Assess the patient for pulse and respirations using standard BLS techniques (both may be slow or difficult to detect); if there are no signs of life, immediately begin CPR.

Table 20-4 Levels of Hypothermia and Typical Clinical Findings

Severity	Core Temperature	Common Clinical Findings
Mild	32–35°C (90–95°F)	Tachypnea, tachycardia, increased BP, confusion, ataxia, dysarthria, shivering, excessive diuresis
Moderate	28–32°C (82–90°F)	Reduced RR, HR, CO, and consciousness; hallucinations; mydriasis; loss of shivering and airway protection
Severe	<28°C (<82°F)	Coma, areflexia, apnea (<24°C), pulmonary edema, oliguria, hypotension, bradycardia, ventricular arrhythmias, asystole (<20°C)
BP = blood pressure; RR = respiratory rate; HR = heart rate; CO = cardiac output.		

- Quickly gather an immediate past history to confirm cold exposure as the precipitating event and rule out other possibilities (e.g., severe intoxication/drug overdose, stroke, brain trauma).
- Recommend measurement of the patient's *core* temperature using a low-temperature probe placed in the esophagus, bladder, or rectum (for accuracy, rectal probes must not be placed in stool).
- Recommend electrolytes (K^+ levels are critical), glucose (to rule out hypoglycemia as the cause), BUN and creatinine (to assess renal function), creatine phosphokinase (to assess for diffuse cellular injury), a coagulation panel (hypothermia inhibits blood coagulation), and a blood alcohol and drug screen.
- Obtain and monitor SpO_2, but note that peripheral vasoconstriction may affect the accuracy of digital probe data—consider using an ear or forehead probe instead.
- Obtain an ABG and assess and apply the values *uncorrected* for temperature (i.e., ventilation should be adjusted to maintain an *uncorrected* pH of 7.40).
- Recommend continuous ECG monitoring (which may show prolonged PR, QRS, and QT intervals, and atrial or ventricular arrhythmias); however, unless VF, VT, or asystole is confirmed, treat the patient according to his or her perfusion status rather than the ECG results, as PEA is a common finding.
- Recommend a chest x-ray (to assess for aspiration pneumonia and pulmonary edema, both of which may be seen in accidental hypothermia).
- Recommend urinary catheterization to monitor fluid balance and assess renal sufficiency.
- Try to minimize patient manipulation, because extensive movement and invasive monitoring can cause cardiac arrhythmias.

Treatment/Decision Making

- Remove any wet clothing, dry the skin, and cover the patient with warm blankets.
- If there are no signs of life, immediately initiate CPR and continue it until the patient has been rewarmed to at least 32–34°C (death should never be declared until after assessing the patient's response to rewarming).
- Provide warm supplemental O_2 sufficient to maintain an SpO_2 above 90% (use either a heated nebulizer with an aerosol mask or high-flow nasal cannula for this purpose).
- If the patient is unresponsive or in cardiopulmonary arrest, insert an oral ET tube and provide ventilation, ideally with warm (40–42°C), humidified O_2 (intubation also helps prevent aspiration); monitor the ECG during intubation because patients with hypothermia are prone to cardiac arrhythmias.
- For patients with VF, VT, or PEA, recommend or implement the applicable ACLS protocol *concurrent with efforts to increase core body temperature* (discussed later in this section); the likelihood of success is greatest when the patient's core temperature is above 30°C.
- Recommend concurrent rewarming appropriate to the severity of hypothermia and the patient's perfusion status:
  - *Mild/moderate hypothermia with a perfusing rhythm*: recommend passive external warming (e.g., warm blankets).

- *Severe hypothermia with a perfusing rhythm*: recommend either active external warming (e.g., forced heated air, heat lamps, or other surface-warming devices) or (better) active internal rewarming using IV solutions heated to 40–42°C, gastric lavage with warm isotonic solutions (no more than 45°C), and heated, humidified O_2 (40–42°C). To avoid aspiration, gastric lavage should not be recommended unless the patient is intubated.
  - *Severe hypothermia and cardiac arrest*: recommend cardiopulmonary bypass if available. If it is not available, recommend hemodialysis, thoracic/pleural lavage with warm isotonic solutions, or full-body immersion in warm water, such as via a Hubbard tank (full-body immersion is obviously not feasible during ACLS protocols).
- If the patient is hypotensive (commonly due to vasodilation), recommend (warmed) IV fluids and, as needed, vasopressors to elevate and maintain blood pressure.
- For patients who were pulseless, upon return of spontaneous circulation (ROSC), recommend continued rewarming to a core temperature of 32–34°C (maintained according to standard ACLS postarrest guidelines).
- For patients requiring mechanical ventilation:
  - Use active, heated humidification, *not* an HME; if the humidifier temperature can be altered, set it to 42–45°C. Note that this method provides only modest rewarming and should never be used alone.
  - Adjust minute ventilation to achieve a normal pH (7.35–7.45) using values uncorrected for the patient's core temperature (i.e., measured at the standard 37°C).
  - Recognize that hypothermia shifts the oxyhemoglobin dissociation curve to the left, increasing the affinity of hemoglobin for O_2 and thus impairing tissue oxygen extraction; this effect is overcome with rewarming but can be mitigated by ensuring that the F_{IO_2} is sufficient to keep the Sp_{O_2} above 90%.
  - If the patient also suffers from aspiration pneumonia (most commonly seen with hypothermia associated with alcohol intoxication/drug overdose), follow the guidelines included here for case management of drug overdose.

CARDIOVASCULAR DISEASE

The NBRC expects candidates to be proficient in the management of common cardiovascular disorders, including congestive heart failure, coronary artery disease (CAD), and valvular heart disease. Because CAD and valvular disorders often involve surgical intervention, you also need to understand the perioperative management of patients undergoing coronary artery bypass grafting (CABG) and valve repair/replacement.

Congestive Heart Failure

Heart failure occurs when the heart's ability to pump blood is not adequate to meet the body's metabolic needs. The most common cause is impaired contractility of the left ventricle (LV), due to CAD, myocardial infarction, dilated cardiomyopathy, valvular heart disease, or hypertension. Right ventricular (RV) failure also can occur, most commonly due to LV failure, RV infarction, pulmonary hypertension, or tricuspid regurgitation.

Signs and symptoms vary according to the severity and progression of the disease. Patients with advanced disease typically exhibit signs and symptoms of fluid retention and pulmonary congestion (thus the term *congestive heart failure*), including dyspnea, orthopnea, and paroxysmal nocturnal dyspnea. Additional findings may include fatigue, chest pain or pressure, and palpitations. If the RV is involved, jugular venous distension, peripheral edema, hepatomegaly, and ascites are common findings. Auscultation may reveal a gallop rhythm (with an S_3 sound and often an S_4 sound) and, in valvular disease, heart murmurs.

As indicated in **Table 20-5**, functional impairment in patients with heart failure is categorized by the level of dyspnea they experience.

With good disease management, even patients with NYHA Class III/IV heart failure can remain relatively stable most of the time. However, patients with heart failure can decompensate and develop acute dysfunction, most typically resulting in pulmonary edema or hypotension/

Table 20-5 New York Heart Association (NYHA) Heart Failure Symptom Classification System

NYHA Class	Level of Impairment
I	No symptom limitation with ordinary physical activity
II	Ordinary physical activity somewhat limited by dyspnea (e.g., long-distance walking, climbing two flights of stairs)
III	Exercise limited by dyspnea with moderate workload (e.g., short-distance walking, climbing one flight of stairs)
IV	Dyspnea at rest or with very little exertion

shock. The following pearls address the basics in the management of stable heart failure and acute decompensation.

Assessment/Information Gathering

- To identify or manage stable CHF:
  - Assess for the signs and symptoms previously noted.
  - Recommend serum electrolytes (fluid balance, sodium levels), BUN and creatinine (renal function), and brain natriuretic peptide (BNP—a hormone useful in diagnosing CHF and its response to treatment).
  - Recommend a chest x-ray; look for cardiomegaly, pulmonary vascular congestion, Kerley B lines, and pleural effusion.
  - Recommend 12-lead ECG; look for indicators suggesting LV or RV hypertrophy or ischemia/CAD (discussed subsequently).
  - If the ECG indicates ischemia/CAD, recommend a stress test, cardiac catheterization, or coronary computed tomographic angiography (CTA) to confirm or exclude CAD as the cause (see the subsequent section on CAD).
  - Recommend an echocardiogram to assess for systolic and diastolic function, hypertrophy, chamber size, and valve abnormalities (discussed subsequently).
- To assess for decompensation/pulmonary edema:
  - Assess for signs of acute decompensation, e.g., sudden onset of restlessness, confusion, diaphoresis, dyspnea, increased work of breathing, tachypnea, tachycardia.
  - Assess peripheral perfusion; look for cool, pale, cyanotic or mottled skin and slow capillary refill.
  - Assess cough and sputum production; look for frothy or pinkish/blood-tinged sputum.
  - Assess breath sounds (marked bilateral crackles and wheezing indicate acute decompensation).
  - Assess for chest pain (its presence suggests acute myocardial ischemia/infarction).
  - Initiate SpO_2 monitoring and obtain an ABG (which typically shows hypoxemia with respiratory alkalosis).
  - Recommend an immediate chest x-ray (which typically reveals bilateral fluffy infiltrates).
  - Recommend cardiac biomarkers (troponin, CK, and CK-MB) to assess for MI.
  - Recommend an echocardiogram (to help determine possible mechanical causes such as cardiac tamponade or valve problems).
  - Do *not* recommend PA catheter insertion unless the patient's diagnosis cannot be confirmed without it or there are unexpected responses to therapy.

Treatment/Decision Making

- To manage stable CHF:
  - Recommend disease management education (Chapter 7), with an emphasis on sodium and fluid restriction, smoking cessation, daily monitoring of BP, weight control, and moderate aerobic exercise.
  - Recommend the following medications for all CHF patients:

- An angiotensin-converting enzyme (ACE) inhibitor (e.g., captopril) or angiotensin receptor blocker (e.g., valsartan)
- A beta blocker (e.g., carvedilol)
  - Depending on the severity of symptoms, additional medications may include digoxin (especially with A-fib), a diuretic (preferably a loop diuretic such as furosemide or torsemide), and an aldosterone antagonist such as spironolactone.
- To manage decompensation/pulmonary edema:
  - Initiate O_2 therapy with the highest F_{IO_2} possible (via nonrebreathing mask at 12–15 L/min or high-flow cannula at 30–40 L/min) to obtain an S_{PO_2} above 90%.
  - Recommend CPAP or BiPAP with 100% O_2 (improves gas exchange and decreases venous return and ventricular preload).
  - Recommend morphine or a benzodiazepine such as lorazepam to reduce anxiety (morphine also may decrease preload via venous dilation).
  - Recommend the appropriate ACLS protocol for any associated arrhythmia or MI.
  - Recommend the following medications (these recommendations assume the patient is *not* hypotensive):
    - A vasodilator such as nitroglycerin, sodium nitroprusside, or nesiritide (to decrease preload and afterload)
    - A rapid-acting loop diuretic such as furosemide or torsemide
  - If the patient *is* hypotensive, recommend an inotropic agent such as dobutamine to maintain a mean arterial pressure of at least 70–75 mm Hg.
  - Recommend intubation and invasive ventilation if the patient develops severe respiratory acidosis on CPAP/BiPAP.
  - In the patient with persistent hypotension and pulmonary edema due to an acute MI, recommend intra-aortic balloon pumping (if available) until angioplasty or cardiac surgery can be performed.

Coronary Artery Disease and Acute Coronary Syndrome

CAD is a pathologic process affecting the coronary arteries, most commonly due to atherosclerosis. Buildup of atherosclerotic plaque narrows the arteries and reduces blood flow to the myocardium, eventually causing ischemia, angina, and infarction. Risk factors include hyperlipidemia (especially elevated low-density lipoprotein [LDL]), diabetes, hypertension, smoking, sedentary lifestyle and obesity, and a family history of CAD.

The primary symptom of CAD is angina pectoris. The angina can vary in severity from that occurring only with strenuous exercise to constant pain at rest. Angina is *stable* if the pattern of discomfort remains unchanged over time; it is *unstable* when abrupt changes occur in the frequency, intensity, or duration of pain or its precipitating factors.

When CAD progresses to cause partial or complete blockage of a coronary artery resulting in unstable angina or a myocardial infarction, the condition is known as *acute coronary syndrome* (ACS). As indicated in **Table 20-6**, the two categories of ACS are defined primarily by the ECG: the ST-segment elevation myocardial infarction (STEMI) type and the non-ST-segment elevation myocardial infarction (NSTEMI)/unstable angina type. Because STEMI-type MI involves complete obstruction of a coronary artery, it is the more serious event and the one generally requiring the most rapid and aggressive response.

Table 20-6 Basic Classification of Acute Coronary Syndrome

Classification	Recognition	Presumed Cause
STEMI or new left bundle branch block (LBBB)	ST-segment elevation in two or more contiguous chest leads (V1-V6)	Complete coronary artery occlusion
NSTEMI/unstable angina	Ischemic ST-segment depression or dynamic T-wave inversion with pain	Partial or intermittent occlusion

The following management pearls address both stable CAD and ACS.

Assessment/Information Gathering

- To identify or assess CAD with stable angina:
  - Assess vital signs including *all peripheral pulses* and the ratio of ankle to brachial BP or ankle–brachial index (values less than 0.90 support the diagnosis of CAD).
  - Auscultate the carotid arteries, listening for bruits (indicating atherosclerosis).
  - Obtain a patient history, to include current symptoms, risk factors, and family history; assess for chest pain and palpitations, shortness of breath, fatigue, and limited tolerance for exertion.
  - Recommend a 12-lead ECG to identify the presence and severity of myocardial ischemia; *note that a normal ECG does not exclude CAD.*
  - Recommend the following lab tests: electrolytes, fasting glucose (to assess for diabetes/diabetes control), lipid panel (total cholesterol, high-density lipoprotein [HDL], LDL, and triglycerides), and C-reactive protein (an inflammatory marker whose level increases in atherosclerotic disease).
  - Recommend a chest x-ray.
  - Recommend stress echocardiography or radionuclide stress testing (imaging with thallium-201 or technetium-99m) to identify the presence and magnitude of ischemia and myocardial infarction.
  - Recommend either coronary arteriography/cardiac catheterization (the gold standard for diagnosing CAD) or minimally invasive computed tomography angiography to help identify the exact location and extent of coronary artery blockage.
- To identify or assess for ACS:
  - Assess for centralized chest pain, pressure, fullness, or "squeezing" sensation; pain may radiate to the jaw, shoulder, arm, and/or back. *Note that some patients with MI may be asymptomatic.*
  - Measure SpO_2 and vital signs, and assess for hypotension and the potential for cardiogenic shock.
  - Assess for dyspnea, diaphoresis, nausea, lightheadedness, confusion, and syncope.
  - Auscultate the lungs and listen for crackles (indicating CHF/pulmonary edema).
  - Recommend 12-lead ECG; look for ST-segment deviation (±1 mm or greater) or T-wave inversion in multiple chest leads.
  - Recommend electrolytes, coagulation panel, and *serial measurement* of creatine phosphokinase (CK), CK-MB, and troponin (cardiac biomarkers whose levels increase with MI). *However, do not delay treatment to wait for lab results!*
  - Recommend a chest x-ray.

Treatment/Decision Making

The nature and urgency of treatment provided to patients with CAD varies according to the severity of their disease process. In general, patients with stable angina are managed conservatively using a comprehensive disease management protocol, whereas those presenting with acute coronary syndrome receive more urgent care.

To Manage CAD with Stable Angina (Including Post-MI)

- Recommend participation in a cardiac rehabilitation program that provides smoking cessation (Chapter 7), encourages regular exercise (30 min/day of moderate activity), and assists with weight control and healthy dieting (low saturated fat, high fiber).
- If the patient is diabetic, recommend careful blood glucose control via hemoglobin A_{1c} monitoring.
- Recommend pharmacologic therapy (see **Table 20-7** for contraindications):
  - An antiplatelet drug (e.g., low-dose aspirin, warfarin, clopidogrel)
  - An antianginal drug—nitroglycerin (sublingual, tab, spray) for relief, a beta blocker (e.g., metoprolol), a calcium-channel blocker (e.g., nifedipine), a long-acting nitrate (e.g., isosorbide extended release), or ranolazine for control

Table 20-7 Contraindications to Drug Classes Used in Acute Coronary Syndrome

Drug Class	Contraindications
Nitrates	Hypotension (systolic BP < 90 mm Hg) or evidence of RV infarction
Fibrinolytics	Active bleeding, intracranial hemorrhage, ischemic stroke, severe hypertension
Beta blockers	Hypotension, shock, bradycardia, uncompensated CHF, asthma

- For patients with CAD and high LDL levels, a statin (e.g., atorvastatin [Lipitor])
- For patients with stable angina but significant limitations to activity (NYHA Class III/IV heart failure), recommend either elective percutaneous coronary angioplasty or coronary artery bypass grafting (CABG)

To Manage Acute Coronary Syndrome/MI

- Support the ABCs (airway, breathing, circulation) as needed; be prepared to implement the applicable ACLS protocol.
- Initially recommend that all patients with suspected ACS (STEMI or NSTEMI) receive:
  ○ Aspirin (or clopidogrel if aspirin is contraindicated)
  ○ Nitroglycerin, unless contraindicated (Table 20-7)
  ○ A beta blocker such as metoprolol, unless contraindicated (Table 20-7)
  ○ O_2 to maintain SpO_2 above 90%
  ○ Morphine for pain
- Recommend a chest x-ray.
- For STEMI, new LBBB, or likely MI with cardiogenic shock: if available, recommend emergency revascularization via either percutaneous coronary angioplasty (PCA) or CABG within 90 minutes; if not available, recommend immediate fibrinolytic/thrombolytic therapy using a tissue plasminogen activator (t-PA) such as alteplase or reteplase.
- For initially responsive NSTEMI: recommend conservative management with antianginal therapy, antiplatelet therapy, and antithrombin therapy (heparin, either unfractionated or low molecular weight)—*not* fibrinolytic therapy; followed by a stress test and—if needed—diagnostic angiography.
- For worsening NSTEMI (rising CK/troponin, new ECG changes, refractory angina, serious arrhythmias, hemodynamic instability, onset of heart failure): recommend urgent revascularization via either PCA or CABG.

As noted in Table 20-7, several problems can contraindicate administration of some common drug classes used to treat CAD. Do not recommend any agent in these drug classes when the patient has or is suspected of having a contraindicated condition.

Valvular Heart Disease

Valvular heart disease—especially that affecting the aortic and mitral valves—can cause significant disability that normally requires surgical correction. **Table 20-8** summarizes the four most common left heart valve abnormalities that RTs are likely to encounter.

In regard to assessment and information gathering, note that the clinical findings in valvular heart disease are often similar to those in CHF. For this reason, echocardiography should be recommended in all patients exhibiting signs and symptoms of heart failure. Specifically, both two-dimensional (2D) and Doppler echo are indicated if a valve problem is suspected. Two-dimensional echocardiography provides real-time analysis of chamber and valve mechanical function, while the Doppler method allows measurement of actual blood flow.

In terms of treatment and decision making, note that with minor exceptions, cardiac valve disorders require surgical intervention to repair or replace the damaged tissue. Consequently, as an RT your involvement with valvular heart disease most often will occur in the perioperative setting.

Cardiac Surgery

Cardiac surgery is associated with significant pulmonary complications, even among patients with healthy lungs. Typically, a diminished postoperative FRC increases the likelihood of atelectasis,

Table 20-8 Common Heart Valve Problems

	Aortic Valve		Mitral Valve	
	Stenosis	**Regurgitation**	**Stenosis**	**Regurgitation**
Description	Narrowing of aortic valve, impeding LV emptying	Leakage of blood from aorta back into LV during diastole	Narrowing of mitral valve, impeding LV filling	Leakage of blood from LV back into LA during systole
Cause(s)	Congenital anomaly or valve calcification, rheumatic heart disease, hypercholesterolemia	Congenital anomaly, infective endocarditis, long-standing hypertension, rheumatoid arthritis	Rheumatic disease, calcification, infective endocarditis	Connective tissue weakening (myxomatous degeneration), chordae tendineae rupture, CAD, rheumatic disease, infective endocarditis, cardiomyopathy
Effects	Over time, back-pressure causes LV hypertrophy, leading to either diastolic failure or ischemia (O_2 demand exceeds supply)	LV volume and pressure overload, causing dilation and hypertrophy	Back-pressure increases pressure in and dilates LA, predisposing patient to A-fib and embolization; also can cause pulmonary congestion, edema, RV failure	LV volume overload and dilation leads to heart failure; increased LA volumes leads to A-fib and embolization; high pulmonary pressures can cause pulmonary congestion, edema, RV failure
Signs and Symptoms	Harsh systolic murmur at base of heart; exertional dyspnea, angina syncope	Soft diastolic murmur, fatigue, palpitations, wide pulse pressure, bounding pulses	Accentuated first heart sound and P2 if pulmonary hypertension; exertional dyspnea, fatigue, angina, plus signs of RV failure	Pansystolic murmur (starts at S_1, extends into S_2); dyspnea, PND, orthopnea fatigue, and palpitations caused by A-fib
Diagnosis	*2D and Doppler echo:* confirms presence and severity	*ECG:* LV hypertrophy; *2D and Doppler echo:* confirms presence and severity	*Chest x-ray:* LA dilation and pulmonary congestion without cardiomegaly; *ECG:* LA dilation, A-fib, and (advanced) RV hypertrophy; *2D and Doppler echo:* confirms presence and severity	*Chest x-ray:* LA dilation with cardiomegaly; *2D and Doppler echo:* confirms presence and severity
Treatment	Valve replacement	*Medical:* vasodilators to reduce backflow; *Surgical:* valve repair or replacement	*Medical:* diuretics, beta- and calcium-channel blockers, digoxin for A-fib; anticoagulants (emboli); *Surgical:* balloon valvotomy, commissurotomy, or valve replacement	*Medical:* vasodilators to reduce afterload; *Surgical:* valve repair or replacement

LV = left ventricle; LA = left atrium; CAD = coronary heart disease; A-fib = atrial fibrillation; PND = paroxysmal nocturnal dyspnea.

while the reduced vital capacity and impaired airway clearance due to pain and analgesia make the patient prone to secretion retention and pneumonia. Moreover, fluid imbalances and the general inflammatory response to surgery often increase capillary leakage and lung water, further aggravating $\dot{V}/\dot{Q}$ inequalities and worsening hypoxemia. To help avoid or minimize these problems, initial postoperative respiratory care aims to restore the FRC and maintain adequate gas exchange via mechanical ventilation with PEEP. Subsequent efforts involve weaning and extubation, followed by rigorous bronchial hygiene therapy.

With the advent of new anesthesia strategies and minimally invasive techniques, including "off-pump" and robotically assisted cardiac surgery, there has been a dramatic decrease in the frequency of postoperative pulmonary complications as well as the need for lengthy ventilatory support. Both achievements depend in part on the integral role that RTs play in managing cardiac surgery patients, as summarized in the following management pearls.

Assessment/Information Gathering

Ideally, patient assessment should occur before surgery, and subsequently upon admission to the postoperative unit, with continuous monitoring taking place while the patient is receiving care.

- Via chart review and patient interview, assess the patient preoperatively for the following postoperative risk factors (all likely to increase complications/ICU length of stay):
  - *Demographics*: advanced age (75 years or older), female gender
  - *Degree of cardiac dysfunction*: NYHA Class III or IV, low ejection fraction (less than 40%), prior CABG or current valve disorder, prior MI, need for preoperative intra-aortic balloon pump
  - *Comorbidities*: COPD, CHF, diabetes, hypertension, cerebrovascular disease, renal impairment, obesity, smoking history
  - *Operative factors*: emergency (nonelective) procedure, cardiopulmonary bypass (versus "off-pump"), left main coronary artery graft, multiple vessel grafts, valve repair/replacement, expected lengthy procedure, ASA class greater than III (**Table 20-9**)
- Recommend bedside spirometry for any patient with a history of lung disease or smoking; measure FVC, slow vital capacity, and IC.
- To help reduce postoperative complications, provide *preoperative* patient education, to include discussion of airway and ventilator management, as well as training in the selected bronchial hygiene/airway clearance methods.
- After surgery, on admission to the postsurgical unit or placement on a ventilator:
  - Initiate continuous pulse oximetry and capnography.
  - After the patient has been on the ventilator for 20 minutes, obtain a blood gas analysis and compute the $P(_{A}-_{a})O_2$ and P/F ratio (usually on 100% O_2).

Table 20-9 Physical Status Classification Developed by the American Society of Anesthesiologists

Class	Patient Characteristics
I	No organic, physiologic, biochemical, or psychiatric disturbance; localized pathologic process for which operation is to be performed; no systemic disturbance
II	Mild-to-moderate systemic disturbance caused by the condition to be treated surgically or by other pathophysiologic processes
III	Severe systemic disturbance or disease from whatever cause, with the potential for perioperative complications
IV	Severe systemic disorders that are already life-threatening, not always correctable by operation
V	Moribund with little chance of survival
E	Emergency operation (the letter "E" is placed beside the numeric classification to indicate increased risk and poorer physical condition associated with an emergency procedure)

- Recommend 5-lead ECG telemetry monitoring (including leads II and V5 for detecting ischemia), ideally with computerized ST-segment analysis.
- Recommend hemodynamic monitoring, ideally to include direct radial arterial pressures (use the right side for aortic surgery) and CVP (do *not* recommend routine use of a PA catheter).
- Recommend careful monitoring of fluid output via urinary catheter, chest tube drainage, and NG tube.
- Recommend a postsurgical chest x-ray to assess for ET tube position and vascular line placement and to evaluate the patient's lung fields for lung expansion/atelectasis, infiltrates, pneumothorax, pleural effusion, or pulmonary edema.
- Where feasible, recommend point-of-care ABG testing (to minimize blood loss).
- Recommend antiembolism stockings (reduces the risk of DVT and pulmonary embolism).

Treatment/Decision Making

Most patients who undergo cardiac surgery are provided with ventilatory support immediately after transfer from the OR. Initial ventilator settings vary by institutional protocol, but generally include the following elements:

- *Mode*: full ventilatory support (pressure or volume control A/C or normal-rate SIMV with pressure support)
- *Tidal volume*: 8–10 mL/kg with plateau pressure of 30 cm H_2O or less
- *Rate*: to provide $P_{ET}CO_2$ (capnography) of 30–40 torr, normalize pH
- *FIO_2*: match the operating room %O_2 or initially provide 100% O_2 to obtain $P(A\text{-}a)O_2$; immediately titrate down to maintain the SpO_2 above 90% with PEEP
- *PEEP*: initially 8–10 cm H_2O

Ideally, these patients should be weaned from ventilatory support and extubated within 2 to 6 hours after leaving the OR—a strategy known as the *fast-track* approach. Early extubation and spontaneous breathing decreases intrapleural pressure, which in most patients increases LV end-diastolic volume, ejection fraction, and cardiac output. Of course, not all patients can or should be fast-tracked. Thus the first step is deciding who is ready to wean, followed by implementation of a rapid weaning and extubation protocol.

- Assess the patient to determine if he or she is ready to fast-track. Example criteria in fast-track protocols include the following:
  - Patient meets respiratory and acid–base criteria:
    - Patient is spontaneously breathing with $\dot{V}E$ < 12 L/min
    - FIO_2 ≤ 0.50 with SpO_2 ≥ 90%
    - pH 7.35–7.50 with arterial HCO_3 > 21 mmol/L
  - Patient meets neurologic criteria:
    - Can move all extremities/lift head and legs off of bed on command
    - Nods appropriately to questions
    - Has intact cough reflex
  - Patient meets hemodynamic criteria:
    - Blood pressure is within an acceptable range (e.g., MAP > 75 mm Hg or systolic BP 100–120 mm Hg) without vasoactive drug support
    - No evidence of major bleeding; chest tubes drainage < 50–100 mL/hr
    - Heart rate < 120/min with no significant arrhythmias
    - Cardiac index > 2.0 L/min/m²; ejection fraction > 40%
    - CVP < 17 mm Hg
- For patients meeting fast-track criteria for whom sedation has been discontinued, follow a standard spontaneous breathing trial protocol (Chapter 10) using CPAP or CPAP + pressure support (to maintain FRC):
  - Judge weaning to be successful if the patient remains hemodynamically stable with an acceptable pattern of breathing (e.g., RSBI < 100) and no signs of distress.

- ○ If the weaning attempt is unsuccessful, try again every 30–60 minutes until the patient can maintain adequate oxygenation and ventilation without hemodynamic compromise for at least 30 minutes with pressure support of 5 cm H_2O or less.
  - ○ Recommend extubation or (if the protocol allows) extubate the patient if the patient is stable for at least 30 minutes without signs of distress.
  - ○ Be prepared for reintubation or provision of noninvasive ventilation should the patient deteriorate after ET tube removal.
- As soon as possible after successful extubation:
  - ○ Recommend that the patient sit up in a chair and begin to ambulate.
  - ○ Recommend initiation of appropriate bronchial hygiene and airway clearance therapy, to include at least deep breathing and directed coughing (Chapters 9 and 10); helping patients with median sternotomies splint their incisions (using a "cough pillow") can facilitate effective coughing.
  - ○ Continue to monitor the patient for signs of atelectasis or pneumonia (progressive hypoxemia, dyspnea, decreased breath sounds, dull percussion note, fever), even after transfer to a step-down unit.

NEUROMUSCULAR DISORDERS

Neuromuscular disorders commonly encountered by RTs include those for which acute muscle weakness/paralysis is the major presenting symptom (such as myasthenia gravis and Guillain-Barré syndrome), and chronic disorders in which a slow but progressive decline in muscle function eventually results in respiratory insufficiency and failure (such as muscular dystrophy and amyotrophic lateral sclerosis). Rarely encountered by RTs (but one of the disorders cited by the NBRC for this CSE disease management category) is tetanus, which is covered briefly here for completeness.

Neuromuscular Disorders with Acute Manifestations (Guillain-Barré Syndrome and Myasthenia Gravis)

Guillain-Barré syndrome (GBS) is an acute inflammatory neuropathy affecting the spinal root and peripheral nerves. Inflammation destroys the myelin sheaths surrounding the nerves, causing acute muscle weakness and diminished reflexes. GBS often occurs following viral or bacterial infections, especially *Campylobacter jejuni* (diarrhea) and cytomegalovirus (URI) infections. GBS also has been reported to develop after certain immunizations.

Myasthenia gravis is an autoimmune disease in which excessive anti-acetylcholine receptor (anti-AchR) antibody blocks the acetylcholine receptors at the myoneural junction, causing a characteristic progressive loss of muscle strength with repeated use (*fatigability*). Once diagnosed, the condition typically is recurrent, with fluctuating episodes of weakness followed by periods of remission. A severe episode of weakness, termed a *myasthenic crisis*, can involve life-threatening respiratory muscle weakness. Myasthenic crises commonly are triggered by viral infections, surgery, childbirth, or drug-related issues.

Because one of these acutely presenting neuromuscular conditions often appears on the CSE and because candidates frequently confuse the two, we have summarized our case management pearls in the form of a comparative table (**Table 20-10**).

Muscular Dystrophy

Muscular dystrophies constitute a group of more than 30 inherited diseases that cause progressive muscle weakness and loss, eventually resulting in the inability to walk, swallowing difficulty, respiratory muscle insufficiency, and respiratory failure. The most common variant is Duchenne-type muscular dystrophy (DMD), an X-linked recessive trait disorder that occurs almost exclusively in males. Diagnosis of DMD is based on patient history and physical findings, and is confirmed by genetic testing or protein analysis of muscle tissue, which will demonstrate an absence of the dystrophin protein.

Table 20-10 Case Management Pearls: Guillain-Barré Syndrome Versus Myasthenia Gravis

Guillain-Barré Syndrome	Myasthenia Gravis
Assessment/Information Gathering I: History and Clinical Signs and Symptoms	
• History of recent febrile illness	• History of painless muscle weakness that worsens with repeated use
• Rapidly progressing *ascending* symmetrical muscle weakness/paralysis	• *Descending* and often episodic muscle weakness/paralysis
• Sensory dysesthesias (pain or discomfort to touch)	• Ptosis (drooping eyelids)
• Decreased or absent deep tendon reflexes	• Ophthalmoplegia/diplopia (weakness of eye muscles, double vision)
• Dysautonomia (rapid, wide fluctuations in BP, frequent cardiac arrhythmias)	• Dysphagia (indicating bulbar muscle involvement), loss of gag reflex
• Dysphagia (indicating bulbar muscle involvement), loss of gag reflex	• Normal deep tendon reflexes
• Dyspnea, often progressing to respiratory insufficiency	• Respiratory distress (advanced/untreated)
Assessment/Information Gathering II: Diagnostic Tests to Recommend and Characteristic Findings	
• Lumbar puncture to gather cerebral spinal fluid: increased protein, low WBC	• Antibody tests: ↑ anti-acetylcholine receptor (anti-AchR) antibody
• Electromyography (EMG) and nerve conduction studies (NCS): slowing or blockage of nerve conduction	• EMG/NCS: decreased amplitude of muscle action potential with repeated stimulation
• Antibody tests: ↑ antiganglioside antibodies	• Positive tensilon (edrophonium) test: dramatic improvement in muscle strength within 1 minute of administration*
• Liver enzymes: ↑ AST, ALT	• CT or MRI scan: may show presence of a thymoma (thymus gland tumor)
• Serology−positive for *C. jejuni* or CMV	• Breath sounds: normal unless aspiration and/or pneumonia due to loss of upper airway reflexes (indicated by basilar crackles and wheezes)
• Breath sounds−normal unless aspiration and/or pneumonia due to loss of upper airway reflexes (indicated by basilar crackles and wheezes)	• Spirometry: ↓ VC, ↓ MIP/NIF, ↓ MEP
• Spirometry: ↓ VC, ↓ MIP/NIF, ↓ MEP	• Blood gases: if respiratory involvement, acute respiratory acidosis; hypoxemia only if aspiration and/or pneumonia due to loss of upper airway reflexes
• Blood gases: if respiratory involvement, acute respiratory acidosis; hypoxemia only if aspiration and/or pneumonia	• Chest x-ray: normal unless aspiration and/or pneumonia
• Chest x-ray: normal unless aspiration and/or pneumonia	

Treatment/Decision Making I: General Medical/Surgical Treatment to Recommend	
• Vital signs, SpO$_2$, and ECG monitoring (dysautonomia requires continuous HR, BP and arrhythmias monitoring)	• Vital signs and SpO$_2$ monitoring; close observation if myasthenic crisis
• Plasmapheresis (plasma exchange)	• Acetylcholinesterase inhibitor therapy, such as pyridostigmine (Mestinon)
• IV immunoglobulin therapy	• Immunosuppressant therapy, such as hydrocortisone or azathioprine (Imuran)
• Analgesics for dysesthesia (NSAIDs, opioids)	• Plasmapheresis (plasma exchange)
• Fluids/Trendelenburg positioning for severe hypotension (for patients who are sensitive to vasoactive medications)	• IV immunoglobulin therapy
• Deep vein thrombosis (DVT) prophylaxis for immobility	• Thymectomy (especially if thymoma is present)
• Physical rehabilitation during recovery stage	• DVT prophylaxis for immobility
	• Physical rehabilitation during recovery stage

Treatment/Decision Making II: Respiratory Management to Implement/Recommend	
• Implement VC, NIF monitoring every 8 hours	• Implement VC, NIF monitoring every 8 hours
• Provide O$_2$ therapy as needed to keep SpO$_2$ > 90%	• Provide O$_2$ therapy as needed to keep SpO$_2$ > 90%
• Recommend intubation and mechanical ventilation if:	• Recommend intubation and mechanical ventilation if:
- VC < 1.0 L or < 15 mL/kg	- VC < 1.0 L or < 15 mL/kg
- MIP/NIF < −25 cm H$_2$O, MEP < 40 cm H$_2$O	- MIP/NIF < −25 cm H$_2$O, MEP < 40 cm H$_2$O
- Inability to cough, swallow, and protect the airway	- Inability to cough, swallow, and protect the airway
- ABG evidence of respiratory failure	- ABG evidence of respiratory failure
- Aspiration pneumonia with severe hypoxemia	- Aspiration pneumonia with severe hypoxemia
• Recommend trach if:	• Recommend trach if:
- Severe weakness, especially if bulbar involvement	- Severe weakness, especially if bulbar involvement
- Likely need for mechanical ventilation > 10 days	- Likely need for mechanical ventilation > 10 days
• Implement rigorous infection control/VAP protocol	• Implement rigorous infection control/VAP protocol

↑ = increased; ↓ = decreased; ALT = alanine aminotransferase; AST = aspartate aminotransferase; BP = blood pressure; CMV = cytomegalovirus; HR = heart rate; MEP = maximum expiratory pressure; MIP = maximum inspiratory pressure; NIF = negative inspiratory force; NSAID = nonsteroidal anti-inflammatory drug; VAP = ventilator-associated pneumonia; VC = vital capacity.

*A patient who worsens when given tensilon likely is having a cholinergic—not myasthenic—crisis (due to *excessive* acetylcholine at the myoneural junction). Other symptoms include diaphoresis, bronchorrhea, bronchospasm, and miosis. Atropine is the treatment.

Assuming an early diagnosis, DMD typically progresses through four stages: (1) normal respiratory function; (2) adequate ventilation but ineffective cough; (3) adequate daytime ventilation but inadequate nighttime ventilation; and (4) inadequate daytime and nighttime ventilation. During each stage, the role of the RT varies according to the functional limitations experienced by the patient. For this reason, the DMD management pearls presented here follow this four-stage progression. Note that other chronic neuromuscular diseases such as amyotrophic lateral sclerosis follow a pattern similar to DMD and, therefore, require similar treatment and decision making.

Assessment/Information Gathering

- Stage 1: Normal respiratory function
  - Recommend annual visits to a physician and routine immunizations (pneumococcal vaccination at 2 years old, annual influenza vaccine beginning at 6 month of age).
  - Establish baseline respiratory function (i.e., SpO_2, FVC, FEV_1, peak cough flow, MIP and MEP); *reassess at every subsequent visit (over the patient's entire lifetime)*.
- Stage 2: Adequate ventilation, ineffective cough
  - Recommend biannual visits to a pulmonologist after age 12, after confinement to a wheelchair, or after the patient's VC drops below 80% predicted; follow up on respiratory function measures.
  - Recommend annual polysomnography for sleep-disordered breathing.
  - Recommend assessment for dysphagia.
  - Recommend annual chest x-ray.
- Stage 3: Adequate daytime ventilation, inadequate nighttime ventilation
  - Recommend quarterly visits to the pulmonologist; follow up on respiratory function measures and dysphagia.
  - Measure awake $P_{ET}CO_2$.
- Stage 4: Inadequate daytime and nighttime ventilation
  - Recommend quarterly visits to the pulmonologist; follow up on respiratory function measures and dysphagia.
  - Implement continuous monitoring of SpO_2 with regular assessment of $P_{ET}CO_2$.

Treatment/Decision Making

- Stage 1: Normal respiratory function
  - Begin patient/caregiver education in disease management, with emphasis on preventive care (e.g., immunizations, regular visits to doctor), airway clearance strategies, and monitoring respiratory function.
- Stage 2: Adequate ventilation, ineffective cough
  - Train and have caregivers implement an airway clearance regimen such as manually assisted coughing or mechanical insufflation–exsufflation (Chapter 9) once peak cough flow is less than 270 L/min (4.5 L/sec) or MEP is less than 60 cm H_2O.
  - Train and have caregivers incorporate manual volume recruitment/deep lung inflation into the airway clearance regimen when FVC is less than 40% predicted or less than 1.25 L (in adults); avoid incentive spirometry, which generally is not effective in patients with respiratory muscle weakness.
- Stage 3: Adequate daytime ventilation, inadequate nighttime ventilation
  - Recommend/initiate nocturnal noninvasive positive-pressure ventilation (NPPV) for respiratory insufficiency and/or sleep-disordered breathing. Criteria include:
    - Signs and symptoms of hypoventilation (fatigue, dyspnea, headache, lack of concentration, hypersomnolence)
    - $SpO_2 < 95\%$ (air) or $P_{ET}CO_2 > 45$ torr while awake
    - Apnea–hypopnea index > 10/hr or at least four O_2 desaturation events/hr (ODI $\geq$ 4)
  - Avoid simple CPAP because it does not overcome hypoventilation, and ***do not*** recommend negative-pressure ventilation because it can cause upper airway obstruction in these patients.
  - Provide the patient and caregivers with the training needed to manage ventilatory support in the home (Chapter 17).

- Stage 4: Inadequate daytime and nighttime ventilation
  - Recommend/initiate daytime NPPV when the patient's $P_{ET}CO_2$ is more than 50 torr, when the SpO_2 remains below 92% while the patient is awake, or when ventilatory support is required to relieve persistent dyspnea.
  - Use oral/mouthpiece interfaces for daytime NPPV; some patients with DMD also can use a mouthpiece while sleeping.
  - Recommend invasive ventilation via tracheostomy if NPPV is contraindicated, if it is not feasible due to paralysis/weakness of the muscles controlling swallowing (bulbar weakness), or if the patient/caregivers express preference for the invasive route.
  - Provide the patient and caregivers with the training needed to manage continuous ventilatory support in the home (Chapter 17).

Hypoxemia can occur in patients with DMD. When this condition is due to hypoventilation, the appropriate treatment is to lower the P_{CO_2} (which raises the P_{O_2}) via assisted ventilation, not administering O_2. Likewise, if the hypoxemia is due to mucus plugging or atelectasis, O_2 therapy will merely mask the underlying problem. In these cases, the best management approach is rigorous application of the selected airway clearance regimen, with the goal being restoration of an SpO_2 of 92% or greater.

Tetanus

Tetanus is a neuromuscular disorder caused by wound exposure to a toxin produced by *Clostridium tetani*, an anaerobic bacterium found in the soil. The tetanus toxin blocks the inhibitory motor and autonomic neurons in the spinal cord, resulting in intense muscle spasms/rigidity as well as sympathetic overactivity. The toxin does not affect sensory neurons, so patients remain fully aware and typically experience severe pain associated with the muscle spasms.

Fortunately, tetanus is rare in developed countries due to widespread immunization. However, because you might encounter cases of tetanus among those individuals who have not been immunized, the following pearls should help guide management should a patient with this condition present to your hospital.

Assessment/Information Gathering

- Look for a recent history (typically 4 days to 2 weeks) of either a contaminated penetrating wound (including unsterile needle punctures by illicit drug users) or a necrotic or anaerobic infection (e.g., infected umbilical stumps, septic abortions, anaerobic periodontal infections, chronic diabetic ulcers).
- Assess for the following symptoms:
  - *Trismus* (intense spasms of the masseter muscle, commonly called "lockjaw")
  - Dysphagia and abnormal gag reflex (insertion of a tongue blade causes the patient to bite down instead of gagging)
  - Spasms of the facial muscles, causing unnatural expressions such as an odd grin (called *risus sardonicus*)
  - Neck stiffness progressing to *opisthotonus* (severe spasm in which the head and heels arch or "bow" backward in extreme hyperextension)
  - Rigid abdominal wall
  - Sympathetic overactivity—for example, irritability, restlessness, sweating, tachycardia, and reflex spasms in response to minimal external stimuli such as noise, light, or touch
  - Electromyography (EMG)—continuous discharge of motor units
- No laboratory or imaging tests can confirm the diagnosis; however, the presence of serum antitoxin levels greater than 0.01 U/mL can help rule out a diagnosis of tetanus.
- Recommend a toxicology screen for drug-induced dystonias or strychnine poisoning and a neurology assessment for other causes of seizures.

Treatment/Decision Making

- Upon diagnosis, recommend immediate IM administration of tetanus immunoglobulin.
- If the wound is contaminated, recommend that it be cleansed and debrided.
- Recommend an antibiotic such as metronidazole (Flagyl) to control further *C. tetani* growth.

- If ventilation and upper airway function are compromised, recommend intubation, mechanical ventilation, and intensive care.
- Because intubation may cause severe reflex laryngospasm, recommend rapid-sequence intubation with succinylcholine.
- Recommend IV administration of a benzodiazepine (e.g., midazolam) to provide sedation and control spasms.
- If benzodiazepine administration fails to control spasms, recommend a nondepolarizing neuromuscular blocking agent such as vecuronium or pancuronium (with ventilatory support); magnesium sulfate also can be recommended to reduce spasms and autonomic overactivity.

PEDIATRIC PROBLEMS

Whether your hospital has specialized inpatient units or outpatient clinics for managing pediatric disorders is no matter to the NBRC. In its "hospital," RTs must be able to help manage a variety of acute and chronic childhood disorders. These include croup (laryngotracheobronchitis), epiglottitis, bronchiolitis, childhood asthma, and cystic fibrosis.

Croup (Laryngotracheobronchitis) and Epiglottitis

Croup is a *viral* infection of the upper airway that occurs most commonly in children 6 months to 3 years of age. It is most often caused by the parainfluenza virus, adenovirus, respiratory syncytial virus (RSV), or influenza A and B. Infection causes inflammation and swelling of *subglottic* tissue, including the larynx, trachea, and larger bronchi.

Epiglottitis is a *bacterial* infection of the upper airway that occurs most commonly among children 2 to 8 years old. Prior to immunizations against *Haemophilus influenzae*, this organism was the most common cause. Today *Staphylococcus aureus* and Group A *Streptococcus*–associated epiglottitis is more commonplace. Infection causes acute inflammation and swelling of the epiglottis, aryepiglottic folds, and arytenoids, which if not treated can progress to airway obstruction and death in hours.

Because one of these acutely presenting pediatric airway disorders often appears on the CSE and because candidates frequently confuse the two, we have summarized our case management pearls in the form of a comparative table (**Table 20-11**).

Bronchiolitis

Bronchiolitis is a viral respiratory tract infection, primarily affecting infants younger than 2 years old. Respiratory syncytial virus (RSV) causes most bronchiolitis infections, with the parainfluenza virus and adenoviruses also being responsible for some cases. Inflammation in the bronchioles causes edema and excessive mucus production, which can lead to airway obstruction, air trapping, and atelectasis. Most cases are self-limiting and treated on an outpatient basis. More severe cases may require hospitalization.

Assessment/Information Gathering

- Assess for age-related diagnosis (younger than 24 months) and seasonal occurrence (predominantly November to March).
- Look for an immediate prior history (1 to 3 days) of cold-like upper respiratory tract symptoms (e.g., nasal congestion, mild cough), followed by worsening respiratory distress.
- Assess for signs of lower respiratory tract infection, including cough, wheezing, crackles, tachypnea (respiratory rate greater than 60–70/min), grunting, nasal flaring, intercostal retractions, mild fever, and possible cyanosis.
- Assess for risk factors indicating likelihood of severe disease or need for hospitalization, including age younger than 12 weeks, a history of prematurity, underlying chronic lung disease, congenital heart disease, or an immune deficiency syndrome.
- Assess SpO_2.
- Because the diagnosis typically is based on history and physical findings alone, do *not* routinely recommend imaging studies, lab work, or PFTs; a chest x-ray *may* be considered if a hospitalized infant does not improve after standard treatment.

Table 20-11 Case Management Pearls: Croup Versus Epiglottitis

Croup	Epiglottitis
Assessment/Information Gathering I: History and Clinical Signs and Symptoms	
• Determine age (infant/toddler)	• Determine age (toddler to school age)
• Obtain or review the history of initial cold-like symptoms with possible low-grade fever that progresses to more severe symptoms (often at night), including hoarseness, barking cough, and inspiratory stridor (with severe stridor, intercostal retractions may appear)	• Obtain or review the history of abrupt onset of acute illness with high fever (typically up to 40°C [104°F]), and sore throat/difficulty swallowing (often with drooling), accompanied by stridor (with possible retractions) and labored breathing
• Confirm physical findings as above plus assess for agitation; in more severe cases, look for significant tachypnea and tachycardia; lethargy, hypohypotonia, and cyanosis are late signs	• Confirm physical findings as above plus assess for restlessness, irritability, and extreme anxiety; the child also may prefer sitting upright and leaning forward; as obstruction worsens, breath sounds may decrease; as with croup, lethargy, hypotonia, and cyanosis are late signs of impending respiratory failure
	• Determine immunization status (*H. influenzae*)
Assessment/Information Gathering II: Diagnostic Tests to Recommend	
• Diagnosis based mainly on typical age, history, and physical exam findings	• Diagnosis based mainly on typical age, history, and physical exam findings
• Recommend lateral neck x-ray, looking for characteristic subglottic "steeple sign"	• Recommend lateral neck x-ray, looking for characteristic "thumb sign" indicating a swollen epiglottis
	• To confirm diagnosis, recommend visualizing the inflamed epiglottis via nasal fiberoptic laryngoscopy (a skilled operator is essential!)
	• To help substantiate the presence of a bacterial infection, recommend a CBC and differential, looking for elevated WBC, with left shift (↑ bands)
Treatment/Decision Making I: General Medical/Surgical Treatment to Recommend	
• Recommend close respiratory and cardiac monitoring, including SpO2	• Recommend close respiratory and cardiac monitoring, including SpO2
• Recommend adequate hydration	• Minimize procedures that could precipitate airway compromise, such as venipuncture and upper airway manipulation
• Recommend an antipyretic for fever	• Recommend an antipyretic for fever
• Recommend systemic corticosteroids (oral or IM); aerosolized budesonide is an option	• Recommend mild sedation for comfort and to reduce anxiety
• Do *not* recommend antibiotics or viral serology; lab tests are of limited value	• Recommend a broad-spectrum antibiotic (after the airway is secure) such as a cephalosporin, with treatment to continue for 7–10 days
• If the patient is admitted to the hospital, recommend droplet precautions	

(Continues)

493

Table 20-11 Case Management Pearls: Croup Versus Epiglottitis (*Continued*)

Croup	Epiglottitis
Treatment/Decision Making II: Respiratory Management to Implement/Recommend	
• Initiate supplemental O_2 therapy as needed to keep $SpO_2 > 90\%$	• Initiate supplemental O_2 therapy as needed to keep $SpO_2 > 90\%$
• Recommend or administer aerosolized racemic epinephrine (0.25–0.50 mL 2.25% solution with 3.0 mL saline), repeated up to three times as needed	• If acute respiratory arrest occurs, ventilate the child with 100% O_2 via manual resuscitator and call for intubation
• If repeat racemic epinephrine treatments fail to relieve symptoms, recommend heliox via high-flow cannula or nonrebreathing mask	• Recommend fiberoptic–assisted nasotracheal intubation under controlled conditions (e.g., rapid-sequence intubation)
• If symptoms persist for more than 4 hours after initial treatment, recommend hospital admission with close monitoring of respiratory status	• If intubation cannot be accomplished and airway obstruction persists or worsens, recommend cricothyroidotomy
• In the rare situation where obstruction worsens, consciousness decreases, or respiratory acidosis develops, recommend intubation and mechanical ventilation	

Treatment/Decision Making

- Recommend hospitalization if the patient meets the following criteria:
  - Exhibits persistent/worsening respiratory distress (tachypnea, nasal flaring, retractions, grunting) or episodes of apnea with cyanosis or bradycardia.
  - Needs supplemental O_2 to maintain $SpO_2 > 90\%$
  - Requires continuous maintenance of airway clearance (using bulb suctioning)
  - Exhibits significant restlessness or lethargy
  - Is dehydrated and unable to maintain oral feedings sufficient to prevent dehydration
- Recommend the hospitalized infant be placed under contact and respiratory (droplet) isolation precautions.
- Initiate supplemental O_2 to maintain the SpO_2 above 90%.
- Recommend nasal suctioning as needed, before feedings, and prior to aerosol therapy.
- Recommend repeated clinical assessment to detect deteriorating respiratory status.
- For patients with more severe disease or those with reported episodes of apnea with cyanosis and bradycardia, recommend continuous cardiac and respiratory rate monitoring.
- Do *not* recommend routine bronchodilator therapy (most wheezing is due to edema, not bronchospasm); if wheezing and respiratory distress persist, recommend a trial of inhaled racemic epinephrine or albuterol and continue the therapy only if there is objective evidence of a positive response.
- Do *not* recommend corticosteroids.
- Do *not* recommend ribavirin.
- Do *not* recommend antibiotics unless a coexisting bacterial infection is confirmed.
- Recommend hospital discharge when the infant meets the following criteria:
  - Is breathing at a rate less than 60–70/min with no signs of distress
  - Has an SpO_2 of 92% or higher on room air
  - Is taking oral feedings and is adequately hydrated
- Recommend family education to help prevent recurrent respiratory infections:
  - Avoid infant/child exposure to secondary smoke.
  - Limit infant/child exposure to sick siblings and settings likely to spread infections (e.g., daycare programs).
  - Implement proper hand decontamination, respiratory hygiene, and cough etiquette (Chapter 5).
- Recommend the monoclonal antibody palivizumab (Synagis) for prophylaxis against RSV for *high-risk infants*—that is, those born prematurely, and those with either chronic lung disease or congenital heart disease.

Childhood Asthma

Asthma is a chronic inflammatory disease characterized by airway inflammation, intermittent airflow obstruction, and bronchial hyperresponsiveness. Asthma can affect most age groups, but is more prevalent in children and young adults.

Diagnosis requires documenting recurrent episodes of airflow obstruction that are at least partially reversible. In addition, other causes of airflow obstruction with similar symptoms need to be excluded before a definitive diagnosis can be made. These differential diagnoses include allergic rhinitis, foreign body aspiration, vocal cord dysfunction, bronchiolitis, bronchiectasis, bronchopulmonary dysplasia, cystic fibrosis, and gastroesophageal reflux.

RTs may be involved in two types of asthma treatment: long-term outpatient management and management of acute exacerbations requiring ED or hospital admission.

Assessment/Information Gathering (Long-Term Management)

The goal of asthma outpatient management is control of the disease, to include preventing recurrent symptoms and minimizing medication use. Achieving this goal requires careful assessment of disease control, regular monitoring of symptoms, and a step-based approach to treatment.

Table 20-12 summarizes the National Asthma Education and Prevention Program guidelines for assessing asthma control in children 5–11 years old.

Table 20-12 Classification of Asthma Control in Children 5–11 Years Old

Components of Control	Well Controlled	Not Well Controlled	Very Poorly Controlled
Symptoms	≤ 2 days/week but not multiple times per day	> 2 days/week or multiple times on ≤ 2 days/week	Throughout the day
Nighttime awakenings	≤ 1×/month	≥ 2×/month	≥ 2×/week
SABA use for symptom control	≤ 2 days/week	> 2 days/week	Several times per day
Interference with normal activity	None	Some limitation	Extremely limited
Lung function	FEV_1 or PF > 80% predicted* FEV_1% > 80%	FEV_1 or PF 60–80% predicted* FEV_1% 75–80%	FEV_1 or PF < 60% predicted* FEV_1% < 75%

FEV_1 = forced expiratory volume in 1 second; FEV_1% = ratio of FEV_1/FVC; PF = peak expiratory flow; SABA = short-acting b-agonist.
*Predicted normal *or* personal best.
Adapted from: National Asthma Education and Prevention Program. *Expert panel report 3 (EPR3): guidelines for the diagnosis and management of asthma.* Bethesda, MD: U.S. Department of Health and Human Services; 2007. Note that the control elements/definitions vary somewhat for children younger than 5 years old. See the complete report for details.

Key management pearls in assessing children for asthma include the following:
- Recommend or obtain a family history with a focus on close relatives having asthma, allergic disorders, sinusitis, eczema, or nasal polyps.
- Look for a history of recurrent episodes of wheezing, coughing (usually unproductive), and shortness of breath, commonly occurring at night.
- Assess onset, duration, and pattern of symptoms, as well as any aggravating factors such as exercise, cold air, or smoke exposure.
- Recommend assessment for conditions presenting with similar symptoms such as bronchiolitis or foreign body aspiration.
- Recommend a chest x-ray (to help rule out conditions with similar symptoms).
- Recommend spirometry (FEV_1, FEV_1/FVC, peak flow) to establish baseline values and "personal bests."
- Recommend eosinophil counts and IgE levels (to assess for ectopic asthma).
- In the older child for whom a diagnosis is in doubt, recommend bronchial provocation testing (Chapter 11) or expired nitric oxide analysis (Chapter 2).

Treatment/Decision Making (Long-Term Management)

Recommend or implement a comprehensive disease management program involving both the child and key family members (Chapter 7):

- Control of environmental factors and coexisting conditions that can aggravate asthma (e.g., sinusitis, gastroesophageal reflux)
- Regular monitoring of symptoms
- Use of action plans to deal with acute exacerbations (Chapter 7)
- Careful selection and implementation of drugs and delivery approaches
- Step-based drug treatment consistent with the level of disease control

Table 20-13 summarizes the step-based drug treatment regimen for childhood asthma recommended by the National Heart, Lung, and Blood Institute's National Asthma Education and Prevention Program. Step 1 is the norm for well-controlled asthma with intermittent symptoms. Higher steps may be required for persistent asthma to maintain good control. Step ups are considered whenever the patient's asthma becomes inadequately controlled.

Table 20-13 Step-Based Approach to Drug Therapy for Childhood Asthma

Step	Preferred Drug Regimen
1	Short-acting β-agonist as needed (see Table 10-14; dosages vary for children)
2	Add a low-dose inhaled corticosteroid (see Table 10-14; dosages vary for children)
3	Add LABA, LTRA, or theophylline to the low-dose inhaled corticosteroid or step up to a medium-dose inhaled corticosteroid
4	Medium-dose inhaled corticosteroid + LABA
5	High-dose inhaled corticosteroid + LABA
6	High-dose inhaled corticosteroid + LABA + oral systemic corticosteroid

LABA = long-acting β-agonist (e.g., salmeterol or formoterol); LTRA = leukotriene receptor antagonist (e.g., montelukast or zafirlukast).
Adapted from National Asthma Education and Prevention Program. *Expert panel report 3 (EPR3): guidelines for the diagnosis and management of asthma.* Bethesda, MD: U.S. Department of Health and Human Services; 2007. Note that the treatments by step vary somewhat for children younger than 5 years old. See the complete report for details.

Note that *a short-acting beta-agonist should always be available as needed to relieve symptoms.* Patients can take up to 3 doses at 20-minute intervals. However, use more often than 2 days per week indicates inadequate control and the need for a step up in treatment.

Decision making in long-term outpatient asthma management is based on assessing the patient's level of control:

- If the patient's asthma is well controlled (Table 20-12):
  - Recommend maintaining the current drug regimen/step and having the patient follow up with the doctor in 1 to 6 months.
  - If the patient's asthma remains well controlled for 3 months or longer, recommend a step *down* in the drug regimen.
- If the patient's asthma becomes not well controlled (Table 20-12):
  - Assess the patient's compliance with the drug regimen, inhaler technique, and control of environmental factors and coexisting conditions.
  - If the patient's compliance is confirmed and environmental factors and coexisting conditions are under control, recommend a step *up* in the drug regimen and reevaluation by the doctor in 2–6 weeks.
- If the patient's asthma becomes very poorly controlled (Table 20-12):
  - Assess the patient's compliance with the drug regimen, inhaler technique, and control of environmental factors and coexisting conditions.
  - If the patient's compliance is confirmed and environmental factors and coexisting conditions under control:
    - Recommend a short course of oral systemic corticosteroids.
    - Recommend a step *up* in the drug regimen and reevaluation by the doctor in 2 weeks.

Assessment/Information Gathering (Acute Exacerbation)

Acute exacerbations of asthma can vary substantially in terms of their severity. Because the severity of the exacerbation determines the initial treatment approach, RTs must be able to quickly assess the patient on a number of clinical indicators. **Table 20-14** applies these measures to categorize asthma exacerbations by level of severity.

In assessing the severity of the patient's exacerbation, two important points should be emphasized:

- Early on, the patient's arterial blood gas typically reveals respiratory alkalosis with mild to moderate hypoxemia; *normalization of the pH ("the cross-over point") usually indicates a rising $Paco_2$ and progression toward respiratory acidosis and failure.*
- The progression to life-threatening respiratory failure is marked by a rapid decline in status, typically manifested by the development of drowsiness, bradypnea, bradycardia, decreased breath sounds, and fatigue.

Table 20-14 Assessing the Severity of Asthma Exacerbation

Assessment	Severity		
	Moderate	Severe	Life-Threatening
Breathlessness	Dyspnea at rest; talks in phrases	Dyspnea at rest; talks in words	Limited effort indicating fatigue
Sensorium/behavior	Alert/may be agitated	Alert/usually agitated	Drowsy or confused
Respiratory rate	Tachypnea	Tachypnea	Bradypnea possible
Work of breathing/ respiratory distress	May show accessory muscle use with retractions	Usually shows accessory muscle use with retractions	May exhibit thoraco-abdominal paradox
Heart rate/pulse	Tachycardia with pulsus paradoxus	Tachycardia with pulsus paradoxus	Bradycardia (indicating fatigue)
Breath sounds	Prominent expiratory wheezing	Prominent inspiratory + expiratory wheezes	Absence of wheezing ("silent chest")
FEV_1 or PF (% predicted)	$\geq 40\%$	25–40%	< 25% (if able to perform)
Pao_2/Sao_2 (air)	≥ 60 torr/90%	< 60 torr/90%	< 60 torr/90%
$Paco_2$/pH	< 35–40 torr/↑pH	> 40 torr/N or ↓ pH	> 45–50 torr/↓ pH

Treatment/Decision Making (Acute Exacerbation)

Once the severity of the exacerbation is determined, the appropriate management begins. **Table 20-15** outlines the recommended initial treatment regimens for patients presenting to the ED suffering an acute worsening of asthma symptoms, according to their severity.

After initial management, you reassess the patient and implement or recommend further action based on the response to therapy. For the patient being managed for moderate or severe symptoms, the following guidelines apply:

- Recommend discharge from the ED to home if:
  - The patient's symptoms are relieved by treatment.
  - The FEV_1 or PEF is restored ($\geq 70\%$ predicted/personal best).
  - The response is sustained for at least an hour without further intervention.
- Recommend hospital admission to a medical unit if:
  - Mild to moderate symptoms continue despite appropriate treatment.
  - The FEV_1 or PEF is not adequately restored (40–69% predicted/personal best).

Table 20-15 Initial Emergency Management of Asthma Exacerbations

Moderate	Severe	Life-Threatening
• O_2 to achieve $Sao_2 \geq 90\%$ • SABA by SVN or MDI + valved holding chamber; up to 3 doses in first hour • If no immediate response, recommend oral steroids	• O_2 to achieve $Sao_2 \geq 90\%$; consider heliox if available • High-dose SABA plus ipratropium by SVN or MDI + valved holding chamber, every 20 minutes or CBT for 1 hour • Oral steroids • Trial application of NPPV*	• Intubation and mechanical ventilation with 100% O_2 • Inhaled SABA + ipratropium • IV steroids • IV $MgSO_4$
CBT = continuous bronchodilator therapy; SABA = short-acting beta-agonist. *In the patient with severe symptoms whose $Paco_2$ is rising, a trial of noninvasive positive-pressure ventilation (NPPV) may forestall further deterioration. Successful application requires that the patient be conscious and cooperative and not have any contraindications (Chapter 10). If the patient has already progressed to life-threatening respiratory failure, application of NPPV may merely delay needed intubation and invasive support.		

- Recommend admission to the ICU if:
  - Severe symptoms continue despite appropriate treatment.
  - The patient is drowsy or confused.
  - The FEV$_1$ or PEF remains below 40% predicted
  - The Paco$_2$ indicates hypercapnia.

Should the patient require intubation and mechanical ventilation, the following guidelines apply:

- Initially use control mode ventilation (*no patient triggering*).
- Ensure adequate oxygenation.
  - Set the initial Fio$_2$ to 1.0 (100% O$_2$).
  - Titrate Fio$_2$ down to maintain Spo$_2$ > 90%.
- Avoid further air trapping/hyperinflation.
  - Apply a low minute volume.
    - Set the rate at *low end* of the age-appropriate range (about 15/min for school-age children).
    - Set V$_T$ to 6–8 mL/kg (predicted body weight).
    - Keep the plateau pressure ≤ 30 cm H$_2$O.
    - Accept a high Paco$_2$ as long as the pH > 7.2 (permissive hypercapnia).
  - Provide an I:E ratio of 1:4 or 1:5.
    - Maintain an age-appropriate low rate.
    - Use high flows to shorten the inspiratory time.
    - Use of external PEEP to treat air trapping in asthma is controversial and should not routinely be recommended; consider it only if auto-PEEP can be accurately measured, is contributing to hyperinflation, and is not alleviated using the low V̇E and low I:E ratio strategies.
- Controlled ventilation with low rates, volumes, and I:E ratios, together with permissive hypercapnia, typically requires neuromuscular blockade (which also will facilitate intubation) and heavy sedation (always used in combination with pharmacologic paralysis).

For patients being discharged from the ED or hospital, it is important to provide the patient and family with guidance on how to prevent relapses. To that end, the patient and family should be educated as follows:

- Referred to seek follow-up asthma care within a month
- Provided with instructions for all prescribed medications
- Assessed for proper technique using the prescribed inhaler(s)
- Trained to follow an action plan if symptoms worsen

Cystic Fibrosis

Cystic fibrosis (CF) is a genetically inherited autosomal recessive disease that is more common in white persons than in individuals of other ethnic backgrounds. CF affects the exocrine glands, causing chronic respiratory infections and gastrointestinal dysfunction, including pancreatic enzyme insufficiency. End-stage lung disease is the principal cause of death in persons with CF. Definitive diagnosis is based on genetic testing.

Assessment/Information Gathering

For the patient not already confirmed by genetic testing to have CF:

- Obtain a patient history, looking for the following findings:
  - Chronic cough with sputum production
  - Recurring respiratory infections
  - History of sinusitis
  - History of bowel obstruction or steatorrhea (fatty stool)
  - Failure to thrive/retarded growth

- Conduct or review a physical examination, looking for the following findings:
  - Abnormal breath sounds (e.g., wheezes, crackles, rhonchi)
  - Failure to thrive/retarded growth
    - Body weight below the lower limit of normal
    - BMI < 19
  - Presence of nasal polyps
  - Digital clubbing
  - Signs of pancreatic insufficiency
    - Steatorrhea (fatty stool)
    - Abdominal distension and flatulence
    - Weight loss/fatigue
- Recommend a sweat chloride test (considered positive for CF if > 60 mmol/L).
- Recommend a chest x-ray, looking for the following findings:
  - Hyperinflation (due to air trapping)
  - Peribronchial thickening
  - Infiltrates with or without lobar atelectasis
  - Right ventricular hypertrophy (advanced cases)
  - Bronchiectasis (best confirmed via high-resolution CT scan)
- Recommend spirometry and lung volume measurements (to make the diagnosis and to establish a patient baseline for assessing disease progression), looking for the following findings:
  - Decreased FEV_1 and FEV_1/FVC (obstruction)
  - Increased RV/TLC ratio (air trapping)
  - Decreased TLC and VC (late stage only, indicating lung scarring/fibrosis)
- Recommend sputum Gram stain as well as culture and sensitivity, looking for the following pathogens:
  - *Pseudomonas aeruginosa, Haemophilus influenzae, Staphylococcus aureus, Burkholderia cepacia, Escherichia coli,* or *Klebsiella pneumoniae.* The presence of *P. aeruginosa* supports a diagnosis of CF.

If the patient is being seen in the clinic or ED for acute respiratory distress, obtain the following information:

- Recent history:
  - Development of fever
  - Increase in productive cough with purulent sputum
  - Increased fatigue, weakness, or poor appetite/weight loss
  - New-onset or increased hemoptysis
- Physical assessment:
  - Labored breathing with intercostal retractions and use of accessory muscles
  - Severe wheezing, rhonchi, or rhonchial fremitus
- Diagnostic tests:
  - New infiltrate on chest x-ray
  - Labs: leukocytosis; low Na^+, Cl^-, and K^+; hypochloremic metabolic acidosis
  - ABG/pulse oximetry: moderate hypoxemia, SpO_2 < 90% on room air

Treatment/Decision Making

For the immediate treatment of the CF patient in respiratory distress:

- Minimize the patient's contact with other CF patients and apply applicable transmission-based precautions.
- Provide supplemental O_2 to maintain an SpO_2 above 90%.
- To relieve airway obstruction, implement or recommend a combined aerosol drug and airway clearance regimen that includes the following elements:
  - An aerosolized bronchodilator (e.g., albuterol), followed by
  - Aerosolized dornase alfa (Pulmozyme) or hypertonic saline, followed by

- Appropriate airway clearance therapy (to include directed coughing), followed by
- If *P. aeruginosa* colonization or infection is confirmed, an aerosolized antibiotic:
  - Tobramycin (TOBI): via breath-enhanced nebulizer (e.g., Pari LC) or DPI (TOBI Podhaler)
  - Polymyxin E (Colistin): via breath-enhanced nebulizer (e.g., Pari LC)
  - Aztreonam (Cayston): via mesh nebulizer (e.g., Altera)
- Assess the effectiveness of this regimen by noting the patient's subjective response plus changes in SpO_2, sputum production, breath sounds (may clear or increase due to movement of secretions into the larger airways), spirometry (FEV_1), and chest x-ray.
  - Recommend oral, IV, and/or inhaled antibiotics (above) specific to the colonizing organism(s).

Once the patient is stabilized and the diagnosis confirmed, recommend implementation of a comprehensive disease management program:

- Annual influenza immunizations
- A high-energy/high-fat diet with increased salt intake, pancreatic enzyme replacement, and vitamin supplements
- Regular exercise activity (improves airway clearance and reduces exacerbations)
- Patient education:
  - Medication usage, including proper sequencing and inhaler technique(s)
  - Airway clearance techniques (including adjustments to fit the patient's lifestyle)
  - Use of action plans to respond to worsening signs and symptoms
  - Infection control, including proper hand hygiene, containment of respiratory secretions, avoidance of direct contact with other patients with CF, and proper cleaning and disinfection of reusable home care equipment
- Clinic visits every 2–3 months:
  - Assessment of growth and development, nutritional status, and BMI
  - Lung function (FEV_1 and SpO_2)
  - Collection of sputum sample for Gram stain as well as culture and sensitivity
  - Assessment of therapy effectiveness in retarding disease progression
  - Counseling regarding psychosocial issues
- PA and lateral chest x-rays every 2–4 years

NEONATAL PROBLEMS

In the NBRC "hospital," all RTs are expected to be familiar with perinatal care, including the care delivered in the delivery room and the neonatal intensive care unit (NICU). To ensure success on CSE problems in this area, in this section we cover delivery room management (including meconium aspiration), apnea of prematurity, infant respiratory distress syndrome, bronchopulmonary dysplasia, and critical congenital heart defects.

Delivery Room Management

Typically, RTs will be called to the delivery room to assist with neonatal management after high-risk deliveries, especially those involving births occurring prior to 35 weeks' gestation. The focus in these cases is on rapid assessment and protocol-based resuscitation and stabilization.

Assessment/Information Gathering

- Immediately after birth, assess the neonate's heart rate, respiratory rate, muscle tone, reflexes, and color—that is, the basic parameters included in the Apgar score (Chapter 2); also assess for meconium staining.
- Repeat the Apgar score at 5 minutes; if it is less than 7, repeat the assessment every 5 minutes for up to 20 minutes (never delay action for an infant needing support).
- If the neonate remains cyanotic or exhibits severe pallor and/or is given supplemental O_2, assess the SpO_2, ideally via the right hand (preductal SpO_2). In normal infants breathing room air immediately after birth, the preductal SpO_2 typically ranges from 60–70%. The SpO_2 may take 5–10 minutes to "normalize" (exceeding 85%).

Table 20-16 Silverman-Anderson Index for Assessing Respiratory Distress

Feature	Score		
	0	1	2
Chest/abdominal movement	Synchronized	Lag on inspiration	See-saw movement
Intercostal retractions	None	Just visible	Marked
Xiphoid retractions	None	Just visible	Marked
Nasal flaring	None	Minimal	Marked
Expiratory grunting	None	Stethoscope only	Naked ear

- After the infant has been adequately stabilized and transferred to the nursery, recommend a thorough exam (at 10–20 hours after birth) using the Ballard assessment to estimate gestational age and identify any potential developmental abnormalities. Also after stabilization, the newborn's respiratory status should be continuously observed for delayed development of respiratory distress or hypoxemia.

Respiratory distress can be evaluated using an objective system such as the Silverman-Anderson scale (**Table 20-16**). A score of 0 on this index indicates no respiratory distress, scores of 1 to 6 indicate mild to moderate distress, and a score of 7 or greater indicates impending respiratory failure.

In terms of late development of hypoxemia, look for the appearance of central cyanosis in room air or a preductal Sp_{O_2} that does not quickly normalize or falls back below 90%.

Treatment/Decision Making

- If a near-term baby (37 or more weeks' gestation) cries, begins breathing, and exhibits good muscle tone immediately after birth, there is no need for resuscitation. Instead, dry the infant, place in skin-to-skin contact with the mother, cover with dry linen to keep warm, and continue to observe breathing, activity, and color.
- If after clearing the airway the newborn exhibits apnea, gasping, or labored breathing or a heart rate less than 100/min, immediately apply positive-pressure ventilation (PPV).
- For meconium-stained babies:
  - With normal respiratory effort, muscle tone, and heart rate (> 100/min), do not intubate; instead, clear secretions and meconium from the mouth and nose and continue to monitor.
  - With depressed respiratory effort, poor muscle tone, or a low heart rate (< 100/min), recommend ET intubation and tracheal suctioning immediately after delivery (ideally within 5 seconds); if no meconium is suctioned, do not repeat.
  - If meconium is retrieved via initial ET suctioning and the heart rate exceeds 100/min, recommend repeat suctioning. If the heart rate is less than 100/min, administer PPV and consider resuming suctioning later.
- During resuscitation, assess heart rate, respirations, and Sp_{O_2}, ideally via the right hand (preductal Sp_{O_2}).
- If supplemental O_2 is needed, target the following Sp_{O_2} levels:

1 min	60–65%
2 min	65–70%
3 min	70–75%
4 min	75–80%
5 min	80–85%
10 min	85–95%

- If the heart rate is less than 60/min, initiate chest compressions and recommend intubation (to coordinate compressions with PPV).
  - Deliver compressions on the lower third of the sternum to a depth of about one-third the AP diameter of the chest.

- Maintain a 3:1 ratio of compressions to ventilations, giving 90 compressions and 30 breaths per minute (½ second per event, 120 events per minute)
- Continue chest compressions and ventilation until the heart rate is 60/min or greater.
- If the heart rate remains less than 60/min despite adequate ventilation with O_2 and chest compressions, recommend epinephrine administration.
- If after stabilization an infant develops a Silverman-Anderson score greater than 5, recommend transfer to intensive care for further assessment and management.
- If after stabilization an infant develops central cyanosis in room air or has a preductal SpO_2 that does not quickly normalize or falls back below 90%, recommend transfer to intensive care for further assessment and management.

Apnea of Prematurity

Apnea of prematurity is a developmental disorder affecting infants born at less than 37 weeks' gestation. Although likely caused by "physiologic immaturity" of respiratory control (central apnea), some premature infants also exhibit airway obstruction (obstructive apnea). By definition, the apnea episodes must be recurrent and either last for more than 20 seconds or be accompanied by cyanosis, a 4% or greater fall in SpO_2, or bradycardia. In general, the incidence of apnea of prematurity varies inversely with gestational age and birth weight, with nearly all infants born at less than 28 weeks' gestation or weighing less than 1,000 g being affected. The incidence of apneas typically decreases over time, often resolving by 34–36 weeks' postconceptual age.

Assessment/Information Gathering

- Look for recurrent episodes of apnea with or without desaturation or bradycardia during the first 2 to 3 days after birth in any spontaneously breathing infant born at less than 37 weeks' gestational age (events are typically identified and recorded by cardiorespiratory monitors).
- Assess the infant and the record to rule out other common causes of apnea, including hypoxemia, anemia, sepsis, unstable thermal environment (hypothermia or hyperthermia), administration of opiates to the mother before birth or the infant postnatally, intracranial hemorrhage, congenital upper airway anomalies (e.g., choanal atresia), seizures, and electrolyte or acid–base disturbances.

Treatment/Decision Making

- Recommend that the infant be cared for in the prone position.
- Recommend continuous apnea monitoring for respirations and heart rate (Chapter 2).
- Recommend continuous pulse oximetry if episodes of desaturation occur with the apnea.
- When a confirmed episode of apnea occurs, intervene immediately if the infant exhibits cyanosis or severe pallor; otherwise, wait 10 seconds to see if the apnea "self-corrects."
- If an apnea episode does not self-correct within 10 seconds of alarm notification, progressively follow these steps:
  1. Stimulate the infant by tickling or flicking the feet or stroking the abdomen.
  2. If there is no response, briefly suction the oropharynx, and then repeat the stimulation.
  3. If there is still no response, slightly extend the neck to minimize airway obstruction.
  4. If there is still no response, apply bag and mask ventilation using the O_2% that the infant was receiving prior to the episode (*not* 100%).
  5. If there is still no response, consider either intubation and mechanical ventilation or nasal noninvasive positive-pressure ventilation (NPPV).
- Recommend daily dosing of caffeine until the infant is at least 33 weeks' postconceptual age or has infrequent events that do not resolve spontaneously (apnea monitoring should continue for a further week after medication is stopped).
- If the infant has frequent apnea episodes requiring stimulation despite caffeine administration, recommend or implement either nasal CPAP at 4–6 cm H_2O or a high-flow nasal cannula at 1–6 L/min, adjusted empirically to reduce the frequency of events.

Infant Respiratory Distress Syndrome

Infant respiratory distress syndrome (IRDS; previously called hyaline membrane disease) is a common disorder in premature infants. In these infants, the lungs have not yet completed development and, therefore, lack sufficient quantities of pulmonary surfactant. The lack of normal surfactant increases surface tension, making the alveoli prone to collapse. The resulting atelectasis causes shunting and severe hypoxemia that does not respond to O_2 therapy. The severe hypoxemia, in turn, causes pulmonary vasoconstriction and hypertension, which can lead to circulatory disturbances and extrapulmonary right-to-left shunting. The high surface tension also decreases lung compliance and increases the work of breathing.

Assessment/Information Gathering

- Assess the history and look for evidence of prematurity (less than 37 weeks' gestation), low birth weight (less than 1,500 g), and related maternal risk factors such as diabetes (Chapter 1).
- Assess for prior measurement (at 35 weeks' gestation) of lecithin/sphingomyelin (L/S) ratio (less than 2) and absence of phosphatidyl glycerol as indicators of pulmonary immaturity.
- Observe for signs of progressive respiratory distress shortly after birth, including tachypnea (more than 60 breaths/min), subcostal and intercostal retractions, expiratory grunting, decreased breath sounds, nasal flaring, and cyanosis in room air (signs may not appear for a few hours).
- Recommend a chest x-ray, looking for low lung volume with diffuse reticulogranular ("ground-glass") appearance and air bronchograms.
- Recommend an ABG, looking for respiratory acidosis with severe hypoxemia.
- In terms of the differential diagnosis, transient tachypnea of the newborn (TTN) is generally seen in more mature infants (i.e., term or late preterm infants) compared to RDS.
- Recommend appropriate cultures to rule out an infectious cause, such as streptococcal pneumonia or sepsis.
- Recommend a hyperoxia test to rule out a critical congenital heart defect (CCHD) as the cause of the cyanosis and respiratory distress (CCHDs are described later in this chapter).
- Recommend an echocardiogram if extrapulmonary shunting (e.g., PDA) is suspected.

Treatment/Decision Making

- For women at risk of giving birth between weeks 24 and 34 of pregnancy, recommend corticosteroid administration prior to birth ("antenatal steroids" enhance lung maturation and reduce the risk of RDS, brain hemorrhage, and death).
- For spontaneously breathing infants with clinical and x-ray findings indicating IRDS, recommend or implement early prophylactic surfactant therapy using the "intubation–surfactant–extubation" approach (i.e., the infant is briefly intubated after birth, is administered surfactant, and then is immediately extubated and placed on nasal CPAP at 4–6 cm H_2O).
- A high-flow nasal cannula at 1–6 L/min is an alternative to nasal CPAP; CPAP levels vary with flow and leakage and are judged empirically by patient response.
- Recommend maintenance of a neutral thermal environment using an incubator or radiant warmer (Chapter 4).
- Provide sufficient F_{IO_2} to maintain the Pa_{O_2} between 50 and 70 torr or the Sp_{O_2} between 85% and 92%.
- Recommend intubation and mechanical ventilation for any infant less than 27 weeks' gestational age whose mother did not receive antenatal steroids or if the infant
  - Is apneic
  - Is unable to maintain an adequate airway
  - Exhibits increased work of breathing (grunting, retractions, flaring) on CPAP
  - Cannot maintain a pH greater than 7.25 on CPAP

- When mechanical ventilation is required, to avoid volutrauma, recommend or implement permissive hypercapnia by using volume-controlled ventilation with low tidal volumes (4–5 mL/kg corrected) and letting the $Paco_2$ rise as long as the pH remains greater than 7.20.
- Aim for early extubation to nasal CPAP in the following circumstances:
  - The infant exhibits adequate respiratory drive.
  - Mean airway pressure is 7 cm H_2O or less.
  - Satisfactory oxygenation can be maintained on 35% O_2 or less.
- Do not recommend high-frequency ventilation (it does not offer any benefit over conventional ventilation).
- Do not recommend inhaled nitric oxide (INO) therapy unless the IRDS is accompanied by pulmonary hypertension of the newborn (PPHN).

Bronchopulmonary Dysplasia

Bronchopulmonary dysplasia (BPD) is a syndrome defined primarily by the long-term need for supplemental O_2 among premature infants (less than 32 weeks' gestation) for at least 28 days after birth. Within this broad definition, three levels of BPD are recognized, all based on assessing the infant's status at 36 weeks' postconceptual age:

- *Mild*: infant can maintain satisfactory oxygenation breathing room air.
- *Moderate*: infant needs supplemental O_2, but no more than 30% to maintain satisfactory oxygenation,
- *Severe*: infant needs more than 30% O_2 to maintain satisfactory oxygenation.

BPD is associated with prolonged treatment with O_2 and positive-pressure ventilation, especially in premature or low-birth-weight (less than 1,250 g) infants and those being managed for infant respiratory distress syndrome. Pathological changes are complex and include airway inflammation, bronchial smooth muscle and arteriole hypertrophy, bronchomalacia, interstitial edema, alveolar hypoplasia, capillary obliteration, and pulmonary fibrosis.

Assessment/Information Gathering

- Evaluate for the presence and severity of BPD using the 36-week assessment guidelines described previously.
- Assess for risk factors: prematurity, low birth weight, IRDS, mechanical ventilation, high Fio_2 needs or maintenance of Spo_2 more than 95%, sepsis, and patent ductus arteriosus.
- Conduct or review a physical examination, looking for tachypnea, retractions, crackles, and expiratory wheezing.
- Recommend or review a chest x-ray, which will typically show decreased lung volumes with diffuse areas of both atelectasis and hyperinflation with possible evidence of fibrosis or pulmonary interstitial emphysema.
- Obtain an arterial blood gas analysis, which typically indicates respiratory acidosis with hypoxemia.
- Recommend an echocardiogram to detect pulmonary hypertension and cor pulmonale (due to pulmonary vasoconstriction, arteriole hypertrophy, and capillary obliteration).

Treatment/Decision Making

The best way to reduce the impact of BPD is to prevent it. To help prevent BPD, recommend or implement the following measures for high-risk infants:

- The lowest level of supplemental O_2 needed to maintain an Spo_2 in the 88–92% range, with slightly higher levels acceptable for infants who are 33 weeks' or more postconceptual age
- Prophylactic surfactant treatment using the "intubation–surfactant–extubation" approach described for IRDS
- Prophylactic vitamin A administration (decreases the risk of BPD development in extremely low-birth-weight infants)
- Early (before the infant is a few days old) prophylactic caffeine administration (decreases the incidence of BPD and the duration of PPV)

If the infant is already intubated and receiving PPV with O_2, recommend the following measures:

- Select volume-controlled ventilation, not pressure-controlled ventilation.
- Implement permissive hypercapnia to avoid volutrauma by using low tidal/minute volumes; this requires letting the $Paco_2$ rise as long as the pH remains greater than 7.20.
- Wean the infant to nasal CPAP as soon as possible, accepting $Paco_2$ levels as high as 60–65 torr as long as they remain stable and the pH can be kept at or above 7.3.
- Do *not* recommend nitric oxide unless persistent pulmonary hypertension of the newborn is a coexisting diagnosis.
- Do *not* recommend high-frequency ventilation (it does not offer any benefit over conventional modes).

Other considerations to recommend:

- Ensuring adequate calorie intake (infants with BPD have higher than normal calorie needs).
- Restricting fluids and providing diuresis (using hydrochlorothiazide and spironolactone, not Lasix) may provide some benefit.
- Administering a β_2 bronchodilator such as albuterol to help alleviate episodic bronchospasm, should it occur.
- Performing a tracheotomy on infants likely to need continued ventilator support beyond 48 weeks' postconceptual age.

Corticosteroids were once a mainstay of therapy for BPD. However, due to their severe side effects in premature infants (including development of cerebral palsy), their routine use is no longer recommended. Some neonatologists will still consider corticosteroids in the most severe cases, with current evidence favoring the use of hydrocortisone over dexamethasone.

Most infants with BPD improve gradually over time. Complete weaning off supplemental O_2 can take weeks to months, often is conducted in the home, and may requires a calibrated low-flow meter (capable of accuracy to ±0.25 L/min).

Critical Congenital Heart Defects

A critical congenital heart defect (CCHD) is a structural abnormality in the circulatory system of an infant that is apparent at birth, causes right-to-left shunting with cyanosis and hypoxemia, and normally requires surgical correction early in life. CCHDs include the classic "five T's"—tetralogy of Fallot, total anomalous pulmonary venous return, transposition of the great arteries, tricuspid atresia, and truncus arteriosus—as well as hypoplastic left heart syndrome and pulmonary atresia with intact septum.

In several of these defects, survival depends on maintenance of pulmonary blood flow through an open ductus arteriosus. In fact, as long as the ductus arteriosus remains patent in these patients, major symptoms may not always be apparent. Unfortunately, if CCHD is not recognized and corrected before discharge, infants with these "ductal-dependent" defects can develop life-threatening cardiogenic shock when the ductus closes. For this reason, early detection of these defects is essential.

Assessment/Information Gathering

- Recommend and perform pulse oximetry screening for CCHDs on all infants 24 hours after birth (see **Figure 20-1** for the screening protocol).
- Conduct or review the physical examination, looking for the following findings:
  - Presence of central cyanosis or persistent pallor. Note that cyanosis generally requires an Spo_2 less than 80%; however, even at these levels cyanosis may not be apparent in dark-skinned infants or those with anemia.
  - Abnormal cardiovascular findings, including abnormal heart rate, precordial activity, and sounds; pathologic murmurs; and weak or absent peripheral pulses.
  - Abnormal respiratory findings, including tachypnea, labored breathing at rest, coughing, wheezing, and increased distress when feeding.
- For cyanotic infants, assess the Pao_2 after 10 minutes of breathing 100% O_2 (the hyperoxia test):
  - $Pao_2 < 150$ torr on 100% O_2: *intracardiac* R-L shunt/CCHD likely
  - $Pao_2 > 150$ torr but < 200 torr: ambiguous results
  - $Pao_2 > 200$ torr: *pulmonary* R-L shunt (e.g., RDS, PPHN)

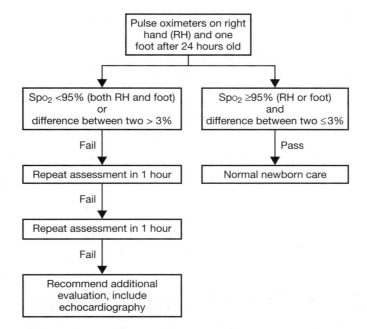

Figure 20-1 Basic Pulse Oximetry Screening Protocol for CCHD. Screening should be performed after 24 hours of life or as late as possible if early discharge is planned. The infant *passes* the screen if while breathing room air *both* the right hand and the foot SpO_2 are 95% or greater, with the difference between them being 3% or less. The infant *fails* the screen if *any* SpO_2 is less than 90% on initial assessment or if two additional measurements (for a total of three) confirm either a low SpO_2 at both measurement sites or more than a 3% difference between them. Infants failing the screen should undergo further assessment to confirm CCHD, including echocardiography.

- Recommend a chest x-ray, which may reveal a tell-tale heart shape:
  - "Snowman" with total anomalous pulmonary venous return
  - "Boot" with pulmonary atresia, tetralogy of Fallot, and tricuspid atresia
  - "Egg on string" with transposition of the great arteries
- Recommend an ECG to detect axis deviation:
  - Right axis deviation indicating right ventricular hypertrophy: transposition of great arteries, total anomalous pulmonary venous return, tetralogy of Fallot
  - Left axis deviation indicating left ventricular or biventricular hypertrophy: truncus arteriosus, transposition of great arteries, tricuspid atresia
- If available, recommend neonatal 2D and Doppler echocardiography for infants who test positive for CCHD on the pulse oximetry screening or hyperoxia test; these imaging modalities provide definitive detection of CCHD and other cardiac anomalies.

Treatment/Decision Making

- Recommend surgical correction for any infant with a confirmed CCHD.
- If an infant with a suspected or confirmed CCHD presents with or develops cardiogenic shock, treat according to the neonatal resuscitation protocol (Chapter 15).
- If an infant with a confirmed ductal-dependent defect exhibits severe cyanosis with evidence of heart failure and pulmonary edema, recommend IV prostaglandin E_1 (PGE_1 or alprostadil) to dilate the ductus arteriosus; be prepared for apnea and hypotension as possible side effects.
- If the infant in heart failure exhibits systemic hypotension or low cardiac output, recommend an inotropic agent such as dopamine.

Table 20-17 Effect of Ventilator Settings on Pulmonary Vascular Resistance and Blood Flow

Ventilator Setting	Increases PVR/Decreases Pulmonary Blood Flow	Decreases PVR/Increases Pulmonary Blood Flow
Minute ventilation	Low ($\uparrow$ Paco$_2$, $\downarrow$ pH)	High ($\downarrow$ Paco$_2$, $\uparrow$ pH)
Inspired O$_2$ concentration	Low (e.g., 18% by adding N$_2$)	High
Peak/mean airway pressure	High	Low
PEEP	High	Low
I:E ratio	High	Low

- For infants requiring mechanical ventilation, the neonatologist may request changes in ventilator settings to alter vascular resistance and blood flow through the pulmonary circulation; **Table 20-17** summarizes how key ventilator settings can affect pulmonary vascular resistance and blood flow.

OTHER MEDICAL OR SURGICAL CONDITIONS

A variety of other medical and surgical conditions can appear on the CSE. Here we focus on two of the most common disorders you may be expected to help manage: drug overdose and poisonings and obesity–hypoventilation syndrome.

Drug Overdose and Poisonings

Harmful accidental or intentional abusive exposure to various drugs or chemicals is a common occurrence that often requires supportive respiratory care. With so many different harmful agents potentially involved, it is impossible to cover all of the responses needed to deal with every specific substance. Instead, we focus on the general aspects of drug overdose and poisoning management.

Assessment/Information Gathering

Symptoms of drug overdose and poisoning vary according to the specific substance involved and the route by which it enters the body. Given this enormous variability in presentation, resuscitation and stabilization of the patient comes first, with in depth symptom assessment and identification of the specific offending substance of secondary importance (see the discussion of treatment and decision making).

Nonetheless, general knowledge of the diagnostic process in cases of suspected drug overdose or poisonings can help direct therapy, especially when considering antidote treatment. To that end, the following guidelines apply when assessing a patient for harmful exposure to drugs or chemicals:

- If available, try to determine what the patient ingested, injected, or was exposed to, including when and how much.
- Quickly assess the patient's level of consciousness and vital signs, looking for key clusters of symptoms (called "toxidromes") that might indicate the offending agent's general category or classification (**Table 20-18**).
- Obtain an ABG to assess for hypoxemia, hypercapnia, and acid–base imbalances.
- Recommend or conduct CO-oximetry to measure HbCO levels (carbon monoxide poisoning).
- Recommend serum electrolytes and calculation of the anion gap (look for high-anion-gap metabolic acidosis in salicylate, methanol, and ethylene glycol poisoning).
- Recommend urinalysis to identify the presence of offending drugs or drug by-products.
- Recommend a quantitative toxicology screen to measure serum levels of common agents such as acetaminophen, salicylates, ethanol/methanol, barbiturates, and cyclic antidepressants.
- Recommend an ECG if the patient is unstable or is suspected of having ingested any drugs with potential cardiac toxicity (e.g., digoxin).

Table 20-18 Categories of Drugs or Poisons and Their Typical Symptoms

Drug Category	Example Agents	Symptoms
Narcotic	Opiate analgesics (morphine, heroin, oxycodone)	Depressed level of consciousness, respiratory depression, miosis
Sedative/hypnotic	Barbiturates, benzodiazepines	Depressed level of consciousness, respiratory depression, hyporeflexia
Adrenergic/sympathomimetic	Ecstasy, amphetamines, methamphetamines	CNS stimulation, mydriasis, hypertension, tachycardia, seizures
Cholinergic/parasympathomimetic	Neostigmine, organophosphates (insecticides), chemical warfare nerve agents (e.g., sarin)	Salivation, lacrimation, urination, defecation, GI upset, and emesis ("SLUDGE"); bradycardia, fasciculations, confusion, miosis
Anticholinergic	Atropine, anticholinergic bronchodilators (e.g., tiotropium), diphenhydramine (Benadryl), bupropion (Zyban)	Dry skin, hyperthermia, mydriasis, tachycardia, delirium, thirst

Treatment/Decision Making

- Always prioritize the ABCs (airway, breathing, circulation) in managing drug overdoses or poisonings.
- Recommend intubation for any overdose/poisoning patient who is obtunded or any patient for whom upper airway control is suspect or aspiration is a concern.
- Provide supplemental O_2 as needed to maintain the SpO_2 above 90% (administer 100% O_2 for suspected carbon monoxide poisoning).
- Unless there is evidence of cardiac depression, recommend fluids to treat hypotension.
- If the patient is obtunded and exhibits miosis and respiratory depression, *assume* opioid overdose and recommend naloxone administration.
- For patients suspected of orally ingesting an overdose of drugs, recommend gastric lavage or activated charcoal administration (*both require airway protection*).
- In cases of salicylate or barbiturate overdose, recommend alkaline diuresis via bicarbonate administration.
- Recommend hemodialysis for *life-threatening* ingestions of alcohols, amphetamines, salicylates, barbiturates, and lithium.
- Once the drug or chemical agent is identified, recommend the appropriate reversing agent or antidote (**Table 20-19**).

Obesity–Hypoventilation Syndrome

The obesity–hypoventilation syndrome (OHS) is defined as obesity (BMI > 30 kg/m²) accompanied by chronic hypoventilation leading to daytime hypercapnia and hypoxemia ($PaCO_2$ > 45 torr and

Table 20-19 Reversing Agents or Antidotes for Selected Drugs and Chemicals

Category or Drug	Reversing Agent
Opioid narcotics	Naloxone (Narcan)
Acetaminophen	N-acetylcysteine
Benzodiazepines	Flumazenil (Romazicon)
β-Adrenergic blockers	Glucagon
Calcium-channel blockers	Calcium chloride, glucagon
Carbon monoxide	100% O_2, hyperbaric O_2
Cyanide	Nitrites, hydroxocobalamin, sulfanegen TEA
Organophosphates	Atropine, pralidoxime

$PaO_2 < 70$ mm Hg). Most patients with OHS also exhibit sleep-disordered breathing, due primarily to obstructive sleep apnea (OSA). Definitive diagnosis requires excluding any coexisting pulmonary, neuromuscular, neurologic, or hormonal condition that maybe causing ventilatory impairment, such as COPD, kyphoscoliosis, central sleep apnea, and hypothyroidism.

In OHS, excessive fatty tissue restricts chest-wall movement, reduces lung volumes (restrictive pattern), decreases both thoracic and lung compliance, and increases the work of breathing (along with O_2 consumption and CO_2 production). Many patients with this syndrome also exhibit a blunted ventilatory response to hypercapnia.

Assessment/Information Gathering

- Measure the patient's height and weight, and compute the body mass index to document obesity (BMI > 30 kg/m²).
- Obtain an ABG to document hypercapnia (usually compensated respiratory acidosis) and hypoxemia breathing room air.
- Review or obtain a patient history, looking for fatigue, exertional dyspnea, and findings consistent with OSA (e.g., loud snoring, witnessed obstructive apneas, excessive daytime sleepiness, morning headaches).
- Obtain an objective measure of daytime sleepiness using the Epworth Sleepiness Scale (Chapter 1).
- Recommend a polysomnography exam for any patient with OHS and symptoms of OSA and/or an Epworth Sleepiness Scale score of 10 or higher.
- Obtain an objective measure of dyspnea using the Borg Scale or equivalent measure (Chapter 2).
- Review or conduct a physical exam, to include inspection of the airway (Chapter 2) and assessment for hypertension and signs of cor pulmonale/heart failure such as peripheral edema and a loud P_2 heart sound.
- Recommend spirometry and lung volume measure to confirm the presence and assess the magnitude of pulmonary restriction (the typical pattern to look for: decreased TLC, IC, FRC, and FVC, but normal FEV_1/FVC).
- Recommend measurement of MIP/MEP to confirm abnormal respiratory mechanics and respiratory muscles' weakness or impairment.
- Recommend a complete blood count (to assess for secondary polycythemia) and a thyroid screen to identify hypothyroidism.

Treatment/Decision Making

- When a patient with OHS presents to the ED with acute-on-chronic hypercapnic respiratory failure, quickly assess the patient:
  - If pH is less than 7.25 and the patient is obtunded with signs of hemodynamic instability, implement appropriate resuscitation measures (ABCs) and consider intubation, mechanical ventilation, and admission to intensive care.
  - If pH is greater than 7.25 and the patient remains conscious and is otherwise stable, recommend noninvasive positive-pressure ventilation (NPPV or BiPAP) and supportive care.
- For stable but symptomatic patients with OHS:
  - Recommend an initial trial of CPAP (successful treatment may require pressures of 12–14 cm H_2O).
  - If the patient remains hypercapnic on CPAP, recommend NPPV.
  - For outpatient management, follow the basic disease management guidelines in Chapter 7 and the home care principles in Chapter 17.
- For stable patients with OHS who remain hypoxemic on CPAP, or if warranted by overnight oximetry data, implement or recommend supplemental nocturnal O_2 administration in addition to CPAP or NIPPV.
- For long-term resolution of OHS, recommend a managed weight-loss program using appropriate diet therapy and medications; if that proves ineffective in sustaining weight loss over time, recommend bariatric surgery.

Test-Taking Tips and Techniques

Craig L. Scanlan

To perform well on the NBRC written exams (CRT and written registry or WRRT), you first must know the subject matter. However, to pass these exams, you also need good test-taking skills. **Figure A-1** offers our simple two-part "formula" for success on these exams.

Our simple formula reveals why many knowledgeable candidates fail their NBRC written exam. Typically, such individuals do poorly because they lack the test-taking skills needed to translate their mastery of the subject matter into consistently correct answers. The common refrain "I'm no good at taking tests" is a symptom of this problem. Fortunately, this condition is treatable. With good guidance and practice, everyone can develop good test-taking skills. The purpose of this appendix is to help you become a better test-taker. By doing so, you will improve your odds of passing the NBRC written exams.

HOW TO FAIL YOUR NBRC EXAM

It might seem strange to begin with instructions on how to fail your test. In fact, knowing why people fail NBRC exams can actually help you avoid failure. Of course, the most common reason why candidates perform poorly on these exams is lack of content knowledge. Other causes of failure include the following:

- Taking the test "cold" or unprepared
- Memorizing as many practice questions and answers as possible
- Reviewing everything you ever learned in school
- Cramming the night before the exam
- Letting anxiety get the best of you
- Not finishing the test

It always amazes us how some candidates insist on taking NBRC exams without proper preparation. Of course, some do so because they plan poorly and run out of time. Others take the test "cold" because they are overly confident. Last and most foolish are those who take these exams without preparation just to "see how they will do." By not preparing, you risk wasting both your time and your money should you fail. Although we do advocate "gambling" on specific test questions, taking an NBRC exam without any preparation is a very bad bet that you are likely to lose. As indicated in our formula for success, you cannot pass these tests without good knowledge of their content. And good knowledge of the subject matter comes only with good preparation, as provided in Chapters 1–17 of this text.

Another common cause of failure is the misguided strategy of memorizing hundreds of practice questions and answers. As mentioned in this text's Introduction, this strategy is a waste of your time. Instead, you should use practice questions and answers to help identify concepts that you know and those that you still need to work on.

$$\boxed{\begin{array}{c}\text{Passing the}\\\text{NBRC exam}\end{array}} = \boxed{\begin{array}{c}\text{Knowledge of}\\\text{subject matter}\end{array}} + \boxed{\begin{array}{c}\text{Good test-}\\\text{taking skills}\end{array}}$$

Figure A-1 Formula for Success on the NBRC Exams

We also know of candidates who prepare by surrounding themselves with all the books and lecture notes they acquired in school. Many of these folks simply do not know where to begin, and most will feel overwhelmed by the sheer volume of study materials. Such a strategy typically causes anxiety and confusion, which lead to poor exam performance. To avoid the problems associated with this strategy, you first need to remember that the NBRC exams do *not* test for isolated facts or the "book knowledge" covered in school. Instead, *these exams assess your job-related knowledge and skills*. Thus, instead of reviewing everything taught in school, your time is better spent focusing on the specific test content as defined by the NBRC and as covered in this text.

Cramming is probably most common reason candidates fail NBRC exams. Lacking a good study plan and pressed for time, many folks put off preparation until the week *or even the night* before their test date. Besides producing even worse anxiety than trying to review everything ever learned, cramming typically causes loss of sleep in the days leading up to the test. "Dazed and confused" best describes these candidates when they show up to take the test—and "disappointed" when they get their score reports!

Anxiety is another common cause of poor exam performance. More precisely, *overanxiety* can lead to failure. Some anxiety prior to taking a test is not only natural but can actually be beneficial. Like getting "pumped up" before a sports contest, the stress associated with test taking can help motivate you to excel and improve your exam performance.

Last, the surest way to fail any test is not to finish it. Because every question on NBRC multiple-choice exams that you do not complete counts against you, you simply cannot afford to throw away points by omitting answers. To finish these exams in the allotted time, you will need to develop good pacing strategies (described subsequently in this appendix).

HOW TO PASS YOUR NBRC WRITTEN EXAM

Based on our decades of experience working with NBRC candidates, we have developed a three-pronged strategy for passing the CRT and WRRT exams. First, you must fully understand the structure and content of these exams, including the significant differences between them—a strategy we call "know your enemy." Second, in studying for these exams, you need to prepare yourself as if "working" in the idealized setting we call the "NBRC hospital." Last, and most important, you need to develop good test-taking skills—that is, you must become "test-wise."

Know Your Enemy

A common strategy among generals planning a battle is to *know your enemy*. Thinking of your written exam as an adversary to be conquered can help you prepare for your upcoming "battle." In this case, *knowing the enemy means understanding both the structure and the content of the exam you will take and applying this knowledge to your study plan*.

The structure and content of the CRT and WRRT exams are well defined in the current version of the NBRC's *Candidate Handbook and Application*. The current CRT exam consists of 140 graded questions and 20 ungraded items being pre-tested for future use. The current WRRT exam consists of 100 graded questions and 15 ungraded items.*

The content of both exams is based on national survey data describing the common clinical skills performed at entry into the field (CRT exam) or as an advanced practitioner (WRRT exam). Questions on both exams fall into one of three major content sections: (I) Patient Data Evaluation and Recommendations; (II) Equipment Manipulation, Infection Control, and Quality Control; and (III) Initiation and Modification of Therapeutic Procedures. Also on both exams, questions are written at three different cognitive levels: recall, application, and analysis. **Table A-1** compares the current CRT and WRRT exams by the number and level of questions in each of their three major sections.

---

*Beginning in 2015 there will be one written exam with two different cut scores. Candidates attaining the lower score will earn the CRT credential, while those meeting the higher score requirement will be eligible for the CSE. Text updates reflecting these and other NBRC credentialing exam changes can be accessed via the J&B Learning companion website described in Appendix D.

Table A-1 Comparison of CRT and WRRT Exam Structure

Section	CRT Exam Number of Questions	% of Total	% Application or Analysis	Written RRT Exam (WRRT) Number of Questions	% of Total	% Application or Analysis
I	26	18%	58%	28	28%	86%
II	29	21%	83%	12	12%	83%
III	85	61%	78%	60	60%	100%

Careful review of this table demonstrates first that the majority of questions on *both exams* (approximately 60%) assess your ability to initiate and modify therapy (Section III)—but that is where the similarity ends. The CRT exam gives almost twice the weight to equipment questions (Section II) as does the WRRT (21% versus 12%, respectively). Conversely, almost 90% of the WRRT focuses on evaluating patient data and implementing or altering procedures (Sections I and III).

Perhaps more significant is the different level of questioning characterizing these two exams. Overall, 75% of the questions on the CRT exam are at the application or analysis level, with 25% requiring only recall of information. In contrast, 94% of the questions on the WRRT exam are written to assess your ability to apply or analyze information as the basis for action, with a mere 6% focusing on recollection of facts.

To help understand differences in the cognitive level of questions, we will look at three examples covering the same content area, with the correct answers underlined (Subcategory III-E: Evaluate and Monitor the Patient's Objective and Subjective Responses to Respiratory Care).

Recall Example

A-1. An otherwise healthy 25-year-old male patient who took an overdose of sedatives is being supported on a ventilator. Which of the following measures of total static compliance (lungs + thorax) would you expect in this patient?
A. 100 mL/cm H_2O
B. 10 mL/cm H_2O
C. 1 mL/cm H_2O
D. 0.1 mL/cm H_2O

Comments: To evaluate and monitor a patient, you need to know what is normal and what is abnormal. This question tests your ability to recall normal static compliance.

Application Example

A-2. An adult patient receiving volume control A/C ventilation has a tidal volume of 700 mL, a peak pressure of 50 cm H_2O, and a plateau pressure of 40 cm H_2O, and is receiving 5 cm H_2O positive end-expiratory pressure (PEEP). What is this patient's static compliance?
A. 200 mL/cm H_2O
B. 20 mL/cm H_2O
C. 2 mL/cm H_2O
D. 0.2 mL/cm H_2O

Comments: This item tests your ability to apply a formula to a clinical situation (most formula-type questions are at the application level). To answer it correctly, you need to "plug" the correct data into the formula for computing static compliance—that is, compliance (mL/cm H_2O) = tidal volume ÷ (plateau pressure − PEEP).

Analysis Example

A-3. A patient in the intensive care unit with congestive heart failure receiving assist/control ventilation with a set volume of 650 mL exhibits the following data on three consecutive patient–ventilator checks:

Time	Peak Pressure	Plateau Pressure	PEEP
9:00 AM	40	25	8
10:00 AM	50	35	8
11:00 AM	60	45	8

The patient also exhibits diffuse crackles at the bases and some wheezing. Which of the following would you recommend for this patient?
A. <u>A diuretic</u>
B. A bronchodilator
C. A mucolytic
D. A steroid

Comments: This item assesses your ability to analyze monitoring data and apply this information to recommend a treatment approach for this patient. First, you must analyze the data, which should reveal that the patient is suffering from a progressive decrease in compliance (rising plateau – PEEP pressure difference). Second, you need to recognize that in patients with congestive heart failure, the most common cause of a progressive decrease in compliance is the development of pulmonary edema. Last, you need to apply these data and your knowledge of pathophysiology and pharmacology to recommend the correct course of action—in this case, the administration of a diuretic such as Lasix.

What conclusions can you glean from analysis of the NBRC CRT and WRRT content outlines? Key pointers include the following:

- The majority of test questions focus on therapeutic procedures—so you should spend the bulk of your preparation time on this content (Chapters 7–17 of this text).
- Because one-fourth or fewer of the questions included on these exams are based on recall, *you cannot pass either the CRT or WRRT by simply memorizing facts.*
- When preparing for the CRT exam, you need to give substantially more emphasis to equipment than when preparing for the WRRT; conversely, your study plan for the WRRT must stress *analysis* of patient data and use of that information to select, implement, or modify procedures.
- Because these exams focus on job-related skills, it can help to visualize and relate your experiences at the bedside as you prepare for your test.

Working in the NBRC Hospital

Besides the structure and content of the exams, your study plan also should take into account what we refer to as the "NBRC hospital." What is the NBRC hospital? *It is not a place, but rather a state of mind.* You "enter" the NBRC hospital whenever you take an NBRC exam. This hospital may or may not resemble the clinical sites you rotated through as a student or the facility where you currently work. Instead, it represents an idealized institution. What do we mean by *idealized*? We mean that the NBRC hospital's respiratory care department always relies on generally accepted standards in the field, based in part on current nationally recognized practice guidelines. In addition, the NBRC hospital respiratory care department's "procedure manual" covers a broad variety of clinical skills performed by RTs throughout the United States. For these reasons, when working in the NBRC hospital, you may be expected to know and do more or do things differently from the way they are done in your facility.

For example, in your facility, a separate electrocardiogram (ECG) department may be responsible for taking 12-lead ECGs and maintaining the related equipment. Perhaps nurses, physician assistants, or residents are the ones responsible for obtaining 12-lead ECGs in your special care units or the emergency department. In the NBRC hospital, however, you should be able to obtain a 12-lead ECG, interpret the basic findings, and even troubleshoot the device should it not function properly.

Another potential distinction characterizing the NBRC hospital is the level of independent judgment you are expected to exercise. In many hospitals, RTs—especially new graduates—are limited in what they can do without physician approval. However, a quick review of the current CRT and WRRT content outlines reveals that the single most important subsections in the therapeutic procedures section call for the RT to *independently* modify or recommend modifications to these procedures based on the patient's response. Indeed, this expectation goes well beyond making adjustments to simple "floor therapy." For example, on both the CRT and the WRRT, you will be asked to apply your knowledge to alter key mechanical ventilation parameters, such as the oxygen concentration (FIO_2) and the PEEP level. In these cases, the NBRC hospital typically gives you the freedom to make your own choices, without being constrained by the need for physician approval. This is especially true if the scenario involves protocol-based care. Only if the question clearly limits your discretion (as when a protocol boundary is reached) should you consider not exercising your independent judgment.

So how do you prepare to "work" in the NBRC hospital? We recommend the following:

- Treat the NBRC exam content outlines as your departmental procedure manual, focusing in particular on those things you either do not do or do not frequently perform in your facility.
- Use the pre-test and post-test questions included in this text to help you identify how the practices in the NBRC hospital differ from what you have learned in your training or experience.
- When given the opportunity, do not be afraid to exercise your independent judgment and modify a procedure when changes in the patient's status warrant it.

Develop Test-Wiseness

Students and NBRC examination candidates who consistently do well on tests have two things going for them. First, *they know the content and are confident in that knowledge*. In addition, these high performers have a "secret weapon" in their back pocket—the ability to apply knowledge of test design and specific reasoning skills to improve their exam scores. We call this ability *test-wiseness*.

How does test-wiseness work? **Table A-2** demonstrates the difference between a test-unaware and a test-wise candidate on a hypothetical NBRC written exam. Both candidates are comfortable enough with the content to "know cold" or be absolutely sure about their answers to half the questions on the exam (70 items). Both have to guess at the remaining 70 questions. Unfortunately, the test-unaware candidate does no better than chance on these questions, getting about one in four correct, resulting in a failing score of 88/140, or 63%. In contrast, the test-wise candidate applies knowledge of test design and question reasoning skills to get half of these questions correct, resulting in an overall score of 105/140, or 75%—sufficient to pass the exam.

Table A-2 Hypothetical Impact of Test-Wiseness on Exam Performance

Candidate Response and Performance	Test-Unaware Candidate		Test-Wise Candidate	
	Questions Answered	Questions Correct	Questions Answered	Questions Correct
"Knows cold"	70	70	70	70
Guesses at	70	18	70	35
Raw score		88		105
Percentage		63%		75%
Result		FAIL		PASS!

Fortunately, test-wiseness is a skill that anyone can learn. It entails both techniques related to multiple-choice questions in general and specific rules of thumb applicable to NBRC-like questions. By developing this skill, you not only will improve your exam scores, but will also increase your command over testing situations in general. The added benefits are increased confidence and decreased anxiety when taking tests.

General Tips for Multiple-Choice Items

To become test-wise, you first must develop a good understanding of the structure of NBRC-type multiple-choice questions. Based on this knowledge, there are several general option selection strategies that you can apply to increase your odds of correctly answering individual questions. In addition, because so many candidates have concerns regarding the questions requiring computations, we discuss the special category of math problems.

The Anatomy of Multiple-Choice Items

The NBRC written exams consist entirely of multiple-choice questions. Most of these are the simple "one best answer" type, but a small percentage currently use the multiple-true format, also known as complex multiple-choice items.

The first skill in becoming test-wise is to understand the various parts of these questions and to use that knowledge to improve your odds of identifying the correct answer. **Table A-3** summarizes the key elements common to most NBRC written exam questions, with **Figure A-2** providing a "dissected" example.

Scenario A question scenario briefly describes a clinical situation. We recommend that you thoroughly review the scenario before even looking at the stem or question options (note that sometimes the scenario and the stem are combined and must be reviewed together). When assessing the scenario, look for the following critical information:

- The location or setting (e.g., ICU, outpatient clinic, patient's home)
- The available resources (e.g., equipment that is being used or is at hand)
- The patient's general characteristics (e.g., age, size, disease process, mental status)
- Any relevant objective data (e.g., from ABGs, PFTs)
- Any relevant subjective information (e.g., signs and symptoms)

Assume that all the information in the scenario is there for a reason. As you assess the scenario, note in particular the patient's characteristics and any and all *abnormal* data or information, especially laboratory results. As an example, based on your assessment of the scenario in Figure A-2, you should extract the following critical information:

1. The patient:
   a. Weighs 80 kg (about 176 lbs), which is appropriate for his height (76 inches)
   b. Has aspiration pneumonia (often a cause of hypoxemia)
2. The equipment is a ventilator capable of volume-control

Table A-3 Elements Common to NBRC Multiple-Choice Questions

Question Element	Description
Scenario	Brief description of the clinical situation
Stem	The statement that asks the question or specifies the problem
Options	Possible answers to the question or solutions to the problem
Keyed response	The option that answers the question correctly (the correct answer)
Distractors	The remaining incorrect options (wrong answers)

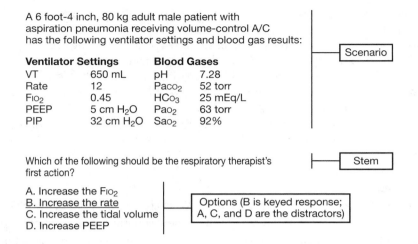

A 6 foot-4 inch, 80 kg adult male patient with
aspiration pneumonia receiving volume-control A/C
has the following ventilator settings and blood gas results: —— Scenario

Ventilator Settings		Blood Gases	
V_T	650 mL	pH	7.28
Rate	12	$Paco_2$	52 torr
F_{IO_2}	0.45	HCO_3	25 mEq/L
PEEP	5 cm H_2O	Pao_2	63 torr
PIP	32 cm H_2O	Sao_2	92%

Which of the following should be the respiratory therapist's
first action? —— Stem

A. Increase the F_{IO_2}
B. Increase the rate
C. Increase the tidal volume
D. Increase PEEP

Options (B is keyed response;
A, C, and D are the distractors)

Figure A-2 The Key Elements in a Typical NBRC-Like Question. In this example,
the scenario and the stem are separate. The scenario and stem may be combined in many
cases.

3. In terms of the objective data:
   a. The set tidal volume is about 8 ml/kg, toward the high end of the acceptable range
   b. The PIP (32 cm H_2O) is also at the high end of the acceptable range for lung protection
   c. The F_{IO_2} is at an acceptably safe level
   d. The blood gas is abnormal:
      i. The primary/most severe problem is acute respiratory acidosis
      ii. Oxygenation is adequate (Sao_2 > 90%)

Stem The stem asks the question or directs your action. In Figure A-2, the stem asks which action
the RT should take first. As with the scenario, you always must read the stem carefully. The stem
often contains key words or phrases that may help you choose the correct answer. **Table A-4**
describes common key words or phrases that you should look for in question stems and suggests
what to do when you encounter them.

In our sample question in Figure A-2, the stem contains the key word *first*. This priority clue
directs you to choose the action *most immediately* needed. Based on our analysis of the blood gas

Table A-4 Key Words or Phrases Found in Question Stems

Type of Clue	What to Look for	What to Do
Priority	Words such as *first, initially, best, priority, safest, most,* and *least*	Put a value on each available option and then place them in rank order
Sequence	Words such as *before, after,* and *next*	Apply procedural knowledge or logic to place the options in proper sequence
Negative polarity	Words such as *not, except, contraindicated, unacceptable,* and *avoid*	Switch from being concerned with what is correct or true to what is false; consider each option to be a true/false question and select the one that is false
Absolutes	Key words such as *always* and *never*	Find the only option that would be correct in every case every time
Verbal associations	Word or phrase in the stem that is identical or similar to a word in the correct answer	Select the option that includes wording similar to that found in the stem

data, we identified the primary/most severe problem as being acute respiratory acidosis. The keyed response or right answer, therefore, should be one that best corrects this problem. Given that correction of respiratory acidosis requires an increase in the patient's minute ventilation, there are two possible options that would achieve that end—that is increasing the rate or increasing the tidal volume. Which to choose? Based on analysis of the scenario, the choice should be clear. An increase in tidal volume would further increase the PIP and the risk of lung damage, making option B (*Increase the rate*) the best choice among the alternatives.

In addition to the general clues described in Table A-4, be on the lookout for other key words or phrases. For example, compare the wording of the following two question stems related to endotracheal intubation:

Stem Wording A	**Stem Wording B**
Which of the following assessment procedures would help determine proper positioning of an endotracheal tube in a patient's trachea?	Which of the following assessment procedures would confirm proper positioning of an endotracheal tube in a patient's trachea?

Note that the two stems are identical except for the verb. Question stem A specifies "help determine," while B specifies "confirm." This tiny variation in wording makes a huge difference in the likely best answer for these two questions. Whereas there are many potentially good answers for A (e.g., breath sounds, capnography, tube insertion length, esophageal detection device, chest x-ray), there is only one consistently correct response for B (i.e., chest x-ray).

Although you should always be on the lookout for key words or phrases in NBRC test items, we also recommend that you avoid reading anything into your exam questions. When you read too much into a test item, you usually end up answering a question differently than intended by the exam writers. Read all questions as is. Do not be led astray by either overanalyzing or oversimplifying any question. Last, avoid drawing any assumptions beyond those supported by the facts at hand. *The simplest interpretation is generally the correct one.*

You also might want to consider a useful strategy that many good test-takers employ. Good test-takers frequently paraphrase the question in their own words and then anticipate the answer— *before looking at the options available.* In the days of pencil-and-paper testing, this meant actually covering up each question's options with scratch paper or the test-taker's hand. Such a strategy can help minimize any confusion that a question's options may cause, especially the distractors. In general, this technique works best when you can quickly and confidently identify the answer in your head.

Options Options are the possible answers to a question. The good news is that every NBRC exam item has only four options, labeled A through D. Also good news for well-prepared candidates is that a substantial portion of these questions will be straightforward and relatively easy to answer. Indeed, if you understand and can apply the information being tested, you will often recognize the correct answer immediately.

The bad news is that not even the smartest candidate knows all the correct answers. Indeed, we believe that, on average, most candidates will be forced to guess on between one-third to one-half of the exam questions. If the best you can do on these questions is to guess randomly at their answers, you will get only approximately 25% of them correct. To do better, you will need to apply our recommended option selection strategies.

Option Selection Strategies

To do well on the NBRC written exams, you need to thoughtfully examine each question's options. *When you are sure of the correct response, select it and move on.* In contrast, if the correct response is not immediately apparent to you, you will need to apply specific skills to analyze the available options before selecting an answer.

First, do not panic when you encounter questions that appear difficult or unfamiliar to you. All exam candidates will encounter dozens of such questions when they take this test. Instead of getting flustered, get resourceful. Whenever you encounter a difficult question, you need to rise to the challenge and use the strategies we provide here to select the most logical answer.

Useful general option selection strategies include the following:

- Always look for the best option, not just a correct one. As demonstrated in our prior example (Figure A-2), two or more options may be correct, but one likely is the "most" correct in *the particular circumstances or with the specific patient described.*
- When you are unsure of the correct option, switch from finding the right answer to finding the wrong answer(s).
- Eliminate options you know to be incorrect; each time you can eliminate a true distractor, you dramatically increase your chances of answering the question correctly.
- When in doubt, give each option a "true–false" test as compared with the stem (the true statement is usually the most plausible answer).
- Be wary of options that are totally unfamiliar to you; more often than not, unfamiliar options are distractors.
- If you encounter a "double negative" in a stem and option, remember that it creates the equivalent positive statement.
- Avoid impulsively selecting an option simply because it provides correct information, as an option can provide correct information but still be the wrong choice because it does not answer the question asked.

If these selection strategies do not help, you will need to apply more specific reasoning skills to identify the correct answer. These skills involve identification of absolutes and qualifiers, dealing with equally plausible options, weighing two options that are opposite to each other, addressing duplicate facts appearing in options, finding the most general or global option, and dealing with a range of option values. In addition, if the question involves using basic math skills, a few key strategies can help you succeed whenever you need to perform computations.

Absolutes (Specific Determiners) As with question stem's, some options may include absolutes or specific determiners. You know an option includes a specific determiner when you find words such as *always, never, all, every, none,* and *only.* These key words indicate that the option has no exceptions. Question A-4 provides an illustrative example.

A-4. Which of the following is true regarding patients in the early stages of an asthmatic attack?
  A. They all exhibit respiratory alkalosis.
  B. They always have moderate hypoxemia.
  C. <u>They have decreased expiratory flows.</u>
  D. They never respond to beta-adrenergic agents.

In this hypothetical example, options A, B, and D all contain specific determiners or absolutes. More often than not, options that use absolutes are false. Generally, you should avoid choosing any option that *must* be true or false every time, in every case, or without exception. In this case, applying this strategy helps you easily zero in on the correct answer (C), the only one not containing an absolute.

Because specific determiners are easy to identify, the NBRC minimizes their use on its exams. Thus you should not expect to encounter these options frequently. Also note that some absolutes, especially those founded in rules or standards, may be a correct option. For example, most would agree that the statement "You always must properly identify the patient before treatment" holds without exception in general patient care situations. For this reason, if the scenario and stem are addressing policies, procedures, rules, or standards, you may need to allow for absolutes. In contrast, *if the question involves a patient in unique clinical circumstances, few, if any, absolutes pertain.*

Qualifiers A qualifier is the opposite of a specific determiner. Qualifiers represent a conditional or "hedge" word or phrase such as *usually, probably, often, generally, may, frequently,* and *seldom.* Qualifiers may appear either in the question stem or in one or more options. Question A-5 is a good example of the use of qualifiers.

A-5. A patient's advanced directive:
   A. Is usually obtained at the time of admission
   B. Can be found in the physician's progress notes
   C. Represents a guideline, not a legal requirement
   D. Cannot be altered after it is written and signed

Options that contain qualifiers usually represent good choices. In this example, only option A contains a qualifier and is, in fact, the correct option. As with absolutes, note that the NBRC minimizes the use of qualifiers in its exam questions, especially in question options. Nonetheless, you need to be on the lookout for these key words and apply the appropriate strategy when needed.

Equally Plausible Options As previously demonstrated (see Figure A-2), NBRC questions often contain two very similar or equivalent options. Question A-6 provides a different example.

A-6. An intubated patient is receiving volume control ventilation. The patient's condition has not changed, but you observe higher peak inspiratory pressures than before. Which of the following is the most likely cause of this problem?
   A. There is a leak in the patient–ventilator system.
   B. The endotracheal tube cuff is deflated or burst.
   C. The endotracheal tube is partially obstructed.
   D. The endotracheal tube is displaced into the pharynx.

Note that options A and B are equivalent because a deflated or burst endotracheal (ET) tube cuff represents a leak in the patient–ventilator system. Usually when two items are very similar to each other and nothing in the scenario helps differentiate between them, they are distractors and should be eliminated from consideration. Then make your choice from among the remaining two options (in this case, option C is the correct choice). By doing so, you immediately improve your odds of correctly answering this question from 25–50%. As noted previously, this is exactly what test-wise candidates do.

What if three of the options are very similar to each other? In this case, apply the "Odd Man Out" strategy, as applicable in answering Question A-7.

A-7. Over a 3-hour period, you note that a patient's plateau pressure has remained stable, but her peak pressure has been steadily increasing. Which of the following is the best explanation for this observation?
   A. The patient's airway resistance has increased.
   B. The patient is developing atelectasis.
   C. The patient's compliance has decreased.
   D. The patient is developing pulmonary edema.

In this example, options B, C, and D are similar, in that they all correspond to a decrease in the patient's compliance. When this occurs, turn your attention to the different or "Odd Man Out" option, which is most likely the correct one (option A in this example).

Opposite Options Another very common way NBRC item writers create distractors is to include a pair of direct opposites among the options—what we call "mirror-image options." Question A-8 is an NBRC-like item with mirror-image options.

A-8. You are assisting with the oral intubation of an adult patient. After the ET tube has been placed, you note that breath sounds are decreased on the left compared with the right lung. What is the most likely cause of this condition?
   A. The tip of the tube is in the right mainstem bronchus.
   B. The cuff of the endotracheal tube has been overinflated.
   C. The endotracheal tube has been inserted into the esophagus.
   D. The tip of the tube is in the left mainstem bronchus.

In general, when you encounter two options that are opposites, chances are the correct choice is one of the two. In this example, options A and D are literally mirror images of each other, and one of them is likely the correct answer. Referral back to the scenario (breath sounds decreased on the left compared to the right) should help you decide which of these two responses is correct (A).

It is important to note that there are exceptions to this strategy. Although you will encounter them less frequently, some questions may include mirror-image options as distractors, meaning that *both* are incorrect choices. In these cases, the item writer is using option opposites to divert your attention from the correct answer, as in Question A-9.

A-9. A patient receiving long-term ventilatory support exhibits a progressive weight gain and a reduction in the hematocrit. Which of the following is the most likely cause of this problem?
   A. Leukocytosis
   B. Chronic hypoxemia
   C. Water retention
   D. Leukocytopenia

In this example, leukocytosis and leukocytopenia are polar opposites. Is one of them the correct choice, or are they both distractors? To make this decision often requires referring back to the scenario or the stem (they are combined in this question). Logically, both leukocytosis and leukocytopenia are more often the result of abnormal processes (such as infection) and less often the *cause* (a key word in the stem) of such processes. Here, these two options are more likely both being used as distractors and should be eliminated. Now, by selecting from the two remaining two options, your odds of correctly answering this question have improved to 50-50. If you also remember that chronic hypoxemia tends to increase—and not decrease—the hematocrit, you can now be almost certain of selecting the correct option (C).

Duplicate Facts in Options Item writers often create options that include two or more similar or identical statements among the choices. Question A-10 is a good example of this question design.

A-10. In reviewing the PFT results of a 67-year-old smoker with an admitting diagnosis of emphysema and chronic bronchitis, you would expect which of the following general findings?
   A. Increased airway resistance and decreased lung compliance
   B. Increased airway resistance and increased lung compliance
   C. Decreased airway resistance and decreased lung compliance
   D. Decreased airway resistance and increased lung compliance

This question's options contain two contrasting sets of statements: increased/decreased resistance and increased/decreased compliance. When you encounter this type of question and are unsure of the answer, you should try to identify any statement that you know is *either* true or false. Once you do so, you usually can eliminate at least two options as being distractors. In this example, if you know that patients with emphysema and chronic bronchitis typically have high airway resistance, then you can immediately eliminate options C and D. Alternatively, if you know that patients with emphysema do *not* have decreased lung compliance, then you can eliminate options A and C. Either way, you have doubled the likelihood of selecting the correct answer (B).

Global Options Question options often include a mix of general and specific statements, as in Question A-11.

A-11. In instructing a patient how to breathe during a small-volume nebulizer drug treatment, the respiratory therapist coaches the patient to hold his breath at the end of each inspiration. The purpose of this maneuver is to improve:
   A. Drug delivery
   B. Particle stability
   C. Aerosol penetration
   D. Inertial impaction

In this example, option A is the most general or global alternative, while options B through D are much more specific. Candidates who are test-wise know that global statements are more likely to be the correct option than choices that are very specific or limited in focus, because the most global option usually includes the most information. In this question, particle stability, aerosol penetration, and inertial impaction are all factors that *fall under the broader concept of enhanced drug delivery*, making option A the best choice here.

Options Constituting a Range Some test questions, especially those focusing on recall, provide options representing a range of values, typically from early to late, or from big to small. Question A-12 is a good example.

A-12. You obtain an SpO_2 measurement on a patient of 80%. Assuming this is an accurate measure of hemoglobin saturation, what is the patient's approximate PaO_2?

    A. 40 torr
    B. <u>50 torr</u>
    C. 60 torr
    D. 70 torr

When item writers create questions like this one, they often try to hide or mask the correct choice by placing it within a set of higher and lower values. In these cases, you should consider eliminating the highest and lowest values, choosing an option in the middle. Following this logic for this question would result in eliminating options A and D, giving you a 50-50 shot at the correct answer to this question (B). Of course, this strategy should be applied only when you do not know the answer. Those familiar with the "40-50-60/70-80-90" rule of thumb might recognize its application to this question and immediately know that 80% saturation roughly corresponds to a PaO_2 of 50 torr.

Math Problems

Typically, the NBRC written exams will include a small number of questions that require a simple calculation to obtain the correct answer. To help you prepare for these questions, Appendix C reviews common cardiopulmonary calculations that are likely to appear on these exams. Here we provide more general guidance in regard to selecting options when presented with questions involving math.

Because many candidates lack confidence in their math skills, they tend to panic when confronted with a question that requires computation. This response generally is unwarranted because the math skills tested on the NBRC exams are rather basic and typically involve no more than one or two computational steps. Thus there is really no reason to get anxious over these questions.

To improve your confidence in approaching math questions and help you consistently select the correct answers, we recommend the following:

- Always set up the problem before you begin to solve it; use the scratch paper provided at the testing center to write out the applicable formula, *being sure to set it up properly to solve for the value being requested.*
- After setting up the formula, try *estimating* or "*ballparking*" the answer without calculating it; prior estimation can help you avoid making formula or computational errors.
- After doing the computation, do it a second time to confirm that you get the same answer.
- Do not immediately select an answer that matches your calculation; most math question distractors are based on common computation errors. Instead, reread the problem, recheck your formula, and if necessary redo your math.
- If you are completely stumped, "choose from the means and not the extremes." If you do not know the applicable formula or cannot come up with a good estimate, toss out the high and low numbers and select one near the middle.

Question A-13 illustrates using math problem strategies to arrive at the correct answer.

A-13. A portable spirometer requires that you enter the patient's height in centimeters to derive normal values. The patient tells you that she is 5 feet 6 inches tall. Which value would you enter into the device?

A. 26 cm
B. 66 cm
C. <u>168 cm</u>
D. 186 cm

First, you should set up the problem. This represents a straight unit conversion, from English to metric units (inches to centimeters). All such problems are based on a simple formula that requires knowledge of the applicable conversion factor:

Measurement (X units) × conversion factor = measurement (Y units)

In this case, the X units are inches, the Y units are centimeters, and the conversion factor is 2.54 cm/inch. Thus the proper setup of the formula for this problem is

Measurement (inches) × 2.54 cm/in = measurement (cm)

Slightly complicating this problem is your need to convert 5 feet 6 inches to inches. Because there are 12 inches to a foot, the patient is (5 × 12) + 6, or 66 inches tall. Note that the numeric value 66 appears among the distractors. Including a value derived in an intermediate step as a distractor is a common ploy used by item writers. You can avoid succumbing to this ploy by completing all computations before comparing your answer to those provided.

Now that you are sure you have set up the correct formula to answer the question, estimate the answer before you compute it. The answer should be about 2½ times greater than the patient's height in inches, 66 inches. Twice 66 is *about* 130 and half of 66 is *about* 33, so the answer should be *about* 130 + 33 or 163 cm. Based on estimation alone, answer C, 168 cm, looks very good. Based on estimation, you also can eliminate option A because it is *less than* the patient's height in inches. Based on the setup of your formula, that would be impossible. Indeed, option A (26 cm) is lurking there to catch those who set up the formula improperly or use the wrong conversion factor. You would get 26 cm as the answer if you mistakenly *divided* the patient's height in inches by 2.54 instead of multiplying by this factor.

Last, after doing the initial computation, do not immediately select the answer. Instead, recompute the answer after rereading the question and rechecking the setup of your formula.

What if you do not know the exact formula or factor to use? Ideally, your estimated answer will allow you to eliminate at least some of the distractors and improve your odds of answering the question correctly. If elimination does not help, apply our last-ditch "choose from the means and not the extremes" strategy.

Specific Tips for Common NBRC-Type Items

Applying general option selection strategies will go a long way toward improving your NBRC written exam score. To boost your score even more, we have developed several item response guidelines that apply specifically to common NBRC question formats. By learning to apply these guidelines when you encounter these question formats, you will increase your likelihood of passing the exam!

The Triple S Rule

The "Triple S" rule is the most basic of all principles we recommend you apply to answering NBRC-type questions. Put simply, if a patient gets worse when you are giving therapy, *Stop, Stabilize,* and *Stay.* In other words, stop what you are doing, try to stabilize the patient, and stay until help arrives. Question A-14 is a good example of the Triple S rule.

A-14. During postural drainage of the left lower lobe, a patient complains of acute chest pain. Which of the following should you do?
- **A.** Give the patient supplemental oxygen
- **B.** Continue the treatment with the bed flat
- **C.** Ask the nurse to administer pain medication
- **D.** <u>Discontinue the treatment and monitor the patient</u>

A corollary to the Triple S rule is to *never start* therapy if the patient is exhibiting abnormal signs or symptoms that could be worsened by your action. Instead, as illustrated in Question A-15, you should always contact the physician.

A-15. A 45-year-old patient with asthma is prescribed 0.5 mL of albuterol (Proventil) in 3 mL normal saline via small-volume nebulizer. Before initiating therapy, you note from chart review that the patient is severely hypertensive and has been experiencing episodes of superventricular tachycardia. Which of the following should you do?
- **A.** Administer the treatment as ordered
- **B.** <u>Postpone the treatment and notify the physician</u>
- **C.** Dilute the albuterol with extra normal saline
- **D.** Decrease the amount of albuterol administered

Act First, Ask Questions Later

With all the emphasis that teachers place on assessing patients, students often forget that sometimes you should act first, and only then gather information. The best examples are always emergency situations, where any delay for information gathering may cause harm to the patient. Question A-16 provides a good example of this principle.

A-16. A patient is admitted to the emergency department comatose with suspected smoke inhalation. After confirming airway patency, which of the following should you do *first*?
- **A.** Measure the Spo_2
- **B.** <u>Initiate 100% oxygen</u>
- **C.** Obtain an arterial blood gas
- **D.** Request a STAT chest x-ray

In this scenario, getting more information is important, but the first priority is to ensure adequate oxygenation. Given that the patient is suspected of having a smoke inhalation injury, 100% O_2 should be administered immediately, without waiting for more information.

Question A-17 also illustrates this principle, which emphasizes that your patient's safety and welfare must always be your first priority.

A-17. You are called to the bedside of a patient by her ICU nurse to check the attached volume ventilator. You note that both the low-volume and high-pressure limit alarms are sounding on each breath. What should your first action be?
- **A.** <u>Disconnect the patient and manually ventilate with 100% O_2</u>
- **B.** Call the attending physician for further patient information
- **C.** Check the patient's chart for the original ventilator orders
- **D.** Ask the nurse about how recently the patient was suctioned

In this example, the patient is in danger, as evident by the ventilator alarms. Although options B, C, and D might help you understand the cause of the problem, they waste valuable time and ignore the immediate needs of the patient. Because your first priority always must be the patient's safety and welfare, option A is the best answer for this question.

If It Ain't Broke, Don't Fix It!

Another of our "top ten" principles is to *leave well enough alone*—that is, "If it ain't broke, don't fix it!" Typically this principle will show up on an NBRC exam as a situation in which patient data indicate normal parameters, but you are given the option to change things. *Don't.* Question A-18 illustrates application of this item response guideline.

A-18. A 60-kg (132-lb) COPD patient is receiving volume control SIMV with a V_T of 450 mL at a rate of 10/min and an F_{IO_2} of 0.35. Blood gases are as follows: pH = 7.36; $Paco_2$ = 61 torr; HCO_3 = 36 mEq/L; Pao_2 = 62 torr. Which of the following changes would you recommend at this time?

A. Increase the SIMV rate
B. Increase the F_{IO_2}
C. <u>Maintain the current settings</u>
D. Increase the V_T

As previously emphasized, the scenario in this question includes vital information, specifically that the patient has COPD. As is common in such patients, the blood gas indicated *fully compensated respiratory acidosis,* so even though the Pco_2 is high, we don't want to alter ventilation. What about oxygenation, that is the low Pao_2? That too is to be expected in patients with COPD. In fact, raising the F_{IO_2} could depress the patient's respiratory drive. If it ain't broke, don't fix it—maintain the current settings (option C).

Back Off Bad!

Exam candidates love to complain about NBRC questions with "two right answers." Of course, according to the NBRC, there is only one best answer for each question. One perfect example of this type of question is the "double effect" scenario. Typically, a patient who is receiving multiple therapies at the same time either worsens or improves. At least two different changes could help the situation—which do you choose? Question A-19 is a good example.

A-19. A 30-kg (66-lb) child is receiving volume control SIMV. The following data are available:

Ventilator Settings	Blood Gases
F_{IO_2} 0.45	pH 7.38
Mandatory rate 18	$Paco_2$ 42 torr
Total rate 23	Pao_2 110 torr
V_T 250 mL	HCO_3 23 mEq/L
PEEP 12 cm H_2O	BE 0 mEq/L

Based on these data, which of the following should you do?

A. Decrease tidal volume
B. <u>Reduce the PEEP</u>
C. Decrease the rate
D. Lower the F_{IO_2}

In this scenario, the child's acid–base status and Pco_2 are normal, so no change in ventilation is warranted. The Pao_2 is above normal (hyperoxia) and can be safely lowered if the patient's hemoglobin is acceptable. You can lower the Pao_2 by either lowering the PEEP level *or* lowering the F_{IO_2}. Both answers are right! Which do you choose?

Actually, there is only one correct answer. In this case, an F_{IO_2} of 0.45 presents little or no danger to the patient, but a PEEP of 12 cm H_2O is definitely hazardous. Decrease the PEEP first! The lesson is that when confronted with two or more possible changes in therapy, both of which would have the same good effect, first change the therapy that poses the greatest potential harm to the patient—*back off bad!*

Data Just Don't Jive

Given the number and variety of instruments used to measure and monitor a patient's physiologic status, it is no wonder that the NBRC will test your ability to recognize and deal with conflicting data—in other words, numbers that "just don't jive" with each other. Question A-20 is a good example.

A-20. The following data are obtained for a patient:

Blood Gas Analyzer	CO Oximeter
pH 7.35	Oxyhemoglobin 97%
$Paco_2$ 28 torr	Carboxyhemoglobin 1%
HCO_3 14 mEq/L	Methemoglobin 1%
BE −10 mEq/L	Hemoglobin 13.8 g/dL
Pao_2 40 torr	
Sao_2 73%	

You should do which of the following?
A. Report the Sao_2 value as 73%
B. Report the Sao_2 value as 97%
C. Recommend administration of bicarbonate
D. <u>Recalibrate the instruments and repeat the analysis</u>

In this example, careful inspection of the data indicates a large discrepancy between the ABG analyzer's Pao_2 and Sao_2 (40 torr and 73%) and the actual oxyhemoglobin reported by the oximeter (97%). *One of these readings must be wrong.* Unfortunately, because no additional information is provided (patient or equipment status), the only good option is to recalibrate the instruments and repeat the analysis. At the same time, you should probably give the patient supplemental oxygen (just to be sure) while re-analyzing the sample.

Errors, Errors Everywhere!

A little-known NBRC exam specification requires that candidates be able to "verify computations and note erroneous data" (Section III-A). Usually the NBRC will offer one or two questions that confirm your ability to "check your math" or to recognize plainly incorrect data. Common math error questions focus on equations you use frequently in clinical practice, such as the alveolar air equation and the calculation of compliance or airway resistance on ventilator patients. Also common are errors in reported lab values, as evident in Question A-21.

A-21. The results of an arterial blood gas analysis for a patient who is breathing 100% oxygen follow:

Blood Gases
pH 7.27
$Paco_2$ 44 torr
HCO_3 23 mEq/L
BE +1
Pao_2 598 torr
Sao_2 100%

Which of the following is the likely problem?
A. Respiratory acidosis
B. Large physiologic shunt
C. Metabolic acidosis
D. <u>Laboratory error</u>

Whenever one option (here D) includes the possibility of an error, check out the numbers! First, the Pao_2 of 598 torr on 100% O_2 is not only possible, but near normal (based on the alveolar air equation). In contrast, the acid–base values are *not* consistent with the underlying relationship that determines pH (the Henderson-Hasselbalch equation). In this case, both the $Paco_2$ and HCO_3 are normal. With both these values being within the normal range, the pH also would have to be close to normal, which it clearly is not (pH = 7.27). The only possibility here is a laboratory error.

Don't Know What You're Missing!

In addition to using conflicting or erroneous data in its questions, the NBRC likes to give candidates questions with missing data. These questions are designed to "trap" those individuals who are inclined to act on insufficient information, while rewarding those who carefully review the data. Question A-22 illustrates this type of question.

A-22. A doctor asks you to assess if a 75-kg (165-lb) patient with a neuromuscular disorder who is receiving volume control SIMV is ready for weaning. You obtain the following data during a bedside ventilatory assessment:

Spontaneous tidal volume	250 mL
Minute ventilation	10 L/min
Vital capacity	750 mL
Maximum inspiratory pressure (MIP)	–28 cm H_2O

Based on this information, which of the following would you recommend?
A. Begin a spontaneous breathing T-piece trial
B. <u>Postpone weaning and reevaluate the patient</u>
C. Begin weaning using a pressure support protocol
D. Begin weaning by decreasing the SIMV rate

In this question, many candidates would observe that the patient's vital capacity and MIP are borderline adequate, and conclude that the patient is ready for weaning. *Wrong!* In this case, the minute ventilation and tidal volume data suggest a major problem, *but this becomes clear only after identifying and deriving the missing data*—the spontaneous breathing rate (spontaneous rate = 10 L/min ÷ 0.25 L/breath = 40 breaths/min). This yields a rapid shallow breathing index of 40/0.25 = 160, which is far above the threshold value of 100 that indicates a potential weaning problem and likely weaning failure. Based on discovery and analysis of the missing data, you would recommend postponing weaning and reevaluating the patient.

This type of question should make it clear that when given a problem with numeric information, you should *always* review the numbers to see what, if anything, is missing. Then see if you can derive the missing data from the available numbers. Often this is the key to solving these problems.

Jump Back, Jack!

Often the NBRC presents you with a situation in which things go bad (e.g., the patient's condition worsens, equipment fails). Just as often, *your* action immediately preceded things going bad. In these cases, the corrective action is usually to reverse course and *undo* what you have done—*jump back, Jack!* Question A-23 illustrates this principle.

A-23. A surgeon orders an increase in PEEP from 6 to 10 cm H_2O for a postoperative patient receiving mechanical ventilation. After you adjust the PEEP setting, you note a rapid fall in the patient's arterial blood pressure. Which of the following actions would you recommend to the surgeon?
A. Increase the Fio_2 by 10%
B. Administer a vasopressor
C. <u>Return the PEEP to 6 cm H_2O</u>
D. Obtain a STAT blood gas

One of the adverse effects of PEEP is decreased cardiac output (due to increased pleural pressure and decreased venous return). A rapid drop in a patient's blood pressure indicates decreased cardiac output. Whenever an adverse response to therapy occurs, your first consideration should be to stop the therapy and restore the patient to his or her prior state; in this case, return the PEEP to its initial level of 6 cm H_2O.

KISS It!

The KISS principle is straightforward: Keep It Simple, Stupid! When taking an NBRC test, this means that the simplest solution to a problem is often the best. Question A-24 is a good example of the KISS principle.

A-24. Manual ventilation of a patient with a self-inflating bag-valve-mask device fails to inflate the patient's chest adequately. You should do which of the following?
  A. Intubate and mechanically ventilate the patient
  B. Switch to a gas-powered resuscitator with mask
  C. <u>Reposition the patient's head, neck, and mask</u>
  D. Insert a laryngeal mask airway (LMA)

In this sample troubleshooting question, most of the options might help resolve the problem. However, option C is the simplest and should at least be tried before moving on to more aggressive options. The lesson here is that whenever one of the options is relatively simple and could provide the solution to the problem at hand, it is probably the correct answer.

Gas Goes In, Gas Comes Out

Almost every NBRC exam includes two or more questions testing your ability to differentiate between leaks and obstructions in equipment, their sources, and their correction. A basic rule of thumb is that *leaks prevent pressure buildup, and obstructions cause pressure buildup*. The classic example is the simple bubble humidifier. Block the tubing outlet while gas is flowing and the pressure pop-off should sound (an obstruction). If the pressure pop-off does not sound, there is a system leak. A similar example is the leak test you perform on a ventilator circuit.

Identifying sources of leaks is simple—any mechanical connection (e.g., tubing, nebulizer/humidifier caps, exhalation valves) is a potential source for leakage, as is the patient's airway (e.g., mouthpiece, mask, tracheal tube/cuff). To correct a leak, tighten the connection, fix or replace the component, or provide a better airway seal. Question A-25 provides a good example of a "leaky" question.

A-25. When checking a ventilator, you discover that the set PEEP level cannot be maintained. Which of the following might be causing this problem?

  1. Leak in the tubing
  2. Faulty exhalation valve
  3. Leak around the airway cuff
  4. Loose humidifier connection
      A. 1 and 2
      B. 1 and 3
      C. 2 and 4
      D. <u>1, 2, 3, and 4</u>

According to our rule of thumb, this is definitely a leak scenario. Because any mechanical connection or the patient's airway can be the source of a leak, *all* of the cited problems could be the cause, making D the correct response.

Obstructions can be more challenging to identify, in part because an obstruction can be complete or partial and because "obstruction" during mechanical ventilation can involve any factor that raises airway pressure (increased resistance or decreased compliance). Correcting or overcoming an obstruction must address the underlying cause. Question A-26 illustrates this type of question.

A-26. At the bedside of a patient receiving volume control A/C ventilation, you suddenly observe the simultaneous sounding of the high-pressure and low-volume alarms. Which of the following is the most likely cause of this problem?

A. A leak in the ET tube cuff
B. A mucus plug in the ET tube
C. Ventilator circuit disconnection
D. Development of pulmonary edema

Because this scenario deals with volume control ventilation, it is best to rely first on a tried-and-true alarm rule of thumb to identify this problem as being an obstruction:

If the alarm combination is:	Then the problem is:
High pressure/low volume	An obstruction
Low pressure/low volume	A leak

The problem in Question A-26 is that two options involve "obstruction"—the mucus plug and the decreased compliance associated with the development of pulmonary edema. Which to choose? In this case, our prior advice on dissecting the question should help. Note the key word *suddenly* in the stem. Although pulmonary edema can develop relatively quickly, it would not change airway pressures suddenly. In contrast, a mucus plug can cause a sudden rise in airway pressure, making B the best choice and correct answer.

Love Those Multiple Trues!

Students tend to hate multiple-true-type questions (the ones with all those answer combinations!). The fact is that most multiple-true questions are easier to answer than simple "ABCD" questions (probably the reason that the NBRC is slowly phasing them out). Why? Because more than any other type of question, multiple trues improve your odds of being correct when you have only partial knowledge of the answer. Question A-27 demonstrates this important item response concept.

A-27. Which of the following would facilitate clearance of pulmonary secretions in a patient with cystic fibrosis?

1. Pulmozyme (DNase)
2. Flutter valve
3. Atropine sulfate
4. Hypertonic saline
  A. 1 and 3
  B. 2 and 4
  C. 1, 2, and 4
  D. 2, 3, and 4

Most candidates will recognize Pulmozyme (DNase) as a proteolytic agent that might facilitate clearance of pulmonary secretions. Based on this partial knowledge, you can eliminate options B and D because they do not include Pulmozyme. Alternatively, if based on your partial knowledge you recognize that atropine can dry airway secretions, you can eliminate options A and D because both include this drug. Note that either of these partial-knowledge approaches immediately improves your odds of getting this question correct from 1 out of 4 (for pure guessing) to 50-50. Then all you need to know is that either hypertonic saline *or* a flutter valve can also help, and you can be sure to get this item right!

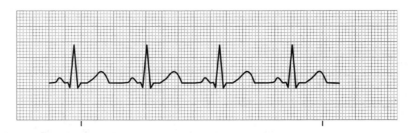

Figure A-3 ECG Rhythm Observed on Monitor.

Source: Garcia T, Miller GT. *Arrhythmia recognition: the art of interpretation.* Sudbury, MA: Jones and Bartlett; 2004.

Treat the Patient, Not the Monitor!

A favorite NBRC "trick" question is to place you in a scenario where patient and monitor data conflict, but action is required. Common forms of this type question include (1) pulse oximetry data (good) versus bedside assessment of the patient's oxygenation (bad), and (2) ECG (good) versus bedside assessment of the patient's perfusion (bad). Question A-28 is a good example.

A-28. During a short pause from resuscitation of a child in the emergency department, you cannot palpate a carotid pulse but observe a regular rhythm on the ECG monitor (**Figure A-3**):

Which of the following actions should you take at this time?
A. <u>Resume cardiac compressions and ventilation</u>
B. Discontinue compressions and monitor the patient
C. Recommend cardioversion at 100 joules
D. Recommend epinephrine administration

In Question A-28, the likely problem is pulseless electrical activity (PEA). Remembering that the ECG represents only electrical activity and that a patient with no pulse requires resuscitation should make this a "no-brainer." However, more than one-third of those candidates taking our practice exams decide to go against their better judgment (and their training) and instead treat the monitor. Test smart by not joining that group!

Order in the House

All NBRC entry-level exams assess your ability to sequence multiple therapies or coordinate your therapy with that of other health professionals. Most of these questions rely on simple common sense—for example, do not perform postural drainage immediately after a patient has eaten!

As a special case, you will often be asked in which order to perform combinations of therapy aimed at either getting drugs (e.g., steroids, antibiotics) in or getting secretions out of the airway. In these situations, apply the following rule of thumb:

1. Open 'em up
2. Thin 'em down
3. Clear 'em out

"Open 'em up" means first open the airways, using a bronchodilator. "Thin 'em down" means you should next use hydrating or mucolytic agents (e.g., bland aerosols, Mucomyst, Pulmozyme, hypertonic saline) to decrease the viscosity of secretions. "Clear 'em out" means applying airway clearance methods to remove the secretions (e.g., directed coughing, postural drainage, suctioning). Last, administer any other drugs designed for pulmonary deposition (e.g., antibiotics, steroids). Question A-29 illustrates this approach.

A-29. A physician has ordered albuterol (Proventil), DNase (Pulmozyme), and tobramycin for inhalation (TOBI) for a patient with cystic fibrosis who also receives postural drainage 3 times a day. You should administer these therapies in which of the following sequences?
A. DNase, albuterol, tobramycin, postural drainage
B. <u>Albuterol, DNase, postural drainage, tobramycin</u>
C. Postural drainage, albuterol, DNase, tobramycin
D. tobramycin, DNase, albuterol, postural drainage

Give Me a V; Give Me an O!

Typically the NBRC includes at least a half-dozen questions testing your ability to modify ventilator settings properly based on a blood gas report. You simply cannot afford to get many of these questions wrong.

First, you need to be able to interpret blood gases properly (Chapters 1 and 11). Just as important, however, is the need to differentiate between problems of ventilation ("Give Me a V") and problems of oxygenation ("Give Me an O"). This is the secret for slam-dunking these questions.

To help you out in this area, we recommend that you draw a line or mark or circle to separate the blood gas report's ventilation/acid–base data from its oxygenation data. As an example:

Blood Gases

pH 7.22

$Paco_2$ 65 torr

HCO_3 26 mEq/L

BE +1

– – – – – – – – –

Pao_2 70 torr

Sao_2 93%

Once you have drawn the line, *separately* assess (1) ventilation/acid–base status and then (2) the adequacy of oxygenation. In most cases, the NBRC will limit the problem to one or the other— that is, a problem of ventilation *or* a problem of oxygenation.

If the problem is mainly one of ventilation (as in the preceding data), either increase or decrease the ventilation, as appropriate. If the problem is mainly oxygenation, you will need to either raise or lower the Fio_2 or adjust PEEP/CPAP. Question A-30 is an example.

A-30. A 90-kg (198-lb) patient is being ventilated in the postanesthesia care unit following upper abdominal surgery. Ventilator settings and arterial blood gas data are below:

Ventilator Settings		Blood Gases
Mode	Vol Ctrl SIMV	pH 7.51
V_T	600 mL	$Paco_2$ 31 torr
Set rate	14/min	HCO_3 24 mEq/L
Total rate	14/min	BE +1
Fio_2	0.40	Pao_2 115 torr
PEEP	5 cm H_2O	Sao_2 99%

Which of the following should you recommend?
A. Increase the Fio_2
B. <u>Decrease the rate</u>
C. Decrease the tidal volume
D. Discontinue the PEEP

Here the problem is clearly one of ventilation, *not* oxygenation. In this case, the patient is being hyperventilated (respiratory alkalosis) and the minute ventilation should be decreased. Because the tidal volume is acceptable (approximately 6–7 mL/kg), you should recommend decreasing the rate.

Alternatively, you may identify the primary problem as one of oxygenation, as evident in Question A-31.

A-31. A 45-year-old, 70-kg (154-lb) male with a diagnosis of bilateral pneumonia is receiving volume control SIMV. Ventilator settings and arterial blood gas data are below.

Ventilator Settings		Blood Gases
Mode	Vol Ctrl SIMV	pH 7.35
VT	700 mL	$Paco_2$ 45 torr
Set rate	6/min	HCO_3 23 mEq/L
Total rate	10/min	BE –1
Fio_2	0.65	Pao_2 51 torr
PEEP	5 cm H_2O	Sao_2 86%

Which of the following should you recommend?
A. <u>Increase PEEP</u>
B. Increase the rate
C. Increase the Fio_2
D. Add an inspiratory plateau

Because the Pao_2 is less than 60 torr and the Sao_2 is less than 90%, hypoxemia is present. Therefore option A or C could potentially improve oxygenation (a good example of a "double effect" item). Which option you choose depends on the underlying cause of the patient's hypoxemia.

To determine the cause and treatment of hypoxemia, we recommend you use the "60/60" rule, as described in Chapter 13. In this case, the patient's Pao_2 is less than 60 torr and the Fio_2 is greater than 0.60, so according to the 60/60 rule, the cause of the patient's hypoxemia is physiologic shunting. When the cause of hypoxemia is physiologic shunting, increasing the Fio_2 will do little good and may potentially do harm (oxygen toxicity). Instead, you need to open up unventilated alveoli by adding or increasing PEEP/CPAP.

Who's in Charge Here?

Some questions check whether you know who prescribes respiratory care and who needs to be contacted should a change in care be needed and no protocol exist to manage the patient. Question A-32 also tests your knowledge of what to do before initiating therapy on a patient.

A-32. A nurse tells you that his patient is scheduled to start chest physiotherapy four times a day this morning and that he would like you to get started before the patient goes to radiology for a CT scan. Which of the following should you do *first*?
A. Auscultate and percuss the patient's chest
B. Initiate therapy after reviewing the x-ray
C. Interview the patient to obtain a history
D. <u>Confirm the doctor's order in the chart</u>

Similar questions will ask what to do if you believe a change in therapy is needed, or if the patient asks specific questions regarding his or her diagnosis or prognosis (contact the doctor). Remember, all respiratory care is provided by physician prescription, and (without a protocol) only the physician can change the order.

TAKING YOUR TEST

Good preparation for any test should also involve consideration of how to take the exam, that is strategies to use just before and during actual test administration. Here we provide a few additional pointers specifically applicable to taking NBRC written exams.

Be Familiar with the Exam Format

Our "know your enemy" guideline applies not just to the content of the NBRC written exams, but also to their format. Fortunately, by the time most candidates actually sit for the CRT or WRRT exam, they will have taken dozens of similar tests, usually in school. Indeed, most programs require that students pass a CRT-like exam to graduate. You probably already know most of what to expect on the real thing.

As most candidates are aware, all NBRC exams are administered by computer at selected testing centers throughout the United States. The NBRC test software presents one question at a time on the computer screen. As depicted in **Figure A-4**, each question appears at the top of the screen with the four answer options immediately below. A function bar appears below each question. This bar contains several important buttons and text boxes, and their functions are described in the figure. If you choose to provide comments on specific test questions, the NBRC will apply this information when determining if test score adjustments are needed. For this reason, if you believe that the question you are trying to answer is flawed, be sure to provide a comment that explains why.

To select an option as your answer, you either click your mouse over the corresponding letter (A, B, C, or D) or type in that letter using the keyboard. To change your option choice, simply click on or key in a different letter. Your responses are not registered until you exit the exam for scoring, so you can change your answer to any question at any time during the exam period.

Strategies to Employ During the Test

The following strategies should help you perform at your best level when taking an NBRC written exam:

- Get comfortable.
- Answer all questions.
- Budget your time.
  - Monitor your pace.
  - Answer easy questions first.

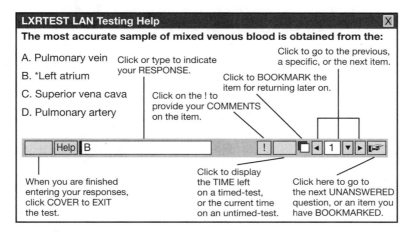

Figure A-4 NBRC Computer-Based Testing Screen.

Courtesy of the National Board for Respiratory Care.

- ○ Bookmark difficult items and return to them later.
- ○ Use all the available time.
- • If in doubt, reconsider your answers.

Getting comfortable might seem difficult when taking a high-stakes exam, but the preparation this text provides—especially the strategies reviewed in this chapter—should help allay your test anxiety. Moreover, just like an athlete with pre-game "butterflies in the stomach," once you get down to the task at hand, you will get into the needed rhythm.

Because your score on an NBRC written exam is based on the number of items you get correct, it is essential that you answer all questions. To do so, you need to develop a good pace and budget your time properly.

Budgeting your time is the single most important strategy when taking a test. On average, the NBRC gives you a little more than a minute for each question. To keep on pace, you need to be aware of your progress. However, rather than constantly checking the clock, we recommend that you check your progress every 20 to 30 minutes, with the goal of completing, on average, one question per minute. For example, if you check your progress at 1 hour into the exam, you should have completed about 60 questions.

To further maximize your use of time, you should answer the easy questions first and save the difficult ones for last. However, even if a question appears straightforward, do not rush through it. Spend enough time on each item to read it carefully and apply the strategies we recommend here to select your answer. By the same token, you should not linger too long on any one question. In general, if you feel stumped on a question or know that more than a minute has elapsed, bookmark the item and return to it later.

After completing all the easy questions, use the remaining time to review and answer all your bookmarked items. If you must guess, apply the option selection strategies outlined in this chapter to better your odds of selecting the correct answer.

If time remains after you have answered all the questions, review those items about which you were most unsure. *If an answer was a guess, do not hesitate to reconsider your choice.* Note that this advice is contrary to what most students are taught (i.e., "your first guess is best"). Research consistently indicates that changing answers on multiple-choice exams is more likely to boost your score than to lower it.

After you finish the exam, clicking on the COVER button on the function bar will take you to a "cover page," which summarizes how many questions you have answered and how much time you have used. If you have completed all questions and are satisfied with your answers, you can EXIT the exam from this cover page. After exiting the exam, the testing center provides you with your score report. If you have followed the guidance we provide throughout this text, we are confident you will receive a passing score.

APPENDIX B · Cardiopulmonary Calculations

NBRC exams do not have a separate major section assessing your computation skills. Instead, common calculations can be embedded anywhere throughout these tests. Typically, these calculations are few in number and require only basic math skills. Unfortunately, too many candidates simply "write off" these questions, assuming that without access to a calculator they will get most of them wrong. Of course, giving up on *any* NBRC exam questions simply lowers your probability of passing. Even if you lack confidence in your math skills, you simply cannot afford to concede any questions involving computations. The good news is that the computations you will likely encounter on the NBRC exams are predictable and relatively simple. With the preparation we provide here, you should be able to obtain high scores on these items.

For organizational purposes, this appendix presents the common calculations you may see on the NBRC exams by functional category, such as computations involving ventilation or those related to oxygenation. For each calculation, we provide the applicable formula, an example computation, and one or more "ballpark rules." A ballpark rule is simply a way to help estimate the answer or the range within which the answer should fall. Our guidance is to always check your answer against the applicable rule before committing to it. If your answer is inconsistent with the ballpark rule, review the problem, the formula, and your computation.

VENTILATION CALCULATIONS

Likely calculations regarding ventilation include the minute volume, tidal volume, physiologic deadspace, deadspace to tidal volume ratio, and alveolar ventilation. Also possible are conversions between CO_2 percentages and partial pressures. **Table B-1** provides the formulas for these parameters, example calculations, and "ballpark" rules to help you estimate or verify your computations.

OXYGENATION CALCULATIONS

Likely calculations regarding oxygenation include the inspired and alveolar P_{O_2}, the A-a gradient, percent shunt, P/F ratio, and arterial O_2 content. **Table B-2** provides the formulas for these parameters, example calculations, and "ballpark" rules to help you estimate or verify your computations.

CALCULATIONS INVOLVING PULMONARY MECHANICS

Likely calculations regarding pulmonary mechanics include static compliance and airway resistance of patients receiving ventilatory support. **Table B-3** provides the formulas for these parameters, example calculations, and "ballpark" rules to help you verify your computations.

PULMONARY FUNCTION CALCULATIONS

Likely calculations related to pulmonary function testing include lung volumes and capacities, forced expiratory volume (time) as a percentage of FVC, the percent change in a value, and the percent predicted compared to normal. **Table B-4** provides the formulas for these parameters, example calculations, and "ballpark" rules to help you estimate or verify your computations.

Table B-1 Computation Formulas and Example Problems for Ventilatory Parameters

Parameter/Formula	Example
Minute Volume ($\dot{V}E$)	
$\dot{V}E = f \times VT$ *Ballpark rule*: At normal rates of breathing, the computed minute volume for adults will generally be in the 4–10 L/min range.	*Problem B.1* A patient has a tidal volume of 400 mL and is breathing at 14/min. What is her minute volume? *Solution*: $\dot{V}E = f \times VT$ $\dot{V}E = 14$ breaths/min $\times 400$ mL/breath $\dot{V}E = 5{,}600$ mL/min or 5.6 L/min
Tidal Volume (VT)	
$VT = \dot{V}E \div f$ *Ballpark rule*: Recheck your calculations if for an adult you obtain a $VT < 100$ mL or > 1000 mL.	*Problem B.2* A patient has a minute volume of 8.25 L/min and is breathing at a rate of 22/min. What is his average tidal volume? *Solution*: $VT = \dot{V}E \div f$ $VT = 8.25$ L/min $\div 22$ breaths/min $VT = 0.375$ L/breath $= 375$ mL
Physiologic Deadspace (VD)	
$VD = VT \times \dfrac{Paco_2 - P\overline{E}co_2}{Paco_2}$ where VD = physiologic deadspace, VT = tidal volume, $Paco_2$ = arterial Pco_2, and $P\overline{E}co_2$ = mixed expired Pco_2 *Ballpark rules*: (1) Unless the patient has a trach (which lowers VD), VD will be ≥ 1 mL/lb PBW and usually less than 70% of the tidal volume; (2) large $Paco_2 - P\overline{E}co_2$ differences (> 15–20 torr) indicate large deadspace volume.	*Problem B.3* A patient has a tidal volume of 450 mL, an arterial Pco_2 ($Paco_2$) of 60 torr, and a mixed expired Pco_2 ($P\overline{E}co_2$) of 30 torr. What is the patient's deadspace? *Solution*: $VD = VT \times \dfrac{Paco_2 - P\overline{E}co_2}{Paco_2}$ $VD = 450$ mL $\times [(60 - 30)/60]$ $VD = 450$ mL $\times [30/60]$ $VD = 225$ mL
Deadspace to Tidal Volume Ratio (VD/VT)	
$VD/VT = VD \div VT$ or (if given VD/VT) $VD = VD/VT \times VT$ *Ballpark rule*: Unless the patient has a trach (which lowers VD), VD/VT will generally be in the range of 0.30–0.70.	*Problem B.4* A 6-foot-tall, 170-lb patient with normal lungs has a tidal volume of 600 mL. What is his deadspace to tidal volume ratio? *Solution*: With normal lungs, assume that $VD = 1$ mL/lb body weight $VD = 1$ mL/lb $\times 170$ lb $= 170$ mL $VD/VT = 170 \div 600 = 0.28$ *Problem B.5* A 5-foot-tall, 105-lb patient has a deadspace to tidal volume ratio of 0.40 and a tidal volume of 500 mL. What is her deadspace volume? *Solution*: $VD = VD/VT \times VT$ $VD = 0.40 \times 500$ mL $= 200$ mL

Alveolar Ventilation ($\dot{V}_A$)	
$\dot{V}_A = f \times (V_T - V_D)$	**Problem B.6**
Ballpark rules: (1) Unless otherwise stated, assume normal deadspace = 1 mL/lb; (2) $\dot{V}_A$ must always be less than the minute volume and in proportion to the V_D/V_T ratio—that is, $\dot{V}_E - (V_D/V_T \times \dot{V}_E)$	A 6-foot, 4-inch-tall, 200-lb man with normal lungs has a tidal volume of 680 mL and is breathing at a rate of 15 breaths/min. What is his approximate alveolar ventilation?
	Solution:
	Assume normal deadspace 1 mL/lb $\times$ 200 lb = 200 mL
	$\dot{V}_A = f \times (V_T - V_D)$
	$\dot{V}_A = 15 \times (680 - 200)$
	$\dot{V}_A = 15 \times 480$
	$\dot{V}_A = 7{,}200$ mL/min or 7.2 L/min
Convert End-Tidal CO_2% ($F_{ET}CO_2$) to $P_{ET}CO_2$	
$P_{ET}CO_2 = F_{ET}CO_2 \times (P_B - 47)$	**Problem B.7**
Ballpark rule: A normal $F_{ET}CO_2$ ranges between 4% and 6%; 5% $F_{ET}CO_2$ is equivalent to a $P_{ET}CO_2$ of 36 torr.	A patient at sea level has an end-tidal CO_2 concentration ($F_{ET}CO_2$) of 0.043. What is her BTPS-corrected end-tidal P_{CO_2} ($P_{ET}CO_2$)?
	Solution:
	Sea level $P_B = 760$ mm Hg
	Correction for BTPS = -47 mm Hg
	$P_{ET}CO_2 = F_{ET}CO_2 \times (P_B - 47)$
	$P_{ET}CO_2 = 0.043 \times (760 - 47)$
	$P_{ET}CO_2 = 0.043 \times 713$
	$P_{ET}CO_2 = 30.7$ mm Hg (torr)

Table B-2 Computation Formulas and Example Problems for Oxygenation Parameters

Parameter/Formula	Example
Inspired P_{O_2} (P_{IO_2})	
$P_{IO_2} = F_{IO_2} \times P_B$	**Problem B.8**
Ballpark rule: At sea level with an F_{IO_2} of 1.0, the $P_{IO_2} = 760$ torr; therefore, with an F_{IO_2} of 0.50, the $P_{IO_2} = 1/2 \times 760 = 370$ torr.	You are transporting a patient on 40% O_2 in an unpressurized airplane cabin at 8,000 ft altitude ($P_B = 565$ mm Hg). What is his P_{IO_2}?
	Solution:
	$P_{IO_2} = F_{IO_2} \times P_B$
	$P_{IO_2} = 0.40 \times 565$ mm Hg
	$P_{IO_2} = 226$ mm Hg (torr)
Alveolar P_{O_2} (P_{AO_2})	
$P_{AO_2} = F_{IO_2} \times (P_B - 47) - (1.25 \times P_aCO_2)$	**Problem B.9**
Ballpark rules: (1) Maximum P_{AO_2} at sea level breathing room air ≈ 130 torr and breathing 100% $O_2 \approx 680$ torr; (2) estimate normal P_{AO_2} as $6 \times O_2$%—for example, you would expect a patient breathing 50% O_2 to have a P_{AO_2} of about 300 torr.	A patient breathing 60% O_2 at sea level has a P_aCO_2 of 28 torr. What is her alveolar P_{O_2} (P_{AO_2})?
	Solution:
	Sea level $P_B = 760$ mm Hg
	$P_{AO_2} = F_{IO_2} \times (P_B - 47) - (1.25 \times P_aCO_2)$
	$P_{AO_2} = 0.60 \times (760 - 47) - (1.25 \times 28)$
	$P_{AO_2} = 428 - 35$
	$P_{AO_2} = 393$ mm Hg (torr)

(Continues)

Table B-2 Computation Formulas and Example Problems for Oxygenation Parameters (*Continued*)

A-a Gradient [P(A-a)O$_2$]	
$P(\text{A-a})O_2 = P_{AO_2} - P_{aO_2}$ *Ballpark rules:* (1) When breathing 100% O$_2$, the P(A-a)O$_2$ typically ranges between 50 and 60 torr for normal subjects, but may rise to more than 600 torr when severe shunting is present; (2) compare to % shunt, with about 5% shunt per 100 torr P(A-a)O$_2$.	*Problem B.10* A patient breathing 100% O$_2$ at sea level has a PaO$_2$ of 250 torr and a PaCO$_2$ of 60 torr. What is her A-a gradient or P(A-a)O$_2$? *Solution:* Sea level P$_B$ = 760 mm Hg $P_{AO_2} = F_{IO_2} \times (P_B - 47) - (1.25 \times P_{aCO_2})$ $P_{AO_2} = 1.0 \times (760 - 47) - (1.25 \times 60)$ $P_{AO_2} = 713 - 75 = 638$ mm Hg (torr) $P(\text{A-a})O_2 = P_{AO_2} - P_{aO_2}$ $P(\text{A-a})O_2 = 638 - 250$ $P(\text{A-a})O_2 = 388$ mm Hg (torr)
Percent Shunt Estimate	
$\% \text{ shunt} = \dfrac{P(\text{A}-\text{a})O_2 \times 0.003}{\left[P(\text{A}-\text{a})O_2 \times 0.003\right] + 5}$ *Ballpark rule:* There is about a 5% shunt for every 100 torr P(A-a)O$_2$.	*Problem B.11* What is the estimated percent shunt of the patient in Problem B.10? *Solution:* $\% \text{ shunt} = \dfrac{P(\text{A}-\text{a})O_2 \times 0.003}{\left[P(\text{A}-\text{a})O_2 \times 0.003\right] + 5}$ $\% \text{ shunt} = \dfrac{388 \times 0.003}{\left[388 \times 0.003\right] + 5}$ $\% \text{ shunt} = \dfrac{1.164}{6.164}$ $\% \text{ shunt} = 0.189 = 19\%$
Arterial PO$_2$ to FIO$_2$ Ratio (P/F Ratio)	
$PaO_2/F_{IO_2} = PaO_2 \div F_{IO_2}$ *Ballpark rule:* Expect P/F ratios > 500 for patients with normal lung function; P/F ratios < 300 signify acute lung injury.	*Problem B.12* What is the P/F ratio of a patient breathing 50% O$_2$ with a PaO$_2$ of 68 torr? *Solution:* $PaO_2/F_{IO_2} = PaO_2 \div F_{IO_2}$ $PaO_2/F_{IO_2} = 68 \div 0.50$ $PaO_2/F_{IO_2} = 136$

(*Continues*)

Arterial O_2 Content (CaO_2)	
CaO_2 = (O_2 bound to Hb) + (dissolved O_2) CaO_2 = (total Hb $\times$ 1.36 $\times$ SaO_2) + (0.003 $\times$ PaO_2) *Ballpark rule*: If the SaO_2 > 75% (as is typically the case for arterial blood), the computed CaO_2 value in mL/dL will always be a bit larger than the total Hb present but never more than 40% larger—for example, with a total Hb of 8 g/dL and an SaO_2 of 90%, you would expect a CaO_2 between 8 and 11 mL/dL.	*Problem B.13* A patient has a hemoglobin concentration of 10 g/dL, a PaO_2 of 50 torr, and an SaO_2 of 80%. What is his total arterial O_2 content (CaO_2)? *Solution*: O_2 bound to Hb = (total Hb $\times$ 1.36 $\times$ SaO_2) O_2 bound to Hb = (10 $\times$ 1.36 $\times$ 0.80) O_2 bound to Hb = 10.9 mL/dL Dissolved O_2 = 0.003 $\times$ PaO_2 Dissolved O_2 = 0.003 $\times$ 50 Dissolved O_2 = 0.15 mL/dL CaO_2 = (O_2 bound to Hb) + (dissolved O_2) CaO_2 = 10.9 + 0.15 = 11.05 mL/dL

Table B-3 Computation Formulas and Example Problems for Pulmonary Mechanics Parameters

Parameter/Formula	Example
Static Compliance (C_{LT})	
$$C_{LT} = \frac{V_T}{P_{plat} - PEEP}$$ where C_{LT} = static compliance of the lungs and thorax, V_T = the corrected tidal volume, P_{plat} = the plateau pressure during a volume hold, and PEEP = the baseline airway pressure *Ballpark rule*: Expect to see the C_{LT} range from 100 mL/cm H_2O (normal) to 10 mL/cm H_2O (severe reduction in compliance, such as might occur in ARDS).	*Problem B.14* A patient receiving volume-limited ventilation with a tidal volume of 700 mL and 8 cm H_2O PEEP has a peak pressure of 42 cm H_2O and a plateau pressure of 35 cm H_2O. What is her static compliance? *Solution*: $$C_{LT} = \frac{V_T}{P_{plat} - PEEP}$$ $$C_{LT} = \frac{700}{35 - 8}$$ C_{LT} = 26 mL/cm H_2O
Airway Resistance (R_{AW})	
$$R_{AW} = \frac{PIP - P_{plat}}{\dot{V}}$$ where R_{AW} = airway resistance (cm H_2O/L/sec), PIP = peak inspiratory pressure, P_{plat} = the plateau pressure during a volume hold, and $\dot{V}$ = inspiratory flow in liters/second *Ballpark rule*: Normal R_{AW} for orally intubated patients ranges from 10 to 15 cm H_2O/L/sec; expect higher computed values in patients with airway obstruction.	*Problem B.15* A patient receiving volume-controlled ventilation with a tidal volume of 400 mL, inspiratory flow of 75 L/min, and 6 cm H_2O PEEP has a peak pressure of 45 cm H_2O and a plateau pressure of 30 cm H_2O. What is her airway resistance? *Solution:* Convert 75 L/min to L/sec: 75 L $\div$ 60 = 1.25 L/sec $$R_{AW} = \frac{PIP - P_{plat}}{\dot{V}}$$ $$R_{AW} = \frac{45 - 30}{1.25}$$ R_{AW} = 12 cm H_2O/L/sec

Table B-4 Computation Formulas and Example Problems for Selected Pulmonary Function Parameters

Parameter/Formula	Example
Volumes/Capacities	
Most common formulas: VC = TLC – RV VC = IRV + TV + ERV TLC = FRC + IC TLC = IRV + TV + ERV + RV RV = FRC – ERV RV = TLC – VC FRC = RV + ERV FRC = TLC – IC *Ballpark rule*: Verify the selected formula by drawing and labeling a graph of lung volumes and capacities before computation.	*Problem B.16* A patient has a FRC of 3,800 mL, a tidal volume of 400 mL, and an expiratory reserve volume of 1,300 mL. What is her residual volume? *Solution*: RV = FRC – ERV RV = 3,800 – 1,300 RV = 2,500 mL
Forced Expiratory Volume (Time) Percent	
$FEV_t\% = \dfrac{FEV_t}{FVC} \times 100$ where FEV_t = the forced expiratory volume at time t (typically 1, 3, or 6 seconds) *Ballpark rule:* A patient with normal pulmonary function should have a $FEV_1\% > 75\%$ and a $FEV_3\% > 95\%$.	*Problem B.17* A patient has a forced vital capacity of 4.5 L and a FEV_3 of 4.0 L. What is his $FEV_3\%$? *Solution*: $FEV_3\% = \dfrac{FEV_3}{FVC} \times 100$ $FEV_3\% = \dfrac{4.0}{4.5} \times 100$ $FEV_3\% = 89\%$
Percent Change Value	
$\%\ change = \dfrac{post - pre}{pre} \times 100$ where pre is the pretreatment value and post is the post-treatment value for the parameter being measured *Ballpark rule:* If post > pre, then computed % change must be positive; for FEV_1, the improvement must be at least 12–15% to be considered significant.	*Problem B.18* A patient has a FEV_1 of 2.4 L before bronchodilator treatment and a FEV_1 of 2.7 L after treatment. What percent change in FEV_1 occurred? *Solution*: $\%\ change = \dfrac{post - pre}{pre} \times 100$ $\%\ change = \dfrac{2.7 - 2.4}{2.4} \times 100$ $\%\ change = 12.5\%$
Percent Predicted Value	
$\%\ predicted = \dfrac{actual}{predicted} \times 100$ where actual is the patient's measured value and predicted is the patient's predicted normal value for that parameter *Note*: When monitoring for changes over time for some measures such as peak flow, we substitute the patient's personal best value for the predicted value. *Ballpark rule*: If actual < predicted, then computed % predicted must be < 100%.	*Problem B.19* In the pulmonary lab, you measure a patient's forced vital capacity as 3.25 L. Her predicted normal FVC is 3.82 L. What percent of predicted normal is her FVC? *Solution*: $\%\ predicted = \dfrac{actual}{predicted} \times 100$ $\%\ predicted = \dfrac{3.25}{3.82} \times 100$ $\%\ predicted = 85\%$ of normal

CARDIOVASCULAR CALCULATIONS

Likely calculations regarding cardiovascular parameters include heart rate (from an ECG), pulse pressure, mean pressure, stroke volume, cardiac output, and cardiac index. **Table B-5** provides the formulas for these parameters, example calculations, and "ballpark" rules to help you estimate or verify your computations.

EQUIPMENT CALCULATIONS

Likely calculations regarding equipment include cylinder duration of flow, air-entrainment ratios, total output flows for air-entrainment devices, suction catheter sizes, and pressure conversions. **Table B-6** provides the formulas for these parameters, example calculations, and "ballpark" rules to help you estimate or verify your computations.

FORMULAS AND EXAMPLE PROBLEMS FOR MECHANICAL VENTILATION TIME AND FLOW PARAMETERS

Likely calculations regarding mechanical ventilation involve time or flow parameters. In general, these calculations will apply only to volume or pressure control modes. **Table B-7** provides the formulas for these parameters, example calculations, and "ballpark" rules to help you estimate or verify your computations.

DRUG CALCULATIONS

Likely pharmacology-related calculations include dilution and dosage problems. **Table B-8** provides the generic formulas for these problems, example calculations, and "ballpark" rules to help you estimate or verify your computations.

Table B-5 Computation Formulas and Example Problems for Cardiovascular Parameters

Parameter/Formula	Example
Heart Rate (from ECG)	
For regular rhythms: HR = 60 ÷ R-R (sec) where HR is the heart rate and R-R is the R-to-R interval on an ECG rhythm strip *Ballpark rule*: Approximate HR = 300 ÷ R-R span in large (5-mm = 0.2-sec) boxes.	*Problem B.20* On an ECG strip, a patient has a regular rhythm with an R-R interval of 10 mm (two large boxes). What is the heart rate? *Solution*: ECG recording speed = 25 mm/sec = 0.04 sec/mm 10 mm × 0.04 sec/mm = 0.40 sec 60 sec/min ÷ 0.40 sec = 150/min
Pulse Pressure	
Pulse pressure = systolic – diastolic *Ballpark rules*: (1) Compare to normal resting value of about 40 mm Hg (up to 100 mm Hg is normal during exercise); (2) expect high values with atherosclerosis, hyperthyroidism, and aortic regurgitation; expect low values with CHF or shock.	*Problem B.21* A patient's arterial blood pressure is 165/90 mm Hg. What is her pulse pressure? *Solution*: Pulse pressure = systolic – diastolic Pulse pressure = 165 – 90 = 75 mm Hg

(Continues)

Table B-5 Computation Formulas and Example Problems for Cardiovascular Parameters (*Continued*)

Mean Blood Pressure Estimate	
Mean pressure = [systolic + (2 × diastolic)] ÷ 3 *Ballpark rule*: The mean pressure will be a bit less than halfway between the systolic and diastolic pressures.	*Problem B.22* A patient's arterial blood pressure is 100/70 mm Hg. What is his mean arterial pressure? *Solution*: Mean pressure = [systolic + (2 × diastolic)] ÷ 3 Mean pressure = [100 + (2 × 70)] ÷ 3 Mean pressure = [100 + 140] ÷ 3 Mean pressure = 80 mm Hg
Cardiac Output (CO)	
CO = (HR × SV) ÷ 1000 where CO = cardiac output in L/min, HR = heart rate, and SV = average left ventricular stroke volume in mL *Ballpark rules*: (1) Compare to a "normal" output of 70 × 70 = 4,900 or 4.9 L/min (HR = 70/min and SV = 70 mL); (2) for adult patients, expect to see the computed CO range between 3 and 10 L/min (normal 4–8 L/min).	*Problem B.23* A patient has a left ventricular stroke volume of 60 mL and a heart rate of 105 beats/min. What is her cardiac output? *Solution*: CO = (HR × SV) ÷ 1,000 CO = (105 × 60) ÷ 1,000 CO = 6,300 ÷ 1,000 = 6.3 L/min
Cardiac Index (CI)	
CI (L/min/m^2) = CO ÷ BSA where CO = cardiac output in L/min, and BSA = body surface area in m^2 (usually provided to you and based on the DuBois formula/nomogram) *Ballpark rules*: (1) For adults, the normal cardiac index will always be less than the cardiac output— about half as much for the average-size adult; (2) compare the computed value to the normal range of 2.5–5.0 L/min/m^2.	*Problem B.24* A patient has a cardiac output of 6.1 L/min and a body surface area of 2.3 m^2. What is his cardiac index? *Solution*: CI = CO ÷ BSA CI = 6.1 ÷ 2.3 CI = 2.65 L/min/m^2
Stroke Volume (SV)	
SV = CO ÷ HR where SV = average left ventricular stroke volume in mL, CO = cardiac output in mL/min, and HR = heart rate *Ballpark rule*: Compare to the normal range of 60–130 mL.	*Problem B.25* A patient has a cardiac output of 4.0 L/min and a heart rate of 80. What is her stroke volume? *Solution*: First convert CO in L/min to mL/min 4.0 × 1,000 = 4,000 mL/min SV = CO ÷ HR SV = 4,000 ÷ 80 SV = 50 mL

Table B-6 Formulas and Example Problems for Equipment-Related Computations

Parameter/Formula	Example
Cylinder Duration of Flow	
Time to empty (min) $= \dfrac{\text{psig} \times \text{factor}}{\text{flow}}$ where psig is the cylinder pressure in pounds per square inch gauge, factor is the cylinder factor (below), and flow is the flow in L/min Gas D E G H/K O_2, air 0.16 0.28 2.41 3.14 He/O_2 0.14 0.23 1.93 2.50 *Ballpark rule*: A full E cylinder at 10 L/min will last about 1 hour; a full H cylinder at 10 L/min will last about 10 times longer (10 hours).	*Problem B.26* How long will an E cylinder of oxygen with a gauge pressure of 800 psi set to deliver 5 L/min take to become empty? *Solution*: Time to empty $= \dfrac{\text{psig} \times \text{factor}}{\text{flow}}$ Time to empty $= \dfrac{800 \times .28}{5}$ Time to empty (min) $= 45$ minutes *Note*: It is common practice to change out a cylinder at least 15–30 minutes before its contents are fully exhausted.
Air-Entrainment Ratio (Air to O_2 Ratio)	
Air:O_2 ratio $= \dfrac{100 - \%O_2}{\%O_2 - 21}$ *Note*: This formula is the same as the "magic box" that appears in many textbooks. *Ballpark rule*: 60% O_2 is achieved with an air to O_2 ratio of about 1:1; lower O_2% values mean higher ratios, and higher O_2% values mean lower ratios.	*Problem B.27* What is the air to O_2 ratio for a 35% air-entrainment mask? *Solution*: Air:O_2 ratio $= \dfrac{100 - \%O_2}{\%O_2 - 21}$ Air:O_2 ratio $= \dfrac{100 - 35}{35 - 21}$ Air:O_2 ratio $= \dfrac{65}{14}$ Air:O_2 ratio $= 4.6{:}1 \cong 5{:}1$
Air-Entrainment Device Total Output Flow	
Total flow $=$ input flow $\times$ (air $+ O_2$ ratio parts) *Ballpark rule*: For a given input flow, the lower the %O_2 setting of the air-entrainment device, the higher its total output flow. For example, with an input flow of 10 L/min, an air-entrainment nebulizer set to 60% O_2 (1:1 ratio) will deliver 20 L/min, but when set to 28% O_2 (10:1 ratio), it will deliver 110 L/min.	*Problem B.28* Assuming an input O_2 flow of 8 L/min for the air-entrainment mask in Problem B.27, what would be the total flow delivered to the patient? *Solution*: Total flow $=$ input flow $\times$ (air $+ O_2$ ratio parts) Total flow $= 8 \times (5{+}1)$ Total flow $= 48$ L/min
Suction Catheter Size Estimation	
Catheter size (Fr) $= 1.5 \times$ ET tube ID where catheter size is in French units (Fr) and endotracheal tube internal diameter (ET tube ID) is in millimeters. *Ballpark rule:* Multiply the ET tube ID by 2 and use the next-smallest-size French catheter.	*Problem B.29* A patient has an 8-mm ID tracheostomy tube. Which size suction catheter should you use? *Solution*: Catheter size (Fr) $= 1.5 \times$ ET tube ID Catheter size (Fr) $= 1.5 \times 8 = 12$ Fr

(Continues)

Table B-6 Formulas and Example Problems for Equipment-Related Computations (*Continued*)

Pressure Conversions	
The two conventional pressure units commonly used in respiratory care are cm H_2O and mm Hg (torr). A third unit is the kilopascal (kPa), which is the SI unit of pressure. To convert from a conventional unit to an alternative unit, *multiply it* by its conversion factor (see the table below). To convert from an alternative unit back to a conventional unit, *divide it* by the factor.	*Problem B.30* You record a patient's cuff pressure as 30 cm H_2O. What pressure is this in mm Hg? *Solution*: cm $H_2O = 1.363 \times$ mm Hg mm Hg = cm $H_2O \div 1.36$ mm Hg $= 30 \div 1.36 = 22$ mm Hg

Conventional Unit	Alternative Unit	Conversion Factor
mm Hg (torr)	cm H_2O	1.363
cm H_2O	kilopascal (kPa)	0.098
mm Hg (torr)	kPa	0.133

Ballpark rule: 1 kilopascal equals about 10 cm H_2O or 10 mm Hg.

Table B-7 Common Mechanical Ventilation Time and Flow Parameters

Parameter/Formula	Example
Total Cycle Time (Seconds per Breath)	
Total cycle time (sec) $= \dfrac{60}{f}$ where f = set frequency or rate of breathing in breaths per minute *Ballpark rule*: Total cycle time also equals the sum of the inspiratory and expiratory times (if known).	*Problem B.31* An infant is receiving control mode ventilation at a rate of 40 breaths per minute. What is the total cycle time? *Solution*: Total cycle time $= \dfrac{60}{f}$ Total cycle time $= \dfrac{60}{40}$ Total cycle time $= 1.5$ sec
Inspiratory to Expiratory Time Ratio (I:E Ratio)	
I:E ratio $= 1 : \dfrac{T_E}{T_I}$ where T_E = the expiratory time in seconds and T_I = the inspiratory time in seconds *Ballpark rule*: Unless it is clear that the patient is receiving inverse ratio ventilation ($T_I > T_E$), the I:E ratio normally will be less than 1:1 (e.g., 1:2, 1:3).	*Problem B.32* A patient on pressure control ventilation has an inspiratory time of 2 seconds and an expiratory time of 3 seconds. What is his I:E ratio? *Solution*: I:E ratio $= 1 : \dfrac{T_E}{T_I}$ I:E ratio $= 1 : \dfrac{3}{2}$ I:E ratio $= 1 : 1.5$

(Continues)

Inspiratory Time (T$_I$)

T_I (seconds) = total cycle time $-T_E$

or

$$T_I \text{ (seconds)} = \frac{\text{total cycle time}}{\text{sum of I:E ratio parts}}$$

Ballpark rule: When the I:E ratio is less than 1:1, T_I will always be shorter than T_E.

Problem B.33

A patient on volume control ventilation has an I:E ratio of 1:4 and a set rate of 20 per breaths/min. What is her inspiratory time?

Solution:

First compute total cycle time $= 60 \div 20 = 3$ seconds

$$T_I = \frac{\text{total cycle time}}{\text{sum of I:E ratio parts}}$$

$$T_I = \frac{3}{(4+1)}$$

$T_I = 0.6$ second

Expiratory Time (T$_E$)

T_E (seconds) = total cycle time $-T_I$

Ballpark rule: When the I:E ratio is less than 1:1, T_E will always be longer than T_I.

Problem B.34

Compute the expiratory time of the patient in Problem B.33.

Solution:
T_E = total cycle time $-T_I$

$T_E = 3 - 0.6 = 2.4$ seconds

Percent Inspiratory Time (%T$_I$ or "Duty Cycle")

$$\%T_I = \frac{T_I}{\text{total cycle time}}$$

Ballpark rule: The %T_I and I:E ratio are related as indicated in the following table. For I:E ratios less than 1:1, the %T_I = 100 ÷ (sum of I:E parts).

I:E Ratio	%T$_I$
1:4	20%
1:3	25%
1:2	33%
1:1.5	40%
1:1	50%
1.5:1	60%
2:1	67%

Problem B.35

Solution:

Compute the %T_I of the patient in Problem B.33.

Solution:

$$\%T_I = \frac{T_I}{\text{total cycle time}}$$

$$\%T_I = \frac{0.6}{3} = 0.20 = 20\%$$

Ventilator Flow (Volume Control Ventilation)

$$\dot{V} = \frac{\dot{V}_E}{\%T_I}$$

where $\dot{V}$ is the inspiratory flow in L/min, $\dot{V}_E$ is the minute volume in L/min, and %T_I is the percent inspiratory time (as a decimal)

Ballpark rule: A simple alternative that works as long as inverse ratio ventilation is not being used is to multiply the sum of the I:E parts by the minute volume.

Problem B.36

Which inspiratory flow is needed for a patient receiving volume-controlled ventilation at a rate of 15 breaths/min and an I:E ratio of 1:3, with a tidal volume of 600 mL?

Solution:

First compute the minute volume in L/min:

$\dot{V}_E = 15 \times 600 = 9{,}000 \text{ mL} = 9.0 \text{ L}$

Next compute the %T_I:

$\%T_I = 100 \div (3 + 1) = 25\% = 0.25$

$$\dot{V} = \frac{\dot{V}_E}{\%T_I} = \frac{9.0}{0.25}$$

$\dot{V} = 36$ L/min

Table B-8 Formulas and Example Problems for Drug Dilution and Dosage Computations

Formula	Example
Dilution	
$V_1 \times C_1 = V_2 \times C_2$ where V_1 is the original volume, C_1 is the original concentration, V_2 is the new volume, and C_2 is the new concentration *Ballpark rule*: Doubling the volume halves the concentration of the solute.	*Problem B.37* A doctor orders 5 mL of 10% acetylcysteine (Mucomyst) via small-volume nebulizer TID for a patient with thick secretions. The pharmacy stocks only 20% acetylcysteine in multidose vials. How many milliliters of the 20% acetylcysteine would you administer to the patent for each treatment? *Solution*: $V_1 \times C_1 = V_2 \times C_2$ $V_2 = \dfrac{V_1 \times C_1}{C_2}$ $V_2 = \dfrac{5\ mL \times 10\%}{20\%}$ $V_2 = 2.5$ mL (mixed with 2.5 mL normal saline for total nebulizer volume of 5 mL)
Dosage Computations	
mg/mL = $10 \times$ % concentration mg/mL % concentration = $\dfrac{mg/mL}{10}$ mL = $\dfrac{dosage\ (mg)}{concentration\ (mg/mL)}$ *Ballpark rule*: A 1% solution contains 10 mg/mL of solute; a 0.5% solution contains half as much (5 mg/mL) and a 2% solution twice as much (20 mg/mL).	*Problem B.38* A doctor orders 2 mL of a 0.5% solution of a bronchodilator via SVN. How many milligrams of the drug are you administering? *Solution*: mg/mL = $10 \times$ % concentration mg/mL = 10×0.5 mg/mL = 5 mg/mL 5 mg/mL $\times$ 2 mL = 10 mg *Problem B.39* A doctor orders 40 mg of a 0.25% solution of a bronchodilator for continuous nebulization, to be diluted with 200 mL normal saline. How many milliliters of the bronchodilator solution would you mix with the saline solution? *Solution*: First compute the mg/mL in the 0.25% bronchodilator solution: mg/mL = $10 \times$ % concentration mg/mL = 10×0.25 mg/mL = 2.5 mg/mL Next compute the mL bronchodilator solution required: mL = $\dfrac{dosage\ (mg)}{concentration\ (mg/mL)}$ mL = $\dfrac{40\ mg}{2.5\ mg/mL}$ mL = 16 mL

APPENDIX C Selected Sources

GENERAL SOURCES

Books

Butler TJ. *Laboratory exercises for competency in respiratory care.* 3rd ed. Philadelphia, PA: F. A. Davis; 2013.

Cairo JM. *Pilbeam's mechanical ventilation: physiological and clinical applications.* 5th ed. St. Louis, MO: Elsevier-Mosby; 2012.

Cairo JM, Pilbeam SP. *Mosby's respiratory care equipment.* 8th ed. St. Louis, MO: Elsevier-Mosby; 2009.

Des Jardins T, Burton GG. Clinical *manifestations and assessment of respiratory disease.* 6th ed. St. Louis, MO: Mosby-Elsevier; 2011.

Gardenhire DS. *Rau's respiratory care pharmacology.* 8th ed. St. Louis, MO: Elsevier-Mosby; 2011.

Hess DR, MacIntyre NR, Mishoe SC, et al, eds. *Respiratory care: principles and practices.* 2nd ed. Burlington, MA: Jones & Bartlett Learning; 2012.

Heuer AJ, Scanlan CL, eds. *Wilkin's clinical assessment in respiratory care.* 7th ed. St. Louis, MO: Elsevier-Mosby; 2013.

Hodgkin JE, Celli BR, Connors G, eds. *Pulmonary rehabilitation: guidelines to success.* 4th ed. St. Louis, MO: Elsevier-Mosby; 2008.

Kacmare RM, Stoller JK, Heuer AJ, eds. *Egan's fundamentals of respiratory care.* 10th ed. St. Louis, MO: Elsevier-Mosby; 2012.

Mottram C. *Ruppel's manual of pulmonary function testing.* 10th ed. St. Louis, MO: Elsevier-Mosby; 2013.

Wilkins RL, Dexter JR, Gold PM. *Respiratory disease: a case study approach to patient care.* 3rd ed. Philadelphia, PA: F. A. Davis; 2007.

Guidelines and Consensus Statements

American Association for Respiratory Care

Evidence-Based Guidelines

American Association for Respiratory Care Evidence-Based Clinical Practice Guideline. Inhaled nitric oxide for neonates with acute hypoxic respiratory failure. *Respir Care.* 2010;55:1717–1745.

American Association for Respiratory Care Evidence-Based Clinical Practice Guideline. Care of the ventilator circuit and its relation to ventilator-associated pneumonia. *Respir Care.* 2003;48:869–879.

American Association for Respiratory Care Evidence-Based Clinical Practice Guideline. Weaning and discontinuing ventilatory support. *Respir Care.* 2002;47:69–90.

Expert Panel Guidelines

American Association for Respiratory Care Clinical Practice Guideline. Surfactant replacement therapy: 2013. *Respir Care.* 2013;58:367–375.

American Association for Respiratory Care Clinical Practice Guideline. Humidification during invasive and noninvasive mechanical ventilation: 2012. *Respir Care.* 2012;57:782–788.

American Association for Respiratory Care Clinical Practice Guideline. Capnography/capnometry during mechanical ventilation: 2011. *Respir Care*. 2011;56:503–509.

American Association for Respiratory Care Clinical Practice Guideline. Incentive spirometry—2011. *Respir Care*. 2011;56:1600–1604.

American Association for Respiratory Care Clinical Practice Guideline. Endotracheal suctioning of mechanically ventilated patients with artificial airways 2010. *Respir Care*. 2010;55:758–764.

American Association for Respiratory Care Clinical Practice Guideline. Providing patient and caregiver training—2010. *Respir Care*. 2010;55:765–769.

American Association for Respiratory Care Clinical Practice Guideline. Infant/toddler pulmonary function tests—2008 revision and update. *Respir Care*. 2008;53:929–945.

American Association for Respiratory Care Clinical Practice Guideline. Bronchoscopy assisting—2007 revision and update. *Respir Care*. 2007;52:74–80.

American Association for Respiratory Care Clinical Practice Guideline. Long-term invasive mechanical ventilation in the home—2007 revision and update. *Respir Care*. 2007;52:1056–1062.

American Association for Respiratory Care Clinical Practice Guideline. Oxygen therapy in the home or alternate site health care facility—2007 revision and update. *Respir Care*. 2007;52:1063–1068.

American Association for Respiratory Care Clinical Practice Guideline. Removal of the endotracheal tube—2007 revision and update. *Respir Care*. 2007;52:81–93.

American Association for Respiratory Care Clinical Practice Guideline. Application of continuous positive airway pressure to neonates via nasal prongs, nasopharyngeal tube, or nasal mask—2004 revision and update. *Respir Care*. 2004;49:1100–1108.

American Association for Respiratory Care Clinical Practice Guideline. Metabolic measurement using indirect calorimetry during mechanical ventilation—2004 revision and update. Care. *Respir Care*. 2004;49:1073–1079.

American Association for Respiratory Care Clinical Practice Guideline. Nasotracheal suctioning—2004 revision and update. *Respir Care*. 2004;49:1080–1084.

American Association for Respiratory Care Clinical Practice Guideline. Resuscitation and defibrillation in the health care setting—2004 revision and update. *Respir Care*. 2004;49:1085–1099. (Retired)

American Association for Respiratory Care Clinical Practice Guideline. Transcutaneous blood gas monitoring for neonatal and pediatric patients—2004 revision and update. *Respir Care*. 2004;49:1069–1072.

American Association for Respiratory Care Clinical Practice Guideline. Bland aerosol administration—2003 revision and update. *Respir Care*. 2003;48:529–533. (Retired)

American Association for Respiratory Care Clinical Practice Guideline. Intermittent positive pressure breathing—2003 revision and update. *Respir Care*. 2003;48:540–546.

American Association for Respiratory Care Clinical Practice Guideline. In-hospital transport of the mechanically ventilated patient—2002 revision and update. *Respir Care*. 2002;47:721–723.

American Association for Respiratory Care Clinical Practice Guideline. Oxygen therapy for adults in the acute care facility—2002 revision and update. *Respir Care*. 2002;47:717–720.

American Association for Respiratory Care Clinical Practice Guideline. Pulmonary rehabilitation. *Respir Care*. 2002;47:617–625. (Retired)

American Association for Respiratory Care Clinical Practice Guideline. Selection of an oxygen delivery device for neonatal and pediatric patients—2002 revision and update. *Respir Care*. 2002;47:707–716. (Retired)

American Association for Respiratory Care Clinical Practice Guideline. Blood gas analysis and hemoximetry—2001 revision and update. *Respir Care*. 2001;46:498–505.

American Association for Respiratory Care Clinical Practice Guideline. Body plethysmography—2001 revision and update. *Respir Care*. 2001;46:506–513. (Retired)

American Association for Respiratory Care Clinical Practice Guideline. Capillary blood gas sampling for neonatal and pediatric patients. *Respir Care*. 2001;46:506–513.

American Association for Respiratory Care Clinical Practice Guideline. Exercise testing for evaluation of hypoxemia and/or desaturation—2001 revision and update. *Respir Care*. 2001:46:514–522. (Retired)

American Association for Respiratory Care Clinical Practice Guideline. Methacholine challenge testing—2001 revision and update. *Respir Care*. 2001;46:523–530. (Retired)

American Association for Respiratory Care Clinical Practice Guideline. Static lung volumes—2001 revision and update. *Respir Care.* 2001;46:531–539. (Retired)

American Association for Respiratory Care Clinical Practice Guideline. Selection of device, administration of bronchodilator, and evaluation of response to therapy in mechanically ventilated patients. *Respir Care.* 1999;44:105–113. (Retired)

American Association for Respiratory Care Clinical Practice Guideline. Single-breath carbon monoxide diffusing capacity—1999 update. *Respir Care.* 1999;44:539–546. (Retired)

American Association for Respiratory Care Clinical Practice Guideline. Suctioning of the patient in the home. *Respir Care.* 1999;44:99–104. (Retired)

American Association for Respiratory Care Clinical Practice Guideline. Selection of a device for delivery of aerosol to the lung parenchyma. *Respir Care.* 1996;41:647–653. (Retired)

American Association for Respiratory Care Clinical Practice Guideline. Spirometry—1996 update. *Respir Care.* 1996;41:629–636. (Retired)

American Association for Respiratory Care Clinical Practice Guideline. Training the health-care professional for the role of patient and caregiver educator. *Respir Care.* 1996;41:654–657. (Retired)

American Association for Respiratory Care Clinical Practice Guideline. Assessing response to bronchodilator therapy at point of care. *Respir Care.* 1995;40:1300–1307. (Retired)

American Association for Respiratory Care Clinical Practice Guideline. Discharge planning for the respiratory care patient. *Respir Care.* 1995;40:1308–1312. (Retired)

American Association for Respiratory Care Clinical Practice Guideline. Management of airway emergencies. *Respir Care.* 1995;40:749–760. (Retired)

American Association of Respiratory Care and Association of Polysomnography Technologists. Clinical Practice Guideline. Polysomnography. *Respir Care.* 1995;40:1336–1343. (Retired)

American Association of Respiratory Care Clinical Practice Guideline. Selection of an aerosol delivery device for neonatal and pediatric patients. *Respir Care.* 1995;40:1325–1335. (Retired)

American Association for Respiratory Care Clinical Practice Guideline. Neonatal time-triggered, pressure-limited, time-cycled mechanical ventilation. *Respir Care.* 1994;39:808–816. (Retired)

American Association for Respiratory Care Clinical Practice Guideline. Directed cough. *Respir Care.* 1993;38:495–499. (Retired)

American Association for Respiratory Care Clinical Practice Guideline. Use of positive airway pressure adjuncts to bronchial hygiene therapy. *Respir Care.* 1993;38:516–521. (Retired)

American Association for Respiratory Care Clinical Practice Guideline. Patient–ventilator system checks. *Respir Care.* 1992;37:882–886. (Retired)

American Association for Respiratory Care Clinical Practice Guideline. Sampling for arterial blood gas analysis. *Respir Care.* 1992;37:891–897. (Retired)

American Association for Respiratory Care Clinical Practice Guideline. Postural drainage therapy. *Respir Care.* 1991;36:1418–1426. (Retired)

American Association for Respiratory Care Clinical Practice Guideline. Pulse oximetry. *Respir Care.* 1991;36:1406–1409. (Retired)

American Association of Sleep Medicine

American Association of Sleep Medicine. Practice parameters for the indications for polysomnography and related procedures: an update for 2005. *Sleep.* 2005:28:499–519.

Kushida CA, Chediak A, Berry RB, et al. Clinical guidelines for the manual titration of positive airway pressure in patients with obstructive sleep apnea. *J Clin Sleep Med.* 2008;4:157–171.

Morgenthaler TI. Practice parameters for the use of autotitrating continuous positive airway pressure devices for titrating pressures and treating adult patients with obstructive sleep apnea syndrome: an update for 2007. *Sleep.* 2008;31:141–147.

American College of Chest Physicians

Dolovich MB, Ahrens RC, Hess DR, et al. Device selection and outcomes of aerosol therapy: evidence-based guidelines. *Chest.* 2005;127:335–371.

Mehta AC, Prakash UB, Garland R, et al. Consensus statement: prevention of flexible bronchoscopy-associated infection. *Chest.* 2005;128:1742–1755.

Society of Critical Care Medicine

Society of Critical Care Medicine. Clinical practice guidelines for the management of pain, agitation, and delirium in adult patients in the intensive care unit. *Crit Care Med*. 2013;41:263–306.

Society of Critical Care Medicine and American Society for Parenteral and Enteral Nutrition. Guidelines for the provision and assessment of nutrition support therapy in the adult critically ill patient. *Crit Care Med*. 2009;37:1–30.

Warren J, Fromm RE, Orr RA, et al. Guidelines for the inter- and intrahospital transport of critically ill patients. *Crit Care Med*. 2004;32:56–62.

American College of Radiology

Aquino SL, Kahn A, Batra PV, et al. *Expert panel on thoracic imaging: routine chest radiograph*. Reston, VA: American College of Radiology; 2006.

American Heart Association

American College of Cardiology and American Heart Association Task Force on Practice Guidelines, Committee on Exercise Testing. *2002 guideline update for exercise testing*. Bethesda, MD: Author; 2002.

American Heart Association. 2010 guidelines for cardiopulmonary resuscitation and emergency cardiovascular care. *Circulation*. 2010;122(suppl 3):S640–S946.

American Society of Anesthesiologists

American Society of Anesthesiologists. Practice guidelines for management of the difficult airway: an updated report by the American Society of Anesthesiologists Task Force on Management of the Difficult Airway. *Anesthesiology*. 2013;118:251–270.

American Society of Anesthesiologists. Practice guidelines for postanesthetic care: an updated report by the Task Force on Postanesthetic Care. *Anesthesiology*. 2013;118:291–307.

American Society of Anesthesiologists. Practice guidelines for pulmonary artery catheterization: an updated report by the American Society of Anesthesiologists Task Force on Pulmonary Artery Catheterization. *Anesthesiology*. 2003;99:988–1014.

American Thoracic Society/European Respiratory Society

American Thoracic Society. *Pulmonary function laboratory management and procedure manual*. 2nd ed. New York: Author; 2005.

American Thoracic Society and European Respiratory Society. Standardisation of spirometry. *Eur Respir J*. 2005;26:319–338.

American Thoracic Society and European Respiratory Society. Interpretative strategies for lung function tests. *Eur Respir J*. 2005;26:948–968.

American Thoracic Society and European Respiratory Society. Standardisation of the single-breath determination of carbon monoxide uptake in the lung. *Eur Respir J*. 2005;26:720–735.

American Thoracic Society and European Respiratory Society. General considerations for lung function testing. *Eur Respir J*. 2005;26:153–161.

American Thoracic Society and European Respiratory Society. Standardized procedures for the online and offline measurement of exhaled lower respiratory nitric oxide and nasal nitric oxide. *Am J Respir Crit Care Med*. 2005;171:912–930.

American Thoracic Society and European Respiratory Society. Standardisation of the measurement of lung volumes. *Eur Respir J*. 2005;26:511–522.

American Thoracic Society. ATS statement: guidelines for the six-minute walk test. *Am J Respir Crit Care Med*. 2002;166:111–117.

Clinical and Laboratory Standards Institute

Clinical and Laboratory Standards Institute. *Pulse oximetry*. 2nd ed. (Document POCT11-A2). Wayne, PA: Author; 2011.

Clinical and Laboratory Standards Institute. *Procedures for the handling and processing of blood specimens*. 4th ed. (Document H18-A4). Wayne, PA: Author; 2010.

Clinical and Laboratory Standards Institute. *Blood gas and pH analysis and related measurements.* 2nd ed. (Document C46-A2). Wayne, PA: Author; 2009.

Clinical and Laboratory Standards Institute. *Procedures and devices for the collection of diagnostic capillary blood specimens.* 6th ed. (Document 1104-A6). Wayne, PA: Author; 2008.

Clinical and Laboratory Standards Institute. *Statistical quality control for quantitative measurement procedures: principles and definitions.* 3rd ed. (Document C24-A3). Wayne, PA: Author; 2006.

Clinical and Laboratory Standards Institute. *Protection of laboratory workers from occupationally acquired infections.* 3rd ed. (Document M29-A3). Wayne, PA: Author; 2005.

Clinical and Laboratory Standards Institute. *Procedures for the collection of arterial blood specimens.* 4th ed. (Document H11-A4). Wayne, PA: Author; 2004.

Clinical and Laboratory Standards Institute. *A quality management system model for health care.* 2nd ed. (Document HS01-A2). Wayne, PA: Author; 2004.

Clinical and Laboratory Standards Institute. *Reference and selected procedures for the quantitative determination of hemoglobin in blood.* 3rd ed. (Document H15-A3). Wayne, PA: Author; 2000.

Centers for Disease Control and Prevention

Centers for Disease Control and Prevention. Guidelines for preventing health-care–associated pneumonia, 2003: recommendations of CDC and the Healthcare Infection Control Practices Advisory Committee. *MMWR.* 2004;53(RR03):1–36.

Centers for Disease Control and Prevention. *Interim recommendations for infection control in health-care facilities caring for patients with known or suspected avian influenza.* Atlanta, GA: Author; 2004.

Centers for Disease Control and Prevention. *Public health guidance for community-level preparedness and response to severe acute respiratory syndrome (SARS), Version 2, Supplement I: infection control in healthcare, home, and community settings.* Atlanta, GA: Author; 2004.

Centers for Disease Control and Prevention. Guidelines for environmental infection control in health-care facilities: recommendations of CDC and the Healthcare Infection Control Practices Advisory Committee. *MMWR.* 2003;52(RR-10):1–48.

Centers for Disease Control and Prevention. Guideline for hand hygiene in health-care settings: recommendations of the Healthcare Infection Control Practices Advisory Committee and the HICPAC/SHEA/APIC/IDSA Hand Hygiene Task Force. *MMWR.* 2002;51(RR16):1–44.

Healthcare Infection Control Practices Advisory Committee. *Guidelines for the prevention of intravascular catheter-related infections, 2011.* Atlanta, GA: Centers for Disease Control and Prevention; 2011.

Healthcare Infection Control Practices Advisory Committee. *Guideline for disinfection and sterilization in healthcare facilities, 2008.* Atlanta, GA: U.S. Department of Health and Human Services, Centers for Disease Control and Prevention; 2008.

Healthcare Infection Control Practices Advisory Committee. *2007 guideline for isolation precautions: preventing transmission of infectious agents in healthcare settings.* Atlanta, GA: Centers for Disease Control and Prevention; 2007.

U.S. Department of Health and Human Services

U.S. Public Health Service. *Clinical practice guideline: treating tobacco use and dependence: 2008 update.* Rockville, MD: Author; 2008.

CHAPTER-SPECIFIC SOURCES

Chapter 2

Carter W, Harkins, DK, O'Connor, R, et al. *Taking an exposure history.* Atlanta, GA: U.S. Department of Health and Human Services, Agency for Toxic Substances and Disease Registry; 2000.

Fuhrman TM. Be aware of advanced directives. *NBRC Horizons.* 2004;30:2.

Joint Commission. *The Joint Commission guide to patient and family education.* 2nd ed. Chicago, IL: Author; 2007.

MacIntyre NR. Respiratory monitoring without machinery. *Respir Care.* 1990;35:546–553.

Chapter 4

Ferguson GT, Enright PL, Buist AS, Higgins MW. Office spirometry for lung health assessment in adults: a consensus statement from the National Lung Health Education Program. *Chest.* 2000;117:1146–1161.

McCoy R. Oxygen-conserving techniques and devices. *Respir Care.* 2000;45:95–103.

Chapter 5

Collins SE, Klompas M, Classen D, et al. Strategies to prevent ventilator-associated pneumonia in acute care hospitals. *Infect Control Hosp Epidemiol.* 2008;29(S1):531–540.

Institute for Clinical Systems Improvement. *Prevention of ventilator-associated pneumonia.* 5th ed. Bloomington, MN: Author; 2011.

Occupational Safety and Health Administration. *Pandemic influenza preparedness and response guidance for healthcare workers and healthcare employers.* Washington, DC: U.S. Department of Labor; 2009.

Chapter 6

Emergency Care Research Institute. Minimum requirements for ventilator testing. *Health Devices.* 1998;27:363–364.

National Institute for Occupational Safety and Health. *NIOSH spirometry training guide* (NIOSH Publication No. 2004-154c). Atlanta, GA: Centers for Disease Control and Prevention; 2003.

Chapter 7

American Association for Respiratory Care. *Guidelines for preparing a respiratory care protocol (RC protocol).* n.d.

American Association for Respiratory Care. Respiratory care standard abbreviations and symbols. *Respir Care.* 1997;42:637–642.

Fiore MC, Baker TB, Jaén CR, et al. *Treating tobacco use and dependence: 2008 update.* Rockville, MD: U.S. Department of Health and Human Services, Public Health Service; 2008.

Institute for Safe Medication Practices. *List of error-prone abbreviations, symbols and dose designations.* Horsham, PA: Author; 2008.

Institute of Medicine. *The computer-based patient record: an essential technology for health care.* Washington, DC: National Academy Press; 1991.

Mallin R. Smoking cessation: integration of behavioral and drug therapies. *Am Fam Phys.* 2002;65:1108–1114.

Piper ME, Fox BJ, Fiore MC. (2001). Strategies for smoking cessation. *Pul Crit Care Update.* 2001;15: Lesson 13.

University of California San Diego, Respiratory Services. *Respiratory care patient-driven protocols.* 3rd ed. Dallas, TX: Daedalus Enterprises; 2008.

Weed LL. *Medical records, medical education, and patient care: the problem-oriented record as a basic tool.* Chicago, IL: Year Book Medical Publishers; 1970.

Chapter 8

Hess DR. Tracheostomy tubes and related appliances. *Respir Care.* 2005;50:497–510.

Chapter 9

Boitano LJ. Management of airway clearance in neuromuscular disease. *Respir Care.* 2006;51:913–922.

Chatburn RL. High-frequency assisted airway clearance. *Respir Care.* 2007;52:1224–1235.

Lapin C. Airway physiology, autogenic drainage, and active cycle of breathing. *Respir Care.* 2002;47: 778–779.

Lester MK, Flume PA. Airway-clearance therapy: guidelines and implementation. *Respir Care.* 2009; 54:733–738.

Chapter 10

American Association for Respiratory Care, Protocol Committee, Subcommittee on Adult Critical Care. *Adult respiratory ventilator protocol* (Version 1.0a). 2003.

National Heart, Lung, and Blood Institute and ARDS Clinical Network. Mechanical ventilation protocol summary. 2008. Retrieved from www.ardsnet.org/.

Weiner P, McConnell A. Respiratory muscle training in chronic obstructive pulmonary disease: inspiratory, expiratory, or both? *Curr Opin Pul Med.* 2005;11:140–144.

Chapter 12

Burns SM, ed. *AACN protocols for practice: noninvasive monitoring* (2nd ed.). Sudbury, MA: Jones and Bartlett; 2006.

Chapter 14

American Association for Respiratory Care. Guidelines for preparing a respiratory care protocol (RC protocol). n.d. Retrieved from www.aarc.org (Protocol Resources; members only area).

American College of Chest Physicians, Respiratory Care Section Steering Committee. Position paper: respiratory care protocols. Chicago, IL: American College of Chest Physicians; 1992. Retrieved from www.aarc.org (Protocol Resources; members only area).

Des Jardins T, Burton GG, Tietsort J. *Respiratory care case studies: the therapist driven protocol approach.* St. Louis, MO: Mosby-Yearbook; 1997.

Orens D, Kester L, Ford R, et al. Strategies for measuring protocol outcomes. n. d. Retrieved from www.aarc.org (Protocol Resources; members only area).

Vines D. Quality in acute care protocols. 2003. Retrieved from www.aarc.org (Protocol Resources; members only area).

Chapter 15

Hazinski MF, Samson R, Schexnayder S, eds. *Handbook of emergency cardiovascular care for healthcare providers.* Chicago, IL: American Heart Association; 2010.

Kaveh J, Bradford BW, McDonald KM, Wachter RM. *Making health care safer: a critical analysis of patient safety practices.* Evidence Report/Technology Assessment #43 (AHRQ Publication 01-E058). Rockville, MD: Agency for Healthcare Research and Quality; 2001.

Quenot JP, Milési C, Cravoisy A, et al. Intrahospital transport of critically ill patients (excluding newborns): recommendations of the Société de Réanimation de Langue Française (SRLF), the Société Française d'Anesthésie et de Réanimation (SFAR), and the Société Française de Médecine d'Urgence (SFMU). *Ann Intens Care.* 2012;2:1–6.

Chapter 16

Crosby ET. Airway management in adults after cervical spine trauma. *Anesthesiology.* 2006;104:1293–1318.

Eastern Association for the Surgery of Trauma. Emergency tracheal intubation immediately following traumatic injury. *J Trauma Acute Care Surg.* 2012;73:S333–S340.

Chapter 17

American Thoracic Society and European Respiratory Society. Statement on pulmonary rehabilitation. *Am J Respir Crit Care Med.* 2006;173:1390–1413.

Ries AL, Bauldoff GS, Carlin BW, et al. Pulmonary rehabilitation: joint ACCP/AACVPR evidence-based clinical practice guidelines. *Chest.* 2007;131(5 suppl):4S–42S.

Chapter 20

Alberta Medical Association Clinical Practice Guideline Working Group. *Guideline for the diagnosis and management of croup.* Edmonton, Alberta, Canada: Author; 2008.

Alberta Medical Association Clinical Practice Guideline Working Group. *Guideline for the investigation of the poisoned patient.* Edmonton, Alberta, Canada: Author; 2006.

American Academy of Pediatrics. Clinical practice guideline: diagnosis and management of bronchiolitis. *Pediatrics.* 2006;118:1774–1793.

American Academy of Pediatrics. Clinical practice guideline: diagnosis and management of childhood obstructive sleep apnea syndrome. *Pediatrics.* 2012;130:576–584.

American Academy of Pediatrics, Committee on Fetus and Newborn. Apnea, sudden infant death syndrome, and home monitoring. *Pediatrics.* 2003;111:914–917.

American Association of Neuroscience Nurses. *Clinical practice guideline: nursing management of adults with severe traumatic brain injury.* Chicago, IL: Author; 2008.

American College of Cardiology and American Heart Association. Guideline for the diagnosis and management of chronic heart failure in the adult. *J Am Coll Cardiol.* 2009;53:1343–1382.

American College of Chest Physicians. Diagnosis and management of lung cancer: ACCP evidence-based clinical practice guidelines (2nd edition). *Chest.* 2007;132(3 suppl):1S–19S.

American College of Physicians, American College of Chest Physicians, American Thoracic Society, and European Respiratory Society. Diagnosis and management of stable chronic obstructive pulmonary disease: a clinical practice guideline update. *Ann Intern Med.* 2011;155:179–191.

American Thoracic Society. Respiratory care of the patient with Duchenne muscular dystrophy: an official ATS consensus statement. *Am J Respir Crit Care Med.* 2004;170:456–465.

American Thoracic Society. Guidelines for the management of adults with community-acquired pneumonia: diagnosis, assessment of severity, antimicrobial therapy, and prevention. *Am J Respir Crit Care Med.* 2001;163:1730–1754.

Centers for Disease Control and Prevention, DMD Care Considerations Working Group. The respiratory management of patients with Duchenne muscular dystrophy. *Pediatr Pulmonol.* 2010;45:739–748.

Consortium for Spinal Cord Medicine. Early acute management in adults with spinal cord injury. *J Spinal Cord Med.* 2008;31:403–479.

Eastern Association for the Surgery of Trauma. Management of pulmonary contusion and flail chest: a practice management guideline. *J Trauma Acute Care Surg.* 2012;73:S351–S361.

European Respiratory Society and European Society for Clinical Microbiology and Infectious Diseases. Guidelines for the management of adult lower respiratory tract infections. *Clin Microbiol.* 2011;17(suppl 6):E1–E59.

European Society of Cardiology Committee for Practice Guidelines. Guidelines for the diagnosis and treatment of pulmonary hypertension. *Eur Heart J.* 2009;30:2493–2537.

Howard JE, ed. *Myasthenia gravis: a manual for the health care provider.* St. Paul, MN: Myasthenia Gravis Foundation of America; 2008.

Institute for Clinical Systems Management. *Diagnosis and treatment of respiratory illness in children and adults.* 4th ed. Bloomington, MN: Author; 2013.

Institute for Clinical Systems Management. *Diagnosis and treatment of chest pain and acute coronary syndrome (ACS).* 8th ed. Bloomington, MN: Author; 2012.

Institute for Clinical Systems Management. *Heart failure in adults.* 11th ed. Bloomington, MN: Author; 2011.

Kair LR, Leonard DT, Anderson JM. Bronchopulmonary dysplasia. *Pediatr Rev.* 2012;33:255–264.

Kempainen RR, Brunette DD. The evaluation and management of accidental hypothermia. *Respir Care.* 2004;49:192–205.

Kemper AR, Mahle WT, Martin GR, et al. Strategies for implementing screening for critical congenital heart disease. *Pediatrics.* 2011;128:e1–e8.

Lisboa T, Ho L, Filho GT, et al. Guidelines for the management of accidental tetanus in adult patients. *Rev Bras Ter Intensiva.* 2011;23:394–409.

Mlcak RP, Suman OE, Herndon DN. Respiratory management of inhalation injury. *Burns.* 2007;33:2–13.

National Heart, Lung, and Blood Institute, National Asthma Education and Prevention Program. *Expert panel report 3 (EPR3): guidelines for the diagnosis and management of asthma.* Bethesda, MD: Author; 2007.

Olson AL, Zwillich C. The obesity hypoventilation syndrome. *Am J Med.* 2005;118:948–956.

Panitch HB. Respiratory issues in the management of children with neuromuscular disease. *Respir Care*. 2006;51:885–895.

Piper AJ, Grunstein RR. Obesity hypoventilation syndrome: mechanisms and management. *Am J Respir Crit Care Med*. 2011;183:292–298.

Rao PS. Diagnosis and management of cyanotic congenital heart disease. *Indian J Pediatr*. 2009;76:297–308.

Skeie GO, Apostolski S, Evoli A, et al. Guidelines for treatment of autoimmune neuromuscular transmission disorders. *Eur J Neurol*. 2010;17:893–902.

Zhao J, Gonzalez F, Mu D. Apnea of prematurity: from cause to treatment. *Eur J Pediatr*. 2011;170:1097–1105.

What's Online

To supplement this text, Jones & Bartlett Learning provides a companion website to further support your preparation for the NBRC exams.

ACCESSING THE COMPANION WEBSITE

To access the companion website for this text, point your browser to **go.jblearning.com /respexamreviewCWS**.

Each new text includes an access code for the Navigate Companion Website. Online access to the Navigate Companion Website may also be purchased separately. For more information, or to purchase individual access, visit **go.jblearning.com/respexamreview**.

If you need assistance acquiring an access code, please contact our Customer Service Department at 1-800-832-0034.

ONLINE RESOURCES

Companion website resources include chapter post-tests, mock CRT and WRRT exams, practice clinical simulation problems, selected Web resources, and updated content with corresponding self-assessment exercises.

Chapter Post-Tests

To help confirm your mastery of the applicable NBRC topical content, the website provides post-tests for each of the 17 chapters in Section I of the text. Upon completing each chapter post-test, you will receive both your overall score and individual question feedback. You also can send a copy of your post-test scores to your professor.

A post-test score of 80% or higher indicates that you are adequately prepared for the applicable section of the NBRC written exams. If you score less than 80%, you should first review the question feedback provided with each post-test and continue to review the applicable chapter content. In addition, you may want to access and review the Web resources associated with the applicable NBRC topic, as described subsequently.

Mock CRT and WRRT Exams

Also available on the companion website are two mock exams: a 140-question CRT-like mock exam and a 100-question WRRT-like mock exam. To further assist you in preparing for the actual NBRC versions, upon completing each mock exam you will be provided with your overall score as well as individual question feedback. As with the chapter post-tests, you can send a copy of your score report to your professor. We recommend that you use your mock exam scores and feedback to identify areas needing further review and study before taking the applicable NBRC exam.

CSE Practice Problems

The companion website also provides access to seven clinical simulation problems—one example each representing the current seven NBRC disease management categories. These practice problems are designed to give you experience with the CSE format and help you apply the case management and CSE test-taking skills reviewed in Chapters 18 and 19.

Upon completion of each problem, you will receive summary Information Gathering and Decision-Making scores as well as feedback regarding the adequacy of your pace through the simulation. Also provided with each problem is an answer key with case pointers and follow-up resources specific to the disease or disorder requiring management. If you score poorly on any individual practice problem or consistently have difficulty with either information gathering or decision making, we recommend you review the test-taking skills in Chapter 19 and the corresponding disease management "pearls" provided in Chapter 20. You also may want to access and review the follow-up resources provided with each practice problem and the Web-based disease management guidelines provided on the companion website. Then retake or review the applicable practice problem while using the section map and key as your guide.

Web Resources

The companion website provides access to two sets of regularly updated Web resources, provided courtesy of RTBoardReview.com. The first set provides links to selected Web resources organized by NBRC exam topic (corresponding to content covered in the 17 chapters that make up Section I of this text). The second set provides links to selected disease management guidelines, corresponding to the current categories of disorders covered on the NBRC CSE. These resources are particularly useful when you continue to have difficulty understanding either topical content or patient management practices after taking chapter post-tests or practice simulation problems.

Updated Mock Exam, Topical Content, and Practice Exercises

The NBRC has announced major changes to its credentialing exams, effective January 2015. These changes will affect both the testing process and the scoring methods, as well as exam contents.

Regarding the testing process and scoring methods, beginning in 2015 there will be one therapist written exam with two different cut scores. Candidates attaining the lower score will earn the CRT credential, while those meeting the higher score requirement will be eligible for the CSE. Also changing will be the structure of the CSE, which beginning in 2015 will include twice as many problems as the current exam, with each simulation having about half as many sections.

In terms of content changes, the single 2015 written exam will be based on a new content outline derived from a recently conducted national job analysis survey. Examples of potential new content include exchanging artificial airways, recommending pulmonary vasodilators, and assisting in withdrawal of life support. Examples of potential new areas of disease management include bariatric surgery, pulmonary hypertension, lung transplantation, and geriatric care.

To accommodate these changes, in October 2014 the companion website to this text will provide a revised two-level written exam covering any and all new topical content defined by the NBRC. In addition, website users will be able to access details on each new topic, with accompanying example questions to help assess content mastery. Over time, additional CSE practice problems will be offered, including those addressing any new disease management categories or disorders defined by the NBRC.

RTBoardReview.com

This text evolved from an online review program originally developed at the University of Medicine and Dentistry of New Jersey in 1999 and later made available commercially at **RTBoardReview.com**.

Since its inception, the RTBoardReview online program has helped thousands of learners prepare for and pass the NBRC exams. Online options range from mock written practice exams, up to in depth comprehensive topical reviews covering the full range of NBRC CRT, WRRT, and CSE exam content. Other major features include the following:

- Available 24 hours/7 days—prepare anywhere and anytime, at your convenience
- Immediate scoring/feedback on all practice quizzes and mock exams
- Explanations of the correct answers for every quiz or mock exam question
- Online access to experienced teachers to answer your test- or content-related questions, with bilingual support for Spanish-speaking exam takers
- One-time fee guarantee—participate until you pass the applicable exam
- Individual guidance for those needing to retake any NBRC exam (requires submission of NBRC score reports)

For those who already have purchased and are using this text to prepare for the NBRC exams, the best use of RTBoardReview would be to gain additional testing experience beyond that provided on the Jones & Bartlett Learning companion website (Appendix D). Depending on the RTBoardReview course option selected, these additional assessment opportunities can be used to further confirm mastery of specific NBRC topical content or to gain practice with additional CRT- or WRRT-like mock exams. Because RTBoardReview maintains a pool of more than 4,000 validated test questions and weights its written exam topics according to published NBRC test specifications, enrollees can be sure that each quiz or mock board exam they take will contain a unique set of questions that closely parallels the content and concepts covered on the actual NBRC exams. Also available on RTBoardReview are additional practice simulation problems helpful in preparing for the NBRC Clinical Simulation Exam (CSE). As with its written exams, RTBoardReview simulations have been designed specifically to meet published test specifications, including coverage of both the NBRC's current disease management categories and applicable topical content.

Purchasers of this text qualify for discounted enrollment fees for all RTBoardReview courses. For more details on RTBoardReview and to obtain your enrollment discount, please go to the course home page at **RTBoardReview.com**.

To receive an RTBoardReview enrollment discount, you will need to supply either a copy of your printed invoice/receipt for this text or the original (tear-out) of Appendix E (i.e. this page)
For more details, go to RTBoardReview.com.

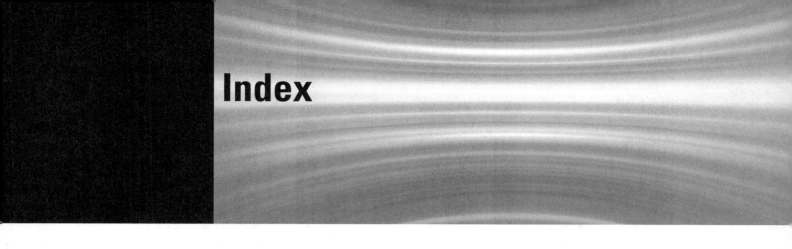

Index

Note: Page numbers followed by *f*, or *t* indicate material in figures, or tables, respectively.

A

AARC. *See* American Association for Respiratory Care
abbreviations, 195*t*
abdominal distension, 33
abdominal tenderness, 33
abdominal thrust, 240, 241
ABG. *See* arterial blood gas
ability to cooperate, assessing, 36
abnormal patterns, common, 10, 11*t*
abnormal red blood cells (RBCs), 7
A/C mode. *See* assist/control mode
Acapella device, 242, 243*f*
accidental extubation, 222
accuracy, defined, 176*t*
acetylcysteine (Mucomyst), 250, 284*t*, 286
acid–base balance, 9
acid–base disorders, 382*t*
acid–base status, 301–302
acidosis, metabolic, 327, 302*t*
ACLS. *See* Advanced Cardiac Life Support
acrocyanosis, 25
ACS. *See* acute coronary syndrome
active humidifiers, 111
acute airway obstruction, medications for, 364*t*
acute asthma, 19
acute bacterial infection, 7
acute cardiogenic pulmonary edema, 271
acute coronary syndrome (ACS)
    contraindications to drug classes used in, 483*t*
    coronary artery disease and, 481–483
    managing, 483
acute exacerbation, 497–499
acute lung injury, 288
acute manifestations, neuromuscular disorders with, 487, 488*t*–489*t*

acute myocardial infarction, 287
acute phase of SCI management, 474–475
acute respiratory distress syndrome (ARDS), 500
    high-frequency oscillation ventilation (HFOV), 276
    inhaled nitric oxide therapy, 339
    patient positioning, 211*t*
    procedure associated hypoxemia, 288–289
    protocol, 275–276, 280–281
    x-ray findings, 18, 297*t*–298*t*
ADDCs. *See* automated drug dispensing cabinets
adequate respiratory support
    common errors to avoid, 289
    deep breathing/muscle training, 257–259
    disease-specific ventilator protocols, 275–276
    elevated baseline pressure (CPAP, PEEP, EPAP, P low Plow), 270–273
    endotracheal instillation, 286–287
    high-frequency ventilation, 276–278
    hypoxemia, 287–289
    IPPB therapy, 259–262, 260*t*, 261*f*
    mechanical ventilation, 259–269
    medications, 281–287
    noninvasive ventilation, 262, 269–270, 269*t*
    ventilator graphics, 273–275
    weaning procedures, 279–281
Adrenalin, 282*t*
adrenergic + anticholinergic combinations, 283*t*
adrenergic/sympathomimetic drugs, 509*t*
adult cardiac arrest, ACLS algorithm for, 394*f*

adult orotracheal intubation, 214
adult resuscitation protocols, 393
adults
    altering the pH and Paco$_2$, 268*t*
    ventilatory support of, 267*t*
Advair Diskus (trade name), 284*t*
advance directive, 18, 41
Advanced Cardiac Life Support (ACLS), 392–395
    algorithm for adult cardiac arrest, 394*f*
    medication, 394*t*
advanced-stage emphysema, LVRS in, 468–469
adventitious breath sounds, 34, 313, 314*t*
adverse reactions, 196, 197
Aerobid (flunisolide), 284*t*
aerosol drug therapy, modifications for, 335, 336*t*
aerosol drug-delivery systems, 114–120
    advantages and disadvantages of, 116*t*
    assembly and use, 117, 118*t*–119*t*
    selection, 115, 117, 117*f*
    troubleshooting, 119, 120*t*
    in ventilator circuits, 132
aerosol mask, airway appliances, 230*t*
aerosol medications
    bronchopulmonary secretions administration of, 250–251, 250*t*
    bland aerosols, 249–250
    descriptions of, 281–286
    patient response to treatment, 334–335, 335*t*
aerosol-generating procedures, 171
age group, heart rate reference ranges, 31
agitation, 313
air compressors, 100–101
air contamination error, 177*t*

air transport, 398, 400, 401
air-entrainment devices,
    105–106, 105t
air-entrainment masks, 103t, 111t
air-entrainment nebulizers,
    103t, 111t
air-leak syndromes, 276
air-mix modes, 261
airway
    assessment, 25
    care plans, 382t
    common errors to avoid, 232
    complications, x-ray
        findings, 297t
    edema, medications for, 364t
    endotracheal intubation,
        213–216
    esophageal–tracheal
        Combitube, 226–228, 227f
    extubation, 231–232
    home care, 436
    humidification, 228–231
    inspection, 27t
    interfaces, IPPB devices, 260
    laryngeal mask airways, 125t,
        222, 224–226, 224f, 225t
    management techniques, 169,
        474, 477
    nasopharyngeal airways, 124t,
        210, 212–213
    obstruction, 314
    oropharyngeal airways, 124t,
        210–212, 212t
    patient positioning, 210, 211t
    pressures, assessing
        end-expiratory pause
            pressure, 320–321
        inspiratory pause or plateau
            pressure, 318–320
        mean airway pressure, 321
        PIP, 317–318
    tracheal airway cuff
        management, 220–221
    tracheal airways, 221–222
    tracheotomy, 216–219
airway pressure release ventilation
    (APRV), 262, 265t, 266, 267f
airway resistance, 13, 86, 88t, 317,
    319–320
airway suctioning, 134
alarm systems, monitoring and,
    314, 316t–317t, 345–348, 346t,
    348t, 372, 372t
albuterol, 7, 282t
alkalosis, metabolic, 302
Allen's test, 298, 299f
altitude, effect of, 401t
Alupent (metaproterenol), 282t
alveolar minute ventilation, 50
alveolar pressure, 320–321

alveolar ventilation, 369
alveolar–arterial O₂ tension
    gradient, 302, 303
alveolar–capillary diffusion, 56
ambulatory care settings. See
    home care
American Association for
    Respiratory Care (AARC)
    abbreviations and symbols,
        194, 195t
    guidelines, 451
    patient-ventilator system
        checks, 195, 196t
    requirements for documenting
        protocols, 201
American Society of
    Anesthesiologists, 485t
American Thoracic Society
    (ATS), 85
    Breathlessness Scale, 37, 38t
Amidate (etomidate), 366t
analgesics, 363, 366t
analyte, 176t
analytical errors, 176t, 179, 180t
anemia, 7
aneroid manometers, 138,
    139t, 140
angina pectoris, 481
angiography, 12t
anteroposterior (AP)
    projection, 298
anti-acetylcholine receptor (anti-
    AchR) antibody, 487
anti-AchR antibody. See
    anti-acetylcholine receptor
    antibody
antibiotics, 85, 286
anticholinergic bronchodilators,
    283t
anticholinergic drugs, 509t
antidotes, 509t
anti-infective agents, 285t, 286
antipsychotics, 365, 366t
antiseptic, defined, 161t
AP projection. See anteroposterior
    projection
Apgar score, 16, 28
apical pulse, 31
apnea monitoring, 60,
    439–441, 441t
apnea of prematurity
    assessment/information
        gathering, 503
    treatment/decision making, 503
appropriate resuscitation measures
    (ABCs), 510
APRV. See airway pressure release
    ventilation
ARDS. See acute respiratory
    distress syndrome

arterial blood gas (ABG), 89,
    181, 298
    analysis, radial arterial puncture
        for, 298
    interpretation
        acid–base status, 301–302
        oxygenation evaluation,
            302–304
    obtaining samples, 298–299
    point-of-care testing, 148
    results, 9–11
arterial blood pressure, 463t
arterial catheter system,
    indwelling, 299, 300f
arterial line insertion, key
    elements, 299
arterial lines, 90, 298
    obtaining blood samples, 300t
arterial oxygenation, 367
arterial puncture, 301
    sampling, 298
artificial airways, 123
    common errors to avoid, 232
    endotracheal intubation,
        213–216
    esophageal–tracheal
        Combitube, 226–228, 227f
    extubation, 231–232
    humidification, 228–231
    indications for, 124t–125t, 360t
    laryngeal mask airways, 222,
        224–226, 224f, 225t
    modifications relating to
        management, 342, 343t
    nasopharyngeal airways, 210,
        212–213
    obstruction, 347
    oropharyngeal airways,
        210–212, 212t
    patient positioning, 210, 211t
    recommending insertion and/or
        modifications, 359, 361t
    selection, use, and
        troubleshooting of,
        124t–125t
    tracheal airway cuff
        management, 220–221
    tracheal airways, 221–222
    tracheotomy, 216–219
aspirated foreign bodies, 47
aspiration, 83, 168
assessment, patient
    apnea monitoring, 60
    arterial blood gas results,
        9–11
    bedside assessment of
        ventilation, 49–51
    bedside spirometry, 53–55
    blood gases and related
        measures, 59–60

cardiopulmonary exercise testing, 66–68
cardiopulmonary status
  auscultation, 33–34
  inspection, 25–27
  palpitation, 30–33
  percussion, 33
chest radiograph, review and interpret, 44–46
common errors to avoid, 18
exhaled nitric oxide analysis, 56–59
hemodynamic monitoring, 68–76, 90
imaging studies, 11, 44–46
integrating physical examination findings, 34
lung mechanics and ventilator graphics, 51
maternal data, 14–16
monitoring data, 11–14
neonatal inspection, 27–30
overnight pulse oximetry, 61–62
oxygen titration with exercise, 68
patient history, 5
patient interview, 34–44
patient learning needs, assessing, 41–44
PEFR, 51–53
perinatal and neonatal data, 16
pulmonary function laboratory studies, conducting, 55–56
pulmonary function testing results, 7–9
6-minute walk test, 63–65
titration of CPAP or BiPAP during sleep, 62–63
twelve-lead ECG, 47–49
assessment/information gathering
  bronchopulmonary dysplasia, 505
  bronchiolitis, 492
  burns/smoke inhalation, 476
  cardiac surgery, 485–486
  critical congenital heart defect, 506–507
  cystic fibrosis, 499–500
  chest trauma, 470
  childhood asthma, 495–498
  congestive heart failure, 480
  coronary artery disease and acute coronary syndrome, 481
  delivery room management, 501–502
  drug overdose and poisonings, 508–509
  head trauma, 472

hypothermia, 477–478
IRDS, 504
muscular dystrophy, 490
obesity–hypoventilation syndrome, 510
spinal cord injury, 473–474
tetanus, 491
assist/control (A/C) mode, 346
  mechanical ventilation, 262, 263t
asthma, 202–203, 202t
  breath sounds, 34
  bronchial hygiene techniques, 238t
  childhood, 495–499
  medications, 286, 364t
  percussion, 33
  pulmonary function lab studies, 56
  pulmonary rehabilitation, 430
  sputum, 28t
asystole, 393
atelectasis, 33
  bronchial hygiene techniques, 238t
  IPPB therapy, 333–334, 334t
  palpation, 32
  percussion, 33
  PMI shift, 31
  trachea shifts, 31
  x-ray findings, 18, 297t
atrial fibrillation, 31, 311, 311f, 421t
atrial flutter, 311, 312f, 421t
atropine, 286
Atrovent (ipratropium), 283t
ATS. See American Thoracic Society
auscultation, 7, 33–34, 313, 479
autoclaving, 162
auto-CPAP, 62, 63
autogenic drainage, 241
automated drug dispensing cabinets (ADDCs), 200–201
auto-PEEP. See end-expiratory pause pressure
avian/bird influenza, 169
Azmacort (triamcinolone), 284t
Aztreonam (cayston), 285t

B
Babinski reflex, 463t
bacterial infection, 7
bacteriostatic, defined, 161t
bag-valve-mask resuscitator systems (BVMs), 121, 122, 163
BAL. See bronchoalveolar lavage
Ballard tools, 19, 29
barbiturates, 366t
barotrauma, 350

basic life support (BLS), 391–392, 392t
"beaked" pressure–volume curve, 350, 350f
beclomethasone (Vanceril, Beclovent), 283t
beclovent, 283t
bedside assessment of ventilation, 49–51
bedside ECG monitors, 145
bedside pulmonary function devices, 140–145
  mechanical respirometers, 140, 143, 143f
  portable electronic spirometers, 143–145, 144f, 145t
bedside spirometry, 53–55, 87t
benzodiazepines, 366t, 492
beta-adrenergic bronchodilators, 2, 281, 282t–283t, 285
bias, 176t
  quality control tests, 179
bi-level positive airway pressure, 17, 62–63, 262, 265t, 268t, 269, 439t
biohazardous materials, infection control, 164–165
biological indicators, 164t
biopsies, 83
BiPAP. See bi-level positive airway pressure
bite block/tube holder, 211
  endotracheal intubation, 215t
bitolterol, 282t
Bivona Fome-Cuf tube, 221
bland aerosol therapy, 229, 230t, 249–250, 334–335, 335t, 435
blanket orders, 193
blood flow, ventilator settings on, 508, 508f
blood gases, 9t
  analysis, 89t, 177t
  analyzers, 178t
  hemoximetry, 177t
  point-of-care testing, 148–149, 149t
  quality control, 175–180
  and related measures, 59–60
  results, 9–11
blood, handling, 164–165
blood pressure, 34, 90
blood tests, 85, 86t. See also blood gases
  abnormal RBCs, 7
  coagulation studies, 5t
  differential WBC, 7
  point of care tests, 180–181
  recommending, 312
"blown cuff," 221
BLS. See basic life support

blunt chest trauma, 470, 471t
body fluids, 165
body surface area (BSA), 475
Borg Scale, 37
Bourdon gauge, 100
BPD. *See* bronchopulmonary dysplasia
brachial arteries, 31
bradycardia, 31, 60, 309, 310, 311f
breast implants, 46t
breath sounds, 34, 313
breathing circuits, 123, 127–134, 372, 373
    dual-limb circuits, 128, 128f
    single-limb circuits, 128–129, 129f
breathing difficulties, assessing, 37–38
breathing reserve, 67
breathing techniques and exercises, 257–258, 431, 432t
Bricanyl (terbutaline), 283t
bronchial challenge tests, 313t
bronchial hygiene therapy
    modifying, 341, 341t–342t
    patient instruction, 239–241
    protocol, 237, 238f
    recommending and modifying, 359
bronchial obstruction, 7
bronchial provocation, 88t
bronchiectasis, 27, 430
bronchiolitis, 492, 495
    National Guideline Clearinghouse for, 451, 452f
bronchitis, 304
bronchoalveolar lavage (BAL), 85
bronchodilator, 250–251, 250t, 282t–283t, 334
    assessment, 56
    spirometry, 87t
bronchoprovocation studies, 312
bronchopulmonary dysplasia (BPD), 276
    assessment/information gathering, 505
    levels of, 505
    treatment/decision making, 505–506
bronchopulmonary hygiene techniques, 239–241
bronchopulmonary secretions
    aerosol therapy, 249–251
    bronchial hygiene therapy, 237, 238f, 238t
    common errors to avoid, 251
    handheld mechanical percussors and vibrators, 242

hygiene techniques, 239–241
    mechanical devices to facilitate clearance, 241–245
    postural drainage, percussion, and vibration techniques, 237, 239, 239t, 240f
    selecting best approach, 237, 238f, 238t
    suctioning equipment, 245–249
bronchoscopy, 83, 364t, 416–418
    processing of, 153–154
BSA. *See* body surface area
bubble humidifier, 111, 114t
budesonide (Pulmicort), 284t, 286
Bunnell LifePulse, 277
burns, 475–477
    phases of, 476
BVMs. *See* bag-valve-mask systems

C
CAD. *See* coronary artery disease
calibration, 176t, 177–178
Campylobacter jejuni (diarrhea), 487
capillary blood gas sampling, 301
capillary refill, 33
capnography, 13–14, 90, 187, 306, 308, 308t
capnometers/capnographs, 187–188
carbon dioxide (CO_2), measuring, 13
carbon monoxide diffusing capacity (DLCO), 87t
carbon monoxide (CO) poisoning, 14, 89, 287, 325
carboxyhemoglobin (HbCO), 89
cardiac arrest, severe hypothermia and, 479
cardiac arrhythmias, 31, 34
cardiac dysrhythmias, 310
cardiac index (CI), 73, 73t
cardiac murmurs, 34
cardiac output (CO), 11, 73t, 74, 75, 463t
cardiac rehabilitation program, 482
cardiac rhythm monitoring, 310–312
cardiac surgery, 483–487
cardiac valve replacements (prostheses), 46t
cardiogenic pulmonary edema, 271
cardiopulmonary calculations, Fick equation, 74
cardiopulmonary exercise testing, 66–68
cardiopulmonary status assessment, 25–27
    auscultation, 33–34

palpitation, 30–33
percussion, 33
cardiovascular disease
    cardiac surgery, 483–487
    congestive heart failure, 479–481
    coronary artery disease and acute coronary syndrome, 481–483
    valvular heart disease, 483
cardiovascular disorders
    cases involving, 463
    information, 463t
cardioversion, 421–422
cardioverters/defibrillators, 46t
CareFusion (Sensormedics) 3100A, U.S., 277
carotid arteries, 31
case manager, interacting with, 442
CASS. *See* continuous aspiration of subglottic secretions
catheters, 45
    indwelling, 70
    x-rays, appearance on, 46
Cayston (Aztreonam), 285t
CCHD. *See* critical congenital heart defect
CDC. *See* Centers for Disease Control and Prevention
cell washings, 83
Centers for Disease Control and Prevention (CDC)
    avian or bird influenza, 169
    central line bundle, 168
    equipment, infection control, 161
    severe acute respiratory syndrome (SARS), 169–171
    standard precautions, 165–166, 170
    VAP bundle, 168–169
Centers for Medicare and Medicaid Services (CMS), 175
central cyanosis, 25
central venous catheter, 46t, 68
central venous monitoring, 91t
central venous pressures (CVP), 14, 463t
cervical cord injuries, 473
CF. *See* cystic fibrosis
chemical indicators, 164t
chest auscultation, 313
chest cuirass, 437
chest radiographs, 297–298
chest trauma, 396, 403t, 470–472
chest tube insertion, 420–421
chest x-rays, 84t, 462t
    appearance of medical devices, 46

opacities, 18
overview, 11
patient response to care, 297–298
recommending, 83
review and interpret, 44–46
Cheyne-Stokes breathing, 472
CHF. *See* congestive heart failure
childhood asthma, 495–499
children, classification of asthma control in, 495, 496*t*
chloride, electrolyte, 363*t*
chlorpromazine (Thorazine), 366*t*
cholinergic/parasympathomimetic drugs, 509*t*
chronic airway obstruction, medications for, 364*t*
chronic bronchitis, 56, 468, 469*t*
chronic hypercapnia, 287
chronic hypoventilation, 92
chronic hypoxemia, 7
chronic obstructive pulmonary disease (COPD), 202–203, 202*t*, 258, 468–470
    ABG abnormalities, 11*t*
    breath sounds, 34
    cough and sputum, 27
    clinical simulation exam, 450*t*
    inspiratory muscle training technique (IMT), 259
    medications for, 364*t*
    overnight pulse oximetry, 61
    palpation, 31
    percussion, 33
    pulmonary rehabilitation, 430
chronic phase of spinal cord injury management, 475
chronic respiratory infections, 499
CI. *See* cardiac index
circulatory failure, 25
cisatracurium (Nimbex), 365, 366*t*
clamps, 46
cleaning, defined, 161*t*
clinical data, erroneous, 18
Clinical Laboratory Improvement Act (CLIA) program, 175
Clinical Simulation Exam (CSE)
    analysis between information gathering and decision making, 460–463
    computer testing format and option scoring, 457–459
    decision-making guidance. *See* decision-making guidance, CSE
    differential diagnoses, examples of, 460*t*
    disease management categories and cases appear on, 449, 450*t*
IG *vs.* DM sections, 452–454
information gathering guidance. *See* information gathering guidance, CSE
    National Guideline Clearinghouse, 451, 452*f*
    options scoring scale, 458*t*
    pacing, 467
    preparation
        content, 447–452, 451*f*
        CRT and WRRT exams, 447–449
    structure, 452–455
closed head traumatic brain injury, 472
closed-suction system, 247*f*
Clostridium tetani, 491
CMS. *See* Centers for Medicare and Medicaid Services
CO. *See* cardiac output
CO analyzers, 140
CO_2 detectors, 414
CO poisoning. *See* carbon monoxide poisoning
coagulation studies, 5*t*
"code blue," 333
codeine, 366*t*
coefficient of variation (CV), 176*t*
Colistin (polymyxin E), 285*t*, 286
colorimetric CO_2 detector, 215*t*, 414
Combivent, 283*t*
common abnormal patterns, 10, 11*t*
common errors to avoid, 171
    adequate respiratory support, 289
    artificial airways, 232
    bronchopulmonary secretions, 251
    emergency care, 405–406
    equipment, 154
    medical records, 18, 206
    patient response to care, 325
    pertinent clinical information, 77
    procedure recommendations, 92–93
    quality control (QC) procedures, 189
    rehabilitation and home care, 443
    respiratory care plan
        appropriateness of, 386–387
        patient response, 374
    special procedures, 425
    therapeutic procedures, patient response and, 351
common heart valve problems, 483, 484*t*
common hemodynamic parameter reference values, 14, 15*t*
communication
    common errors to avoid, 206
    computer technology, 199–201
    educating the patient and family
        health (disease) management, 202–203, 202*t*
        smoking cessation education, 203–204, 204*t*–206*t*
    patient care orders, 193–194
    planned therapy and goals, 201, 201*t*
    results of therapy, 194–198, 195*t*–197*t*, 198*f*
metabolic acidosis, 327
respiratory alkalosis, 328
complete heart block, 34
comprehensive disease management program, 496, 501
comprehensive disease management protocol, 482
compressed oxygen cylinders, 434
computer testing format, CSE, 457–459
computerized medical records, 199–201
computerized tomography (CT), 462*t*
    angiography, 462*t*
    scan, 12*t*
computerized ventilators, 183, 186
congenital diaphragmatic hernia, 276
congestive heart failure (CHF), 34, 297*t*, 364*t*, 479–481
consolidation, 19
contaminated sharps, 164–165
"continue previous medications," blanket orders, 193
continued metabolism error, 177*t*
continuous aspiration of subglottic secretions (CASS), 248
continuous positive airway pressure (CPAP), 108, 132
    appropriate use of, 127*t*
    Auto-CPAP, 62, 63
    devices for, 123, 127–134
    elevated baseline pressure, 271–273
    home care, 438, 441, 441*t*
    mechanical ventilation, 262, 264*t*
    titration during sleep, 62–63
control charts, defined, 176*t*
control media, 178

control mode ventilation, 345–346
    mechanical, 262, 263t
control valve, 129
CO-oximetry, 14, 89, 89t, 175–180,
    304–305, 305t
COPD. See chronic obstructive
    pulmonary disease
coronary artery bypass (CABG)
    surgery, 452, 453f
coronary artery disease (CAD), 66
    and acute coronary syndrome,
        481–483
corticosteroids, 281, 283t–284t, 286
cough
    care plans, 382t
    etiquette, 165, 166t
    phases of, 240
    production, 27
    types of, 27
cough assist, 244, 244f, 245
cough-related training techniques,
    239–241
counseling and behavioral
    therapies, smoking cessation,
    204, 205t–206t
CPAP. See continuous positive
    airway pressure
crackles, 7, 314t
creatine kinase, 8t
crepitus, 32
critical congenital heart defect
    (CCHD), 504
    assessment/information
        gathering, 506–507
    basic pulse oximetry screening
        protocol for, 507f
    treatment/decision making,
        507–508
cromolyn sodium, 282t, 284t
croup (laryngotracheobronchitis),
    47
    and epiglottitis, 492, 493t–494t
croupette, oxygen therapy
    enclosure, 107t
CRT exam, 447–449
    self-assessment of written exam
        topical scores, 449t
CSE. See Clinical Simulation Exam
CT. See computerized tomography
cuff leaks, 221
cuff pressures, 220
culture and sensitivity (C&S), 85
CV. See coefficient of variation
CVP. See central venous pressures
cyanide poisoning, 287
cylinders, gas, 99–100
cystic fibrosis (CF), 285t, 286, 430,
    451, 451f
    assessment/information
        gathering, 499–500

bronchial hygiene
    techniques, 238t
    treatment/decision making,
        500–501
cytologic assessment,
    83, 85
cytomegalovirus (URI)
    infections, 487

D
damping of pulmonary artery
    pressure, 151, 152f
daytime somnolence
    (sleepiness), 92
deadspace, 13
decision-making guidance,
    CSE, 459
    based on physical assessment
        findings, 464
    problems
        involving acid–base
            imbalances, 465, 466t
        involving disturbances of
            oxygenation, 465,
            466t, 467
        with secretions/airway
            clearance, 465, 466t
Decision-Making (DM) sections of
    CSE, 452–454, 454t
decompensation/pulmonary
    edema, assess for,
    480, 481
decontamination, defined, 161t
decreased cardiac contractility, 31
deep breathing/muscle training,
    257–259
deep tendon reflex, 463t
defibrillation, doses for shockable
    rhythms, 395t
definitive diagnosis, 510
delirium, 365
delivery room management
    assessment/information
        gathering, 501–502
    treatment/decision making,
        502–503
demographic data, 6t
dental appliances, 25
deviated septum, 25
diabetes with ketoacidosis, 11t
diagnostic spirometry, ATS
    standards for, 143–144
diagnostic thoracentesis, 92
Dilaudid (hydromorphone),
    363, 366t
diameter index safety system
    (DISS), 99, 135
diaphragm assessment, 33
diaphragmatic (abdominal)
    breathing, 257–258, 431

diazepam (Valium),
    366t, 422t
differential pressure
    pneumotachometer, 144f
differential WBC values, 7
diffusing capacity, 9, 56
diffusion, transcutaneous, 14
diluting agents, 250, 250t
directed coughing, 211t,
    239–241, 341
disaster
    management, 402–405
    respiratory therapist, role
        of, 403t
    triage priorities, 404t
discontinuous sounds, 313
disease management,
    202–203, 202t
    and diagnostic reasoning,
        454–455
    guidelines, 451
disease-specific ventilator
    protocols, 275–276
disinfection
    defined, 161t
    equipment, 162–164
Diskus inhaler (Advair), 284t
DISS. See diameter index safety
    system
DM sections. See Decision-Making
    sections
DMD. See Duchenne-type
    muscular dystrophy
DNR. See do-not-resuscitate
documentation, therapy
    effects, 196
do-not-intubate (DNI) order,
    410, 411t
do-not-resuscitate (DNR), 41,
    410, 411t
Doppler echo, 483
dornase alpha (Pulmozyme),
    250, 285t
DPIs. See dry-powder inhalers
drift, defined, 176, 176t
driving pressure, 317
drug overdose and poisonings
    assessment/information
        gathering, 508–509
    treatment/decision making, 509
drug therapy
    for childhood asthma, step-
        based approach to,
        496, 497t
    recommending initiation and
        modification of, 362,
        364t, 365t
drugs. See also medications
    ACLS, 393
    categories of, 509t

dry-powder inhalers (DPIs), 114
   advantages and disadvantages
      of, 116t
   assembly and operational
      check of, 118t
   optimal technique and
      therapeutic issues, 119t
   troubleshooting, 120t
dual-limb circuits, 128, 128f
Dubowitz tools, 19, 29
Duchenne-type muscular
      dystrophy (DMD), 487
   stages of, 490
dump valve, 129
Duoneb, 283t
durable power of attorney, 41
duty cycle. See percent inspiratory
      time (%I-time)
dysphagia, 491
dyspnea, 37
dysrhythmias, 7
dyssomnias, 16

E
echocardiograms, 14
ECMO. See extracorporeal
      membrane oxygenation
edema
   acute cardiogenic pulmonary
      edema, 271
   gravity-dependent, 32
   medications for, 364t
   peripheral, 11, 364t
   post extubation, 334
   pulmonary, 11, 271,
      298t, 364t
   pulmonary interstitial, 276
   upper airway, 334
educating patient and family
   apnea monitoring
      programs, 440
   assessing learning needs, 41–44
   bronchopulmonary hygiene
      techniques, 239–241
   deep breathing, muscle
      training, 257–259
   health (disease) management,
      202–203, 202t
   home care, 440, 441
   pulmonary rehabilitation
      program, 431
   smoking cessation, 203–204,
      204t–206t
EEG. See electroencephalogram
effective compliance, 319
effusions, 32
ejection fraction, 463t
elastic resistance to ventilation, 86
electrocardiography (ECG, EKG)
   atrial flutter, 311, 312t

ECG leads, appearance on
      X-rays, 46t
   machines, 12-lead,
      145–148, 147f
   monitors, 145, 147f
   premature ventricular
      contraction (PVC),
      311, 312t
   recommending, 90
   simulator, 145
   twelve-lead ECG, 47–49
electroencephalogram (EEG), 463t
electrolyte therapy, 362, 363t
electromyogram (EMG)
   conduction, 463t
electronic drug nebulizers, 116t
electronic medical record
      (EMR), 199
   automated drug dispensing
      cabinets, 200–201
   automated alerts, 200
   security and privacy, 199
mesh nebulizers, electronic 120t
electronic pressure transducers,
      138, 139t, 140
elevated baseline pressure (CPAP,
      PEEP, EPAP, Plow), 270–273
emergency care
   advance directives, 41
   Advanced Cardiac Life Support
      (ACLS), 392–395
   basic life support (BLS), 391–
      392, 392t
   chest tube insertion, 420–421
   common errors to avoid,
      405–406
   disaster management,
      402–405
   medical emergency teams
      (METs), 402
   patient transport, 398–402
   pediatric and neonatal
      emergencies, 395
   pre-test answers and
      explanations, 390–391,
      406–407
   resuscitation devices, 121–123
   tension pneumothorax,
      395–398
EMG conduction. See
      electromyogram conduction
emotional state, assessing, 34
emphysema, 468, 469t
   diffusing capacity, 9
   pulmonary function studies, 56
   tension pneumothorax,
      395–398
   x-ray findings, 297t
empyema, 420
EMR. See electronic medical record

enclosures, O_2 therapy, 106, 107t
   problems with, 109
end-expiratory pause pressure,
      320–321, 321f, 349–350,
      350f, 367
end-inspiratory occlusion
      method, 88
endotracheal instillation,
      medication, 286–287
endotracheal (ET) intubation
   assist
      patient positioning,
         412–413
      patient's vital signs, 414
      rapid-sequence intubation,
         415–416
      RT's role, 410, 411t
      tube insertion, 414
      tube placement, 414–415
   equipment, 213–214,
      214t, 215t
   oral, 222
   patient positioning, 211t
   procedure, 214, 216
endotracheal tube, 46t, 124t
   capnography, 90
   esophageal–tracheal
      Combitube, 226–228, 227f
   extubation, 222, 231–232
   insertion, 83, 213, 214t,
      411t–412t, 414
   modifications, 342, 343t
   placement considerations, 216
   x-rays, appearance on, 46t
end-tidal CO_2, 13
ensuring equipment cleanliness,
      161–164
epiglottis, 47t
epiglottitis, croup
      (laryngotracheobronchitis)
      and, 492, 493t–494t
epinephrine, 282t, 286
Epworth Sleepiness Scale (ESS), 16
equal pressure method, 272
equipment
   aerosol drug-delivery systems.
      See aerosol drug-delivery
      systems
   air compressors, 100–101
   artificial airways, 123, 124t–126t
   bedside pulmonary function
      devices, 140–145
   bronchoscopes, 153–154
   common errors to avoid, 154
   disinfecting, sterilizing, and
      maintaining, 162–164
   ECG monitors, 145, 147f
   gas cylinders, reducing valves,
      flowmeters, and O_2
      blenders, 99–100

equipment (*cont.*)
gas-delivery, 99*t*
hemodynamic monitoring
devices, 151–152,
151*f*, 151*t*
He/O$_2$-delivery systems,
110–111
humidification, 228–231
humidifiers, 111–113, 114*t*,
162, 163
incentive breathing
devices, 121
infection control, 161–164
infection risk categories of, 162*t*
maintenance, VAP and, 169
manometers. *See* manometers
mechanical devices used to aid
airway clearance, 121
mist tents, 111–114
nebulizers, 111, 113–114,
115*t*, 162
noninvasive oximetry
monitoring devices,
149–151
O$_2$, He, CO, and specialty gas
analyzers, 140
oxygen administration devices.
See oxygen administration
devices
pleural drainage systems,
136–138, 137*f*
point-of-care blood gas
analyzers, 148–149, 149*t*
portable oxygen systems, 101
resuscitation devices, 121–123
12-lead ECG machines,
145–148, 147*f*
vacuum/suction systems,
134–136, 135*t*
ventilators, CPAP devices, and
breathing circuits, 123,
127–134
errors, charting, 194, 196, 198
esophageal–tracheal Combitube
(ETC), 125*t*, 224,
226–228, 227*f*
ESS. *See* Epworth Sleepiness Scale
ET intubation. *See* endotracheal
intubation
ETC. *See* esophageal–tracheal
Combitube
etomidate (Amidate), 366*t*
exercise challenge, 313*t*
exercise test information,
selection, 461, 461*t*
exercise tolerance, 37–38, 66, 430
exhaled nitric oxide (FeNO), 88*t*
expiratory pressures, 50*t*
external patient transport, 399–400

extracorporeal membrane
oxygenation (ECMO),
303–304
extra-treatment supportive
interventions for smoking
cessation, 206*t*
extubation, 221, 222,
231–232, 374
eye protection, 166*t*

F
face tent, airway appliances, 230*t*
facial muscles, spasms of, 491
families, education of
apnea monitoring programs,
440, 441
assessing learning needs, 41–44
bronchopulmonary hygiene
techniques, 239–241
deep breathing, muscle
training, 257–259
health (disease) management,
202–203, 202*t*
home care, 440, 441
smoking cessation, 203–204,
204*t*–206*t*
fast-track approach (cardiac
surgery), 486
fatigue, 93
femoral arteries, 31
fenestrated tracheostomy tubes,
123, 126*t*, 218–219, 219*f*
fentanyl (Sublimaze), 363, 366*t*
FET. *See* forced expiratory
technique
fetal lung maturity, 14
fiberoptic bronchoscope, 154
fiberoptic scopes, 412*t*
Fick equation for cardiac
output, 74
FIO$_2$ and/or liter flow, 260,
261, 317
five R's, smoking cessation,
204, 204*t*
Fleisch pneumotachometer, 144*f*
Flonase (fluticasone
propionate), 284*t*
Flovent Rotadisk, 284*t*
flow durations, cylinders, 435*t*
flow resistor, 260*t*
PEP devices, 243*t*
flow waveform, auto-PEEP,
350, 350*f*
flowmeters, 99–100
flow–volume curve, 88*t*
fluid balance, 11–12, 362, 362*t*
fluid columns, 138, 139*t*, 140
flumazenil (Romazicon), 422*t*
flunisolide (Aerobid), 284*t*

fluticasone + salmeterol, 284*t*
fluticasone propionate
(Flonase), 284*t*
Foradil (formoterol), 282*t*
forced expiratory technique
(FET), 241
forced hyperventilation, 268
forced vital capacity (FVC), 53, 183
validity errors occurring during
measurement of, 184*t*
foreign bodies, 45, 47, 83
formoterol (Foradil), 282*t*
41-French version, esophageal–
tracheal Combitube, 226
FRC. *See* functional residual
capacity
frictional opposition to
ventilation, 86
functional capacity, 52
functional residual capacity (FRC),
56, 87*t,* 321
FVC. *See* forced vital capacity

G
gag reflex, 463*t*
gain, defined, 176*t*
galvanic fuel cell, 186
gas analyzers, 178*t,* 186, 188
therapy and diagnostic, 140,
141*t*–142*t*
gas cylinders, 99–100
gas delivery and metering devices,
188–189
gas-delivery equipment, guidelines
for, 99*t*
gas-powered resuscitators,
121, 122
gastric reflux aspiration, 168
GBS. *See* Guillain-Barré syndrome
germicides, defined, 161*t*
gestational age, 29
Glasgow Coma Scale, 36, 36*t*,
463*t*, 472
glossopharyngeal breathing, 432*t*
gloves, 166*t*
gown, 166*t*
gram stain, sputum, 7
gram-negative infection, 364*t*
graphic displays
scalar (time-based),
274*f*, 275*t*
X-Y loop, 274*f*, 275*t*
graphics, ventilator, 273–275
gravity-dependent tissue
edema, 32
guidewire (Seldinger)
technique, 298
Guillain-Barré syndrome (GBS),
487, 488*t*–489*t*

H

Haemophilus influenzae, 492
Haldol (haloperidol), 365, 366*t*
haloperidol (Haldol), 365, 366*t*
hand hygiene, 166*t*
harmful accidental exposure, 508
helium analyzers, 140
head trauma, 472–473
Health Insurance Portability and
    Accountability Act (HIPAA),
    199, 200
health (disease) management,
    202–203, 202*t*
health management programs,
    with asthma/COPD, 202*t*
heart
    cardiac arrhythmia, 31, 34
    cardiac dysrhythmias, 310
    cardiac output, 90
    CI, 73
    exercise testing, 66
    murmurs, 34
    rate, rhythm, and pulse
        strength, 31
    rhythm monitoring, 310–312
    sounds, 34
heart block, 31
heat and moisture exchangers
    (HMEs), 111, 113, 230, 231
heated humidifier, 111, 114*t*
heating wires, 46*t*
heat-sensitive items, 161, 162, 162*t*
heat-tolerant items, 162*t*
helium-oxygen delivery systems,
    110–111
helium–oxygen (heliox) therapy,
    338–339, 339*t*
hemidiaphragms, 44
hemiparesis, 472
hemodynamic assessment, 309
hemodynamic monitoring, 14,
    68–76, 90
    devices, 151–152, 151*f*, 151*t*
hemodynamic parameter reference
    values, common, 14, 15*t*
hemoglobin, blood
    concentration, 14
hemoximetry, *See* CO-oximetry
HEPA filter, ventilator, 131
hepatomegaly, 45*t*
HFJV. *See* high-frequency jet
    ventilation
HFOV. *See* high-frequency
    oscillation ventilation
high pressure cylinders, 433
high-flow devices, oxygen
    administration, 104–106
    troubleshooting, 111*t*
high-flow nasal cannulas, 103*t*,
    106, 106*t*

high-frequency chest wall
    oscillation/compression
    systems, 242
high-frequency jet ventilation
    (HFJV), 276–277
high-frequency oscillation
    ventilation (HFOV), 276
    devices, 129, 130*f*
high-frequency oscillation *vs.* jet
    ventilation, 277*t*–278*t*
high-frequency ventilation, adequate
    respiratory support, 276–278
high-pitched continuous
    sounds, 313
HIPAA. *See* Health Insurance
    Portability and Accountability
    Act
histamine challenge, 313*t*
history of present illness, 6*t*
history window (CSE), 457
HMEs. *See* heat and moisture
    exchangers
home care
    aerosol drug administration,
        435, 436
    airway care and secretion
        clearance, 436
    apnea monitoring,
        439–441, 441*t*
    bland aerosol therapy, 435
    case manager, 442
    common errors to avoid, 443
    documentation, 442–443
    education, patient and family/
        caregivers, 440, 441
    home mechanical ventilation,
        436–438, 441*t*
    home oxygen therapy, 432–433
    infection control, 441–442
    mechanical ventilation,
        436–438, 441, 441*t*
    nasal continuous positive
        airway pressure
        (CPAP), 438
    oxygen therapy, 106, 107*t*
hospital-acquired infections,
    165, 168
"huff cough," 241
humidification equipment, 228
    needs, therapy type,
        228–229, 228*t*
    strategy
        algorithm, 229, 229*f*
        mechanical ventilation,
            230–231, 230*f*
        spontaneously breathing
            patients, 229, 230*t*
humidification systems, 111–113
    comparison of active, 112*f*
    ventilators, 133

humidifiers, 111–113, 114*t*
hydrocodone (Vicodin), 366*t*
hydromorphone (Dilaudid), 363,
    366*t*
hyperinflation, 31, 33, 45*t*, 333
hyperoxia test, 504
hypertension, 11
hypertonic saline, 285
hyperventilation, 19
hypotension, 11, 34
hypothermia, 477–479
hypoventilation, 13, 304*t*
hypoxemia, 62, 287–289, 491
    causes, 304, 304*t*
    interpreting severity of, 10
    patient positioning
        techniques, 288*t*
    procedure-associated, 288–289
    respiratory failure, 266, 276
    treating and preventing,
        287–289

I

ICP. *See* intracranial pressure
ICU psychosis, 365
I:E ratio. *See* inspiratory to
    expiratory time ratio
IG. *See* information gathering
    (CSE)
imaging studies
    airway complications, 297*t*
    medical devices, appearance
        on, 46
    neck radiographs, review
        lateral, 47
    patient record, 11
    recommending, 44–46
implanted cardiac pacemakers, 46*t*
IMT. *See* inspiratory muscle
    training
incentive breathing devices, 121
incentive spirometry (IS), 121,
    258–259, 333, 333*t*
    proper and improper patient
        explanations for, 201*t*
indwelling arterial catheter system,
    299, 300*f*
indwelling catheter, 70, 90
    indications and
        contraindications for, 91*t*
infant respiratory distress
    syndrome (IRDS), 364*t*
    assessment/information
        gathering, 504
    treatment/decision making,
        504–505
infants
    apnea monitor, 439–440
    cardiopulmonary status, 25
    FIO$_2$ measure, 317

infants (*cont.*)
  heliox delivery, 338
  oxygen therapy, 108, 287
  resuscitation, 395
  temperature and humidity, environmental control, 106, 108
infection control
  avian or bird influenza, 169
  biohazardous materials, 164–165
  CDC standard precautions, 165, 166*t*, 167
  common errors to avoid, 171
  ensuring equipment cleanliness, 161–164
  home care, 441–442
  indwelling catheters, 70
  policies and procedures, 165–168
  pre-test answers and explanations, 159–160, 172–173
  severe acute respiratory syndrome (SARS), 169–171
  transmission-based precautions, 166–167, 167*t*
  ventilator-associated pneumonia protocol, 168–169
  ventilators, 134
infections, 27, 47
infectious disease protocols, implement specific, 169–171
inflammation, 7
inflation, of laryngeal mask airways, 225
influenza, medications for, 364*t*
information gathering (IG)
  guidance, CSE, 459, 460–463
    exercise test information, selection, 461, 461*t*
    imaging studies, selection, 462, 462*t*
    laboratory tests, selection, 462, 462*t*
    pulmonary function, selection, 461, 461*t*
    respiratory-related information, selection, 461, 461*t*
  sections, 452–454, 454*t*
inhalation injuries, 476
inhaled corticosteroids, 286
inhaled nitric oxide therapy, 339–340, 340*t*
inherited autosomal recessive disease, 499

initial emergency management of asthma exacerbations, 498, 498*t*
in-line closed reservoir method, 299, 300*f*
INOvent (Ikaria) delivery system, 339
inspection, 6
inspiratory muscle training (IMT), 259
  parameters, 260*t*
inspiratory pause (or plateau) pressure, 318–320
inspiratory pressures, 50*t*
inspiratory resistance breathing, 432*t*
inspiratory time (I-time), 317
inspiratory to expiratory time ratio (I:E ratio), 321, 369–371, 370*t*, 371*t*
instrument analytical errors, and correction, 180*t*
instrument calibration, 177*f*
Intal (cromolyn sodium), 284*t*
intentional abusive exposure, 508
inter-instrumental comparison, 181
intermittent positive-pressure breathing (IPPB), 259
  scalloping of airway pressure during, 261*f*
  therapy, 259–262, 260*t*, 261*f*, 333–334, 334*t*
intermittent ventilatory support, 218
International Standards Organization (ISO) system, trach tube selection, 216, 217*t*
interstitial lung diseases, 68, 430
interviews, patient, 34–44
intra-aortic counterpulsation balloon device (IACB/IABP), 46*t*
intracranial pressure (ICP), 271, 463*t*
intra-hospital patient transport, 398–399
intrapulmonary percussive ventilation (IPV), 242, 341
intrapulmonary shunting, 339
intra-treatment supportive interventions, for smoking cessation, 206*t*
intubation. *See* endotracheal tube
invasive hemodynamic monitoring, 90
invasive mechanical ventilation, 230–231, 230*f*
invasive positive-pressure ventilation, modifications, 344, 345*t*

inverse ratio ventilation (IRV), 370
IPPB. *See* intermittent positive-pressure breathing
ipratropium bromide (Atrovent), 283*t*
IPV. *See* intrapulmonary percussive ventilation
IRDS. *See* infant respiratory distress syndrome
IRV. *See* inverse ratio ventilation
IS. *See* incentive spirometry
ISO system. *See* International Standards Organization system
isolette, 106, 107*t*, 108
I-STAT, Abbott Laboratories, 148

J
jet nebulizers, 113, 115*t*
  operating principles and uses for, 113*t*

K
Kamen-Wilkinson tube, 221
ketamine (Ketalar), 366*t*
Korotkoff sounds, 34

L
lab tests. *See also* blood gases
  abnormal RBCs, 7
  point-of-care testing, 148–149, 149*t*
  point of care tests, 180–181
  pulmonary function laboratory studies, conducting, 55–56
  quality control, 175–180
laboratory blood gas and hemoximetry analyzers, 175–180
laboratory spirometry (FVC volumes and flows), 87*t*
language barriers, 42
Lanz tube, 221
large-volume jet nebulizers, 335
large-volume nebulizers, 163
laryngeal mask airways (LMAs), 125*t*, 222, 224–226, 224*f*, 225*t*, 342, 343*t*
laryngoscope, 215*t*, 412*t*
laryngotracheobronchitis, 334
lateral costal breathing, 257, 258
leak tests, spirometers, 185
"L-E-A-N." *See* lidocaine, epinephrine, atropine, or naloxone
levalbuterol, 282*t*
level of consciousness, 36
Levy-Jennings chart, 178–180, 179*f*, 180*f*
lidocaine, 286

lidocaine, epinephrine, atropine, or naloxone ("L-E-A-N"), 286
life-threatening hematoma, signs of, 472
life-threatening respiratory failure, progression to, 497
light wand, endotracheal intubation, 215*t*
limit valve, 129
linearity, 176*t*
LIP. *See* lower inflection point
liquid oxygen system (LOX), 435
liquid wastes, 165
lithium (Lithobid), 366*t*
living will, 41
LMAs. *See* laryngeal mask airways
local anesthetic, 420
long-term management, 495–497
lorazepam (Ativan), 366*t*, 422*t*
lower inflection point (LIP), 273
low-flow devices, 104, 104*t*, 105*t*, 435
   troubleshooting, 110*t*
low-temperature sterilization, 162
LOX. *See* liquid oxygen system
lung abscess, 27
lung compliance, 13, 319–320
lung fields, x-rays, 46*t*
lung mechanics, 86, 88, 88*t*
   and ventilator graphics, 51
lung tumors, 33
lung volume reduction surgery (LVRS), 430
   in advanced-stage emphysema, 468–469
lungs, care plans, 382*t*
LVRS. *See* lung volume reduction surgery

M

macroglossia, 27*t*
Magill forceps, 215*t*, 414
magnetic resonance imaging (MRI), 12*t*, 462*t*
maintenance, equipment, 162–164
mallampati classification of pharyngeal anatomy, 27*t*
malnutrition, 38
mandatory breaths, volume and pressure control comparison, 266*t*
manometers, 138–140
   types and clinical applications of, 139*t*
   U-tube, 139*f*
manual chest percussion, 6, 240, 341
manual in-line stabilization (MILS), 413*t*
MAP. *See* mean airway pressure

masks, 102*t*, 104
   infection control, 166*t*
   troubleshooting, 110*t*
mast cell stabilizers, 284*t*
maternal data, 14–16
maternal history, 14–16
Maxair (pirbuterol), 282*t*
maximum expiratory pressure (MEP), 50*t*
maximum inspiratory pressure (MIP), 50*t*
maximum voluntary ventilation (MVV), 67, 87*t*
MDIs. *See* metered-dose inhalers
mean (average), defined, 176, 176*t*
mean airway pressure (MAP), 321
mechanical chest percussion, 341
mechanical devices
   aid airway clearance, 121
   clearance, 241–245
mechanical insufflator–exsufflation (MI-E), 244, 244*f*, 245, 341
mechanical respirometers, 140, 143, 143*f*
mechanical ventilation, 473, 477
   airway pressure release ventilation (APRV), 262, 265*t*, 266, 267*f*
   alarms, 345–348, 346*t*, 348*t*
   appropriate use of, 127*t*
   capnography, 90
   circuit, 372, 373
      aerosol drug-delivery systems in, 132
      assembly, 131
      testing/calibration, 131
      troubleshooting, 132–134, 133*t*
   enhancing oxygenation, 367–369
   home care, 436–438, 441*t*
   humidification needs by, 228*t*
   humidification systems, 133
   infection control, 169
   inhaled nitric oxide therapy, 339
   invasive, 230–231, 230*f*
   IPPB therapy, 259–262, 260*t*, 261*f*
   key elements, 262
   lung mechanics measures, 86, 88
   management, record keeping, 195
   modes and techniques modification, 371, 371*t*
   modifications, 342, 344–348, 345*t*–346*t*, 348–350, 348*t*
   noninvasive, 231

noninvasive positive-pressure ventilation, 129
   overview, 123, 127–134
   for patients, 479
   patient–ventilator asynchrony, 364*t*
   pneumothorax, 361
   protocols, 275–276
   quality control, 183–186
   recommending changes in, 365, 366–373
   record keeping, 193–194
   sedative drugs and, 169
   selection, 127*t*
   settings, 262–267, 373
   spontaneous breathing trials, 279
   tension pneumothorax, 395–398
   weaning, 12, 50, 279–281, 350
   weaning from, 50, 279–281, 351, 373–374
mechanical ventilator loops, 325*t*
meconium aspiration, 276
medical devices, appearance on x-rays, 46
medical emergency teams (METs), 402
medical records
   arterial blood gas results, 9–11
   common errors to avoid, 18, 206
   communicating information, 199
   computer technology, 199–201
   educating the patient and family
      health (disease) management, 202–203, 202*t*
      smoking cessation education, 203–204, 204*t*–206*t*
   home care, 442–443
   imaging studies, 11
   maternal and neonatal history, 14–16
   monitoring data, 11–14
   noting and interpreting, patient response to therapy, 196–198, 197*t*, 198*f*
   overview, 3–4
   patient care orders, 193–194
   patient history, 5
   patient progress, pulmonary rehabilitation, 432
   physical exams, 5–7
   planned therapy and goals, 201, 201*t*
   recording therapy and results, 194–198, 195*t*–197*t*, 198*f*

medical records (*cont.*)
  rules for, 194, 195*t*
  therapy administered
      specification, 194–195, 196*t*
medical wastes, 164, 165, 170
medication history, 6*t*
medications
  ACLS, 393
  administering, 281–287
  analgesics, 363, 366*t*
  antipsychotics, 365, 366*t*
  bronchodilators, 250–251, 250*t*,
      281, 334
  edema, 364*t*
  neuroleptics, 365, 366*t*
  neuromuscular blockade, 362,
      363, 365, 366*t*
  paralytics, 365, 366*t*
  sedation, 422*t*
  sedatives, 363, 366*t*
MEP. *See* maximum expiratory
    pressure
meperidine (Demerol), 366,
    366*t*, 422*t*
mesh nebulizers, electronic 120*t*
acidosis, metabolic, 327, 302*t*
alkalosis, metabolic, 302
metaproterenol (Alupent), 282*t*
metered-dose inhalers (MDIs), 114
  advantages and disadvantages
      of, 116*t*
  assembly and operational
      check of, 118*t*
  optimal technique and
      therapeutic issues, 118*t*
  troubleshooting, 120*t*
methacholine challenge test, 56,
    88*t*, 313*t*
methemoglobin, 14, 306–308
METs. *See* medical emergency
    teams
microbiologic assessment, 85
micronephrin, 282*t*
midazolam (Versed), 366*t*, 422*t*
mid-cervical injuries, 473
MI-E. *See* mechanical insufflator–
    exsufflation
mild/moderate hypothermia, 478
MILS. *See* manual in-line
    stabilization
minute volume, 50*t*
MIP. *See* maximum inspiratory
    pressure
misplaced bronchial sounds, 7
mitral stenosis, 34
mixed venous oxygen content, 74,
    75, 463*t*
modes, ventilatory support,
    262–266, 263*t*–265*t*
monitoring data, 11–14

monitors, noninvasive, 187–188
morphine, 363, 366*t*
mouth/jaw trauma, 212
mouthpieces, IPPB devices, 260
mouth-to-valve mask resuscitators,
    121–123
movement disorders, 92
MRI. *See* magnetic resonance
    imaging
mucokinetics, 250*t*, 281,
    284*t*–285*t*, 286
mucolytics, 250, 250*t*, 286, 334
Mucomyst, 250, 284*t*
muscle tone, 463*t*
muscle training, 257–259
muscular dystrophy, 487, 490–491
musculoskeletal weakness,
    bronchial hygiene
    techniques, 238*t*
MVV. *See* maximum voluntary
    ventilation
myasthenia gravis, 487, 488*t*–489*t*
myasthenic crises, 487
myocardial infarction, 7, 287

N
naloxone (Narcan), 422*t*
narcotic drugs, 509*t*
nasal cannulas, 435
  troubleshooting, 110*t*
nasal cavity, 27*t*
nasal continuous positive airway
    pressure (CPAP), 438
nasal intubation, 414
nasal mask, 130*f*, 134
nasal pillows, 130*f*, 134
nasogastric tubes, 46*t*
nasopharyngeal airways, 124*t*, 210,
    212–213, 342, 343*t*
nasotracheal suction catheter,
    patient positioning for
    insertion of, 249*f*
nasotracheal suctioning, 212,
    248–249, 249*f*
National Asthma Education
    and Prevention Program
    guidelines, 495
National Guideline Clearinghouse,
    451, 452*f*
National Heart, Lung, and Blood
    Institute (NHLBI) ARDS
    protocol, 275–276, 371*t*
National Lung Health Education
    Program (NLHEP)
    recommendation, 144, 145*t*
NBRC Clinical Simulation
    Examination (CSE), 458*f*, 468
NBRC exams
  bronchopulmonary
      secretions, 235

communication skills, 199
content, 191
CRT and WRRT, 447–448
CSE and, 454, 454*t*
disorders identified by, 450–451
educating patient and family
    health (disease) management,
      202–203, 202*t*
    smoking cessation, 203–204,
      204*t*–206*t*
equipment, 96
expectation on, 191
patent airway/care of artificial
    airways, 209
patient response to care,
    293, 313
planned therapy and goals,
    patients, 201, 201*t*
respiratory care plan,
    appropriateness of, 379
respiratory care plan, patient
    response, 355
therapeutic procedures, patient
    response, 329
NBRC hospital, 266
nebulizers, 111, 113–114, 115*t*,
    162, 162*t*
  large-volume, 163
  SVNs, 163
neck, 27*t*, 47
  x-rays, 84*t*, 462*t*
needle thoracostomy
  basic procedure for, 398
  defined, 398
negative inspiratory force
    (NIF/MIP), 13
neonatal data, perinatal and, 16
neonatal inspection, 27–30
neonatal intensive care unit
    (NICU), 501
neonatal patients, CSE, 450*t*
neonates, 14
  apnea monitor, 60
  cardiopulmonary status, 28
  FIO$_2$ measure, 317
  inhaled nitric oxide
      therapy, 339
  IRDS, 364*t*
  resuscitation, 395, 397*f*
neurogenic shock, 473
neuroleptics, 365, 366*t*
neurologic abnormalities,
    bronchial hygiene
    techniques, 238*t*
neurologic disorders, 92
  cases involving, 463
  CSE, 450*t*
  information, 463*t*
neuromuscular blockade, 362, 363,
    365, 366*t*

neuromuscular disorders, 13, 33
with acute manifestations, 487, 488t–489t
cases involving, 463
CSE, 450t
information, 463t
muscular dystrophy, 487, 490–491
tetanus, 491–492
neutrophils, 7
New York Heart Association Heart Failure Symptom Classification System, 480t
NHLBI ARDS protocol. *See* National Heart, Lung, and Blood Institute ARDS protocol
NICU. *See* neonatal intensive care unit
NIF. *See* negative inspiratory force; see also maximum inspiratory pressure (MIP)
Nimbex (cisatracurium), 365, 366t
nitric oxide analysis, exhaled, 56–59
nitrogen dioxide (NO_2), 340
NLHEP recommendation. *See* National Lung Health Education Program recommendation
nocturnal oximetry, 61–62
nocturnal seizures, 92
noncomputerized ventilators, operational verification of, 185t
noninvasive blood pressure measurement, 90
noninvasive monitors, 187–188
noninvasive negative pressure devices, 269
noninvasive oximetry monitoring devices, 149–151
pulse oximeters, 149–150, 150t
transcutaneous monitors, 150–151
noninvasive positive-pressure ventilation (NPPV), 123, 129, 130–131, 130f, 231, 269, 338, 348, 348t, 399, 490, 510
indications and contraindications for, 270t
initial settings and basic adjustments, 270t
problems with, 134, 134t
noninvasive ventilation, 262, 269–270
advantages and limitations of, 269t
nonrebreathing mask, 102t, 106

non-ST-segment elevation myocardial infarction (NSTEMI), 481
normal flow *vs.* time waveforms, 324t
normal resonance, 33
normal volume *vs.* time waveforms, 322, 322t–324t
nostrils, 27t
NPPV. *See* nocturnal noninvasive positive-pressure ventilation; noninvasive positive-pressure ventilation; noninvasive ventilation
NSTEMI. *See* non-ST-segment elevation myocardial infarction
nutritional status, 38

O
O_2 analyzers, 140, 186, 186t
O_2 blenders, 99–101
obesity, 34
obesity–hypoventilation syndrome (OHS), 509
assessment/information gathering, 510
treatment/decision making, 510
obstructed airway, 222, 223f
obstructive disorders, 9, 56
obstructive sleep apnea (OSA), 16, 510
occupational history, 39–41
environmental exposures, 6t
O_2-delivery systems, 104, 106, 109–111
troubleshooting, 105t
ODI. *See* oxygen desaturation index
OHS. *See* obesity–hypoventilation syndrome
OI. *See* oxygenation index
one-point calibration, defined, 178
opacities, 18
operational verification, 183
computerized ventilators, 183, 186
opioids, 364t
analgesics, 366t
option scoring, CSE, 457–459
options window (CSE), 457
oral airway, 212
oral care, VAP and, 169
oral cavity, 27t
oral devices, 131, 134
oral endotracheal intubation, 222
oronasal mask, 130f, 134
oropharyngeal airways, 124t, 210–212, 212t, 342, 343t

oropharyngeal suctioning, 245, 246f
orthopnea, 37
OSA. *See* obstructive sleep apnea
overdistension, 350, 350f
overnight oximetry, 92
overnight pulse oximetry, 61–62
oximeters, operational problems with, 187t
oximetry monitoring devices, noninvasive, 149–151
oxycodone (OxyContin), 366t
oxygen
analyzers, 140
concentrators, 433
delivery, 74
demands, 74
therapy, administering, 287–288
therapy enclosures, 106, 107t
problems with, 109
therapy, home care, 432–433
therapy, humidification needs by, 228t
therapy, modifying, 336–337, 337t, 338f
therapy, quality assurance criteria for, 384
therapy, recommending changes in, 365, 367t
titration with exercise, 68
oxygen administration devices, 101–110, 102t–103t
enclosures, O_2 therapy, 106, 107t
high-flow devices, 104–106
infant environmental control via isolette/warmer, 106, 108
low-flow devices, 104, 104t, 105t
selection, 108–109, 108t, 109t
troubleshooting, 109–110, 110t, 111t
oxygen desaturation index (ODI), 61
oxygen titration with exercise, 68
oxygen "wall" humidifiers, 163
oxygenation
care plans, 382t
effect of altitude on, 401t
enhancing, 367–369
oxygenation index (OI), 303–304
oxygenation, monitoring, 89
oxygenation rule of thumb, 304
oxygen-conserving devices, 104
oxyhemoglobin, blood concentration, 14
oxyhoods, 107t, 338

P

PA catheter. *See* pulmonary artery catheter

PA films. *See* posteroanterior films

PA pressure. *See* pulmonary artery pressure

PA wedge pressure (PAWP), 463*t*

pain, assessing, 36

palpitation, 30–33

pancuronium (Pavulon), 365, 366*t*

pandemics, 169

paralytics, 365, 366*t*

paraplegia, 473

partial rebreathing mask, 102*t*

partial thromboplastin time (PTT), 7

partial-thickness burns, 475

passive humidifiers, 113

passover humidifier, 111

past medical history, 6*t*

pathophysiological state, 381, 382*t*, 455

patient agitation, medications for, 364*t*

patient assessment. *See* assessment, patient

patient care
coordinating, 199
problem-oriented approach to, 198, 198*f*

patient care orders, 193–194

patient clinical status, reporting, 199

patient discharge planning, 199

patient education
apnea monitoring programs, 441
assessing learning needs, 41–44
bronchopulmonary hygiene techniques, 239–241
deep breathing/muscle training, 257–259
history, 6*t*
home care, 440, 441
pulmonary rehabilitation programs, 431
smoking cessation, 203–204, 204*t*–206*t*

patient factors, 318*t*

patient "handoff," 199

patient history, 5

patient interviews, 34–44

patient placement, infection control, 166*t*

patient positioning, 210, 211*t*, 359, 360*t*
endotracheal intubation, 412–413

patient records
arterial blood gas results, 9–11

common errors to avoid, 18
home care, 442–443
imaging studies, 11
maternal and neonatal history, 14–16
monitoring data, 11–14
overview, 3–4
patient history, 5
physical examination, 5–7
pre-test and answers, 3–4, 19–20
PTT, 7
sure bets, 18–19

patient refusal of therapy, 195

patient response to care
airway pressures, 317–321
blood tests, 312
breath sounds, 313
bronchial hygiene therapy, 341, 341*t*–342*t*
capnography, 306, 308, 308*t*
cardiac rhythm, 310–312
common errors to avoid, 325, 351
communicating alterations to therapy, 201–202
CO-oximetry, 304–305
FIO$_2$ and/or liter flow, 317
mechanical ventilation, 348–350
modifying treatment techniques, 333–348
noting and interpreting, 196–198, 197*t*, 198*f*
patient-ventilator asynchrony, 314
respiratory care plan. *See* respiratory care plan, patient response
sputum characteristics, 312, 313
terminating treatment, 333
ventilator waveform evaluation, 348–351
ventilatory support, 351
vital signs, 309

patient resuscitation, 166*t*

patient-care equipment, 170

patient-related asynchrony, causes of and corrective actions for, 368*t*

patients
communication with, 201, 201*t*
exacerbation, severity of, 497, 498*t*
intubation and mechanical ventilation for, 499

patient–ventilator asynchrony, 313, 314, 348–349, 348*f*, 364*t*, 366, 367

patient-ventilator system checks, 196*t*

PAWP. *See* PA wedge pressure

PBW range. *See* predicted body weight range

PDPV techniques. *See* postural drainage, percussion, and vibration

PEA. *See* pulseless electrical activity

peak expiratory flow rate (PEFR), 51–53, 87*t*

peak inspiratory pressure (PIP), 272, 317–318

pediatric and neonatal emergencies, 395

pediatric patients, 47, 395, 399
CSE, 450*t*

pediatric problems
bronchiolitis, 492, 495
childhood asthma, 495–499
croup (laryngotracheobronchitis) and epiglottitis, 492, 493*t*–494*t*

pediatric pulseless arrest algorithm, 396*f*

pediatric resuscitation, 395

PEEP, 132, 271–273

PEFR. *See* peak expiratory flow rate

PEP. *See* positive expiratory pressure

percent inspiratory time (%I-time), 369–370

percent shunt, 75–76

percussion, 6, 33, 237, 239, 239*t*, 240*f*, 341

perforated gastrointestinal tract, 45*t*

perinatal and neonatal data, 16

peripheral cyanosis, 25

peripheral edema, 11, 364*t*

peripheral pulse, 31

peripheral pulses, 463*t*

permissive hypercapnia, 373

persistent pulmonary hypertension of the newborn (PPHN), 339

personal action plans, 203

personal protective equipment (PPE), 165, 405

PET scan. *See* positron emission tomography

P$_{ET}$CO$_2$, 306
waveform descriptions, 307*t*

pH, blood gases, 10

pharmacologic therapy, 482–483
for smoking cessation, 204, 205*t*

pharynx, 27*t*

phrenic nerve paralysis, 45*t*

physical examination, 5–7

physical reconditioning exercises, 431
physician's order, 17, 18
physiologic shunting, 75
PIP. *See* peak inspiratory pressure
pipe-shaped Flutter valve, 242, 243*f*
pirbuterol (Maxair), 282*t*
plateau pressure, 18, 318–320
pleural drainage systems, 136–138, 137*f*
pleural effusions
　breath sounds, 34
　chest radiograph, 45*t*
　chest tube insertion, 420–421
　palpation, 31, 32
　thoracentesis, 419
　X-ray findings, 297*t*
pleural friction rub, 314*t*
pleural space, care plans, 382*t*
Pmean. *See* mean airway pressure (MAP)
PMI. *See* point of maximum impulse
pneumonia
　ABG abnormalities, 11*t*
　chest radiograph, 45*t*
　hyperventilation, 19
　medications for, 364*t*
　palpation, 32
　percussion, 33
　sputum Gram stain and culture, 85
pneumosuit, 437
pneumotachometer, 143, 144*f*
pneumothorax
　breath sounds, 33
　chest tube insertion, 420
　palpation, 32
　percussion, 33
　recommending treatment of, 359, 361
　tension pneumothorax, 395–398, 470
　X-ray findings, 298*t*
POCT. *See* point-of-care testing
point of maximum impulse (PMI), 31
point-of-care testing (POCT), 180–181
　blood gas analyzers, 148–149
　troubleshooting, 149*t*
poisonings, drug overdose and. *See* drug overdose and poisonings
poisons, categories of, 509*t*
polarographic analyzers, 186
polycythemia, 7, 9, 25, 92
polysomnogram, 16
polysomnography, 92

popliteal arteries, 31
portable electronic spirometers, 143–145, 144*f*
　NLHEP recommendation, 145*t*
　troubleshooting, 146*t*
portable oxygen systems, 101, 435
positron emission tomography (PET) scans, 12*t*, 84*t*, 462*t*
positioning patients, 359, 360*t*
　minimize hypoxemia, 288*t*
　postural drainage, 211*t*
　prevent VAP, 211*t*
positive expiratory pressure (PEP), 341
　devices, 242–244, 243*f*, 243*t*
positive-pressure ventilation (PPV), 32
　laryngeal mask airways, 226
postanalytical errors, 176*t*
posteroanterior (PA) films, 298
postextubation edema, 334
postextubation stridor, 364
postural drainage, percussion, and vibration (PDPV) techniques, 211*t*, 237, 239, 239*t*, 240*f*, 341
　patient positions for, 239, 240*f*
potassium, electrolyte, 363*t*
PPE. *See* personal protective equipment
PPHN. *See* persistent pulmonary hypertension of the newborn
PPV. *See* positive-pressure ventilation
Praxair Grab 'n Go™, 100
preanalytical errors, 176*t*
　defined, 176, 177*t*
precision, 176, 176*t*
precordium, palpating, 31
predicted body weight (PBW) range, 266
premature newborn, medications for, 364*t*
premature ventricular contraction (PVC), 311, 312, 312*f*
pre-/post-bronchodilator spirometry, 87*t*
pressure control ventilation, and volume control, 346–347
pressure support ventilation (PSV), 264*t*, 269
pressure waveform, irregular patient–ventilator asynchrony, 348, 348*f*
pressure-measuring devices, 138
pressure-reducing valve, 99
pressure-regulated volume control (PRVC), 262, 264*t*
pressure–volume curve, 88, 88*t*
　overdistension, 350, 350*f*
　respiratory system, 273*t*

primary acid–base disturbances, 301
　interpreting, 10
problem-oriented method, charting, 197–198, 197*t*, 198*f*
problem-solving/skills training treatment, for smoking cessation, 205*t*
procedures, recommending. *See* recommending procedures
proficiency testing, 180
progressive neuromuscular disorder, 460
pro-inflammatory mediators, 476
propofol (Diprivan), 366*t*, 422*t*
Proventil (albuterol), 282*t*
provocative concentration, 313
proxy directive, 41
PRVC. *See* pressure-regulated volume control
Pseudomonas aeruginosa, 286
PSV. *See* pressure support ventilation
PTT. *See* partial thromboplastin time
Pulmicort (budesonide), 284*t*, 286
pulmonary angiography, 85*t*
pulmonary artery (PA) catheter, 46*t*, 68, 423–424
　special procedures, 423–424
pulmonary artery monitoring, 91*t*
pulmonary artery (PA) pressure, 71*t*, 339, 340, 463*t*
pulmonary circulation, physiologic shunting, 75
pulmonary edema, 7, 271, 298*t*, 364*t*
pulmonary embolism, 12*t*
pulmonary fibrosis, 9, 13*t*, 56, 430
pulmonary function laboratory studies, conducting, 55–56
pulmonary function, selection, 461, 461*t*
pulmonary function tests (PFTs), 86, 87*t*–88*t*
　equipment, 163–164, 181–186
　　accuracy of, 181–183
　　quality control, 182*t*
　results, 7–9
pulmonary hyperinflation, 34
pulmonary hypertension, 34, 92, 339, 340
pulmonary hypoplasia, 276
pulmonary infiltrates, 83
pulmonary interstitial edema, 276
pulmonary mechanics, 13
pulmonary rehabilitation, 430–432
pulmonary vascular resistance (PVR), 31, 73*t*, 339
　ventilator settings on, 508, 508*f*

Pulmozyme (dornase alfa), 250, 285t
pulse deficit, 31
pulse dose/demand flow systems, 104
pulse oximeters
  considerations in setup of, 150t
  equipment, 149–150
  quality control, 187
  screening protocol for CCHD, 506, 507f
pulse oximetry, 14, 305, 473
  overnight, 61–62
  overview, 89
pulseless electrical activity (PEA), 393
puncture, arterial sampling by, 298
pure control mode, 263t
pursed-lip breathing, 431
PVR. See pulmonary vascular resistance
Pyxis MedStation, 200

Q
QC procedures. See quality control procedures
"quad cough," 240, 475
quality assurance
  patient transport, 399
  respiratory care protocols monitoring and, 385–386
quality control (QC)
  procedures, 174
  common errors to avoid, 189
  gas analyzers, 178t, 186, 188
  gas delivery and metering devices, 188–189
  laboratory blood gas and hemoximetry analyzers, 175–180
  mechanical ventilators, 183–186
  noninvasive monitors, 187–188
  point-of-care analyzers, 180–181
  pre-test answers and explanations, 189–190
  pulmonary function equipment, 181–186
  sure bets, 189
quality-control procedures, 132

R
racemic epinephrine, 282t
radial arterial puncture for ABG analysis, 298
radial artery, 298
radiographic studies
  airway complications, 297t
  medical devices, appearance on, 46

neck radiographs, review
  lateral, 47
  recommending, 83, 84t–85t, 297–298
  review and interpretation, 44–46
radiolucency, 18
rales, 7, 313
range of motion, neck, 27t
rapid response team (RRT), 333, 402
rapid sequence intubation, 415–416, 415f
rapid shallow breathing index (RSBI), 50
rapid weaning and extubation protocol, 486–487
RBCs. See abnormal red blood cells
RDS. See respiratory distress syndrome
reciprocal reasoning, 455
recommending imaging studies, pre-test and answers, 82–83
recommending procedures
  BAL, 85
  blood gas analysis, pulse oximetry, and transcutaneous monitoring, 88–89
  capnography, 90
  common errors to avoid, 92–93
  diagnostic bronchoscopy, 83
  electrocardiography, 90
  hemodynamic monitoring, 90
  lung mechanics, 86, 88, 88t
  overnight oximetry, 91
  polysomnography, 92
  pulmonary function testing, 86, 87t–88t
  radiographic and other imaging studies, 83, 84t–85t
  sleep studies, 91–92
  sputum gram stain, 85
recording therapy and results, 194–198, 195t–197t, 198f
records
  arterial blood gas results, 9–11
  common errors to avoid, 18, 206
  communicating information, 199
  computer technology, 199–201
  educating the patient and family
    health (disease) management, 202–203, 202t
    smoking cessation education, 203–204, 204t–206t

home care, 442–443
imaging studies, 11
maternal and neonatal history, 14–16
monitoring data, 11–14
patient care orders, 193–194
patient history, 5
patient record, 3–4
physical exam, 5–7
planned therapy and goals, 201, 201t
pulmonary function test, 7–9
recording therapy and results, 194–198, 195t–197t, 198f
reducing valves, 99–100
refractory hypoxemia, 271
Relenza (zanamivir), 285t
remote alarm, 347
reportable range, 176, 176t
reservoir cannulas, 104
resistance, airway, 13, 86, 88t, 317, 319
resonance, percussion, 33
respiratory acidosis, 302, 302t
respiratory alkalosis, 19, 302, 302t, 328
respiratory care
  adult resuscitation protocols, 393
  procedures, 196
  VAP, 168
respiratory care plan
  appropriateness of
    changes in therapeutic plan, 383
    common errors to avoid, 386–387
    pathophysiological state, 381, 382t
    post-test, 389
    prescribed therapy and goals, 381
    respiratory care protocols. See respiratory care protocols
    respiratory care quality assurance, 383–384, 383f
    review planned therapy, 381
    sure bets, 387
  explaining to patients, 201
  patient response
    artificial airways, 359, 360t, 361t
    bronchial hygiene therapy, 359
    common errors to avoid, 374
    drug therapy, 362, 364t, 365t
    electrolyte therapy, 362, 363t

fluid balance, 362, 362*t*

mechanical ventilation, 365–373

NBRC exams, 355

oxygen therapy, 365, 367*t*

patient positioning, 359, 360*t*

pneumothorax, 359, 361

post-test, 378

pre-test and answers, 355–358, 375–378

sedation and neuromuscular blockade, 362, 363, 365, 366*t*

sure bets, 374–375

respiratory care protocols

algorithms, examples of, 385, 386*f*

ARDS protocol, 275–276

developing, monitoring, and applying, 385

disease-specific ventilator protocols, 275–276

monitoring and quality assurance, 385–386

respiratory care quality assurance, 383–384, 383*f*

respiratory depression, medications for, 364*t*

respiratory distress, Silverman-Anderson Index for assessing, 502, 502*t*

respiratory distress syndrome (RDS), 286

respiratory home care

aerosol drug administration, 435, 436

airway care and secretion clearance, 436

bland aerosol therapy, 435

case manager, interacting, 442

documentation, 442–443

home mechanical ventilation, 436–438

home O₂ therapy, 432–435, 436*t*

infection control, 441–442

patient and caregivers, education of, 440–441

sleep disorders, treatment of, 438–440

respiratory hygiene, 166*t*

respiratory infections, 405

respiratory monitoring

parameters, 12–13

thresholds, 12, 12*t*

respiratory syncytial virus (RSV), 492

respiratory tract infection, 85

respiratory-related information, selection, 461, 461*t*

respirometers, 185*t*

mechanical, 140, 143, 143*f*

restless leg syndrome, 92

restrictive disorder, 18

"resume preoperative orders," blanket orders, 193

resuscitation

advance directives, 41

devices, 121–123

infants, 395

neonatal, 395, 397*f*

patient positioning, 211*t*

pediatric, 395

retinopathy of prematurity, 287

reversing agents, 509*t*

rhonchi, 7, 313, 314*t*

rhonchial fremitus, 32

right heart failure, 92, 364*t*

risus sardonicus, 491

rocuronium (Zemuron), 366*t*

Romazicon (flumazenil), 422*t*

room-air humidifiers, 163

infection control, 163

RRT. *See* rapid response team

RSBI. *See* rapid shallow breathing index

RSV. *See* respiratory syncytial virus

RTs. *See* respiratory therapists

rule of 300, 48*f*

"Rule of Nines," 475

S

SAHS. *See* sleep apnea–hypopnea syndrome

salmeterol (Serevent), 283*t*, 286

sanitation, defined, 161*t*

sarcoidosis, pulmonary rehabilitation, 430

SARS. *See* severe acute respiratory syndrome

SBTs. *See* spontaneous breathing trials

scalar graphics, 322

scenario window (CSE), 457

SCI. *See* spinal cord injury

secretions

aerosol therapy, 249–251

bronchopulmonary hygiene techniques, 239–241

care plans, 382*t*

clearance, 333–334, 436

excessive, 18

handheld mechanical percussors and vibrators, 242

mechanical devices to facilitate clearance, 241–245

medications for, 364*t*

postural drainage, percussion, and vibration techniques, 237, 239, 239*t*, 240*f*

selecting best approach, 237, 238*f*, 238*t*

suctioning equipment, 245–249

sedative/hypnotic drugs, 509*t*

sedatives, 169, 362, 363, 365, 366*t*, 422*t*

seizures, 212

Seldinger technique, 298

self-contained breathing apparatus (SCBA), 405

self-inflating manual resuscitators, 121

self-management education, 203

sensitivity, inappropriate, 349, 349*f*

Sensormedics HFOV circuit, 131

Sequential Organ Failure Assessment (SOFA), 404–405

Serevent (salmeterol), 283*t*, 286

serum potassium (hypokalemia), 7

set volume, change in, 347

severe acute respiratory syndrome (SARS), 167, 169–171

severity of hypoxemia, interpreting, 10

sharps, 164–166

shift change reporting, 199

shock, 34, 287, 290

shockable rhythms, defibrillation doses for, 395*t*

shunting, physiologic, 75

Silverman-Anderson Index for assessing respiratory distress, 502, 502*t*

simple acid–base disturbances, interpretation of, 10, 10*f*

simulator, ECG, 145

SIMV. *See* synchronous intermittent mandatory ventilation

single-limb circuits, 128–129, 129*f*

types of, 128

sinus infection, 169

6-minute walk test (6MWT), 63–65

60/60 rule of thumb, 304

skin palpation, 32–33

sleep apnea, 25, 271

sleep apnea–hypopnea syndrome (SAHS), 61, 92, 438

sleep disorders, data pertaining to, 16–17

sleep studies, 91–92

sleep, titration of CPAP/BiPAP, 62–63

small-volume nebulizers (SVNs), 114, 163, 436

advantages and disadvantages of, 116*t*

small-volume nebulizers (SVNs)
(cont.)
   assembly and operational
      check of, 118t
   optimal technique and
      therapeutic issues, 119t
   troubleshooting, 120t
smoke inhalation, 89, 475–477
smoking
   cessation, 203–204,
      204t–206t, 430
   history, 40
sniffing position, 413t
snoring, 25, 92
SOAP format, charting, 197, 197t
social history, 6t, 39–41
sodium, electrolyte, 363t
SOFA. See Sequential Organ
   Failure Assessment
soft tissues palpation, 32–33
soft-tissue non-osseous
   injuries, 474
soiled patient-care
   equipment, 166t
solid infectious waste, 164
space-occupying lesions, 31, 44
speaking tracheostomy tubes,
   123, 126
speaking valves, 123, 126t
special procedures, assisting
   physicians
   bronchoscopy, 416–418
   cardioversion, 421–422
   chest tube insertion, 420–421
   endotracheal intubation,
      410–416
   sedation, 422
   thoracentesis, 419–420
   tracheotomy, 418–419
specialty gas analyzers, 140
specialty gas therapy, 337
   heliox therapy, 338–339, 339t
   inhaled nitric oxide therapy,
      339–340, 340t
spinal cord injury (SCI), 473–475
Spiriva (tiotroprium bromide), 283t
spirometers, 53, 55, 143–145, 144f,
   145t, 181, 182f, 183
spontaneous breathing trials
   (SBTs), 279, 280f
spring-loaded threshold
   resistors, 259
sputum, 7, 27, 312, 313
   Gram stain, 85
squeeze-bulb esophageal
   detection device (EDD), 215t
stable angina, managing CAD
   with, 482–483
stable congestive heart failure,
   identify/manage, 480–481

standard deviation, 176, 176t
standard nasal cannulas, 102t, 104
standard pulse oximeters, 304, 305
Staphylococcus aureus, 492
static compliance, 88t, 319
static lung volumes, 55–56
statistical QC, 176, 176t, 178
steam sterilization, 162
STEMI. See ST-segment elevation
   myocardial infarction
sterilization
   defined, 161t
   equipment, 162–164
   procedures, 164t
sternal wires, 46t
steroids, 250, 250t, 286
stoma, 216–219
stopcock method, 299, 300f
stridor, 313, 314t, 364t
stroke, 73t
stroke volume (SV), 73, 73t
ST-segment elevation myocardial
   infarction (STEMI), 481
stylet, 215t, 412t, 414
subcutaneous emphysema, 32
subglottic edema, 334
subglottic secretions, 248, 248f
Sublimaze (fentanyl),
   363, 366t
substance abuse, 41
succinylcholine (Anectine),
   365, 366t
suctioning
   artificial airway, 342, 344t
   assessment, 249
   nasotracheal, 248–249, 249f
   oropharyngeal, 245, 246f
   through tracheal airway,
      245–248, 247f, 247t, 248f
suctioning equipment,
   134–136, 163
   components, 135
   infection control, 163
   overview, 245
   selection, 135t
surfactant preparations, 286
sustained maximal inspiration, 121
SV. See stroke volume
SVNs. See small-volume nebulizers
SVR. See systemic vascular
   resistance
Swan-Ganz catheter (pulmonary
   artery), 299
symbols, 195t
sympathetic overactivity, 491
synchronous intermittent
   mandatory ventilation (SIMV),
   262, 263t
syringes, 46t
systematic arterial pressures, 71t

systematic error, quality control
   tests, 179–181
systemic arterial catheter, 68
systemic arterial monitoring, 91t
systemic vascular resistance
   (SVR), 73t

T
tachycardia, 31, 310, 310f, 421
tachypnea, 13
temperature-regulation,
   ventilators, 133
tension pneumothorax, 45t,
   395–398, 420, 470. See also
   pneumothorax
tents, oxygen, 107t, 109
terbutaline sulfate (Bricanyl,
   Brethaire), 283t
terminating treatment, 333
tetanus, 491–492
tetraplegia, 473
therapeutic procedures, patient
   response
   bronchial hygiene therapy, 341,
      341t–342t
   mechanical ventilation,
      348–350
   modifying treatment
      techniques, 333–348
   terminating treatment, 333
   ventilator waveform evaluation,
      348–351
   ventilatory support, 351
therapeutic thoracentesis, 92
therapy, PEP devices, 242–244,
   243f, 243t
thiopental (Pentothal), 366
37-French version, esophageal–
   tracheal Combitube, 226
thoracentesis, 92, 419–420
thoracic compliance, 319–320
thoracic CT, 84t
thoracic expansion, palpation, 32
thoracic MRI, 84t
thoracic ultrasound, 462t
thoracostomy (chest) tubes, 46t,
   420–421
thorax, 33, 86
Thorazine (chlorpromazine), 366t
threshold resistors, 259
   PEP devices, 243t
tidal volume, 12t, 50t
tiotropium bromide (Spiriva),
   283t, 285t
titration of CPAP, 62–63
TLC. See total lung capacity
tobacco use, 40, 203–204,
   204t–206t
tobramycin (Tobi), 285t, 286
toddlers, 301

Tornalate (bitolterol), 282*t*
total lung capacity (TLC), 56, 87
toxic inhalation, 83
toxidromes, 508
trach mask, airway appliances, 230*t*
trach tubes. *See* tracheostomy tubes
tracheal airway
    cuff management, 220–221
    devices indications, selection, use, and troubleshooting of, 126*t*
    suctioning through, 245–248, 247*f*, 247*t*, 248*f*
    troubleshooting, 221–222
tracheal position
    palpation, 44
    x-rays, 44
tracheostomy buttons, 123, 126*t*, 219
tracheostomy (trach) tubes, 125*t*, 216
    changing tubes, 218
    esophageal–tracheal Combitube, 226–228, 227*f*
    home care, 436
    modifications, 342, 343*t*
    providing care, 217–218
    specialized airways, 218–219, 219*f*
    standard, 216–217, 217*t*
    x-rays
        appearance on, 44
        positioning for, 44
tracheotomy, 216–219, 418–419
transcutaneous monitoring, 14, 89, 89*t*, 150–151, 187, 308
transcutaneous (tc) partial pressures, 150
transillumination of chest, 29–30
transmission-based precautions, 166–167, 167*t*
transport, patient, 308–402
    advantages and disadvantages, 400*t*
transthoracic ultrasound, 85*t*
transtracheal catheter, 435
trauma
    burns/smoke inhalation, 475–477
    chest, 470–472
    head, 472–473
    hypothermia, 477–479
    spinal cord injury, 473–475
traumatic brain injury. *See* head trauma
triamcinolone acetonide (Azmacort), 284*t*
"Triple S Rule," 333

trismus, 491
troubleshooting
    aerosol drug-delivery systems, 119, 120*t*
    artificial airways, 123, 124*t*–125*t*
    bronchoscopes, 153
    electronic mesh nebulizers, 120*t*
    fenestrated tubes, 218–219
    high-flow therapy devices, 111*t*
    heat and moisture exchangers, 231
    home oxygen, 435, 436*t*
    home ventilator, 438, 438*t*
    humidifiers, 114, 114*t*
    laryngeal mask airways, 226
    low-flow therapy devices, 110*t*
    nasopharyngeal airways, 210, 212–213
    nebulizers, 114, 115*t*
    O₂-delivery systems, 105*t*
    oropharyngeal airways, 210–212, 212*t*
    oxygen administration devices, 109–110
    point of care testing analyzers, 149*t*
    portable spirometers, 146*t*
    resuscitation device, 122–123
    of specialty tracheal airway devices, 126*t*
    tracheal airways, 221–222
    vascular lines, 152*t*
    ventilator circuits and interfaces, 132–134, 133*t*
T-tube, airway appliances, 230*t*
tubes
    thoracostomy, 420–421
    x-rays, 44
tumors, 19, 44
turning and rotation protocols, 239
twelve-lead ECG, 47–49
12-lead ECG machines, 145–148, 147*f*
two-dimensional echocardiography, 483
two-point calibration, 178

U
ulnar artery, 298
ultrasonic nebulizers, 113, 115*t*
    operating principles and uses for, 113*t*
unilateral lung disease, patient positioning, 211*t*
upper airway obstruction, 47
upper airway patency, 83
urine output, 463*t*
U-tube manometers, 149*f*

V
vacuum/suction systems, 134–136
Valium (diazepam), 366*t*, 422*t*
valvular heart disease, 483
Vanceril (beclomethasone dipropionate), 283*t*
VAP. *See* ventilator-associated pneumonia
Vaponefrin, 282*t*
vascular lines
    obtaining samples, 298–299
    troubleshooting, 152*t*
vascular pressures, 70, 152
vascular resistance, 74
vasoconstriction, 475
VC. *See* vital capacity
V_D/V_T, 13
vecuronium (Norcuron), 365, 366*t*
venous admixture error, 177*t*
ventilation, 49–51, 89, 121, 122, 262, 269–270, 269*t*. *See also* ventilators
    high frequency, 276–278
    mechanical, weaning, 12
ventilation-perfusion (V/Q), imbalances, 304
ventilator, mechanical. *See* mechanical ventilation
ventilator waveform evaluation, 348–351
ventilator-associated pneumonia (VAP), 85, 210, 248
    bundle, 168–169
    protocol, 168–169
ventilators, 163
    alarms, 314
        cases, 346–347
        settings and monitoring, adjustments to, 345–346, 346*t*, 348, 348*t*
    factors, 318*t*
    graphics, 273–275, 372, 373*t*
    interpretation, 321–322
    lung mechanics and, 51
Ventolin (albuterol), 282*t*
ventricular fibrillation (VF), 393, 393*f*
ventricular hypertrophy, 31
ventricular tachycardia (VT), 393, 393*f*
verbal/telephone orders, 193
VF. *See* ventricular fibrillation
vibrating mesh nebulizers (VMNs), 114
vibration, postural drainage, and percussion techniques, 239
vibrators, 341
vibratory PEP, 243*t*
Vicodin (hydrocodone), 366*t*
vital capacity (VC), 51

vital signs, 5*t*, 309, 309*t*–310*t*
VMNs. *See* vibrating mesh
    nebulizers
vocal fremitus, 32
volume control ventilation,
    pressure control and, 347
volume loss, 349, 349*f*
volume–time waveform, 349, 349*f*
V/Q scan, 85*t*
VT. *See* rapid ventricular
    tachycardia

W
WBC count. *See* white blood cell
    count
weaning, 477
    patient, ventilator alarms case,
        346–347
    ventilatory support, 351, 460

weaning from mechanical
    ventilation, 373–374
    and extubation, 279–281
Western Medica's Oxytote™, 100
wheezes, 313, 314*t*
white blood cell (WBC) count, 7
work of breathing (WOB), 13, 37
Wright respirometer, 143*f*
WRRT exam, 447–449
    self-assessment of written exam
        topical scores, 449*t*

X
x-linked recessive trait
    disorder, 487
Xopenex (levalbuterol), 282*t*
x-rays
    airway complications, 297*t*

medical devices, appearance
    on, 46
neck radiographs, review
    lateral, 47
recommending and reviewing,
    84*t*–85*t*, 297–298
review and interpretation,
    44–46

Y
Yankauer suction tip, 245, 246*f*

Z
zanamivir (Relenza), 285*t*